W9-BLD-819

THE KEY TO EATING WELL AND BEING HEALTHY IS IN YOUR HANDS!

Before you snack, shop, cook, or dine out again, get the scoop on all the foods you love to eat in this completely updated, revised, and expanded guide. Information about food choices can be confusing, because scientific knowledge is constantly evolving. Nolan and Heslin help you translate the often contradictory information into easy, practical, and reliable advice that gets results.

With more than 17,000 listings, this reference book offers nutrition counts for calories, protein, fat, cholesterol, carbohydrates, fiber, and sodium in hundreds of different categories.

THE COMPLETE FOOD COUNTER
4th Edition

Your valuable mealtime companion!

Books by Karen J. Nolan and Jo-Ann Heslin

The Calorie Counter (*Fifth Edition*)

The Complete Food Counter (*Fourth Edition*)

The Ultimate Carbohydrate Counter (*Third Edition*)

The Protein Counter (*Third Edition*)

The Diabetes Counter (*Fourth Edition*)

Books by Annette B. Natow, Jo-Ann Heslin and Karen J. Nolan

The Cholesterol Counter (*Seventh Edition*)

The Fat Counter (*Seventh Edition*)

The Healthy Wholefoods Counter

The Most Complete Food Counter (*Second Edition*)

Books by Annette B. Natow and Jo-Ann Heslin

Eaitng Out Food Counter

Healthy Heart Food Counter

The Vitamin an

l Food Counter

Published by POCKET BOOKS

THE COMPLETE FOOD COUNTER

4th Edition

Karen J. Nolan, Ph.D.

Jo-Ann Heslin, M.A., R.D.

POCKET BOOKS

New York London Toronto Sydney New Delhi

The sale of this book without its cover is unauthorized. If you purchased this book without a cover, you should be aware that it was reported to the publisher as "unsold and destroyed." Neither the author nor the publisher has received payment for the sale of this "stripped book."

Pocket Books
A Division of Simon & Schuster, Inc.
1230 Avenue of the Americas
New York, NY 10020

Copyright © 1999–2009 Annette B. Natow and Jo-Ann Heslin
Copyright © 2012 Karen J. Nolan and Jo-Ann Heslin

A previous edition of this work was published in 1999 by Pocket Books as *The Most Complete Food Counter*.

All rights reserved, including the right to reproduce this book or portions thereof in any form whatsoever. For information, address Pocket Books Subsidiary Rights Department, 1230 Avenue of the Americas, New York, NY 10020.

This Pocket Books paperback edition January 2012

POCKET and colophon are registered trademarks of Simon & Schuster, Inc.

For information about special discounts for bulk purchases, please contact Simon & Schuster Special Sales at 1-866-506-1949 or business@simonandschuster.com.

The Simon & Schuster Speakers Bureau can bring authors to your live event. For more information or to book an event, contact the Simon & Schuster Speakers Bureau at 1-866-248-3049 or visit our website at www.simonspeakers.com.

Manufactured in the United States of America

10 9

ISBN 978-1-4516-2162-4

The authors and publisher of this book are not physicians and are not licensed to give medical advice. The information in this book has been collected for the convenience of the reader. The nutrient values for prepared foods are subject to change and may now differ from listings herein, which are based on research conducted prior to Summer 2011. Such information does not constitute a recommendation or endorsement of any individual, institution, or product, nor is it intended as a substitute for a personalized consultation with your physician. The authors and publisher disclaim any liability arising directly or indirectly from the use of this book.

For our families,
who support us through every project.

ACKNOWLEDGMENTS

For all her continuous support and help, our agent, Nancy Trichter.

For her suggestions and editing skills, Sara Clemence.

For all her patience, comments, and questions—our favorite reviewer, Jean Schwarsin.

Without the tireless cooperation of Stephen Llano and the production department at Pocket Books, *The Complete Food Counter*, 4th Edition, would never have been completed.

A special thank you to our editor, Emilia Pisani, for keeping this project moving forward.

And we would like to thank all of our readers for their suggestions and questions. Your input helps us provide you with the most useful information.

Foods though so numerous and varied in form can be reduced to rather simple terms.

Mary Swartz Rose, Ph.D.
Feeding the Family
The Macmillan Company, 1919

CONTENTS

INTRODUCTION

Everyone loves to talk about food. And everyone has questions about their health. Listen to any group of people and the conversation almost always turns to food—what's the best choice for lunch, the current popular diet, or the latest health report.

We wrote *The Complete Food Counter* to give you answers. It is a handy, easy-to-use, *complete* food and nutrition resource, listing the calorie, protein, fat, cholesterol, carbohydrate, fiber, and sodium values for more than 17,000 foods, along with information on how to get enough of or limit each nutrient listed.

Let's talk about food—it's fun.
Let's talk about nutrition—it's important to your health.

UNDERSTANDING CALORIES

The amount of calories you eat is important—calories count!

Calories are calories, whether they come from apples or chocolate fudge. Every time you eat, you take in calories. All foods have some, except water.

Your body is a machine that uses food calories as fuel. When the amount of fuel you take in equals the amount of fuel you need to run your body, your weight remains constant. There is no extra fuel to store and no deficit to make up. Eat more calories than your body needs, and it will store the extra for future use, in places like your thighs, hips, and waist. Eat too few calories, and your body draws on its fuel reserves to meet demands. Your thighs, hips, and waist get slimmer as the extra fuel gets used up.

Again and again, studies have shown that if you cut calories, you lose weight. It doesn't matter if those calories come from bread, meat, or salad dressing. When you eat too many calories, even from healthy foods, you gain weight. The key to long-term weight control is to burn as many calories as you eat.

AND THE NUMBERS ARE?

On average, we eat 300 more calories a day than we ate 35 years ago—and we weigh 24 pounds more.

Women eat 1,833 calories a day; men eat 2,670.

To find out how many calories you need each day, you need to do two things. First, decide how much you want to weigh. We're not talking about your current weight—what is your target weight? Then, select an activity factor that fits your current activity level.

1. Your target weight is: __________
2. Your activity factor is: __________

   20 = Very active men

   15 = Moderately active men or very active women

   13 = Inactive men, moderately active women, and people over 55

   10 = Inactive women, repeat dieters, seriously overweight people
3. Target Weight × Activity Factor = Calories needed each day.

   For example, if your target weight is 130 and you are a moderately active woman (factor 13), you need about 1,600 to 1,700 calories a day.

130 pounds × 13 = 1,690 calories

If you're trying to lose weight, eating this amount of calories each day would guarantee weight loss, because you are getting only enough calories to support your target weight, not your current heavier weight. Add extra exercise to your regular routine, and the weight will come off even faster.

TRACK YOUR CALORIES

People cut calories by 10% when they keep track of what they eat each day.

30% to 50% of those who keep a food diary change their eating habits permanently.

FAT FACTS

Most Americans over the age of 6 eat 33% of their daily calories as fat. We are actually doing better eating less fat.

The simplistic view that all fats are bad and you should eat less fat is no longer accurate. The more accurate message is:

- Not all fats are bad for you.
- The type of fat you eat may be more important than how much you eat.
- A moderate fat intake can be healthy.

Don't head for the bacon grease just yet. Even though the current research suggests that a moderate fat intake may be healthier, no one is suggesting that a *high* fat intake is good for you. Eating too much fat puts you at risk for:

- Heart disease
- Stroke
- High blood pressure
- High cholesterol
- Cancer
- Obesity
- Diabetes
- Arthritis
- Gout

- Age-related macular degeneration (ARMD), a leading cause of blindness
- Alzheimer's disease, a leading cause of dementia

A high fat diet may even disrupt your body's clock. We all operate on a 24-hour circadian cycle that regulates sleeping, waking, fluid balance, body temperature, heart output, oxygen use, and gland functions. Recent research on animals confirmed that a high fat diet disrupts normal circadian rhythms. When the body's clock is disrupted it throws off our internal signals, including appetite control. Researchers have found a misaligned body clock can increase the risk for obesity and diabetes. Yet another good reason to eat a moderate amount of fat.

Total fat should be 20% to 35% of total calories

Americans have gotten the message that a high fat intake is not good for them, and currently we are eating less fat. Consumption studies show that we eat about 33% of our daily calories as fat. That is close to the upper end of the recommended 20% to 35% of total calories each day.

The following table will help you set your own daily target fat intake. First, select the number of calories you eat each day. Next, select the percentage of fat calories you wish to eat. The chart will give you the grams of fat to aim for daily. If you regularly eat 1,800 calories a day, for example, you should try to eat between 40 grams (20%) and 70 grams (35%) of fat each day. If you aim to eat 20% to 25% of your daily calories as fat, you will be eating a low fat intake. A moderate fat intake is considered 30% to 35%. Either can be part of a healthy eating plan.

DAILY TARGET FAT INTAKE				
CALORIES PER DAY	PERCENTAGE OF FAT CALORIES EACH DAY IN GRAMS			
	20%	25%	30%	35%
1,000	22	28	33	39
1,100	24	31	37	43
1,200	27	33	40	47
1,300	29	36	43	51
1,400	31	39	47	54
1,500	33	42	50	58
1,600	36	44	53	62
1,700	38	47	57	66
1,800	40	50	60	70
1,900	42	53	63	74
2,000	44	56	67	78
2,100	47	58	70	82
2,200	49	61	73	86
2,300	51	64	77	89
2,400	53	67	80	93
2,500	56	69	83	97
2,600	58	72	87	101
2,700	60	75	90	105
2,800	62	78	93	109
2,900	64	81	97	113
3,000	67	83	100	117

CONSIDER THIS

It's been shown over and over again that people have trouble sticking with a lowfat eating plan.

Moderate fat intakes are more satisfying and people find them easier to adopt for the long haul.

Keep in mind that the type of fat you eat is most important.

Saturated fats—eat less of this type of fat. Keep portions small.

Meat, whole milk, cheese, cream, regular or premium ice cream, butter, lard, bacon, sour cream, and pastries.

Monounsaturated fats—use these fats to replace some saturated fat.

Olives, olive oil, canola oil, peanuts, peanut oil, almonds, almond oil, avocados, cashews, hazelnuts, macadamia nuts, pine nuts, and pistachios.

Polyunsaturated fats—eat more of these fats.

Safflower oil, sesame oil, soybean oil, soybeans, corn oil, sunflower oil, grapeseed oil, nuts, seeds, soft margarine, wheat germ, flaxseeds, walnuts, walnut oil, herring, mackerel, tuna, trout, sardines, salmon, bluefish, and oysters.

Trans fats—eat as little as possible of these fats.

Pastries, solid shortening, stick margarine, doughnuts, deep-fried foods, processed cheese, and partially hydrogenated oil.

CONTROLLING CHOLESTEROL

On average, women eat 225 milligrams of cholesterol a day; men eat 307 milligrams daily.

Total Blood Cholesterol

Desirable: less than 200 mg/dl
Borderline high: 200 to 239 mg/dl
High: 240 mg/dl or higher

High cholesterol quietly does damage to your body, building up on the walls of your arteries. Over time, this buildup can cause the arteries to harden and become narrower, a process called *atherosclerosis.* If arteries get narrowed, blood flow to the heart muscle is slowed down and may even be blocked. A blocked artery to the heart can cause a heart attack. A blocked artery to the brain can cause a stroke.

High cholesterol does not cause any symptoms, so the only way you know if your cholesterol level is too high is through a blood test. It's important to know what the results mean, so you know if you need to change your habits.

Total cholesterol is just that—the total amount of cholesterol in a given volume of blood. It is measured as the number of milligrams (mg) of cholesterol in 1 deciliter (dl) of blood, which is slightly less than a half cup. For example, 222 mg/dl = 222 milligrams of cholesterol per deciliter of blood. To make things simpler, your doctor may give you just the number (222) rather than the more complete measurement. To reduce your risk for heart disease, you want your level to be below 200.

YOU SHOULD KNOW

It's wise to fast for at least 8 hours before getting your blood drawn.

Eating a high fat meal within 4 hours of a blood test can affect the results by raising blood fats.

If your number is good—total cholesterol is close to 200—you can eat a moderate cholesterol diet, which contains 300 milligrams of cholesterol or less a day. If your cholesterol number is less than desirable, or if your doctor has prescribed a cholesterol-lowering medication, you should eat a low-cholesterol diet, with less than 200 milligrams a day.

Total cholesterol isn't the only number that matters. To travel through blood, cholesterol, a fatlike substance, is coated with a protein. The combination of fat and protein is called a *lipoprotein*. If your total cholesterol values are high, your doctor will want to know the amount of LDL (low density lipoprotein) cholesterol and HDL (high density lipoprotein) cholesterol as well.

If too much LDL cholesterol—bad cholesterol—circulates in the blood, it can stick to the walls of the arteries leading to the heart and brain. This eventually forms plaque—thick, hard deposits that clog arteries. Experts believe HDL cholesterol—good cholesterol—carries cholesterol away from the arteries and to the liver, where it is broken down and removed from the body. This process is called reverse cholesterol transport, and it helps prevent the growth of plaque. It may be more important to know if your good HDL cholesterol is too low (less than 40 for men and less than 50 for women) than if your LDL cholesterol is too high.

Easy Steps to Lower Cholesterol

- Use liquid vegetable oils—olive, canola, corn, soybean, sunflower, and safflower—instead of butter, lard, shortening, or stick margarines.
- Limit servings of meat, poultry, fish, and shellfish to 3- to 4-ounce portions.
- Use lean cuts of meat and trim off all visible fat.
- Eat poultry without the skin.
- Don't fry in lard or bacon fat.
- Bake, broil, or roast.
- Use more beans and vegetables to make up for smaller servings of meat, fish, and poultry.
- Substitute two egg whites for one egg with yolk.
- Use lowfat or nonfat milk, cheese, yogurt, and ice cream, and fat free sour cream.
- Use soft margarine instead of stick margarines or butter.
- Use lowfat or fat free salad dressings and gravies.
- Eat fiber-rich foods—beans, whole grains, bran, brown rice, dried fruits, fruits, and vegetables.
- Eat more cholesterol-lowering foods—nuts, soyfoods, and antioxidant-rich fruits and vegetables.
- Eat soy, nuts, and flaxseed with natural cholesterol-lowering plant sterols, or foods

fortified with plant sterols—margarines, cereal, chocolate, orange juice, and yogurt.

- If your doctor prescribes a cholesterol-lowering medication, take it daily, even when your cholesterol values return to normal.

PERSPECTIVE ON PROTEIN

The word protein comes from the Greek word protos*—"of prime importance." You cannot live without protein.*

Your body loses millions of cells each day. They are used up, worn out, rubbed off, and even cut off, like your hair or beard. Protein is in almost every cell, tissue, and substance in your body and you need protein to replace these lost or worn-out cells.

You lose protein when your body is stressed—physically or mentally. When it's too hot or too cold, you need extra protein. More protein is needed during heavy sweating. Exercise, fever, surgery, injury, infection, and broken bones all increase your need for protein. Even emotional stress, such as losing your job or taking an exam, causes protein loss.

The protein in your body is very similar to the protein found in food. Both are made up of smaller building blocks called *amino acids.* Your body uses a combination of amino acids to build and repair different parts of the body—muscles, glands, skin, bones—just like the letters in the alphabet are used in different combinations to form words. Active tissues like muscles and glands contain a lot of protein. Less active tissue like fat has far less.

Some amino acids can be made in the body, others cannot. You get amino acids that can't be made in the body from the food you eat. When you eat different foods, you get varying amounts of different amino acids. That is one of the reasons it's important to eat a variety of foods.

CONSIDER THIS

The top 10 sources of protein eaten in the U.S. are: beef, poultry, milk, yeast bread, cheese, fish, eggs, fresh pork, ham, and pasta.

A quick way to estimate your daily protein need is to divide your weight by 2.2. For example, if you weigh 150 pounds, you should be eating approximately 68 grams of protein a day (150 ÷ 2.2 = 68). Most people eat more than their recommended amount. On average, men eat slightly over 100 grams of protein a day; women eat 70 grams.

Almost all foods you eat contain protein, some more and some less. Fruits have very little protein compared to meat, milk, cheese, beans, grains, and vegetables, all of which have more. Whenever you eat a food containing protein, you are providing your body with the amino acids needed to build and repair your body parts.

Meat, fish, and poultry are the most obvious protein sources, but many other foods are excellent sources as well.

PROTEIN EQUIVALENTS

A 1-ounce Serving of Protein = 6 to 8 Grams of Protein

(All the foods listed are equivalent to 1 ounce of protein.)

1 ounce of meat, fish, or poultry
¼ cup canned tuna, salmon, mackerel
1 ounce cheese
¼ cup cottage cheese
¼ cup cooked soybeans
½ cup cooked beans (any variety)
2 tablespoons peanut or other nut butter
1 egg
¼ cup egg substitute powder
1 cup soymilk
2 tablespoons dry milk
¾ cup lowfat yogurt
1 cup lowfat or nonfat milk
¼ cup (1.5 ounces) tofu
¼ cup tempeh
½ cup (2.5 ounces) meat substitute
¼ cup nuts or seeds
¼ cup wheat germ
1 cup cooked pasta

There are thousands of different proteins, and all have very specific functions. Protein:

- Helps form the structure of your body—skin, organs, bones, hair, and muscles.
- Is part of your immune system, fighting infections and viruses.
- Is part of every enzyme in your body.
- Is part of important hormones in your body.

- Helps keep body fluids stable.
- Transports substances and nutrients around the body.
- Helps you lose weight.
- Protects against disease.
- Is a source of energy (calories).

WEIGHT LOSS WISDOM

Recent studies have shown that diets with extra protein are more satisfying and result in greater weight loss.

CONSIDERING CARBOHYDRATES

Most Americans eat half their daily calories as carbohydrates. Most of us eat too much sugar and not enough whole grain breads, cereals, and pasta.

Not too long ago, you were told to eat all the carbohydrates you wanted. In fact, most Americans get 50% or more of their daily calories as carb. Today, however, carbs are being blamed for many of our health concerns, especially obesity. Just as with any other kind of food, if you eat more carbohydrate calories than your body needs for energy, the leftover is stored as fat.

So, how much carb should you be eating?

The National Academy of Sciences' Recommended Dietary Allowance (RDA) for carbohydrate is at least 130 grams a day. The Food and Drug Administration (FDA) has set 300 grams of carb as the Daily Value (DV) for the nutrition facts panel on food labels, the amount recommended for the "typical" American consumer eating 2,000 calories a day.

You can estimate your individual carb intake by first deciding what amount of carb you want to eat each day. Since most Americans get 50% of their calories from carb, let's use 50% as an example. If you eat 1,800 calories a day:

50% of 1,800 calories = 900 carb calories a day

To figure out how many grams of carb to eat each day, you need to know that 1 gram of carb = 4 calories. Continuing to use the example above:

900 carb calories per day ÷ 4 = 225 grams of carb per day

Most food professionals consider a low carb diet one in which 40% or less of your daily calories come from carbohydrates. Now, let's use 40% as an example of a low carb diet. If you eat 1,800 calories a day:

40% of 1,800 calories = 720 carb calories per day
720 carb calories per day ÷ 4 = 180 grams of carb per day

Both examples more than meet the RDA recommendation of at least 130 grams of carbohydrate a day. To make good carb choices, choose more foods that are higher in starch and fiber (complex carbs), and fewer foods that are high in sugar (simple carbs).

SHOP SMART

Over 3,200 new whole grain foods were introduced in 2010.

49% of grocery shoppers report they are buying more whole grain foods rich in complex carbs.

Complex carbohydrates are foods that contain a lot of starch—whole grains, cereals, beans, vegetables—and are rich in vitamins, minerals, and fiber.

Simple carbohydrates are foods that contain a lot of sugar—syrup, jelly, honey, soda, and molasses—and have few, if any, vitamins and minerals, and no fiber. But there are exceptions. Milk, yogurt, fruits, and some vegetables have a lot of natural sugar but are also rich in vitamins and minerals.

SORTING OUT CARBOHYDRATE FOODS

COMPLEX CARBS	SIMPLE CARBS
Bagels	***with natural sugar***
Beans	Fruits
Breads	Fruit juice
Cereals	Honey
Corn	Milk
Crackers	Unsweetened yogurt
Grains	
Pasta	***with added sugar***
Peas	Cake
Popcorn	Candy
Potatoes	Cookies
Pretzels	Fruit drinks
Rice	Jellies/jams
Rolls	Gelatin
Squash	Soda
Tortillas	Sweetened cereal
Vegetables	Sweetened yogurt

FOCUSING ON FIBER

96% of Americans do not eat enough fiber.

This is one carbohydrate all experts agree on: we need to eat more fiber. Why? Fiber aids in losing weight, managing diabetes, relieving constipation, and protecting against certain cancers. It may even lower the risk for heart disease. All this and it's calorie-free!

Fiber is found only in plants, either as the woody part, which helps promote regularity, or as gums and mucilages (the sticky part of plants), which help lower cholesterol. Even though fiber is a carb, your body cannot break it down and use it the way it uses sugar and starch.

But living in your digestive track are trillions of friendly microbes that use fiber as their main source of nourishment. These friendly bacteria have been with you since birth and help protect you against unfriendly bacteria that could make you sick. When you eat enough fiber, your friendly bacteria are well fed and can put up a good fight. When you eat too little fiber, unfriendly invaders can start to take over. Eating enough fiber stimulates your natural resistance against disease and infection.

CHEW ON THIS

Eating fiber-rich foods is smarter than popping fiber supplements.

Fiber-rich foods are also rich in antioxidants, vitamins, and minerals. Supplements are not.

Most of us eat too little fiber. We average about 15 grams a day, far less than we should be eating. The following chart provides daily fiber recommendations. Check to see how much fiber you should be eating each day.

DAILY FIBER RECOMMENDATIONS

Men	
19–50 years	38 grams of fiber
50 and older	30 grams of fiber
Women	
19–50 years	25 grams of fiber
50 and older	21 grams of fiber
pregnant	28 grams of fiber

AGE + 5

Children 2 and older should eat the amount of fiber daily that equals their age + 5.

For a 5-year-old, that would be at least 10 grams of fiber a day (5 years + 5 = 10).

The rule holds until age 19, when adult requirements apply.

Slowly start adding fiber-rich foods to your daily meals—beans, berries, bran, fruits, oatmeal, vegetables, and whole grains. Don't go overboard, because it takes your body a little time to adjust to the extra bulk passing through your digestive tract. And drink plenty of fluids. Fiber soaks up fluids like a sponge. This not only helps you feel fuller longer but also helps form soft, easily passed stools.

Add a Little Fiber to Your Life

- Eat whole fruits and vegetables instead of drinking juices.
- Eat the fiber-rich skins of cucumbers, apples, pears, potatoes, and zucchini.
- Eat more berries—blueberries, blackberries, raspberries, strawberries.
- Choose whole grains—brown rice, cornmeal, barley, cracked wheat, rye, and whole wheat.
- Eat beans and lentils a few times a week.
- Eat whole grain or high fiber cereals like oatmeal, oat flakes, bran, and shredded wheat.
- Eat whole wheat bread, bagels, pasta, pretzels, crackers, and rolls.
- Try soybeans in every form—soynuts, tofu, tempeh, edamame.
- Snack on fig newtons, graham crackers, and popcorn.
- Have vegetarian meals a few times a week.
- Eat dried fruits and raisins.
- Sprinkle ground flaxseed, bran, or whole grain granola onto cereal or yogurt for a healthy crunch.
- Experiment with higher fiber versions of old favorites, like brown rice, buckwheat noodles, or baked sweet potatoes.

- Try some of the new fiber-fortified foods, like high fiber cereal bars and breads.

YOU SHOULD KNOW

High fiber foods have 5 or more grams of fiber in a serving.

A good source of fiber has 2 or more grams of fiber in a serving.

BE SENSIBLE WITH SODIUM

We eat too much sodium.
Americans eat more than 3,400 milligrams a day. Men eat slightly more and women slightly less than this average.

Ever give that salt shaker on your kitchen table a second thought? You should. Once a precious commodity, salt has become all too common in our food supply, to the point where it's estimated we each eat 1¼ to 2½ teaspoons a day—far more than we need.

When people are told to eat less sodium, their first reaction is to empty the salt shaker and stop adding salt in cooking. This may not be the most effective approach. Table salt is made up of 2 minerals—sodium and chloride. One teaspoon of salt—weighing about 6,200 milligrams—contains 2,400 milligrams of sodium; the rest is chloride. Removing the salt shaker from the table will reduce only a fraction of the sodium most of us eat daily, because your daily sodium intake actually comes from:

Salt in processed and restaurant foods	77%
Sodium naturally occurring in food	12%
Salt added in cooking	5%
Salt from the salt shaker	6%

Dumping the salt shaker only reduces your salt intake by slightly more than 10%. Cutting down on processed foods will make a much bigger dent in your sodium intake. What are processed foods? Prepared salad dressing, jarred tomato sauce, canned tuna, marinated fresh meat and poultry, cake mixes, pickles, pretzels, frozen dinners, desserts, canned soup, microwave meals, deli meats, hot dogs—just to name a few.

DID YOU KNOW?

An average dill pickle contains 1,000 milligrams of sodium, two-thirds of your day's supply.

We are a population that loves salty foods—in fact, we often reject foods with less sodium. Research has shown that for some foods, consumers can taste a sodium reduction as small as 8%. When the consumer's traditional brand does not deliver the anticipated taste, the company can lose sales. For this reason, many companies choose to make "silent reductions" in sodium. They simply lower the sodium without touting the change in advertising campaigns. As consumers embrace the newer lower sodium foods, companies may change their advertising approach.

It's not easy to take the salt out of a recipe. Besides enhancing the taste of food, salt is a functional ingredient.

Salt:

- Keeps food from spoiling by creating a hostile environment for microorganisms. Salted meat and fish kept early man from starving.
- Adds texture to foods. It strengthens the gluten (a protein) in bread dough, allowing it to rise without tearing and exploding.

- Provides fermentation control so that baked goods rise at a steady rate in the oven.
- Helps make cheese and sauerkraut.
- Promotes the typical color that develops in ham, bacon, hot dogs, bologna, and sauerkraut.

Despite the challenges, many food companies and restaurant recipe developers are altering products to be lower in sodium.

All of these initiatives are good. As the companies and restaurants lower the salt in products, our desire for very salty foods will shift and we will be more interested in eating lower-sodium choices. Research has shown that even modest daily sodium reductions, as little as 400 milligrams, can produce health benefits.

Ninety-five percent of American adults exceed the recommended upper limit of sodium intake every day, and 90% of adult Americans are at risk for high blood pressure as they get older. A study done by the Centers for Disease Control and Prevention (CDC) estimated that slightly more than 69% of adults belong to an at-risk group that would benefit from keeping their sodium intake under 1,500 milligrams a day. This group includes those diagnosed with high blood pressure, African Americans, and anyone over the age of 40. Most Americans should be watching their sodium.

WHAT THE EXPERTS ARE SAYING

The American Heart Association recommends that people eat no more than 1,500 milligrams of sodium a day.

The 2010 Dietary Guidelines for Americans recommends less than 2,300 milligrams a day and no more than 1,500 milligrams of sodium a day for people over the age of 51, African Americans, and those with high blood pressure or kidney disease.

The Dietary Reference Intakes from the National Academy of Sciences recommend that people eat no more than 2,300 milligrams a day.

How are sodium and high blood pressure connected? The sodium in body fluids causes the body to hold water. Your heart pumps harder to handle the extra fluid. Sodium also appears to stiffen arteries, making them less flexible. Blood pressure goes up, trying to pump blood through these less flexible vessels. When salt intake is lowered, the extra fluid is reduced and the arteries become less stiff, so your heart doesn't have to work so hard.

Giving up salt isn't easy. Many experts believe that healthy adults could do nicely on as little as 500 milligrams of sodium a day. That may be healthy, but would we consider it tasty?

YOU SHOULD KNOW

A high salt intake:

is linked to an increased risk
for heart attack and stroke;
contributes to kidney disease;
may increase the risk for stomach cancer;
increases your risk for osteoporosis.

To Lighten Up on Salt

- Don't add salt to restaurant or take-out foods.
- Use naturally low sodium foods, like fresh fruits and vegetables, or plain frozen vegetables to complement take-out or prepared entrees.
- Check the nutrition label—keep snacks and single-serving foods under 400 milligrams a serving; keep main dishes under 600 milligrams a serving.
- Try some low sodium or "no salt added" choices. You might be pleasantly surprised at the taste.
- Fresh salads are naturally low in sodium; just go easy on the dressing.
- Plain frozen vegetables are lower in sodium than sauced and seasoned varieties.
- Almost all frozen vegetables are lower in sodium than canned vegetables.
- Try baldy pretzels and unsalted nuts.
- Reduce salt in recipes by half. Swapping a ½ teaspoon of salt for 1 teaspoon saves 1,200 milligrams of sodium.
- Rinse canned beans, sauerkraut, vegetables, and tuna to reduce the sodium by almost half.

- Don't add salt when cooking rice, pasta, or hot cereal.
- Use fresh pepper or herbs to flavor food instead of salt.
- When you eat a high salt/sodium choice, balance it with lower sodium choices later in the day.

DID YOU KNOW?

1 teaspoon of table salt = 2,400 milligrams of sodium.

Coarser salts, such as kosher salt and sea salt, average between 1,100 and 1,900 milligrams sodium per teaspoon.

USING YOUR COMPLETE FOOD COUNTER

The Complete Food Counter, 4th edition, lists the portion size, calories, protein, fat, cholesterol, carbohydrate, fiber, and sodium values for more than 17,000 foods. Now you can compare the values in your favorite foods and, when necessary, choose substitutes before you go out to shop or eat. This will save you time and help you decide what to buy.

The counter section of the book is divided into two parts—Part One: Brand Name, Nonbranded (Generic), and Take-Out Foods (page 37); and Part Two: Restaurant Chains (page 567). Each part lists foods or restaurant chains alphabetically.

In Part One, for each category, you will find nonbranded (generic) foods listed first, in alphabetical order, followed by an alphabetical listing of brand-name foods. The nonbranded listing will help you estimate the calories, protein, fat, cholesterol, carbohydrate, fiber, and sodium values when you don't see your favorite brands. They can also help you evaluate store brands. Large categories are divided into subcategories, such as canned, fresh, frozen, and ready-to-eat, to make it easier to find what you're looking for. Some categories have "see" and "see also" references, to help you find related items.

When a dash (-) appears, it means that no analysis was done for fat, cholesterol, protein, carbohydrate, fiber, or sodium for that food. It is not the same as a "0," which means there is no fat, cholesterol, protein, carbohydrate, fiber, or sodium in the food.

Because we eat out so often, over 800 take-out foods are listed in Part One. These are found in the take-out subcategory in many categories throughout this section. Look there for foods you take-out or order in, since those are not nutrition labeled.

Most foods are listed alphabetically. In some cases, though, foods are grouped by category. For example, a tuna sandwich is found in the sandwich category. Other group categories include:

ALCOHOL DRINKS: **Page 38**

Includes all alcoholic beverages and mixed drinks except beer and ale, champagne, and wine, which have their own separate categories.

ASIAN FOOD: **Page 51**

Includes all types of Asian foods except egg rolls and sushi, which are found in the egg rolls and sushi categories.

DELI MEATS/COLD CUTS: **Page 230**

Includes all sandwich meats except chicken, ham, and turkey, which are found in their own separate categories.

DINNER: **Page 232**
Includes all prepared dinners listed by brand name, except pasta dinners, which are found in the pasta dinners category.

NUTRITION SUPPLEMENTS: **Page 358**
Includes all dieting aids, meal replacements, and drinks, except energy bars and energy drinks, which are found in their own separate categories.

SANDWICHES: **Page 450**
Includes popular sandwich, calzone, and panini choices.

SNACKS: **Page 475**
Includes a variety of snack items, such as pork rinds and cheese puffs.

SPANISH FOOD: **Page 504**
Includes all types of Spanish and Mexican foods except salsa and tortillas, which have their own separate categories.

In Part Two, Restaurant Chains, 97 national and regional restaurant, coffee, doughnut, frozen yogurt, ice cream, pizza, sandwich, soup, and sushi chains are listed.

With *The Complete Food Counter*, 4th edition, as your guide, you have at your fingertips the most comprehensive guide to calories and important nutrients in all the foods you eat.

DEFINITIONS

as prep (as prepared): refers to food that has been prepared according to package directions

lean and fat: describes meat with some fat on its edges that is not cut away before cooking, or poultry prepared with skin and fat as purchased

lean only: refers to lean meat that is trimmed of all visible fat, or poultry without skin

not prep (not prepared): refers to food that has not been cooked and may require the addition of other ingredients to prepare

shelf-stable: refers to prepared products found on the supermarket shelves that are not canned or frozen but are packaged and ready-to-eat or ready to be heated but do not require refrigeration

take-out: describes prepared dishes that you purchase ready-to-eat; those included serve as a guide to the calories, protein, fat, cholesterol, carbohydrate, fiber, and sodium in products you may buy.

ABBREVIATIONS

avg	=	average
diam	=	diameter
fl	=	fluid
frzn	=	frozen
g	=	gram
in	=	inch
lb	=	pound
lg	=	large
med	=	medium
mg	=	milligram
oz	=	ounce
pkg	=	package
prep	=	prepared
pt	=	pint
qt	=	quart
reg	=	regular
sec	=	second
serv	=	serving
sm	=	small
sq	=	square
tbsp	=	tablespoon
tr	=	trace
tsp	=	teaspoon
w/	=	with
w/o	=	without
<	=	less than

NOTES

Cals = Calories

All calorie values have been rounded to the nearest calorie

Prot = Protein

All protein values are given in grams (g)

All values have been rounded to the nearest gram

Fat = Total fat

All fat values are given in grams (g)

All values have been rounded to the nearest gram

Chol = Cholesterol

All cholesterol values are given in milligrams (mg)

All values have been rounded to the nearest milligram

Carb = Carbohydrate

All carbohydrate values are given in grams (g)

All values have been rounded to the nearest gram

Fiber = Fiber

All fiber values are given in grams (g)

All values have been rounded to the nearest gram

Sod = Sodium

All sodium values are given in milligrams (mg)

All values have been rounded to the nearest milligram

tr (trace) = less than 0.5 grams of fat, protein, carbohydrate, or fiber, and less than 0.5 milligrams of cholesterol or sodium

- (dash) indicates data was not available
0 (zero) indicates there are no calories, fat, cholesterol, protein, carbohydrate, fiber, or sodium in that food

Discrepancies in figures are due to rounding of values, product reformulation, and reevaluation. The current labeling law allows rounding. Much of the data listed here is analysis data, obtained directly from manufacturers, not from labels; therefore, some values here may differ slightly from those on labels because they have not been rounded.

PART ONE

Brand Name, Nonbranded (Generic), and Take-Out Foods

OUR BEST EATING ADVICE IN A NUTSHELL

Calories*—go easy, don't overdo, keep portions reasonable.*

Protein*—select lean and lowfat choices, eat both animal and vegetable sources.*

Fat*—aim for moderate amounts daily, limit fried foods and fatty add-ons like salad dressing.*

Cholesterol*—aim for 300 milligrams or less a day.*

Carbohydrates*—limit sugars and select more complex starches, like grains and vegetables.*

Fiber*—eat more, use whole grains.*

Sodium*—go easy, cut down on processed foods, eat more whole foods naturally lower in salt.*

FOOD	PORTION	CALS	PROT	FAT	CHOL	CARB	FIBER	SOD
ABALONE								
breaded & fried	1 serv (3 oz)	162	17	6	80	9	tr	980
steamed	1 serv (3 oz)	127	17	3	84	6	0	574
ACAI JUICE								
Arthur's								
Acai Plus	1 bottle (11 oz)	230	2	5	0	45	5	0
Bossa Nova								
Acai Juice Blueberry	8 oz	89	0	0	0	21	0	14
Acai Juice Mango	8 oz	89	0	0	0	23	0	14
Acai Juice Original	8 oz	94	0	0	0	21	0	14
Acai Juice Passion Fruit	8 oz	89	0	0	0	23	0	14
Acai Juice Raspberry	8 oz	89	0	0	0	23	0	13
O.N.E.								
Amazon Acai	1 bottle (11 oz)	157	1	3	0	32	3	28
Zola								
100% Juice	1 box (11 oz)	170	2	2	0	30	1	45
ACEROLA								
fresh	1 (5 g)	2	tr	tr	0	tr	tr	0
ACEROLA JUICE								
juice	1 cup	56	1	1	0	12	1	7
ADZUKI BEANS								
canned sweetened	½ cup	351	6	tr	0	81	–	323
dried cooked w/o salt	½ cup	147	9	tr	0	28	8	9
Arrowhead Mills								
Organic Dried not prep	¼ cup	130	8	0	0	26	5	0
AKEE								
fresh	3.5 oz	223	5	20	0	5	–	–
ALCOHOL DRINKS (*see also* BEER AND ALE, CHAMPAGNE, MALT, WINE)								
7&7	1 serv	178	0	0	0	19	0	21
alabama slammer	1 serv	103	tr	tr	0	7	tr	tr
amaretto sour	1 serv	295	2	tr	0	57	4	98
angel's kiss	1 serv	85	tr	1	5	5	0	4
anisette	1 oz	111	–	0	0	11	0	–
antifreeze	1 serv	177	1	tr	0	31	tr	2

FOOD	PORTION	CALS	PROT	FAT	CHOL	CARB	FIBER	SOD
apricot brandy	1 oz	96	–	0	0	9	0	–
apricot sour	1 serv	164	tr	tr	0	8	tr	5
aquavit	1 oz	65	0	0	–	0	0	–
b 52	1 serv	247	1	4	0	25	0	24
b&b	1 serv	75	0	0	0	0	0	tr
bahama breeze	1 serv	70	tr	tr	0	9	tr	2
bahama mama	1 serv	153	1	tr	0	23	tr	2
bailey's & amaretto	1 serv	184	1	5	0	16	0	29
banana colada	1 serv	376	2	1	0	64	3	4
bay breeze	1 serv	173	1	tr	0	18	tr	2
bend me over	1 serv	242	1	tr	0	32	tr	33
benedictine	1 oz	104	–	0	0	11	0	–
betsy ross	1 serv	206	tr	0	0	5	0	3
black devil	1 serv	220	tr	tr	0	1	tr	43
black russian	1 serv	184	0	tr	0	12	0	3
bloody mary	1 serv	150	1	tr	0	5	1	332
blue whale	1 serv	222	tr	tr	0	23	0	63
bourbon & soda	1 serv (4 oz)	105	0	0	0	0	0	16
bourbon sour	1 serv	166	tr	tr	0	8	tr	5
brandy	2 oz	255	–	–	–	–	–	–
brandy alexander	1 serv	266	1	6	20	12	0	17
brandy sour	1 serv	164	tr	tr	0	8	tr	5
bushwacker	1 serv	286	tr	5	0	27	tr	23
campari	2 oz	245	–	–	–	–	–	–
cherry heering	2 oz	245	–	–	–	–	–	–
coffee liqueur	1 serv (1.5 oz)	175	tr	tr	0	24	0	4
cognac	1 oz	67	0	0	0	tr	0	–
cosmopolitan martini	1 serv	126	tr	tr	0	7	tr	1
creme de almonde	1 oz	102	–	–	–	–	–	–
creme de banana	1 oz	99	–	–	–	–	–	–
creme de cassis	1 oz	82	–	–	–	–	–	–
creme de menthe	1 serv (1.5 oz)	186	0	tr	0	21	0	3
curacao liqueur	1 oz	81	–	0	0	9	0	–
daiquiri	1 serv (2 oz)	112	tr	tr	0	4	tr	3
daiquiri banana	1 serv	277	1	tr	0	32	1	7
daiquiri frozen	1 serv	393	–	2	–	–	–	–
daiquiri frozen pineapple	1 serv	186	1	tr	0	28	2	3
dark & stormy	1 serv	64	0	0	0	0	0	tr

FOOD	PORTION	CALS	PROT	FAT	CHOL	CARB	FIBER	SOD
doctor pepper	1 serv	95	0	0	0	12	0	1
drambuie	2 oz	225	–	–	–	–	–	–
fuzzy navel	1 serv	247	1	tr	0	10	tr	2
gibson	1 serv (4 oz)	254	–	–	–	–	–	–
gin	1 serv (1.5 oz)	110	0	0	0	0	0	1
gin & tonic	1 serv (7.5 oz)	171	0	0	0	16	–	10
gin ricky	1 serv	114	tr	tr	0	1	tr	38
grasshopper	1 serv	275	1	5	15	26	0	13
happy hawaiian	1 serv	434	2	8	0	60	tr	50
harvey wallbanger	1 serv	198	1	tr	0	16	tr	2
head banger	1 serv	165	0	0	0	4	0	tr
hot buttered rum	1 serv (8.8 oz)	316	tr	12	30	4	tr	8
hot toddy	1 serv	188	tr	1	0	13	5	9
hurricane	1 serv	205	tr	tr	0	19	tr	2
kamikaze	1 serv	136	0	0	0	2	0	2
long island iced tea	1 serv	292	tr	tr	0	7	0	33
lynchburg lemonade	1 serv	465	tr	tr	0	85	1	38
mai tai	1 serv	165	tr	tr	0	17	tr	51
manhattan	1 serv	171	tr	tr	0	3	tr	9
margarita	1 serv	173	0	0	0	11	0	3
margarita strawberry	1 serv	106	tr	tr	0	11	1	1
martini	1 serv (3 oz)	206	tr	0	0	2	0	3
martini apple	1 serv	147	tr	tr	0	4	tr	2
martini rum	1 serv	131	tr	0	0	tr	tr	1
mellow yellow	1 serv	95	0	0	0	4	0	0
mexican grasshopper	1 serv	638	1	19	66	52	0	29
mint julep	1 serv	136	tr	tr	0	17	tr	3
mississippi mud	1 serv	496	3	12	45	46	0	46
mudslide	1 serv	566	2	10	0	46	0	65
narragansett	1 serv	168	0	0	0	2	0	5
nutcracker	1 serv	730	2	10	0	64	0	65
old fashioned	1 serv	223	tr	tr	0	4	tr	5
orange crush	1 serv	461	0	tr	0	65	tr	5
pain killer	1 serv	277	1	tr	0	20	tr	5
peppermint pattie	1 serv	344	tr	tr	0	37	0	7
pina colada	1 serv (4.5 oz)	245	1	3	0	32	tr	8

FOOD	PORTION	CALS	PROT	FAT	CHOL	CARB	FIBER	SOD
planter's cocktail	1 serv	105	tr	0	0	3	tr	1
planter's punch	1 serv	233	2	tr	0	34	4	33
presbyterian	1 serv	170	tr	0	0	8	tr	26
purple passion	1 serv	215	tr	tr	0	22	0	14
rob roy	1 serv	171	tr	0	0	3	tr	13
rum	1 serv (1.5 oz)	97	0	0	0	0	0	0
rum boogie	1 serv	134	tr	tr	0	12	tr	3
rum cola	1 serv	209	tr	tr	0	21	tr	8
rum highball	1 serv	170	0	0	0	11	0	9
rum punch	1 serv	448	1	1	0	88	1	12
rum screwdriver	1 serv	166	1	tr	0	16	tr	2
rum sour	1 serv	156	tr	tr	0	8	tr	5
rum swizzle	1 serv	187	0	0	0	15	0	44
rusty nail	1 serv	159	0	0	0	6	0	tr
sake	1 serv (1 oz)	39	tr	0	0	1	0	1
salty dog	1 serv	210	1	tr	0	19	tr	3
scotch & soda	1 serv	104	tr	0	0	tr	tr	38
sea breeze	1 serv	207	tr	tr	0	19	tr	3
sex on the beach	1 serv	190	tr	tr	0	18	tr	2
singapore sling	1 serv (4 oz)	115	–	–	–	–	–	–
slippery nipple	1 serv	142	tr	2	0	11	0	16
sloe gin fizz	1 serv (2.5 oz)	132	0	0	0	4	0	1
snake bite	1 serv	362	0	0	0	22	0	7
southern comfort	1 serv (1.5 oz)	184	–	–	–	–	–	–
tequila	1 serv (1.5 oz)	117	–	–	–	–	–	–
tequila frozen screwdriver	1 serv	159	1	tr	0	17	1	2
tequila gimlet	1 serv	150	tr	tr	0	6	1	3
tequila sour	1 serv	156	tr	tr	0	8	tr	5
tequila stinger	1 serv	221	0	tr	0	14	0	2
tequila sunrise	1 serv (6.8 oz)	232	1	tr	0	24	0	120
tom collins	1 serv (7.5 oz)	121	tr	0	0	3	–	39
vermouth cassis	1 serv	97	tr	tr	0	5	tr	54
vodka	1 serv (1.5 oz)	97	0	0	0	0	0	0

FOOD	PORTION	CALS	PROT	FAT	CHOL	CARB	FIBER	SOD
vodka gimlet	1 serv	150	tr	tr	0	6	1	3
vodka sour	1 serv	138	tr	tr	0	3	tr	1
vodka stinger	1 serv	378	0	tr	0	28	0	4
whiskey	1 serv (1.5 oz)	105	0	0	0	tr	0	0
whiskey sour	1 serv (3.5 oz)	162	tr	tr	0	14	0	65
white russian	1 serv	290	tr	8	31	17	0	12
zombie	1 serv	235	tr	tr	0	10	tr	5
Absolut								
Vodka	1 shot (1.5 oz)	98	–	0	0	0	–	–
Bacardi								
Gold Rum	1 shot (1.5 oz)	98	–	0	0	0	–	–
Capt. Morgan's								
Original Spiced Rum	1 shot (1.5 oz)	86	–	0	0	0	–	–
Crown Royal								
Canadian Whiskey	1 shot (1.5 oz)	96	–	0	0	0	–	–
Jack Daniel's								
Old No.7 Tennessee Whiskey	1 shot (1.5 oz)	98	–	0	0	0	–	–
Jose Cuervo								
Gold Tequila	1 shot (1.5 oz)	96	–	0	0	0	–	–
Seagram's								
Gin	1 shot (1.5 oz)	120	–	0	0	0	–	–
Smirnoff								
Vodka	1 shot (1.5 oz)	96	–	0	0	0	–	–

ALE (*see* BEER AND ALE)

ALFALFA

FOOD	PORTION	CALS	PROT	FAT	CHOL	CARB	FIBER	SOD
sprouts	½ cup	40	1	tr	0	1	tr	1

ALLIGATOR

FOOD	PORTION	CALS	PROT	FAT	CHOL	CARB	FIBER	SOD
cooked	3 oz	126	28	2	57	0	0	66

FOOD	PORTION	CALS	PROT	FAT	CHOL	CARB	FIBER	SOD
ALLSPICE								
ground	1 tsp	5	tr	tr	0	1	tr	1
ALMONDS								
almond butter w/ salt	2 tbsp	203	5	19	0	7	1	144
almond butter w/o salt	2 tbsp	203	5	19	0	7	1	4
almond extract	1 tsp	38	5	tr	0	–	0	–
almond paste	¼ cup	260	5	16	0	27	3	5
chocolate covered	6 pieces (0.6 oz)	102	3	8	1	6	2	8
dry roasted w/ salt	¼ cup	206	8	18	0	7	4	117
dry roasted w/o salt	¼ cup	206	8	18	0	7	4	0
honey roasted	¼ cup	214	7	18	0	10	5	47
jordan almonds	6 (0.7 oz)	99	2	4	0	14	1	3
oil roasted w/ salt	¼ cup	238	8	22	0	7	4	133
oil roasted w/o salt	¼ cup	238	8	22	0	7	4	0
praline	17 pieces (1.4 oz)	210	5	12	0	21	3	45
yogurt covered	6 pieces (0.8 oz)	122	3	8	0	10	1	13
American Almond								
Marzipan	2 tbsp	130	2	5	0	19	1	0
Arrowhead Mills								
Organic Almond Butter Creamy	2 tbsp	200	7	17	0	6	4	0
Back To Nature								
California Sea Salt Roasted	1 oz	160	6	14	0	6	3	95
Barney Butter								
Almond Butter Crunchy	2 tbsp (1.1 oz)	180	6	16	0	7	3	80
Almond Butter Smooth	2 tbsp (1.1 oz)	180	6	15	0	8	3	100
Diamond								
Slivered	¼ cup (1 oz)	170	7	15	0	6	3	0
Fisher								
Roasted & Salted	¼ cup (1 oz)	170	6	15	0	5	3	110
Godiva								
Dark Chocolate Almonds	1 pkg (2 oz)	310	8	24	0	23	5	40
Justin's								
Almond Butter Classic	2 tbsp (1.1 oz)	200	7	18	0	6	4	0

FOOD	PORTION	CALS	PROT	FAT	CHOL	CARB	FIBER	SOD
Almond Butter Maple	2 tbsp (1.1 oz)	190	6	16	0	8	3	65
Love'n Bake								
Almond Paste	2 tbsp	140	4	9	0	13	2	0
Almond Schmear	2 tbsp	140	4	8	0	14	2	0
Roasted Butter	2 tbsp	180	6	16	0	6	3	55
Mrs. May's								
Almond Crunch	1 oz	156	5	13	0	8	3	37
Naturally More								
Almond Butter	2 tbsp	190	9	16	0	8	4	65
Planters								
Chocolate Lovers Dark Chocolate	11 pieces (1.4 oz)	220	4	17	<5	18	3	15
Dry Roasted	23 pieces (1 oz)	160	6	14	0	6	3	150
NUT-rition Bone Health Mix	¼ cup (1.2 oz)	170	4	10	0	19	2	30
Sunkist								
Accents Italian Parmesan	1 tbsp	40	1	4	0	1	0	95
Accents Original Oven Roasted	1 tbsp	40	1	4	0	1	0	70
SunRidge Farms								
Dark Chocolate Cane Sweetened	11 (1.4 oz)	220	4	16	0	19	3	0
ALOE JUICE								
Alo								
Appeal Aloe Vera + Pomelo Pink Grapefruit & Lemon	8 oz	60	0	0	0	15	0	35
Awaken Aloe Vera + Wheatgrass	8 oz	50	0	0	0	15	0	50
Enliven Aloe Vera + 12 Fruits & Vegetables	8 oz	50	0	0	0	13	0	70
Enrich Aloe Vera + Pomegranate & Cranberry	8 oz	70	0	0	0	15	0	35
Exposed Aloe Vera Original	8 oz	60	0	0	0	15	0	45
TropiKing								
Aloe Vera Juice	8 oz	88	0	0	0	22	tr	5
Aloe Vera Juice & Grape	8 oz	100	0	0	0	25	1	30

FOOD	PORTION	CALS	PROT	FAT	CHOL	CARB	FIBER	SOD
Aloe Vera Juice & Pineapple	8 oz	100	0	0	0	25	1	20
Aloe Vera Juice & Pomegranate	8 oz	120	0	0	0	30	1	130
AMARANTH								
leaves cooked	½ cup	14	1	tr	0	3	–	170
uncooked	½ cup (3.4 oz)	365	14	6	0	65	15	20
Arrowhead Mills								
Organic Whole Grain not prep	¼ cup	180	7	3	0	31	7	10
ANCHOVY								
boneless	1 oz	60	8	3	24	0	0	1042
canned in oil drained	1 can (2 oz)	94	13	4	38	0	0	1651
fresh	1 (4 g)	8	1	tr	3	0	0	147
fresh fillets	3 (0.4 oz)	21	2	1	–	tr	–	–
Polar								
Rolled Fillets w/ Capers In Olive Oil	7 pieces (0.6 oz)	40	4	3	15	0	0	970
ANGLERFISH								
raw	3.5 oz	72	15	1	–	0	0	109
ANISE								
seed	1 tsp	7	tr	tr	0	1	tr	0
ANTELOPE								
roasted	4 oz	215	41	4	127	0	0	304
APPLE								
CANNED								
sliced sweetened	½ cup	68	tr	1	0	17	2	3
Glory								
Fried Apples	½ cup	80	0	0	0	21	1	170
Jake & Amos								
Red Spiced Rings	1 (1 oz)	35	0	0	0	9	0	5
Polar								
Fuji	½ cup	50	0	0	0	12	2	20
DRIED								
chopped	½ cup	104	tr	tr	0	28	4	37
cooked w/o sugar	½ cup	73	tr	tr	0	20	3	26
rings	5	78	tr	tr	0	21	3	28

FOOD	PORTION	CALS	PROT	FAT	CHOL	CARB	FIBER	SOD
Bare Fruit								
Chips Cinnamon	1 pkg (0.6 oz)	43	0	0	0	12	2	15
Chukar Cherries								
Cherry Apple Slices	10 (1 oz)	110	0	0	0	28	4	0
Del Monte								
Dried Apples	¼ cup (1.4 oz)	110	1	0	0	27	3	270
Fruit Ripples								
Cinnamon Apple	1 pkg	50	0	0	0	13	1	75
Strawberry Apple	1 pkg	50	0	0	0	13	1	75
Mott's								
Snacks Freeze Dried	1 pkg (0.55 oz)	60	0	0	0	15	3	0
Mrs. May's								
Fruit Chips	1 pkg	35	0	0	0	8	1	0
Nature's Envy								
Apple Chips Original	1 pkg (0.8 oz)	80	0	0	0	20	tr	20
Stoneridge Orchards								
Green Wedges	⅓ cup (1.4 oz)	140	0	0	0	32	1	0
Sun-Maid								
Apples	¼ cup (1.4 oz)	120	1	0	0	29	2	135
FRESH								
apple	1 lg	110	1	tr	0	29	5	2
apple	1 sm	55	tr	tr	0	15	3	1
apple	1 med	72	tr	tr	0	19	3	1
candied	1 med (6.5 oz)	234	2	4	0	52	4	103
candied	1 lg (9.8 oz)	357	3	6	6	79	6	157
candied	1 sm (4.9 oz)	179	2	3	0	40	3	79
w/ skin sliced	1 cup	57	tr	tr	0	15	3	1
w/o skin sliced	1 cup	53	tr	tr	0	14	1	0
Chiquita								
Apple	1 (6.4 oz)	95	0	0	0	25	4	2

FOOD	PORTION	CALS	PROT	FAT	CHOL	CARB	FIBER	SOD
Apple Bites	1 pkg (2.5 oz)	30	0	0	0	8	2	0
Apple Bites w/ Caramel	1 pkg (2.5 oz)	70	0	0	0	17	2	55
Earthbound Farms								
Organic Slices	1 pkg (2 oz)	30	0	0	0	7	1	0
Eastern Select								
Gala	1 (5.5 oz)	80	0	0	0	22	5	0
Mrs. Prindable's								
Caramel Triple Chocolate	¼ apple (1.7 oz)	120	1	6	5	17	1	10
Caramel Walnut	¼ apple (2 oz)	160	2	10	5	17	1	15
Ready Pac								
Apples w/ Caramel Dip	1 pkg (6 oz)	200	2	0	0	52	2	200
Apples w/ Peanut Butter Dip	1 pkg (5.7 oz)	340	12	24	0	28	6	230
Sullivan								
McIntosh	1 (5.4 oz)	80	0	1	0	22	4	0
FROZEN								
sliced w/o sugar	½ cup	42	tr	tr	0	11	2	3
REFRIGERATED								
Country Crock								
Cinnamon Apples	½ cup (4.4 oz)	130	0	3	0	26	1	200
TAKE-OUT								
baked	1 (6 oz)	128	tr	tr	0	42	4	2
baked no sugar	1 (5.6 oz)	136	tr	tr	0	24	4	2
fried apple rings	1 serv (2.7 oz)	91	tr	4	0	15	2	33

APPLE JUICE

FOOD	PORTION	CALS	PROT	FAT	CHOL	CARB	FIBER	SOD
cider	1 cup	117	tr	tr	0	29	tr	7
juice + vitamin C & calcium	1 cup	117	tr	tr	0	29	tr	17
mulled cider	1 serv	265	1	1	0	42	6	12
unsweetened w/o vitamin C	1 cup	117	tr	tr	0	29	tr	7
Apple & Eve								
100% Juice	8 oz	110	1	0	0	26	–	5
Back To Nature								
100% Juice	1 pkg (6 oz)	80	0	0	0	21	–	25

FOOD	PORTION	CALS	PROT	FAT	CHOL	CARB	FIBER	SOD
Fizz Ed.								
Green Apple	1 can (8.4 oz)	100	0	0	0	25	1	30
Izze								
Sparkling Fortified Apple	1 can (8.4 oz)	90	0	0	0	23	–	15
Land O Lakes								
Juice	1 cup (8 oz)	120	0	0	0	29	0	45
Mott's								
100% Natural	1 bottle (14 oz)	200	1	0	0	48	0	35
Nantucket Nectars								
100% Juice Pressed Apple	8 oz	120	0	0	0	30	tr	15
Organic Cloudy Apple	8 oz	120	0	0	0	29	0	30
Ocean Spray								
Juice	8 oz	100	0	0	0	28	–	35
Old Orchard								
Cider 100%	8 oz	120	0	0	0	29	–	25
Healthy Balance Apple	8 oz	30	0	0	0	6	–	9
Organic 100% Juice	8 oz	128	0	0	0	29	–	25
R.W. Knudsen								
Organic 100% Juice	8 oz	120	tr	0	0	30	0	25
Santa Cruz								
Organic	8 oz	120	tr	0	0	30	0	25
Smart Juice								
Organic 100% Juice	8 oz	117	tr	0	0	29	tr	7
Snapple								
100% Juice Green Apple	8 oz	160	0	0	0	41	–	20
Juice Drink Apple	8 oz	110	0	0	0	27	–	5
Tastee								
Cider 100% Juice	8 oz	120	0	0	0	30	–	60
Tree Ripe								
Organic 100% Juice	6 oz	80	0	0	0	21	0	10
Tropicana								
Orchard Style	1 bottle (14 oz)	200	tr	0	0	50	0	20
Walnut Acres								
Organic Juice	8 oz	110	0	0	0	29	0	0

FOOD	PORTION	CALS	PROT	FAT	CHOL	CARB	FIBER	SOD
APPLESAUCE								
sweetened	½ cup	97	tr	tr	0	25	2	4
unsweetened	½ cup	52	tr	tr	0	14	2	2
Beth's Farm Kitchen								
Chunky	2 tbsp (1 oz)	50	tr	0	0	14	1	0
GoGo Squeeze								
Apple	1 pkg (3.2 oz)	60	0	1	0	14	1	3
Apple Banana	1 pkg (3.2 oz)	60	0	tr	0	14	1	3
Apple Cinnamon	1 pkg (3.2 oz)	50	0	tr	0	10	1	3
Apple Peach	1 pkg (3.2 oz)	60	0	tr	0	13	1	3
Mott's								
Healthy Harvest Granny Smith No Sugar Added	1 pkg (3.9 oz)	50	0	0	0	13	1	0
Organic Original	½ cup (4.5 oz)	110	0	0	0	27	1	0
Organic Unsweetened	½ cup (4.3 oz)	50	0	0	0	14	1	0
Single-Serve Cinnamon	1 pkg (4 oz)	100	0	0	0	25	1	0
Musselman's								
Unsweetened	1 pkg (4 oz)	50	0	0	0	12	2	20
Revolution Foods								
Organic Unsweetened	1 pkg (4 oz)	50	0	0	0	13	2	5
Santa Cruz								
Organic	½ cup (4.5 oz)	60	0	0	0	13	2	20
Organic Apple Apricot	1 pkg (4 oz)	60	0	0	0	14	2	17
Organic Apple Blueberry	1 pkg (4 oz)	60	0	0	0	14	2	17
Organic Apple Cherry	½ cup (4.5 oz)	60	0	0	0	15	2	20
APRICOT JUICE								
nectar	6 oz	106	1	tr	0	27	1	6
Ceres								
100% Juice	8 oz	130	0	0	0	32	0	15
Santa Cruz								
Organic Nectar	8 oz	120	0	0	0	29	tr	35
APRICOTS								
canned in heavy syrup	½ cup	91	1	tr	0	23	3	4
canned in juice	½ cup	59	1	tr	0	15	2	5
canned in water	½ cup	33	1	tr	0	8	2	4

FOOD	PORTION	CALS	PROT	FAT	CHOL	CARB	FIBER	SOD
canned in light syrup	½ cup	80	1	tr	0	21	2	5
dried halves	6	51	1	tr	0	13	2	2
dried halves cooked w/o sugar	½ cup	106	2	tr	0	28	3	5
fresh	1	17	tr	tr	0	4	1	0
fresh sliced	½ cup	40	1	tr	0	9	2	1
frozen sweetened	½ cup	119	1	tr	0	30	3	5
Del Monte								
Halves In Heavy Syrup	½ cup (4.5 oz)	100	0	0	0	26	1	10
Elizabeth's Natural								
Turkish Dried	5 (1.8 oz)	90	1	0	0	22	3	10
FruitziO								
Freeze Dried	1 pkg (0.35 oz)	40	0	0	0	9	1	0
Harvest Bay								
Dried	5 (1.4 oz)	60	2	0	0	15	3	6
Mariani								
Ultimate Dried	¼ cup (1.4 oz)	100	1	0	0	24	6	10
S&W								
Whole In Heavy Syrup	½ cup (4.5 oz)	120	tr	0	0	29	1	10
Sunsweet								
Dried	¼ cup (1.4 oz)	130	0	0	0	36	3	25
ARROWHEAD								
corm boiled	1 med	9	1	tr	0	2	–	2
ARROWROOT								
raw	1 root (1.2 oz)	21	1	tr	0	4	tr	9
raw root sliced	1 cup	78	5	tr	0	16	2	31
Bob's Red Mill								
Starch	¼ cup	110	0	0	0	28	1	0
ARTICHOKE								
CANNED								
hearts in oil	1 serv (3 oz)	100	3	7	0	9	4	73
Cento								
Hearts Quartered Marinated	2 pieces	20	0	2	0	2	–	80

FOOD	PORTION	CALS	PROT	FAT	CHOL	CARB	FIBER	SOD
Gertie's Finest								
Tapenade	2 tbsp	29	1	3	0	2	tr	210
Native Forest								
Organic Hearts Quartered	1 serv (4 oz)	35	2	0	0	6	4	390
Polar								
Hearts	2	18	2	0	0	3	2	480
Hearts Quartered Marinated	1 oz	25	1	2	0	5	1	90
Progresso								
Hearts	2	30	1	0	0	7	2	400
Hearts Marinated	2 (1.1 oz)	60	0	5	0	2	0	110
Roland								
Hearts	½ cup (4.6 oz)	50	3	0	0	9	4	380
The Gracious Gourmet								
Artichoke Parmesan Tapenade	2 tbsp (1 oz)	30	1	2	0	3	tr	150
FRESH								
cooked	1 med	60	4	tr	0	13	7	114
hearts cooked	½ cup	42	3	tr	0	9	5	80
Ocean Mist								
Lemon	1 (4.2 oz)	60	4	0	0	13	6	115
FROZEN								
cooked	1 cup	42	3	tr	0	9	5	80
cooked w/o salt	1 pkg (9 oz)	108	7	1	0	22	11	127
C&W								
Hearts	12 pieces (3 oz)	40	2	1	0	7	5	55
TAKE-OUT								
stuffed	1 (8.8 oz)	397	15	14	8	54	10	1037

ASIAN FOOD (*see also* CURRY, DINNER, EGG ROLLS, SAUCE, SOY SAUCE, SUSHI)

FOOD	PORTION	CALS	PROT	FAT	CHOL	CARB	FIBER	SOD
CANNED								
chow mein chicken w/o noodles	1 cup	194	20	8	51	10	2	955
La Choy								
Chow Mein Beef	1 cup	90	8	2	15	11	2	880
Chow Mein Chicken	1 cup (9.3 oz)	100	8	3	20	10	2	1210
Sweet & Sour Noodles	1 cup	150	6	2	20	29	5	790

FOOD	PORTION	CALS	PROT	FAT	CHOL	CARB	FIBER	SOD
Teriyaki Chicken	1 cup (8.6 oz)	120	7	4	20	16	3	1370
FRESH								
wonton wrapper	1 (0.3 oz)	23	1	tr	1	5	tr	46
FROZEN								
Amy's								
Asian Noodle Stir Fry	1 pkg	290	9	7	0	50	4	630
Indian Mattar Paneer	1 pkg (10 oz)	320	11	8	5	54	6	780
Indian Palak Paneer	1 pkg (9.9 oz)	270	10	9	5	38	5	680
Indian Paneer Tikka	1 pkg (9.4 oz)	320	8	18	20	36	5	550
Indian Vegetable Korma	1 pkg (9.4 oz)	310	9	12	0	41	7	680
Thai Stir Fry	1 pkg (9.4 oz)	310	8	11	0	45	5	420
Contessa								
Chow Mein Chicken w/ Sauce not prep	1¾ cups	320	16	3	25	55	3	1060
Curry Chicken w/ Sauce not prep	1¾ cups	240	12	8	25	29	2	330
Fried Rice Chicken w/ Sauce not prep	1¾ cups	260	17	4	100	49	4	680
General Tsao Shrimp w/ Sauce not prep	1¾ cups	270	10	4	35	49	4	930
Kung Pao Shrimp w/ Sauce not prep	1¾ cups	200	10	4	45	30	3	760
Lo Mein Shrimp w/ Sauce not prep	1¾ cups	250	11	10	35	29	2	830
Stir-Fry Beef w/ Sauce not prep	1¾ cups	190	13	3	20	28	4	820
Stir-Fry Chicken w/ Sauce not prep	1¾ cups	160	16	3	25	18	4	870
Stir-Fry Shrimp w/ Sauce not prep	1¾ cups	120	9	3	40	16	2	980
Sweet & Sour Shrimp w/ Sauce not prep	1½ cups	180	9	0	50	40	3	430
Tandoori Chicken w/ Sauce not prep	1⅓ cups	200	15	4	30	27	3	660

FOOD	PORTION	CALS	PROT	FAT	CHOL	CARB	FIBER	SOD
Ethnic Gourmet								
Bhartha Eggplant	1 pkg (11 oz)	300	8	9	0	47	10	650
Dal Bahaar	1 pkg (11 oz)	360	13	8	0	61	8	500
Kaeng Kari Kai	1 pkg (10 oz)	390	20	11	35	54	2	770
Korma Chicken	1 pkg (10 oz)	340	21	9	40	44	3	720
Korma Vegetable	1 pkg (11 oz)	300	8	6	0	52	4	680
Kotopoulo Domato Ke Feta	1 pkg (10 oz)	340	20	11	40	41	5	–
Pad Thai Chicken	1 pkg (10 oz)	410	20	7	25	66	3	830
Pad Thai Shrimp	1 pkg (10 oz)	410	17	7	55	70	3	850
Tandoori Chicken w/ Spinach	1 pkg (10 oz)	170	14	5	30	19	3	840
French Meadow Bakery								
Vegetarian Dal Makhani	1 pkg (12 oz)	370	8	19	20	39	5	340
Glutino								
Gluten Free Chicken Pad Thai Peach	1 pkg (7 oz)	370	17	5	75	65	3	890
Healthy Choice								
Five Spice Beef & Vegetables	1 pkg (10 oz)	310	15	5	30	49	7	600
General Tso's Spicy Chicken	1 pkg (10.7 oz)	310	18	4	30	50	5	500
Helen's Kitchen								
Thai Yellow Curry w/ Tofu Steaks & Vegetables & Basmati Rice	1 pkg (9 oz)	280	12	5	0	30	2	390
Joy Of Cooking								
Lo Mein Vegetable	1 cup (7.7 oz)	220	9	3	15	40	11	870
Kahiki								
Beef & Broccoli	1 pkg (10.9 oz)	360	23	10	50	42	2	1060

FOOD	PORTION	CALS	PROT	FAT	CHOL	CARB	FIBER	SOD
Chicken Fried Rice	1 pkg (10.9 oz)	460	16	10	85	75	2	1090
General Tso's Chicken	1 pkg (10 oz)	400	12	10	20	66	2	1340
Naturals General Tso's Chicken	1 pkg (10 oz)	330	18	5	35	52	3	1080
Naturals Mandarin Orange Chicken	1 pkg (10 oz)	340	17	5	35	58	3	750
Naturals Szechuan Peppercorn Beef	1 pkg (10 oz)	350	19	14	50	35	3	780
Naturals Teriyaki Mixed Vegetables	1 pkg (10 oz)	260	8	2	0	51	4	750
Sesame Orange Chicken	1 pkg (10.9 oz)	420	15	12	25	60	2	1390
Soothing Lettuce Wraps	4 tbsp (2 oz)	90	5	4	10	9	1	310
Tempura Chicken Nuggets	¾ cup (3.5 oz)	230	13	14	40	10	0	470
Tropical Sweet & Sour Chicken	1 pkg (10.9 oz)	490	14	11	25	82	4	910
Organic Classics								
Thai Chicken Curry	1 pkg (10 oz)	420	19	17	40	50	3	510
Tyson								
Meal Kit Chicken Fried Rice	2½ cups	440	27	6	30	69	5	1810
MIX								
Nissin								
Chow Mein Chicken as prep	½ pkg (2 oz)	240	6	9	0	34	2	660
Chow Mein Thai Peanut as prep	½ pkg (2 oz)	270	6	12	0	35	tr	780
SHELF-STABLE								
Healthy Choice								
Fresh Mixers Sesame Teriyaki Chicken	1 pkg (7.9 oz)	380	13	6	20	69	3	600
Fresh Mixers Sweet & Sour Chicken	1 pkg (7.9 oz)	390	12	3	25	78	5	400
Fresh Mixers Szechwan Beef w/ Asian Noodles	1 pkg (6.9 oz)	370	14	6	15	65	4	600
TAKE-OUT								
beef & broccoli	1 cup	221	18	12	54	10	3	399

FOOD	PORTION	CALS	PROT	FAT	CHOL	CARB	FIBER	SOD
beef w/ black bean sauce	1 serv (7 oz)	288	35	14	85	6	1	1373
bo bia roll shrimp	1 (2.5 oz)	82	6	2	15	10	2	49
buddha's delight w/ cellophane noodles fat choi jai	1 serv (7.6 oz)	211	7	4	tr	44	2	772
bun baked red bean	1 (1.1 oz)	102	3	3	8	16	1	54
cha siu bao steamed buns w/ chicken filling	1 (2.3 oz)	160	5	3	15	26	tr	300
chicken masala	1 serv (8 oz)	430	44	25	128	8	0	1165
chicken tandoori	1 serv (4 oz)	156	19	8	49	2	0	480
chicken tikka	1 serv (2.5 oz)	173	24	8	60	1	1	187
chinese garlic chicken	1 cup (5.7 oz)	290	22	19	83	8	1	778
chinese style fried egg noodles w/ seafood & lettuce	1 serv (14 oz)	694	27	37	257	63	8	1563
chow mein beef w/o noodles	1 cup	271	22	15	51	12	3	922
chow mein chicken w/ noodles	1 cup (7.7 oz)	273	19	14	44	20	2	1054
chow mein noodles	1 cup	237	4	14	0	26	2	198
chow mein pork w/o noodles	1 cup	284	22	16	55	12	3	889
chow mein shrimp w/ noodles	1 cup (7.7 oz)	262	15	12	119	24	3	1274
chow mein shrimp w/o noodles	1 cup	154	16	5	92	11	2	737
chow mein vegetable w/o noodles	1 cup	224	5	15	0	16	4	1014
dim sum deep fried beancurd w/ shrimp	1 (1.1 oz)	77	5	6	9	2	1	133
dim sum deep fried yam	1 (2.4 oz)	201	3	12	3	23	2	794
dim sum meat filled	3 pieces (4 oz)	124	13	3	54	11	1	484
dim sum pork hash	1 (1.1 oz)	59	2	3	3	5	0	64
dim sum shrimp	3 (4 oz)	307	10	16	14	31	2	549
dim sum steamed chives & prawns	1 (1.2 oz)	48	3	2	10	5	1	164

FOOD	PORTION	CALS	PROT	FAT	CHOL	CARB	FIBER	SOD
egg foo yung beef	1 patty (6 oz)	243	17	16	336	7	1	243
egg foo yung chicken	1 patty (3 oz)	121	8	8	166	4	1	121
egg foo yung pork	1 patty (3 oz)	125	8	8	166	4	1	120
egg foo yung shrimp	1 patty (3 oz)	153	8	12	184	3	1	483
filipino chicken adobo	1 serv (15 oz)	555	33	26	116	45	1	468
foochow fish ball	1 (1 oz)	36	2	2	6	3	1	163
fried rice	1 cup	333	12	12	103	42	1	834
fried rice beef	1 cup	346	12	14	107	42	1	649
fried rice chicken	1 cup	329	12	12	105	42	1	602
fried rice pork	1 cup	335	12	13	103	42	1	602
fried rice shrimp	1 cup	323	11	12	115	42	1	851
general tsao's chicken	1 cup (5 oz)	296	19	17	66	16	1	844
green beans szechuan style	1 cup	176	4	12	0	16	6	446
indian style fried egg noodles w/ eggs tomato sauce & lime	1 serv (15 oz)	721	29	31	377	80	8	2418
korean spicy shredded chicken	1 serv (5 oz)	258	23	16	30	5	2	816
kung pao beef	1 cup	410	28	30	62	9	2	645
kung pao chicken	1 cup (5.7 oz)	434	29	31	65	12	2	907
kung pao pork	1 cup	460	26	34	60	12	2	862
kung pao shrimp	1 cup (5.7 oz)	345	30	20	191	11	2	791
lemon chicken w/o vegetables	1 serv (6.6 oz)	503	34	28	127	26	1	1327
lo mein beef	1 cup	286	14	11	26	31	3	594
lo mein chicken	1 cup (7 oz)	280	16	9	26	33	3	536
lo mein meatless	1 cup	234	8	6	0	38	3	366
lo mein pork	1 cup	314	13	14	22	34	3	508
lo mein shrimp	1 cup	236	11	7	48	33	4	180
moo goo gai pan chicken	1 cup (7.6 oz)	272	15	19	35	12	3	305
moo shu pork w/o pancake	1 cup	512	19	46	172	5	1	1048
pad thai w/ chicken	1 cup (7 oz)	358	18	15	64	39	2	564

FOOD	PORTION	CALS	PROT	FAT	CHOL	CARB	FIBER	SOD
pad thai w/ shrimp	1 cup (7 oz)	314	11	11	186	40	1	1498
pakhoras	1 (2.5 oz)	163	8	8	0	16	4	470
paneer pakhora	1 (2.2 oz)	183	8	13	16	8	2	125
peking duck w/ pancakes & seafood sauce	1 serv (14 oz)	1871	39	121	189	157	5	1953
pork w/ chinese cabbage	1 serv (4 oz)	120	11	8	25	1	1	219
sesame seed paste bun	1 (2.5 oz)	220	5	6	0	39	2	53
shrimp chips banh phong tom	6 med	214	3	14	21	20	tr	456
shrimp w/ lobster sauce	1 cup	298	35	12	259	8	1	1030
shu mai chicken & vegetable dumplings	6 (3.6 oz)	160	10	5	35	18	1	910
sukiyaki beef	1 cup	165	19	7	130	6	1	654
sukiyaki chicken	1 serv (18 oz)	436	71	8	175	19	4	1048
sweet & sour chicken w/o rice	1 cup	670	45	37	169	36	2	1819
sweet & sour pork w/ rice	1 cup	268	13	6	29	40	2	898
sweet & sour pork w/o rice	1 cup	231	15	8	38	25	2	1209
sweet & sour shrimp	1 cup	480	12	30	70	46	1	2020
szechuan chicken	1 cup (5.7 oz)	180	16	9	42	9	2	616
szechuan shrimp & vegetables	1 cup	159	14	7	94	10	2	629
tempura hawaiian fish tofu vegetable	2 cups	285	11	22	200	13	2	430
tempura vegetable	8 pieces	90	2	6	36	8	1	20
teriyaki beef	1 cup	454	51	19	149	13	tr	1386
teriyaki chicken	¾ cup	399	30	27	92	7	–	2190
teriyaki chicken w/ rice	1 serv (11 oz)	430	19	6	25	77	1	1210
teriyaki shrimp	1 cup	271	39	3	269	14	1	3103
thai style pineapple rice w/ ham & pork floss	1 serv (7.7 oz)	408	13	14	63	60	6	1277
wonton fried meat filled	1 (0.7 oz)	54	3	3	20	5	tr	111
wonton meat & shrimp boiled	1 (0.5 oz)	19	1	1	3	2	tr	48

FOOD	PORTION	CALS	PROT	FAT	CHOL	CARB	FIBER	SOD
ASPARAGUS								
CANNED								
spears	1	3	tr	tr	0	tr	tr	52
spears	1 cup	46	5	2	0	6	4	695
Del Monte								
Spears Extra Long	½ cup	20	2	0	0	3	1	365
Gertie's Finest								
White	1 oz	15	1	0	0	3	1	340
Green Giant								
Spears Extra Long	5 (4.4 oz)	20	2	0	0	3	1	430
McSweet								
Pickled Spears	6 (1 oz)	25	0	0	0	6	0	290
Native Forest								
White	1 serv (4 oz)	20	2	0	0	3	1	550
S&W								
Spears	½ cup (4.4 oz)	20	2	0	0	3	1	365
FRESH								
cooked	½ cup	20	2	tr	0	4	2	13
spears cooked	4	13	1	tr	0	2	1	8
spears raw	4	10	1	tr	0	2	1	1
Alpine Fresh								
Fresh Green	5 spears (3.3 oz)	20	2	0	0	5	2	0
Ocean Mist								
Spears	5 (3.3 oz)	25	2	0	0	4	2	0
FROZEN								
cooked	1 pkg (10 oz)	53	9	1	0	6	5	9
spears cooked	4	11	2	tr	0	1	1	2
C&W								
Spears	7 (3 oz)	20	2	0	0	3	tr	0
Joy Of Cooking								
Tender	½ cup (3.3 oz)	70	2	5	10	4	1	210
Seabrook Farms								
Spears	7 (2.9 oz)	20	3	0	0	3	2	5
ATEMOYA								
fresh	½ cup	94	1	1	–	24	–	2

FOOD	PORTION	CALS	PROT	FAT	CHOL	CARB	FIBER	SOD
AVOCADO								
california mashed	¼ cup	96	1	9	0	5	4	5
california peeled & pitted	1	289	3	27	0	15	12	14
florida mashed	¼ cup	69	1	6	0	5	1	1
florida peeled & pitted	1	365	7	31	0	24	17	6
Cabilfrut								
Hass fresh	⅕ med (1.1 oz)	55	tr	3	0	3	3	0
Calavo								
Fresh	⅕ med (1 oz)	55	tr	5	0	3	3	0
Chiquita								
Fresh	1 (7 oz)	322	4	29	0	17	13	14
Earthbound Farms								
Organic Fresh	⅕ med (1 oz)	55	1	5	0	3	3	0
Simply Avo								
Hass Avocado Pulp	2 tbsp	50	1	5	0	3	2	0
Hass Halves	⅙ pkg (1.1 oz)	50	1	5	0	3	2	0
Wholly Guacamole								
Classic	2 tbsp	50	1	4	0	2	2	75
Organic	2 tbsp	50	1	5	0	2	2	50
Pico De Gallo Style	2 tbsp	40	1	3	0	2	2	85
TAKE-OUT								
guacamole	1 serv (2.2 oz)	105	1	10	0	5	2	187
BACON								
bacon grease	1 tbsp	116	0	13	12	0	0	19
beef breakfast strips cooked	3 strips	153	11	12	40	tr	0	766
gammon lean & fat grilled	4.2 oz	274	35	15	–	0	0	–
pan fried	3 strips	109	6	9	16	tr	0	303
turkey	2 (0.8 oz)	84	7	6	22	1	0	503
Applegate Farms								
Natural Dry Cured Cooked	2 slices (0.5 oz)	60	4	5	10	0	0	290
Organic Turkey	1 slice (1 oz)	35	6	2	25	0	0	200
Boar's Head								
Fully Cooked Slices	3 (0.5 oz)	70	4	6	15	0	0	260

FOOD	PORTION	CALS	PROT	FAT	CHOL	CARB	FIBER	SOD
Butterball								
Turkey Bacon	1 slice (0.5 oz)	25	2	2	10	0	0	135
Dietz & Watson								
Gourmet	2 strips (0.5 oz)	70	4	6	15	1	0	250
Pancetta	⅙ pkg (0.5 oz)	50	2	5	10	0	0	230
Hormel								
Microwave Ready	2 slices (0.5 oz)	80	5	7	20	0	0	300
Real Bits	1 tbsp (7 g)	25	3	2	5	0	0	240
Jimmy Dean								
Lower Sodium	1 slice (0.3 oz)	50	4	4	10	0	0	105
Original	1 slice (0.3 oz)	50	4	4	10	0	0	230
Thick Slice	1 slice (0.5 oz)	80	5	6	15	0	0	320
Organic Prairie								
Uncured Hardwood Smoked	2 strips (2 oz)	270	5	27	35	1	0	620
Uncured Turkey	2 strips (1 oz)	40	7	1	25	0	0	160
Oscar Mayer								
Bacon Bits	1 tbsp (7 g)	25	3	2	5	0	0	220
Hardwood Smoked	2 slices (0.5 oz)	70	4	6	15	0	0	290
Lower Sodium	3 slices (0.5 oz)	70	4	6	10	0	0	170
Ready To Serve	3 slices	70	5	5	15	0	0	220
Uncured	3 slices (0.5 oz)	60	7	5	15	1	0	400
Tyson								
Hickory Thick Cut	2 pieces (0.8 oz)	140	8	11	25	0	0	380

BACON SUBSTITUTES

bacon bits meatless	1 tbsp	33	2	2	0	2	1	124
meatless	1 strip	16	1	1	0	tr	tr	73

FOOD	PORTION	CALS	PROT	FAT	CHOL	CARB	FIBER	SOD
Bob's Red Mill								
Bac'Ums	4 tsp	25	3	1	0	2	0	140
Worthington								
Stripples	2 strips (0.5 oz)	60	2	5	0	2	tr	220

BAGEL

FOOD	PORTION	CALS	PROT	FAT	CHOL	CARB	FIBER	SOD
cinnamon raisin	1 lg (4 in)	244	9	2	0	49	2	287
cinnamon raisin	1 mini	71	3	tr	0	14	1	84
egg	1 lg (4.5 in)	364	14	3	31	69	3	662
low carb	1 (4 oz)	216	12	0	10	42	14	360
oat bran	1 lg (4 in)	227	10	1	0	47	3	451
onion mini	1 (1.4 oz)	100	4	0	0	20	1	90
plain	1 lg (4.5 in)	360	14	2	0	70	3	700
plain	1 med (3.5 in)	289	11	2	0	56	2	561
plain	1 sm (3 in)	190	7	1	0	37	2	368
Enjoy Life								
Nut Gluten Free Classic Original	1 (3 oz)	270	5	7	0	46	3	380
Finagle A Bagel								
Cinnamon Raisin	1 (4 oz)	300	8	1	0	67	5	350
Everything	1 (4 oz)	310	9	3	0	62	5	420
Onion	1 (4 oz)	300	9	1	0	65	4	380
Plain	1 (4 oz)	290	8	1	0	63	4	410
Poppy Seed	1 (4 oz)	310	11	4	0	60	4	409
Sesame	1 (4 oz)	310	10	5	0	60	5	380
French Meadow Bakery								
100% Spelt	1 (3.4 oz)	270	11	2	0	52	8	520
Hemp	1 (3.4 oz)	280	19	8	0	35	13	370
Sprouted Cinnamon Raisin	1 (3.5 oz)	270	15	2	0	50	7	270
Natural Ovens								
Blueberry	1 (3 oz)	250	11	2	0	47	5	270
Brainy	1 (3 oz)	230	11	3	0	40	8	270
Whole Wheat	1 (3 oz)	230	10	3	0	40	8	260
New York Style								
Crisps Natural Whole Wheat	6	120	4	6	0	16	2	180
Crisps Plain	7	140	3	6	0	17	1	70

FOOD	PORTION	CALS	PROT	FAT	CHOL	CARB	FIBER	SOD
Pepperidge Farm								
100% Whole Wheat	1	250	11	2	0	49	6	450
100% Whole Wheat Mini	1 (1.4 oz)	100	4	1	0	20	3	180
Everything	1	260	9	2	0	53	2	400
Plain Mini	1	110	4	1	0	22	1	200
Thomas'								
100% Whole Wheat Mini	1 (1.5 oz)	110	5	1	0	22	3	180
Bagel Holes Plain	3 (1.6 oz)	120	4	1	0	24	1	230
Bagel Thins Everything	1 (1.6 oz)	110	5	1	0	24	5	190
Bagelbread Mini Squares 100% Whole Wheat	1 (2 oz)	150	7	1	0	30	4	240
Udi's								
Gluten Free Plain	1 (3.5 oz)	280	6	9	0	43	3	480
Gluten Free Whole Grain	1 (3.5 oz)	280	7	9	0	43	3	470
BAKING POWDER								
baking powder	1 tsp	2	0	0	0	1	0	488
low sodium	1 tsp	5	tr	tr	0	2	tr	4
Bob's Red Mill								
Baking Powder	1 tsp	5	0	0	0	1	0	590
Calumet								
Double Acting	1/8 tsp	0	0	0	0	0	0	60
Clabber Girl								
Baking Powder	1/8 tsp (0.6 g)	0	0	0	0	tr	–	65
Davis								
Baking Powder	1/8 tsp (0.6 g)	0	0	0	0	tr	–	65
Rumford								
Aluminum Free	1/8 tsp (0.6 g)	0	0	0	0	tr	–	55
BAKING SODA								
baking soda	1 tsp	0	0	0	0	0	0	1259
Bob's Red Mill								
Baking Soda	1/4 tsp	0	0	0	0	0	0	270
BALSAM PEAR (BITTER GOURD)								
leafy tips cooked w/o salt	1 cup	20	2	tr	0	4	1	8
leafy tips raw	1 cup	14	3	tr	0	2	–	5
pods raw sliced	1 cup	16	1	tr	0	3	3	5
pods sliced cooked w/ salt	1 cup	24	1	tr	0	5	3	300
BAMBOO SHOOTS								
canned sliced	1/2 cup	12	1	tr	0	2	1	5

FOOD	PORTION	CALS	PROT	FAT	CHOL	CARB	FIBER	SOD
fresh sliced cooked w/ salt	½ cup	7	1	tr	0	1	1	144
raw sliced	½ cup	20	2	tr	0	4	2	3
La Choy								
Bamboo Shoots	½ cup	10	tr	0	0	2	tr	10
Polar								
Sliced	½ cup	25	1	0	0	3	2	15
BANANA								
baked	1 (4.5 oz)	163	2	tr	0	42	4	1
banana chips	1 oz	147	1	10	0	17	2	2
fresh	1 sm (6 in)	90	1	tr	0	23	3	1
fresh	1 med (7 in)	105	1	tr	0	27	3	1
fresh	1 lg (8 in)	121	1	tr	0	31	4	1
fresh baby	1 extra sm (<6 in)	72	1	tr	0	19	2	1
fresh mashed	½ cup	100	1	tr	0	26	3	1
fresh sliced	1 cup	134	2	1	0	34	4	2
green fried	1 (3.1 oz)	152	1	8	0	21	2	1
green pickled	½ cup	240	1	22	0	11	1	144
green sliced fried	1 cup	323	2	18	0	45	5	2
powder	1 tbsp	21	tr	tr	0	5	1	0
red ripe	1 (7 in)	93	1	tr	0	24	3	1
red ripe sliced	1 cup	134	2	1	0	34	4	2
whole dried	1 piece (1.2 oz)	130	1	1	0	33	2	0
Bob's Red Mill								
Chips	25 (1.4 oz)	210	0	11	0	26	0	1
Brothers-All-Natural								
Crisps	1 pkg (0.58 oz)	66	1	0	0	16	2	0
Chiquita								
Fresh	1 med (4.1 oz)	105	1	0	0	27	3	1
Crispy Green								
Crispy Bananas	1 pkg (0.5 oz)	55	1	0	0	13	2	0
Crunchies								
Freeze Dried Organic	¼ cup (0.3 oz)	32	tr	0	0	9	1	1

FOOD	PORTION	CALS	PROT	FAT	CHOL	CARB	FIBER	SOD
Kopali								
Organic Dark Chocolate Covered	½ pkg (1 oz)	120	1	6	0	19	2	0
Nana Flakes								
100% Natural	1 tbsp (0.2 oz)	22	0	0	0	6	1	tr
Tree Of Life								
Dried Sweetened	½ cup (1.6 oz)	240	1	15	0	27	4	0
TAKE-OUT								
batter dipped fried	1 sm (4 oz)	266	3	15	17	32	3	103
batter dipped fried sliced	1 cup	335	4	19	22	40	3	129
fried dwarf w/ cheese	1 (1.4 oz)	84	1	5	4	10	1	38
fritter	1 (2.3 oz)	197	1	5	0	36	2	103

BANANA JUICE

FOOD	PORTION	CALS	PROT	FAT	CHOL	CARB	FIBER	SOD
R.W. Knudsen								
Sensible Sippers Organic	1 box (4.23 oz)	35	0	0	0	9	–	5
Snapple								
Juice Drink Go Bananas	8 oz	110	0	0	0	28	–	5

BARBECUE SAUCE

FOOD	PORTION	CALS	PROT	FAT	CHOL	CARB	FIBER	SOD
barbecue	2 tbsp	52	0	tr	0	13	tr	392
low sodium	2 tbsp	52	0	tr	0	13	tr	47
Bear-Man								
Black Bear Boogie	2 tbsp	40	0	1	0	8	0	220
Growlin' Grizzly	2 tbsp	60	1	1	0	12	tr	290
Bone Suckin'								
Sauce	2 tbsp	40	0	0	0	10	0	110
Cattlemen's								
Classic	2 tbsp	60	tr	0	0	15	tr	400
Smokehouse	2 tbsp	60	tr	0	0	14	tr	490
Chef Hymie Grande								
Cascabel Express Barbecue Glaze	2 tbsp (1.2 oz)	30	tr	0	0	7	1	15
Polapote Barbecue Glaze	2 tbsp (1.2 oz)	30	tr	0	0	7	2	15
Dave's Gourmet								
Badlands BBQ	2 tbsp (1.1 oz)	40	1	1	–	8	–	100

FOOD	PORTION	CALS	PROT	FAT	CHOL	CARB	FIBER	SOD
Jake & Amos								
Apple Butter Barbecue Sauce	2 tbsp (0.5 oz)	30	0	0	0	7	0	15
Naturally Fresh								
BBQ	2 tbsp	40	0	0	0	10	0	200
OrganicVille								
Original No Added Sugar	2 tbsp (1 oz)	50	0	0	0	13	tr	200
Ribber City								
Kansas City	2 tbsp (1.1 oz)	40	0	0	0	11	0	210
Steel's								
No Sugar Added Gluten Free	2 tbsp (1.3 oz)	24	0	0	0	3	0	200
The Gracious Gourmet								
Spicy Barbeque Glaze	2 tbsp (1 oz)	35	1	1	0	7	0	300
Walden Farms								
Original Calorie Free	2 tbsp (1 oz)	0	0	0	0	0	0	210
World Harbors								
Bar-B	2 tbsp (1.2 oz)	70	0	0	0	16	0	540
Buccaneer Blends Fra Diavlo	2 tbsp (1.2 oz)	45	1	0	0	11	0	260
Buccaneer Blends Honey Mango	2 tbsp (1.3 oz)	60	0	0	0	13	0	260
Buccaneer Blends Sticky Rum	2 tbsp (1.2 oz)	50	0	0	0	13	0	340
BARLEY								
flour	1 cup	511	16	2	0	110	15	6
pearled cooked	1 cup (5.5 oz)	193	4	1	0	44	6	5
pearled uncooked	¼ cup	176	5	1	0	39	8	5
Arrowhead Mills								
Organic Pearled not prep	¼ cup	160	5	1	0	32	8	5
BARRACUDA								
broiled	4 oz	239	27	14	62	tr	0	480
cooked flaked	1 cup	287	32	16	75	1	0	575
poached	4 oz	227	29	11	67	0	0	111
TAKE-OUT								
breaded & fried	4 oz	282	26	17	59	5	tr	432

FOOD	PORTION	CALS	PROT	FAT	CHOL	CARB	FIBER	SOD
BARRAMUNDI								
Australis								
Barramundi	4 oz	90	23	2	55	0	0	40
Crispy Asian Sesame Panko	1 piece (4 oz)	240	20	11	30	24	1	270
Lemon Herb Butter	1 piece (6 oz)	170	30	4	70	3	0	600
BASIL								
fresh chopped	2 tbsp	1	tr	tr	0	tr	tr	0
ground	1 tsp	4	tr	tr	0	1	1	tr
leaves fresh	5	1	tr	tr	0	tr	tr	0
BASS								
breaded baked	4 oz	205	25	7	129	10	1	506
pickled mero en escabeche	2 oz	156	7	14	16	tr	tr	114
striped baked	3 oz	105	19	3	88	0	0	75
striped bass farm raised	4 oz	110	20	3	90	0	0	80
BAY LEAF								
crumbled	1 tsp	2	tr	tr	0	tr	tr	0
BEANS (*see also individual names*)								
CANNED								
baked beans plain	½ cup	119	6	tr	0	27	5	428
baked beans vegetarian	½ cup	119	6	tr	0	27	5	428
baked beans w/ franks	½ cup	184	9	9	8	20	9	557
baked beans w/ pork	½ cup	134	7	2	9	25	7	524
baked beans w/ pork & tomato sauce	½ cup	119	7	1	9	24	5	553
refried beans	½ cup	134	8	1	–	23	–	534
Allens								
Original Baked	½ cup	150	6	1	0	29	8	350
Refried Black Beans No Fat Added	½ cup	120	7	0	0	23	8	500
Amy's								
Organic Refried	½ cup	140	8	3	0	21	6	440
Organic Refried Light In Sodium	½ cup (4.6 oz)	140	7	3	0	21	6	190
B&M								
Baked Original	½ cup (4.6 oz)	180	7	3	<5	31	8	420

FOOD	PORTION	CALS	PROT	FAT	CHOL	CARB	FIBER	SOD
Barbeque Baked	½ cup (4.6 oz)	190	8	1	0	39	9	570
Country Style	½ cup (4.6 oz)	170	7	1	<5	35	7	720
Vegetarian	½ cup (4.6 oz)	160	7	1	0	31	8	380
Bush's								
Honey	½ cup	160	6	1	0	32	6	540
Maple Cured Bacon	½ cup (4.6 oz)	140	6	1	0	28	5	620
Original	½ cup (4.6 oz)	140	6	1	0	29	5	550
Vegetarian Fat Free	½ cup	130	6	0	0	29	5	550
Campbell's								
Pork & Beans	½ cup	140	6	2	5	25	7	440
Gebhardt								
Refried	½ cup	90	6	2	0	16	4	490
Refried Fat Free	½ cup	80	6	0	0	17	5	500
Refried Jalapeno	½ cup	100	6	2	0	17	5	400
Green Giant								
Three Bean Salad	½ cup	80	3	0	0	18	3	470
Hormel								
Kid's Kitchen Microwave Meals Beans & Wieners	1 pkg (7.7 oz)	310	12	13	30	37	7	780
Jake & Amos								
Four Bean Salad	2 tbsp	32	0	0	0	8	0	78
Old El Paso								
Refried Fat Free Spicy	½ cup	100	6	0	0	18	6	570
Pace								
Refried Salsa	½ cup	70	4	0	0	14	4	590
Read								
3 Bean Salad	⅓ cup	60	1	0	0	13	2	300
Rosarita								
Refried	½ cup	120	7	2	0	18	6	310
Refried Black Beans No Fat	½ cup	110	7	0	0	19	8	320
Refried Fat Free	½ cup	100	7	0	0	19	6	510
Refried Vegetarian	½ cup	120	7	2	0	19	7	540
Van Camp's								
Baked Beans Homestyle	½ cup	170	7	1	0	33	6	680
Beanee Weenee BBQ	1 can	260	15	8	30	35	9	940

FOOD	PORTION	CALS	PROT	FAT	CHOL	CARB	FIBER	SOD
Beanee Weenee Original	1 can	240	14	8	40	29	8	990
Beanee Weenee w/ Chili	1 can	240	14	9	45	26	6	990
Pork And Beans	½ cup	110	6	1	0	23	6	390
Wagon Master								
Pork & Beans	½ cup	130	7	1	0	23	9	420
TAKE-OUT								
baked beans	½ cup	191	7	7	6	27	7	534
barbecue beans	3.5 oz	120	4	tr	0	26	–	460
frijoles a la charra w/ pork tomatoes & chili peppers	1 cup	341	14	22	27	23	5	719
refried beans	½ cup	43	2	2	2	5	–	104
three bean salad	1 cup	114	4	5	0	15	5	651

BEAN SPROUTS (see ALFALFA, SPROUTS)

BEAR

FOOD	PORTION	CALS	PROT	FAT	CHOL	CARB	FIBER	SOD
simmered	3 oz	220	28	11	83	0	0	60

BEAVER

FOOD	PORTION	CALS	PROT	FAT	CHOL	CARB	FIBER	SOD
roasted	4 oz	240	39	8	132	0	0	67

BEE POLLEN

FOOD	PORTION	CALS	PROT	FAT	CHOL	CARB	FIBER	SOD
bee pollen	1 tsp (5 g)	16	1	tr	0	2	tr	0
Tree Of Life								
Bee Pollen	1 tsp (7 g)	30	tr	1	0	3	0	30

BEECHNUTS

FOOD	PORTION	CALS	PROT	FAT	CHOL	CARB	FIBER	SOD
dried	1 oz	163	2	14	0	10	–	11

BEEF (see also BEEF DISHES, JERKY, MEATBALLS, VEAL)

FOOD	PORTION	CALS	PROT	FAT	CHOL	CARB	FIBER	SOD
CANNED								
corned beef	1 oz	71	8	4	24	0	0	285
Hormel								
Corned Beef	1 serv (2 oz)	120	15	6	20	0	0	490
Dried Beef	1 oz	50	8	2	25	1	0	1200
Libby's								
Corned Beef	2 oz	120	14	7	40	0	0	490
Potted Meat	¼ cup	120	9	9	40	0	0	410
Roast Beef w/ Gravy	⅔ cup	140	25	4	60	3	0	750
FRESH								
arm pot roast trim 0 fat braised	3.5 oz	297	29	19	95	0	0	47

FOOD	PORTION	CALS	PROT	FAT	CHOL	CARB	FIBER	SOD
arm pot roast trim 1/8 in fat braised	3.5 oz	302	30	19	79	0	0	50
beef crumbles 70% lean pan browned	3 oz	230	22	15	75	0	0	82
bottom round roast trim 0 fat braised	4 oz	253	38	10	112	0	0	50
bottom round roast trim 0 fat roasted	3.5 oz	187	27	8	86	0	0	36
bottom round roast trim 1/2 in fat braised	4 oz	337	22	22	109	0	0	57
bottom round roast trim 1/8 in fat braised	4 oz	280	37	13	86	0	0	49
bottom round roast trim 1/8 in fat roasted	4 oz	247	30	13	85	0	0	40
bottom sirloin butt roast trim 0 fat roasted	3.5 oz	182	27	8	71	0	0	55
brisket flat half trim 1/8 in fat braised	3.5 oz	298	29	19	80	0	0	46
brisket flat trim 0 fat braised	3.5 oz	221	32	9	46	0	0	52
brisket point half trim 0 fat braised	3.5 oz	358	24	29	92	0	0	68
brisket point half trim 1/4 in fat braised	3.5 oz	404	22	22	92	0	0	65
brisket point half trim 1/8 in fat braised	3.5 oz	349	24	27	92	0	0	69
chuck boston cut roast trim 0 fat roasted	3.5 oz	207	26	11	69	0	0	71
chuck boston cut roast trim 1/4 in fat roasted	3.5 oz	242	24	15	75	0	0	67
chuck bottom roast trim 0 fat braised	3.5 oz	334	27	24	104	0	0	65
chuck bottom roast trim 1/4 in fat braised	3.5 oz	345	27	26	104	0	0	64
chuck fillet steak trim 0 fat broiled	4 oz	181	29	6	71	0	0	80
chuck top roast trim 0 fat broiled	4 oz	245	29	13	69	0	0	76
club steak trim 1/2 in fat broiled	4 oz	384	28	29	91	0	0	70

FOOD	PORTION	CALS	PROT	FAT	CHOL	CARB	FIBER	SOD
corned beef brisket cooked	3 oz	213	15	16	83	tr	0	964
crosscut shank trim ¼ in fat stewed	1 serv (6.8 oz)	510	60	28	155	0	0	118
delmonico steak trim ¼ in fat broiled	4 oz	409	27	33	95	0	0	70
entrecote steak trim ½ in fat broiled	4 oz	413	27	33	95	0	0	70
eye round roast trim 0 fat roasted	4 oz	190	33	5	61	0	0	43
eye round roast trim ¼ in fat roasted	4 oz	283	31	17	82	0	0	67
filet mignon roast trim ¼ in fat roasted	4 oz	376	27	29	97	0	0	63
filet mignon roast trim ⅛ in fat roasted	4 oz	367	27	28	96	0	0	65
filet mignon trim 0 fat broiled	4 oz	247	31	13	95	0	0	63
filet mignon trim ⅛ in fat broiled	4 oz	303	30	19	102	0	0	61
ground 70% lean broiled	3.5 oz	273	25	18	82	0	0	81
ground 75% lean broiled	2.5 oz	195	18	13	62	0	0	55
ground 80% lean broiled	3 oz	234	22	15	77	0	0	64
ground 85% lean pan fried	3 oz	197	21	12	73	0	0	67
ground 90% lean pan fried	3 oz	173	21	9	70	0	0	64
ground 95% lean pan fried	3 oz	139	22	5	65	0	0	60
ground lowfat w/ carrageenan raw	4 oz	160	20	7	53	tr	–	70
london broil trim 0 fat broiled	3.5 oz	188	28	8	45	0	0	56
london broil trim ¼ in fat broiled	4 oz	260	35	12	95	0	0	68
new york strip steak trim 0 fat broiled	4 oz	219	33	9	66	0	0	67
oxtails cooked	6 pieces (6.3 oz)	472	56	26	191	0	0	419
porterhouse steak trim 0 fat broiled	1 lb	1252	109	87	304	0	0	295
porterhouse steak trim ¼ in fat broiled	1 lb	1492	102	117	327	0	0	281

FOOD	PORTION	CALS	PROT	FAT	CHOL	CARB	FIBER	SOD
porterhouse steak trim ⅛ in fat broiled	4 oz	337	27	25	80	0	0	73
porterhouse steak trim ⅛ in fat broiled	1 lb	1324	107	99	322	0	0	290
rib eye roast trim ¼ in fat roasted	3.5 oz	365	23	30	85	0	0	64
rib eye steak trim ⅛ in fat broiled	4 oz	221	34	9	81	0	0	70
rib roast trim ¼ in fat roasted	4 oz	406	26	33	95	0	0	71
rib steak trim ¼ in fat broiled	4 oz	388	25	31	93	0	0	71
round tip roast trim 0 fat roasted	4 oz	213	30	9	105	0	0	40
sandwich steaks thinly sliced	1 serv (2 oz)	173	9	15	40	0	0	38
shell steak trim ¼ in fat broiled	4 oz	366	29	27	90	0	0	71
shortribs lean & fat braised	1 serv (7.8 oz)	1060	49	94	212	0	0	113
skirt steak trim 0 fat broiled	4 oz	289	27	19	67	0	0	104
t-bone steak trim 0 fat broiled	4 oz	280	27	18	68	0	0	76
t-bone steak trim ¼ in fat broiled	1 lb	1388	106	103	295	0	0	304
t-bone steak trim ⅛ in fat broiled	1 lb	804	70	56	178	0	0	489
tip round roast trim ⅛ in fat roasted	4 oz	248	31	13	93	0	0	71
top loin steak boneless trim ⅛ in fat broiled	4 oz	299	30	19	100	0	0	61
top round roast trim 0 fat braised	4 oz	237	40	7	102	0	0	51
top round roast trim ¼ in fat braised	4 oz	281	38	13	102	0	0	51
top round roast trim ¼ in fat roasted	4 oz	265	31	15	93	0	0	71
top round steak trim ¼ in fat pan fried	4 oz	314	37	17	110	0	0	77

FOOD	PORTION	CALS	PROT	FAT	CHOL	CARB	FIBER	SOD
top sirloin steak trim ⅛ in fat broiled	4 oz	275	31	16	85	0	0	63
top sirloin steak trim ⅛ in fat pan fried	4 oz	355	33	24	111	0	0	80
tri-tip roast trim 0 fat roasted	3.5 oz	218	26	12	94	0	0	50
tri-tip steak trim 0 fat broiled	4 oz	300	34	17	77	0	0	82
Dietz & Watson								
Prime Rib Seasoned	3 oz	150	20	8	55	0	0	190
Laura's Lean								
Eye Of Round	4 oz	135	25	4	50	0	0	75
Flank Steak	4 oz	140	–	5	55	–	–	85
Ground Beef 92% Lean	4 oz	160	21	9	60	0	0	70
Ground Beef Patties	1 (4 oz)	160	21	9	60	0	0	70
Ground Round 96% Lean	4 oz	140	24	5	60	0	0	85
Ribeye Steak	4 oz	175	–	9	60	–	–	–
Sirloin Steak	4 oz	145	–	5	65	–	–	70
Sirloin Tip	4 oz	130	24	4	60	0	0	65
Strip Steak	4 oz	150	–	5	55	–	–	70
Tenderloin Filet	4 oz	145	–	5	55	–	–	80
Top Round	4 oz	135	25	4	55	0	0	55
Maverick Ranch								
Ground Beef 85% Lean not prep	4 oz	150	22	17	70	0	0	55
Ground Beef 96% Lean not prep	4 oz	130	22	5	60	0	0	75
NY Strip Steak not prep	4 oz	180	22	10	55	0	0	55
Ribeye Steak not prep	4 oz	215	20	15	50	0	0	55
Organic Prairie								
Grass Fed Ground	4 oz	240	21	17	75	0	0	75
Rumba								
Cheekmeat	4 oz	300	18	25	80	0	0	75
Crosscut Hind Shank	4 oz	190	23	10	45	0	0	70
Marrow Bones	4 oz	290	21	22	75	0	0	0
Oxtail	4 oz	260	21	21	75	0	0	65
Short Ribs	4 oz	400	17	36	70	0	0	56
FROZEN								
patty broiled medium	3 oz	240	21	17	80	0	0	65

FOOD	PORTION	CALS	PROT	FAT	CHOL	CARB	FIBER	SOD
READY-TO-EAT								
dried beef smoked chopped	1 oz	37	6	1	13	1	0	352
roast beef spread	¼ cup	127	9	9	40	2	tr	413
Applegate Farms								
Organic Roast Beef	2 oz	80	12	3	35	0	0	320
Healthy Ones								
Deli Roast Beef	2 oz	70	9	2	0	1	0	480
Laura's Lean								
Beef Pot Roast Au Jus	3 oz	110	17	4	45	3	–	380
Oscar Mayer								
Slow Roasted Shaved	¼ pkg (1.8 oz)	60	10	3	30	0	0	520
Tyson								
Beef Strips Seasoned	1 serv (3 oz)	130	18	6	55	1	0	420
TAKE-OUT								
roast beef rare	2 oz	70	12	2	30	0	0	210
BEEF DISHES								
CANNED								
corned beef hash	3 oz	155	10	10	–	9	–	–
Hormel								
Beef Stew	1 pkg (7.5 oz)	150	10	6	25	15	2	890
Corned Beef Hash	1 cup (8.3 oz)	390	21	24	80	22	2	1000
Corned Beef Hash 50% Reduced Fat	1 cup (8.3 oz)	290	21	12	60	24	2	1070
Roast Beef Hash	1 cup (8.3 oz)	390	21	24	70	22	2	790
Roast Beef In Gravy	1 serv (5.8 oz)	130	18	3	40	8	0	740
Libby's								
Corned Beef Hash	1 cup	420	19	24	55	33	3	1230
Hawaiian Corned Beef	2 oz	120	14	7	40	0	0	490
FROZEN								
Quaker Maid								
Sandwich Steaks Pure Beef	1 serv (1.8 oz)	120	8	10	30	0	0	35

FOOD	PORTION	CALS	PROT	FAT	CHOL	CARB	FIBER	SOD
Tyson								
Steak Country Fried	1 (3.2 oz)	310	10	23	25	15	1	710
MIX								
Hamburger Helper								
Beef Pasta as prep	1 cup	270	4	10	54	24	1	816
Cheddar Cheese Melt as prep	1 cup	310	3	12	57	30	tr	385
Cheesy Baked Potato as prep	1 cup	310	2	11	57	30	2	816
Chili Cheese as prep	1 cup	340	4	13	57	33	1	720
Double Cheesy Quesadilla as prep	1 cup	350	3	11	57	36	tr	888
Italian Sausage as prep	1 cup	290	4	10	24	29	1	840
Microwave Singles Cheesy Lasagna	1 pkg	210	8	5	5	33	1	580
Philly Cheesesteak as prep	1 cup	320	4	13	57	27	1	768
Salisbury as prep	1 cup	260	4	10	54	27	1	840
Tomato Basil Penne as prep	1 cup	300	4	10	54	31	1	720
REFRIGERATED								
Hormel								
Beef Tips & Gravy	1 serv (4 oz)	170	21	8	60	4	1	700
Laura's Lean								
Meatloaf w/ Tomato Sauce	1 serv (5 oz)	230	19	8	60	27	–	580
Shredded Beef w/ Barbecue Sauce	1 serv (5 oz)	245	22	5	65	27	–	390
Tyson								
Chuck Roast w/ Vegetables	1 serv (4 oz)	320	18	21	70	14	2	340
Seasoned Meatloaf	1 serv (5 oz)	320	14	23	60	16	0	600
Steak Tips In Bourbon Sauce	1 serv (5 oz)	180	20	5	45	12	0	480
TAKE-OUT								
beef bourguignonne	1 cup	339	36	12	85	10	1	124
beef satay + peanut sauce	2 skewers	253	25	16	62	6	1	433
bool kogi korean marinated beef ribs	4 oz	190	18	10	55	6	0	580
bracciola	1 roll (4.7 oz)	276	27	14	76	8	1	485
bubble & squeak	5 oz	186	2	13	–	16	3	–
bulgoghi korean grilled beef	1 serv (5.2 oz)	256	23	15	67	5	tr	834
chipped beef on toast	1 slice (5 oz)	226	11	10	22	22	1	715

FOOD	PORTION	CALS	PROT	FAT	CHOL	CARB	FIBER	SOD
cornish pasty	1 (8 oz)	847	20	52	–	79	3	–
goulash w/ potatoes	1 cup	298	27	12	66	19	2	437
greek moussaka	1 serv (8.5 oz)	450	24	33	179	12	1	763
irish stew	1 cup (7 oz)	280	23	16	–	10	–	–
kebab indian	1 (5.4 oz)	553	47	40	–	2	–	–
kheena	6.7 oz	781	34	71	–	1	tr	–
koftas	5	280	18	22	–	3	tr	–
meatloaf	1 lg slice (5 oz)	294	23	17	114	9	1	596
pepper steak	1 cup	317	28	20	69	5	1	562
pot roast w/ gravy	1 serv (6 oz)	320	54	10	110	4	0	620
samosa	2 (4 oz)	652	6	62	–	20	2	–
shepherds pie	1 serv (7 oz)	282	16	16	70	20	2	840
sloppy joes	1 serv (9 oz)	398	39	6	67	48	12	88
steak & kidney pie w/ top crust	1 slice (5 oz)	400	21	26	–	23	1	–
stew w/ potatoes & vegetables	1 cup	199	16	5	30	22	3	504
stroganoff	1 cup	394	26	25	69	15	1	1155
swiss steak w/ sauce	1 serv (8 oz)	234	26	10	66	8	1	563
toad in the hole	1 (4.7 oz)	383	10	29	–	23	1	–
BEEFALO								
roasted	4 oz	213	35	7	66	0	0	93
BEER AND ALE								
alcohol free beer	7 fl oz	50	1	tr	–	11	–	3
ale brown	10 oz	77	1	0	0	8	0	–
ale pale	10 oz	88	1	0	0	12	0	–
beer cooler	1 (16 oz)	194	1	0	0	34	1	43
beer light	12 oz can	103	1	0	0	6	0	14
beer regular	12 oz can	153	2	0	0	13	0	14
black & tan	1 serv (12 oz)	146	1	0	0	13	1	18
black velvet	1 (10 oz)	160	1	0	0	8	1	10
boilermaker	1 serv	216	1	0	0	13	1	18
lager	10 oz	80	1	0	0	4	0	–
lager & black	1 (14 oz)	241	1	0	0	39	–	31
mead	1 serv	250	1	0	0	13	1	18
pilsener lager	7 oz	85	1	tr	–	13	–	4

FOOD	PORTION	CALS	PROT	FAT	CHOL	CARB	FIBER	SOD
shandy	1 serv	125	1	0	0	12	1	16
stout	10 oz	102	1	0	0	6	0	–
trojan horse	1 (16 oz)	189	1	0	0	35	–	57
Amstel								
Light	1 bottle (12 oz)	95	–	0	0	5	–	–
Bard's								
Gluten Free	1 bottle (12 oz)	155	–	0	0	14	–	–
Beck's								
Pilsner	1 bottle (12 oz)	138	–	0	0	12	–	–
Bud								
Dry	1 bottle (12 oz)	130	–	0	0	8	–	–
Budweiser								
Beer	1 bottle (12 oz)	145	–	0	0	11	–	–
Bud Light	1 bottle (12 oz)	110	–	0	0	7	–	–
Coors								
Lite	1 bottle (12 oz)	104	–	0	0	5	–	–
Non-Alcohol	1 bottle (12 oz)	66	–	0	0	15	–	–
Original	1 bottle (12 oz)	149	–	0	0	12	–	–
Super Dry	1 bottle (12 oz)	149	–	0	0	11	–	–
Corona								
Extra	1 bottle (12 oz)	149	–	0	0	14	–	–
Guinness								
Draft In A Bottle	1 bottle (12 oz)	128	–	0	0	11	–	–
Extra Stout	1 bottle (12 oz)	174	–	0	0	12	–	–
Heineken								
Beer	1 bottle (12 oz)	150	–	0	0	12	–	–

FOOD	PORTION	CALS	PROT	FAT	CHOL	CARB	FIBER	SOD
Icehouse								
5.0	1 bottle (12 oz)	149	–	0	0	10	–	–
Keystone								
Light	1 bottle (12 oz)	103	–	0	0	5	–	–
Kilarney's								
Red Lager	1 bottle (12 oz)	197	–	0	0	23	–	–
Killian's								
Beer	1 bottle (12 oz)	163	–	0	0	14	–	–
Labatt								
Blue	1 bottle (12 oz)	127	–	0	0	9	–	–
Lowenbrau								
Beer	1 bottle (12 oz)	160	–	0	0	–	–	–
Michelob								
Porter	1 bottle (12 oz)	196	–	0	0	17	–	–
Ultra	1 bottle (12 oz)	95	1	0	0	3	–	–
Miller								
Genuine Draft	1 bottle (12 oz)	143	–	0	0	13	–	–
Lite	1 bottle (12 oz)	96	–	0	0	3	–	–
MDG 64	1 bottle (12 oz)	64	–	0	0	2	–	–
O'Douls								
Non-Alcoholic	1 bottle (12 oz)	65	–	0	0	13	–	–
RedBridge								
Gluten Free	1 bottle (12 oz)	160	–	0	0	16	–	–
Sierra Nevada								
Porter	1 bottle (12 oz)	194	–	0	0	12	–	–

FOOD	PORTION	CALS	PROT	FAT	CHOL	CARB	FIBER	SOD
Smirnoff								
Ice	1 bottle (12 oz)	241	–	0	0	38	–	–
Weinhard's								
Amber Light	1 bottle (12 oz)	135	–	0	0	12	–	–
Blond Lager	1 bottle (12 oz)	161	–	0	0	14	–	–
Hefeweizen	1 bottle (12 oz)	151	–	0	0	12	–	–
Pale Ale	1 bottle (12 oz)	147	–	0	0	13	–	–
BEET JUICE								
juice	7 oz	72	2	0	0	16	–	400
BEETS								
CANNED								
harvard	½ cup	90	1	tr	0	22	3	199
pickled	½ cup	74	1	tr	0	18	3	300
sliced	½ cup	37	1	tr	0	9	2	176
Freshlike								
Pickled Sliced	4 slices (1 oz)	20	0	0	0	4	0	20
Greenwood								
Harvard	1 serv (4.4 oz)	100	1	0	0	27	1	370
Pickled	1 oz	25	0	0	0	6	0	100
Jake & Amos								
Harvard	1 serv (4 oz)	90	1	0	0	23	1	360
Rise 'N Roll								
Pickled Baby Beets	3 (1 oz)	30	0	0	0	7	1	140
S&W								
Sliced	½ cup (4.3 oz)	35	1	0	0	8	2	290
Sliced Pickled	1 oz	15	0	0	0	4	1	50
FRESH								
greens cooked w/o salt	½ cup	19	2	tr	0	4	2	174
sliced cooked	½ cup	37	1	tr	0	8	2	65
whole cooked	2 med (3.5 oz)	44	2	tr	0	10	2	77

FOOD	PORTION	CALS	PROT	FAT	CHOL	CARB	FIBER	SOD

BEVERAGES (*see* ALCOHOL DRINKS, BEER AND ALE, CHAMPAGNE, COFFEE, DRINK MIXERS, ENERGY DRINKS, FRUIT DRINKS, ICED TEA, MALT, MILKSHAKE, SMOOTHIES, SODA, TEA/HERBAL TEA, WATER, WINE, YOGURT DRINKS)

BISCUIT

FOOD	PORTION	CALS	PROT	FAT	CHOL	CARB	FIBER	SOD
FROZEN								
Jimmy Dean								
Snack Size Sausage On A Biscuit	2	400	9	30	40	24	1	650
MIX								
plain as prep	1 (2 oz)	190	4	7	2	27	1	541
Bisquick								
Heart Smart	⅓ cup	140	3	3	0	27	1	430
REFRIGERATED								
plain baked	1 (1 oz)	93	2	4	0	13	tr	325
Pillsbury								
Buttermilk	3 (2.2 oz)	150	4	2	0	29	1	570
Flaky Layers	3 (2.2 oz)	160	4	4	0	28	1	550
Grands! Butter Tastin'	1 (2 oz)	190	4	9	0	24	tr	590
Grands! Buttermilk Reduced Fat	1 (2 oz)	170	4	6	0	26	tr	590
Grands! Golden Wheat Reduced Fat	1 (2.1 oz)	180	4	7	0	27	2	590
Grands! Original	1 (2 oz)	190	4	9	0	24	tr	550
Grands! Original Reduced Fat	1 (2 oz)	170	4	6	0	26	tr	600
Perfect Portions Butter Tastin'	1 (1.9 oz)	190	4	9	0	23	tr	440
TAKE-OUT								
buttermilk	1 lg (2.7 oz)	280	5	13	1	37	1	810
oatcakes	2 (4 oz)	115	3	5	–	16	1	–
plain	1 sm (1.2 oz)	127	2	6	0	17	1	368
tea biscuit	1 (3 oz)	210	5	3	0	30	1	370
w/ egg	1 (4.8 oz)	373	12	22	245	32	1	891
w/ egg & bacon	1 (5.3 oz)	458	17	31	353	29	1	999
w/ egg & ham	1 (6.7 oz)	442	20	27	300	30	1	1382
w/ egg & sausage	1 (6.3 oz)	581	19	39	302	11	1	1141
w/ egg & steak	1 (5.2 oz)	410	18	28	272	21	–	888
w/ egg cheese & bacon	1 (5.1 oz)	477	16	31	261	33	–	1260
w/ ham	1 (4 oz)	386	13	18	25	44	1	1433
w/ sausage	1 (4.4 oz)	485	12	32	35	40	1	1071

FOOD	PORTION	CALS	PROT	FAT	CHOL	CARB	FIBER	SOD
BISON (*see* BUFFALO)								
BLACK BEANS								
dried cooked w/o salt	1 cup (6 oz)	227	15	1	0	41	15	2
Allens								
Black Beans	½ cup	100	6	1	0	19	8	400
Goya								
Black Beans	½ cup (4.3 oz)	90	7	1	0	19	6	460
Tree Of Life								
Organic	½ cup (4.6 oz)	130	8	1	0	24	<6	120
BLACKBERRIES								
canned in heavy syrup	½ cup	118	2	tr	0	30	4	4
fresh	½ cup	31	1	tr	0	7	4	1
unsweetened frzn	½ cup	48	1	tr	0	12	4	1
Cascadian Farm								
Organic frzn	1 cup	80	1	1	0	22	7	0
Oregon								
In Light Syrup	½ cup	120	1	0	0	29	6	10
BLACKBERRY JUICE								
canned	6 oz	65	1	1	0	13	tr	2
Izze								
Sparkling Esque Blackberry	1 bottle (12 oz)	50	0	0	0	12	–	10
BLACKEYE PEAS								
CANNED								
cowpeas	1 cup	184	11	1	0	33	–	718
w/pork	½ cup	199	7	4	17	40	–	840
DRIED								
catjang cooked	1 cup (2.9 oz)	200	14	1	0	35	–	32
cooked	1 cup	198	13	1	0	36	16	6
FRESH								
cowpeas leafy tips chopped cooked	1 cup	12	2	tr	0	1	–	3
cowpeas leafy tips raw chopped	1 cup	10	1	tr	0	2	–	2

FOOD	PORTION	CALS	PROT	FAT	CHOL	CARB	FIBER	SOD
FROZEN								
cowpeas cooked	½ cup	112	7	tr	0	20	–	5
TAKE-OUT								
blackeye peas & pork	1 cup	236	24	5	27	25	8	1303
BLINTZE								
Golden								
Cheese	1 (2.1 oz)	80	6	2	15	13	2	135
Ratner's								
Cheese	1 (2.2 oz)	100	5	2	30	16	0	140
TAKE-OUT								
cheese	1 (2.7 oz)	160	5	9	65	15	tr	240
BLUEBERRIES								
canned in heavy syrup	½ cup	113	1	tr	0	28	2	4
fresh	½ cup	41	1	tr	0	11	2	1
fresh	1 pt	229	3	1	0	58	10	4
frzn unsweetened	½ cup	40	tr	1	0	9	2	1
C&W								
Ultimate	¾ cup	70	0	0	0	16	3	0
Chukar Cherries								
Puget Sound Dried	¼ cup	160	tr	0	0	38	5	0
White Chocolate Covered	3 tbsp (1.4 oz)	223	2	12	8	26	tr	33
De-Lite								
Dried Sweetened	1 oz	86	1	1	0	23	4	4
Emily's								
Dark Chocolate Covered	¼ cup (1.4 oz)	170	1	8	0	27	2	0
LiteHouse								
Glaze	3 tbsp	70	0	0	0	17	0	45
Marie's								
Glaze	2 tbsp	40	0	0	0	10	0	35
Ocean Spray								
Fresh	1 cup	85	1	0	0	21	–	1
Stoneridge Orchards								
Organic Dried Wild Whole	⅓ cup (1.4 oz)	130	1	0	0	33	2	0
Whole Dried	⅓ cup (1.4 oz)	130	0	0	0	33	1	15

FOOD	PORTION	CALS	PROT	FAT	CHOL	CARB	FIBER	SOD
Sunsweet								
Dried	¼ cup (1.4 oz)	140	1	0	0	33	3	0
Tree Of Life								
Dried	¼ cup (1.5 oz)	150	4	0	0	38	4	0
BLUEBERRY JUICE								
Izze								
Sparkling Blueberry	1 bottle (12 oz)	120	0	0	0	33	–	30
Ocean Spray								
Diet	8 oz	5	0	0	0	2	–	50
Tart Is Smart								
Wild Blueberry Concentrate	0.5 oz	35	0	0	0	9	1	0
Walnut Acres								
Organic	8 oz	130	0	0	0	31	tr	15
BLUEFIN								
fillet baked	4.1 oz	186	30	6	88	0	0	90
BLUEFISH								
fresh baked	3 oz	135	22	5	64	0	0	65
BOAR								
wild roasted	3 oz	136	24	4	–	0	0	–
Natural Frontier Foods								
Wild Boar Steaks	1 (4 oz)	170	25	8	70	0	0	95
BOK CHOY (*see* CABBAGE)								
BONITO								
dried	1 oz	50	8	2	13	0	0	14
fresh	3 oz	117	20	4	–	0	0	–
BORAGE								
fresh chopped	1 cup	19	2	tr	0	3	–	71
BOTTLED WATER (*see* WATER)								
BOYSENBERRIES								
frzn unsweetened	½ cup	33	1	tr	0	8	4	1
in heavy syrup	½ cup	113	1	tr	0	29	3	4

FOOD	PORTION	CALS	PROT	FAT	CHOL	CARB	FIBER	SOD
BRAINS								
beef pan fried	3 oz	167	11	13	1696	0	0	134
beef simmered	3 oz	123	10	9	2635	0	0	92
lamb braised	3 oz	123	11	9	1737	0	0	114
lamb fried	3 oz	232	14	19	2128	0	0	133
pork braised	3 oz	117	10	8	2169	0	0	77
veal braised	3 oz	116	10	8	2635	0	0	133
veal fried	3 oz	181	12	14	1802	0	0	150
BRAN								
corn	1 cup (2.7 oz)	170	6	1	0	65	65	5
oat	½ cup (1.6 oz)	116	8	3	0	31	7	2
oat cooked	½ cup (3.8 oz)	44	4	1	0	13	3	1
rice	½ cup (2.1 oz)	187	8	12	0	29	12	3
wheat	½ cup (2 oz)	63	5	1	0	19	12	1
Bob's Red Mill								
Rice Bran	2 tbsp	60	2	3	0	8	3	0
Quaker								
Unprocessed	⅓ cup (0.6 oz)	35	3	1	0	11	8	0
Tree Of Life								
Oat Bran	½ cup (1.6 oz)	120	3	4	0	31	7	0
Organic Wheat Bran	¼ cup (1.1 oz)	190	4	18	0	4	2	0
BRAZIL NUTS								
dried unblanched	1 oz	186	4	19	0	4	–	0
BREAD								
CANNED								
boston brown	1 slice (1.6 oz)	88	2	1	0	19	2	284
B&M								
Raisin Brown Bread	½ in slice (2 oz)	130	3	1	0	29	2	380

FOOD	PORTION	CALS	PROT	FAT	CHOL	CARB	FIBER	SOD
FROZEN								
Cedarlane								
Organic Mediterranean Stuffed Focaccia	1 piece (4 oz)	295	13	10	22	37	1	485
Pepperidge Farm								
Garlic	1 slice (2.5 in)	170	4	7	0	24	2	250
Texas Toast Five Cheese	1 slice	150	4	7	<5	18	1	200
Whole Grain Texas Toast	1 slice	150	4	8	0	14	2	250
MIX								
cornbread	1 piece (2 oz)	188	4	6	37	29	1	467
READY-TO-EAT								
anadama	1 piece (1.1 oz)	87	2	1	1	16	1	272
baguette whole wheat	2 oz	140	6	0	0	29	1	360
cassava	1 piece (3.5 oz)	299	3	1	0	71	3	1187
challah	1 slice (1.4 oz)	115	4	2	20	19	1	197
cinnamon	1 slice (0.9 oz)	69	2	1	0	13	1	177
cracked wheat	1 slice (1.1 oz)	78	3	1	0	15	2	161
cuban bread	1 slice (1.1 oz)	83	3	1	0	16	1	163
french	1 slice (1.1 oz)	88	3	1	0	17	1	195
italian	1 loaf (1 lb)	1255	41	4	0	256	–	2656
navajo fry	1 piece	281	6	10	6	41	–	280
oat bran	1 slice (1.1 oz)	71	3	1	0	12	1	122
oatmeal	1 slice (0.9 oz)	73	2	1	0	13	1	162
pan criollo	1 piece (0.9 oz)	69	2	1	0	13	tr	136
pannetone	1 slice (0.9 oz)	86	2	2	18	15	1	92
pita	1 sm (1 oz)	77	3	tr	0	16	1	150
pita	1 lg (2 oz)	165	5	1	0	33	1	322

FOOD	PORTION	CALS	PROT	FAT	CHOL	CARB	FIBER	SOD
pita whole wheat	1 lg (2.2 oz)	170	6	2	0	35	5	340
pita whole wheat	1 sm (1 oz)	74	3	1	0	15	2	149
pumpernickel	1 slice (0.9 oz)	65	2	1	0	12	2	174
raisin	1 slice (1.1 oz)	88	3	1	0	17	1	125
rye	1 slice (1.1 oz)	83	3	1	0	15	2	211
seven grain	1 slice (1.1 oz)	80	3	1	0	15	2	456
wheat berry	1 slice (0.9 oz)	65	2	1	0	12	1	133
wheat bran	1 slice (1.3 oz)	89	3	1	0	17	1	175
wheat germ	1 slice (1 oz)	73	3	1	0	14	1	155
white cubed	1 cup	93	3	1	0	18	1	238
whole wheat	1 slice (1 oz)	69	3	1	0	13	2	148
Alvarado Street Bakery								
Sprouted Soy Crunch	1 slice (1.2 oz)	90	5	1	0	15	2	160
Sprouted Whole Wheat	1 slice	90	4	1	0	19	3	170
Arnold								
100% Natural Soft Honey Wheat	2 slices (2 oz)	150	6	2	0	28	3	270
Grains & More Double Omega	1 slice	110	5	2	0	19	3	220
Jewish Rye	1 slice	90	2	2	0	17	1	240
Sandwich Thins Multi-Grain	1 (1.5 oz)	100	4	1	0	22	5	230
Sandwich Thins Whole Grain White	1 (1.5 oz)	100	4	1	0	22	5	230
Whole Grains 100% Whole Wheat Double Fiber	1 slice	100	4	2	0	21	5	200
Whole Grains 12 Grain	1 slice (1.5 oz)	110	5	2	0	21	3	170
Whole Grains 15 Grain	1 slice	110	5	2	0	21	3	210
Whole Grains 7 Grain	1 slice	110	4	2	0	22	3	190
Aunt Gussie's								
Gluten Free Focaccia Bread Kalamata Olive	1 piece (2.7 oz)	180	3	2	0	37	4	450

FOOD	PORTION	CALS	PROT	FAT	CHOL	CARB	FIBER	SOD
Gluten Free Focaccia Bread Rosemary	1 piece (2.7 oz)	180	3	2	0	38	4	420
Baker's Inn								
9 Grain	1 slice	100	5	2	0	18	2	210
Cracked Wheat	1 slice	100	4	2	0	18	2	190
Honey White Made w/ Whole Grain	1 slice	110	4	2	0	19	1	250
Honey Whole Wheat	1 slice	100	4	2	0	19	2	250
Potato Made w/ Whole Grain	1 slice	100	4	2	0	18	1	220
Comfort Care								
Cabin Hearth Whole Wheat	1 oz	170	9	3	0	31	4	0
Ecce Panis								
Classic Ciabatta	⅛ loaf (2 oz)	180	6	2	0	36	tr	340
Flatout								
Fold It Flatbread 5 Grain Flax	1 (1.7 oz)	100	9	3	0	17	8	420
Fold It Flatbread Traditional Country	1 (1.8 oz)	140	8	2	0	24	3	380
Light Original	1 (2 oz)	90	9	3	0	16	9	320
Light Sundried Tomato	1 (1.9 oz)	90	9	3	0	17	9	320
Soft & No Crust Garden Spinach	1 (2 oz)	130	7	2	0	25	3	340
The Original	1 (2 oz)	130	7	2	0	24	3	310
Wrap Healthy Grain Harvest Wheat	1 (2 oz)	120	7	3	0	23	6	310
Wrap Healthy Grain Whole Grain White	1 (1.9 oz)	110	8	2	0	21	7	280
Wrap Mini Healthy Grain Harvest Wheat	1 (1 oz)	70	3	1	0	13	3	140
Freihofer's								
100% Whole Wheat	1 slice	90	4	2	0	17	2	160
French Meadow Bakery								
100% Rye Salt Free	1 slice (1.6 oz)	90	2	0	0	23	3	0
100% Spelt	2 slices (2.4 oz)	170	6	1	0	33	4	360
European Sourdough Rye	1 slice (1.7 oz)	90	2	0	0	22	3	220

FOOD	PORTION	CALS	PROT	FAT	CHOL	CARB	FIBER	SOD
Gluten Free Multigrain	1 slice (1.8 oz)	150	4	5	0	23	3	230
Hemp	2 slices (2.4 oz)	200	13	5	0	24	5	270
Kamut	2 slices (3 oz)	170	8	1	0	31	1	330
Men's Bread	2 slices (2.4 oz)	200	15	8	0	17	3	250
Our Daily Bread	2 slices (2.4 oz)	160	10	3	0	24	5	240
Sprouted Cinnamon Raisin	1 slice (1.5 oz)	100	2	1	0	19	3	90
Summer	1 slice (1.2 oz)	90	4	0	0	17	1	170
Gillian's Foods								
Gluten Free Cinnamon Raisin	1 slice (2 oz)	130	5	1	0	25	2	330
Kontos								
Pocket-Less Pita Whole Wheat	1 (2.8 oz)	210	10	2	0	38	4	510
La Tortilla Factory								
Wraps Smart & Delicious Gluten Free Dark Teff	1 (2.3 oz)	180	2	5	5	31	3	320
Wraps Smart & Delicious Gluten Free Ivory Teff	1 (2.3 oz)	180	2	5	0	30	3	320
Martin's								
Potato 100% Whole Wheat	1 slice (1.3 oz)	70	6	1	0	14	4	125
Mrs Baird's								
Acti-Fiber Wheat	2 slices (2.2 oz)	160	5	3	0	30	4	230
Whole Grain Wheat Sugar Free	1 slice (1.1 oz)	70	4	2	0	13	3	130
Natural Ovens								
100% Sweet Whole	1 slice	90	4	2	0	16	4	130
Carb Conscious Original	1 slice	80	8	2	0	9	4	120
Healthy Beginnings Better White	1 slice	110	5	2	0	20	2	180
Healthy Beginnings Honey Wheat	1 slice	120	4	2	0	21	3	170

FOOD	PORTION	CALS	PROT	FAT	CHOL	CARB	FIBER	SOD
Hunger Filler Whole Grain	1 slice	100	5	2	0	15	4	100
Organic Plus Whole Grain & Flax	1 slice	120	4	2	0	22	3	160
Whole Grain Oat Nut Crunch	1 slice	100	5	3	0	15	4	110
Nature's Own								
100% Whole Wheat	1 slice	50	4	1	0	10	2	115
9 Grain	1 slice	120	4	2	0	24	2	190
Hearty Oatmeal	1 slice	100	5	2	0	18	3	170
Wheat Double Fiber	1 slice	10	4	1	0	10	5	150
Wheat Light	2 slices	80	5	1	0	19	5	200
Wheat N' Fiber	1 slice	60	6	1	0	7	2	105
Whole Wheat w/ Organic Flour	1 slice	100	5	2	0	21	3	240
Nature's Pride								
100% Whole Wheat	1 slice (1.5 oz)	110	5	1	0	20	3	210
100% Whole Wheat Double Fiber	1 slice (1.5 oz)	100	4	1	0	20	6	210
Country Buttermilk	1 slice (1.5 oz)	110	4	2	5	21	tr	190
Healthy Multi-Grain	1 slice (1.5 oz)	110	5	9	0	20	3	190
Honey Wheat	1 slice (1 oz)	70	3	1	0	13	tr	120
Nutty Oat	1 slice (1.5 oz)	110	5	2	0	19	2	150
Oroweat								
100% Whole Wheat	1 slice (1.3 oz)	100	4	1	0	19	3	210
Country Potato	1 slice (1.3 oz)	100	3	1	0	20	tr	180
Country Whole Grain White	1 slice (1.3 oz)	90	4	2	0	17	1	170
Double Fiber	1 slice (1.3 oz)	70	4	1	0	16	6	160
Honey Fiber Whole Grain	1 slice (1.3 oz)	80	4	1	0	18	4	170
Russian Rye	1 slice (1 oz)	80	3	1	0	13	tr	200
Seven Grain	1 slice (1.3 oz)	100	3	1	0	20	2	180

FOOD	PORTION	CALS	PROT	FAT	CHOL	CARB	FIBER	SOD
Whole Grain & Flax	1 slice (1.3 oz)	100	4	2	0	17	3	180
Pepperidge Farm								
100% Natural Whole Grain German Dark Wheat	1 slice	100	4	2	0	20	3	210
Breakfast Apple & Grains	1 slice	90	4	2	0	18	3	150
Canadian White	1 slice	100	3	2	0	18	1	180
Carb Style 7 Grain	1 slice	60	5	2	0	8	3	150
Farmhouse Hearty White	1 slice	120	4	2	0	22	1	250
Farmhouse Honey Wheatberry	1 slice	120	4	2	0	22	2	190
Farmhouse Whole Grain White	1 slice (1.5 oz)	110	4	2	0	21	3	180
Fruit & Grain Cranberry Orange	1 slice (1.4 oz)	90	4	2	0	19	3	180
Honey Flax Whole Grain	1 slice (1.5 oz)	100	5	2	0	19	3	120
Hot & Crusty Italian	1 slice (2 in thick)	150	5	2	0	29	1	250
Jewish Rye Whole Grain Seeded	1 slice	70	3	1	0	14	2	190
Light Style 7 Grain	1 slice	45	2	0	0	9	1	90
Light Style Oatmeal	3 slices	140	7	1	0	27	2	260
Party Pumpernickel	5 slices	130	5	2	0	23	3	320
Swirl 100% Whole Wheat Cinnamon Raisins	1 slice (1 oz)	80	3	1	0	13	2	105
Very Thin White	3 slices	120	4	1	0	24	1	250
Vitality Oats & Barley	1 slice (1.5 oz)	120	4	2	0	21	5	110
Whole Grain 100% Soft Whole Wheat Double Fiber	1 slice	100	4	2	0	21	6	170
Whole Grain Soft Honey Oat	1 slice (1.5 oz)	100	5	2	0	19	4	115
Roman Meal								
Muesli	1 slice (1.5 oz)	110	5	2	0	19	2	160
Original Whole Grain	2 slices (2 oz)	130	5	2	0	25	2	250

FOOD	PORTION	CALS	PROT	FAT	CHOL	CARB	FIBER	SOD
Rudi's Organic Bakery								
100% Whole Wheat	1 slice	100	4	1	0	19	3	150
14 Grain	1 slice	90	4	1	0	19	4	150
Artisan Country French	1 slice	100	4	1	0	20	tr	210
Artisan Rosemary Olive Oil	1 slice	100	3	1	0	19	tr	230
Low Carb Right Choice	1 slice	45	4	1	0	7	2	105
Spelt Ancient Grain	1 slice	120	4	3	0	20	2	170
Whole Grain Apple N Spice	1 slice	110	4	1	0	24	5	190
S. Rosen's								
Hawaiian	1 slice	110	3	2	4	21	0	170
Rye Black Bavarian	1 slice	100	3	2	0	19	1	300
Sara Lee								
Soft & Smooth 100% Whole Wheat	1 slice	70	3	1	0	12	2	135
Soft & Smooth Whole Grain White	2 slices	150	6	2	0	28	3	250
Sonoma								
Wraps Organic Multi Grain	1 (2.4 oz)	180	6	7	0	27	6	330
Wraps Organic Wheat	1 (2.4 oz)	190	5	7	0	30	4	380
Wraps Original White Whole Wheat	1 (2.4 oz)	200	6	5	0	33	4	360
Stroehmann								
Dutch Country Twelve Grain	1 slice	100	4	2	0	18	2	180
Potato	1 slice	100	3	2	0	18	1	170
Sun-Maid								
Raisin Cinnamon Swirl	1 slice (1.2 oz)	100	3	2	5	18	1	130
The Baker								
Yoga Bread	1 slice	70	3	1	0	13	2	80
Thomas'								
Breakfast Original	1 slice	90	4	1	0	17	1	190
Sahara Pita Pockets Mini Whole Wheat	1 (1 oz)	70	3	1	0	13	2	150
Swirl Cinnamon Raisin	1 slice	120	3	2	0	21	1	160
Tumaro's								
Wraps Chipotle Chili & Peppers	1 (2.3 oz)	170	4	2	0	34	2	200
Wraps Sun Dried Tomato & Basil	1 (2.3 oz)	170	5	2	0	34	2	210

FOOD	PORTION	CALS	PROT	FAT	CHOL	CARB	FIBER	SOD
Udi's								
Gluten Free Cinnamon Raisin	2 slices (2.1 oz)	160	3	4	0	29	1	220
Gluten Free Whole Grain	2 slices (2 oz)	140	3	4	0	22	1	270
Wonder								
Classic White	1 slice (1 oz)	70	4	1	0	2	0	150
Classic White Sandwich	1 slice (0.9 oz)	60	2	1	0	13	0	135
REFRIGERATED								
Pillsbury								
Italian	⅛ pkg (1.6 oz)	110	4	2	0	21	tr	270
TAKE-OUT								
banana	1 slice (2 oz)	196	3	6	26	33	1	181
chapati as prep w/ fat	1 (1.6 oz)	95	3	2	3	18	3	180
chapati as prep w/o fat	1 (2.5 oz)	141	5	1	–	31	5	–
cornbread	1 piece (2.3 oz)	183	4	6	26	27	2	317
cornstick	1 (1.4 oz)	118	3	4	17	18	1	204
focaccia onion	1 piece (4.6 oz)	282	6	10	0	43	2	536
focaccia rosemary	1 piece (3.5 oz)	251	6	7	0	40	2	535
focaccia tomato olive	1 piece (4.7 oz)	270	6	8	0	42	2	683
garlic bread	1 slice (1 oz)	96	2	4	0	13	1	177
irish soda bread	1 slice (3 oz)	247	6	4	15	48	2	338
italian garlic	1 loaf (11 oz)	990	23	38	0	137	8	1830
naan	1 bread (3.5 oz)	286	7	9	46	43	2	546
papadum fried	1 (6 g)	30	1	2	0	2	tr	125
paratha plain	1 (1.6 oz)	136	3	5	19	19	2	176
poori indian puffed bread	1 piece (1.3 oz)	112	3	4	0	16	2	226
zucchini	1 slice (1.4 oz)	150	2	7	26	19	1	115

FOOD	PORTION	CALS	PROT	FAT	CHOL	CARB	FIBER	SOD
BREADCRUMBS								
dry seasoned	¼ cup	115	4	2	0	21	2	528
fresh	¼ cup	30	1	tr	0	6	tr	77
plain	¼ cup	107	4	1	0	19	1	198
Edward & Sons								
Organic Lightly Salted	⅓ cup	110	7	1	0	21	1	110
Organic Panko	⅓ cup	110	2	1	0	21	1	110
Gillian's Foods								
Plain Gluten Free	¼ cup (1.2 oz)	60	2	1	0	14	1	430
Kikkoman								
Panko	½ cup (1.1 oz)	110	3	1	0	24	tr	40
Krasdale								
Seasoned	¼ cup	120	4	2	0	21	2	350
Progresso								
Garlic & Herb	¼ cup (1 oz)	110	4	2	0	19	1	520
Italian Style	¼ cup (1 oz)	118	4	2	0	20	1	470
Panko Lemon Pepper	¼ cup (1 oz)	120	2	5	0	17	tr	430
Panko Plain	¼ cup (1 oz)	110	2	3	0	19	0	50
Plain	¼ cup (1 oz)	110	4	2	0	20	1	200
Southern Homestyle								
Corn Flake Crumbs	2 tbsp	40	1	0	0	9	0	50
Tortilla Crumbs	2 tbsp	40	1	0	0	9	0	50
BREADFRUIT								
fresh	1 sm (13.5 oz)	396	4	1	0	104	19	8
fried	1 cup	379	2	21	0	52	9	3
raw	1 cup	227	2	1	0	60	11	4
BREADNUTTREE SEEDS								
dried	1 oz	104	2	tr	0	23	–	–
BREADSTICKS								
plain	1 lg	41	1	1	0	7	tr	66
plain	1 sm	21	1	tr	0	3	tr	33
Fattorie & Pandea								
Fornini w/ Sea Salt	5 (1.2 oz)	140	4	5	0	21	1	320
Ferrara								
Slim Thin Torinese Style	6 (0.5 oz)	60	2	1	0	11	0	150

FOOD	PORTION	CALS	PROT	FAT	CHOL	CARB	FIBER	SOD
Pepperidge Farm								
Garlic frzn	1	160	5	5	0	25	1	320
Pillsbury								
Cornbread Twists	1 (1.4 oz)	140	3	6	0	18	0	340
Original Soft	2 (1.8 oz)	140	4	3	0	25	tr	370
Stella D'Oro								
Original	1 (0.3 oz)	40	1	1	0	6	0	40
Roasted Garlic	1	45	1	1	0	7	0	80
Sesame	1 (0.4 oz)	50	2	3	0	6	0	50
Sodium Free	1 (0.3 oz)	40	1	1	0	6	0	0

BREAKFAST BARS (*see* CEREAL BARS, ENERGY BARS)

BROCCOFLOWER

FOOD	PORTION	CALS	PROT	FAT	CHOL	CARB	FIBER	SOD
fresh flowerets cooked	1 cup (2.9 oz)	26	2	tr	0	5	3	214
fresh raw	1 cup (2.2 oz)	20	2	tr	0	4	2	15
head fresh raw	1 lg (18 oz)	158	15	2	0	31	16	118

BROCCOLI

FRESH

FOOD	PORTION	CALS	PROT	FAT	CHOL	CARB	FIBER	SOD
chinese broccoli (gai lan) cooked	1 cup (3 oz)	19	1	1	0	3	2	6
cooked w/o salt chopped	½ cup (2.7 oz)	27	2	tr	0	6	3	32
cooked w/o salt spear 5 in	1 (1.3 oz)	13	1	tr	0	3	1	15
raab cooked	½ cup (3 oz)	28	3	tr	0	3	2	48
raw	1 bunch (1.3 lbs)	207	17	2	0	40	16	201
raw floweret	1 (0.4 oz)	3	tr	tr	0	1	–	3
raw flowers	1 cup (2.5 oz)	20	2	tr	0	4	–	19
raw spear 5 in long	1 (1.1 oz)	11	1	tr	0	2	1	10
BroccoSprouts								
Broccoli Sprouts	½ cup	16	1	0	0	2	1	3
Mann's								
Broccoli Wokly	1 serv (3 oz)	25	3	0	0	4	2	25
Broccolini	8 stalks (3 oz)	35	3	0	0	6	1	25
Ocean Mist								
Rapini Broccoli Rabe Chopped Raw	1 cup	9	1	0	0	1	1	13
Ready Pac								
Microwave Broccoli Rabe as prep	½ cup (3 oz)	30	3	0	0	3	2	50

FOOD	PORTION	CALS	PROT	FAT	CHOL	CARB	FIBER	SOD
FROZEN								
chopped cooked w/o salt	1 cup (6.5 oz)	52	6	tr	0	10	6	20
spears cooked w/o salt	1 cup (6.5 oz)	52	6	tr	0	10	6	44
Birds Eye								
Broccoli & Cheese Sauce	½ cup	90	3	5	5	8	1	490
Steamfresh Cuts	1 cup (3.1 oz)	30	2	0	0	4	2	20
Steamfresh Florets	1 cup (2.3 oz)	30	1	0	0	4	2	20
C&W								
Broccoli & Cheddar Cheese Sauce	1⅓ cups	70	4	3	5	7	2	370
Florets	1 cup	30	1	0	0	4	2	20
Cascadian Farm								
Organic Florets	⅔ cup	20	2	0	0	4	2	20
Dr. Praeger's								
Broccoli Bites	2 (2 oz)	110	3	4	0	17	2	220
Green Giant								
Cuts as prep	⅔ cup	25	1	0	0	4	2	20
Pasta Broccoli & Alfredo Sauce as prep	1 cup	210	9	4	<5	34	3	780
Steamers Broccoli & Cheese Sauce as prep	½ cup	45	2	2	0	7	2	380
Seabrook Farms								
Broccoli Raab	1 cup (2.9 oz)	25	2	0	0	4	2	35
Skyy								
Broccoli Bites	3 (2.8 oz)	180	7	10	10	16	2	330
TAKE-OUT								
batter dipped & fried	3 pieces (1.4 oz)	58	1	4	7	5	1	62
w/ cheese sauce	1 cup (8 oz)	242	12	15	32	16	5	426

BROWNIE

FOOD	PORTION	CALS	PROT	FAT	CHOL	CARB	FIBER	SOD
brownie	1 (2 oz)	227	3	9	10	36	1	175
butterscotch	1 (1.2 oz)	151	2	8	20	19	tr	95
Arrowhead Mills								
Gluten Free as prep	1	160	1	8	21	21	tr	40
Betty Crocker								
Dark Chocolate as prep	1	170	1	7	21	25	tr	100
Fudge Low Fat as prep	1	140	1	3	12	28	1	125
Original Supreme as prep	1	160	1	6	21	26	tr	105
Triple Chunk as prep	1	180	1	8	21	25	1	90

FOOD	PORTION	CALS	PROT	FAT	CHOL	CARB	FIBER	SOD
Walnut as prep	1	170	1	9	21	22	tr	90
Warm Delights Hot Fudge	1 pkg (3 oz)	370	5	12	–	61	3	270
Bob's Red Mill								
Gluten Free as prep	1	140	2	5	0	27	2	180
Duncan Hines								
Chocolate Fudge frzn	1/12 pkg (1.4 oz)	170	2	8	20	23	0	85
Dark Chocolate Chunk Mix as prep	1/16 pkg	170	2	7	15	25	1	110
Milk Chocolate Mix as prep	1/20 pkg	180	2	9	25	23	0	75
Peanut Butter Cup Mix as prep	1/16 pkg	170	2	8	15	23	1	105
Turtle Mix as prep	1/16 pkg	160	2	7	15	23	1	115
Walnut Mix as prep	1/16 pkg	180	2	8	15	24	2	115
Erin Baker's								
Organic Bites	1 (1 oz)	100	2	3	5	18	2	70
Organic Bites Double Chocolate Chip	1 (1 oz)	90	2	2	5	19	2	75
Fiber One								
Chocolate Peanut Butter	1 (0.89 oz)	90	1	35	0	17	5	110
Chocolate Fudge	1 (0.89 oz)	90	1	3	0	18	5	100
Foods By George								
Gluten Free	1/9 pkg (1.5 oz)	180	2	9	40	24	1	45
Foxy's Bake Shop								
Milk Chocolate	½ (1.7 oz)	200	3	11	55	23	0	65
White Chocolate	½ (1.7 oz)	200	3	12	0	23	0	70
French Meadow Bakery								
Gluten Free Fudge	1 (2.82 oz)	350	3	16	55	48	2	240
Glenny's								
100 Calorie 75% Organic	1 (1.45 oz)	100	4	4	–	12	7	85
Hershey's								
Brownie	½ pkg (1.5 oz)	190	2	9	–	28	1	40
Pillsbury								
Traditional Chocolate Fudge	1 (1.4 oz)	150	2	6	0	24	tr	120
Turtle Supreme Bars	1 (1.4 oz)	180	2	9	5	23	tr	100
Uncle Wally's								
Smart Portion	1 (0.9 oz)	80	1	2	10	17	2	75

FOOD	PORTION	CALS	PROT	FAT	CHOL	CARB	FIBER	SOD
VitaBrownie								
Brownie	1 (2 oz)	100	4	2	0	25	10	125
Dark Chocolate Pomegranate	1 (2 oz)	100	3	2	0	21	6	140
BRUSSELS SPROUTS								
CANNED								
Jake & Amos								
Pickled Dill Brussels Sprouts	2 tbsp	10	0	0	0	1	0	217
FRESH								
cooked	6 pieces	45	3	1	0	9	3	26
Ocean Mist								
Brussels Sprouts	4 (2 oz)	40	2	1	0	6	3	25
Select Gourmet								
Fresh	½ cup	35	3	0	0	8	3	21
FROZEN								
cooked	1 cup	65	6	1	0	13	6	23
Birds Eye								
Steamfresh Baby	10 (2.9 oz)	45	3	0	0	8	3	15
Steamfresh Singles Baby	1 pkg (3.2 oz)	50	3	0	0	9	3	20
C&W								
Petite	10 (3 oz)	45	3	0	0	8	3	15
Green Giant								
Baby & Butter Sauce as prep	½ cup	60	3	1	<5	9	3	320
BUCKWHEAT								
groats roasted cooked	1 cup (6 oz)	155	7	1	0	33	5	252
groats roasted uncooked	½ cup	292	11	3	0	61	9	1
Bob's Red Mill								
Organic Kernels	¼ cup	142	5	1	0	31	3	4
BUFFALO (*see also* HOT DOG, JERKY, SAUSAGE)								
burger	3 oz	202	20	13	71	0	0	62
chuck braised	4 oz	205	36	6	118	0	0	61
top round steak broiled	3 oz	313	54	9	153	0	0	74
water buffalo roasted	3 oz	111	23	2	52	0	0	48
High Plains Bison								
Filet Mignon	4 oz	120	23	4	70	1	0	50
Ground	4 oz	190	20	11	50	0	0	60
Pot Roast	4 oz	150	22	7	70	0	0	85

FOOD	PORTION	CALS	PROT	FAT	CHOL	CARB	FIBER	SOD
Ribeye Steak	4 oz	215	21	14	60	1	0	75
Shredded In BBQ Sauce	1 serv (5 oz)	250	22	3	45	34	0	320
Steak Top Sirloin	4 oz	110	25	3	50	0	0	50
Tenderloin Tips	4 oz	120	23	12	70	1	0	50
Natural Frontier Foods								
Burgers	1 (5 oz)	170	22	9	55	0	0	85
Ground	4 oz	170	22	9	55	0	0	85
Steaks	1 (4 oz)	160	28	3	75	0	0	75
BULGUR								
cooked	½ cup	76	3	tr	0	17	4	5
uncooked	½ cup	239	9	1	0	53	13	12
Bob's Red Mill								
From Soft White Wheat	¼ cup	150	4	1	0	32	4	0
Near East								
Whole Grain Wheat Pilaf as prep	1 cup	200	7	4	9	40	8	672
TAKE-OUT								
tabbouleh	1 cup	198	3	15	0	16	4	797
BURBOT (FISH)								
fresh baked	3 oz	98	65	1	65	0	0	106
BURDOCK ROOT								
cooked w/o salt	1 root (5.8 oz)	146	3	tr	0	35	3	7
cooked w/o salt	1 cup	110	3	tr	0	26	2	5
BUTTER								
clarified butter	¼ cup (1.8 oz)	449	tr	51	131	0	0	1
clarified butter	1 tbsp (0.4 oz)	112	tr	13	33	0	0	0
ghee cow's milk	1 tbsp	126	–	14	39	–	0	0
ghee vegetable oil	1 tbsp	126	–	14	0	–	0	0
honey butter	1 tbsp (0.6 oz)	85	tr	6	15	9	0	42
honey butter	¼ cup (2.5 oz)	338	tr	23	62	36	tr	168
light butter whipped salted	1 tbsp (0.3 oz)	48	tr	5	10	0	0	43
stick salted	1 (4 oz)	810	1	92	243	tr	0	651

FOOD	PORTION	CALS	PROT	FAT	CHOL	CARB	FIBER	SOD
stick salted	1 tbsp (0.5 oz)	102	tr	12	31	tr	0	82
stick salted	¼ cup (2 oz)	407	tr	46	122	tr	0	327
stick unsalted	1 tbsp (0.5 oz)	102	tr	12	31	tr	0	2
stick unsalted	1 (4 oz)	810	1	92	243	tr	0	12
stick unsalted	¼ cup (2 oz)	407	tr	46	122	tr	0	6
whipped salted	1 tbsp (0.3 oz)	67	tr	8	21	tr	0	78
whipped salted	¼ cup (1.3 oz)	271	tr	31	83	tr	0	312
Cabot								
Salted	1 tbsp	100	0	11	30	0	0	90
Country Crock								
Spreadable Butter w/ Canola Oil	1 tbsp (0.4 oz)	80	0	9	15	0	0	65
Deerfield								
Creamy	1 tbsp	100	0	11	30	0	0	0
Earth Balance								
Butter Blend Unsalted	1 tbsp	100	0	11	0	0	0	0
Horizon Organic								
European	1 tbsp	100	0	12	30	0	0	0
Land O Lakes								
Light Salted	1 tbsp (0.5 oz)	50	0	6	15	0	0	100
Light Whipped Salted	1 tbsp (0.4 oz)	45	0	5	15	0	0	85
Salted	1 tbsp (0.5 oz)	100	0	11	30	0	0	95
Spreadable w/ Canola Oil	1 tbsp (0.5 oz)	100	0	11	20	0	0	90
Whipped Salted	1 tbsp (0.2 oz)	50	0	6	15	0	0	50
Organic Valley								
European Style	1 tbsp	110	0	12	25	0	0	0
Straus								
Organic European Style Lightly Salted	1 tbsp (0.5 oz)	110	0	12	30	0	0	45
Organic European Style Sweet Butter	1 tbsp (0.5 oz)	110	0	12	30	0	0	0

FOOD	PORTION	CALS	PROT	FAT	CHOL	CARB	FIBER	SOD
BUTTER SUBSTITUTES								
stick	1 stick	811	1	91	99	1	–	1013
Butter Buds								
Granules	1 pkg (2 g)	5	0	0	0	2	–	75
Molly McButter								
Natural Butter	1 tsp (2 g)	5	0	0	0	1	0	180
Sunsweet								
Lighter Bake	1 tbsp	35	0	0	0	9	–	0
BUTTERBUR								
canned fuki chopped	1 cup	3	tr	tr	0	tr	–	5
fresh fuki	1 cup	13	tr	tr	0	3	–	7
BUTTERNUTS								
dried	1 oz	174	7	16	0	3	–	0
BUTTERSCOTCH (*see also* CANDY)								
E. Guittard								
Baking Chips	33 (0.5 oz)	80	tr	5	0	10	0	15
Hershey's								
Chips	1 tbsp (0.5 oz)	80	1	4	–	9	–	35
CABBAGE (*see also* COLESLAW)								
chinese bok choy shredded cooked w/o salt	1 cup	20	3	tr	0	3	2	58
chinese pe-tsai shredded cooked w/o salt	1 cup	17	2	tr	0	3	2	11
green raw shredded	1 cup	19	1	tr	0	4	2	13
green shredded cooked w/o salt	1 cup	34	2	tr	0	8	3	12
japanese pickled	½ cup	22	1	tr	0	4	2	208
red raw shredded	1 cup	22	1	tr	0	5	2	19
red shredded cooked w/o salt	1 cup	44	2	tr	0	10	4	42
savoy shredded cooked w/o salt	1 cup	35	3	tr	0	8	4	35
Aunt Nellie's								
Sweet & Sour Red	2 tbsp (1 oz)	20	0	0	0	5	0	110
Glory								
Country Cabbage	½ cup	25	1	0	0	6	1	350

FOOD	PORTION	CALS	PROT	FAT	CHOL	CARB	FIBER	SOD
Ready Pac								
Ready Fixin's Shredded Red	2 cups (3 oz)	25	1	0	0	6	2	25
TAKE-OUT								
coleslaw w/ pineapple & dressing	1 cup (4.6 oz)	194	1	16	8	14	2	124
creamed	1 cup	158	5	10	6	13	2	610
kimchee	1 cup	32	2	tr	0	6	2	996
stuffed cabbage w/ rice & beef	1 (3.6 oz)	117	9	5	42	9	1	369
sweet & sour red cabbage	4 oz	61	1	3	–	8	3	–
CACAO								
Kopali								
Organic Dark Chocolate Covered Cacao Nibs	½ pkg (1 oz)	140	2	10	0	15	2	0
Navitas Naturals								
Butter	1 tbsp	120	0	14	0	0	0	0
Nibs	1 oz	130	4	12	0	10	9	0
Powder	1 oz	120	5	3	0	18	7	20
Sunfood								
Organic Cacao Beans	1 oz	171	4	13	0	8	6	15
Organic Cacao Nibs	1 oz	171	4	13	0	8	6	15
CACTUS								
fresh cooked w/ fat	1 pad (1 oz)	11	tr	1	0	1	1	84
fresh cooked w/o fat	1 cup (5.2 oz)	22	2	tr	0	5	3	399
pricklypear	1 (3.6 oz)	42	1	1	0	10	4	5
pricklypear fresh	1 cup (5.2 oz)	61	1	1	0	14	5	7
CAKE (*see also* CAKE MIX)								
battenburg cake	1 slice (2 oz)	204	3	10	–	28	1	–
cream puff shell	1 (2.3 oz)	239	6	17	129	15	–	368
crumpet	1 (2.3 oz)	131	4	1	0	31	2	535
dutch honey cake	1 slice (0.8 oz)	70	1	0	0	17	0	25
eccles cake	1 slice (2 oz)	285	2	16	–	36	1	–
madeira cake	1 slice (1 oz)	98	1	4	–	15	1	–
sponge	1 piece (1.3 oz)	110	2	1	39	23	tr	93
sponge cake dessert shell	1 (0.8 oz)	70	1	2	20	12	0	150

FOOD	PORTION	CALS	PROT	FAT	CHOL	CARB	FIBER	SOD
treacle tart	1 slice (2.5 oz)	258	3	10	–	42	1	–
Amy's								
Organic Chocolate	1 slice	170	2	6	0	27	1	130
Toaster Pops Apple	1 (2.1 oz)	150	3	4	0	27	1	110
Aunt Trudy's								
Organic Baklava Soy Nut	1 (1.8 oz)	190	4	6	0	29	2	60
Balocco								
Il Panettone	1 serv (3.5 oz)	380	7	15	120	54	2	75
Bellino								
Pandoro	1 (2.8 oz)	330	7	16	125	39	1	95
Betty Crocker								
Warm Delights Cinnamon Swirl	1 (3.3 oz)	390	4	10	0	72	1	500
Coppenrath								
Mousse Cake Chocolate	1/8 cake (1.8 oz)	140	3	7	40	17	2	55
Mousse Cake Coconut	1/8 cake (1.8 oz)	140	3	8	45	15	2	50
Mousse Duets Chocolate	1 (3.2 oz)	290	5	15	35	32	2	80
Mousse Duets Lemon Chiffon	1 (3.2 oz)	280	3	16	35	31	tr	70
Do Goodie								
Gluten Free Banana Bread	1 slice (2 oz)	150	2	4	35	27	2	170
Gluten Free Cupcake Chocolate	1	290	2	14	15	41	1	125
Gluten Free Cupcake Vanilla	1	290	2	14	15	41	0	125
Earth Cafe								
Cheesecake Vegan Blueberry Thrill	1 slice (2 oz)	193	3	15	0	12	1	67
Cheesecake Vegan Coconut Carob	1 slice (2 oz)	206	3	16	0	13	1	61
Cheesecake Vegan Rockin' Raspberry	1 slice (2 oz)	194	3	15	0	12	2	67
El Monterey								
Cheesecake Bites Caramel	1 (2 oz)	180	2	10	15	23	0	150
Cheesecake Bites Raspberry	1 (2 oz)	200	3	11	20	21	0	150

FOOD	PORTION	CALS	PROT	FAT	CHOL	CARB	FIBER	SOD
Entenmann's								
Cheese Cake Deluxe French	1/6 cake (3.8 oz)	390	6	24	40	39	tr	400
Chocolate Fudge	1/8 cake (2.2 oz)	240	2	10	25	37	2	190
Cinnamon Swirl Buns	1 (3 oz)	320	5	14	35	45	2	230
Danish Twist Cheese	1/8 cake (1.9 oz)	220	3	11	20	27	tr	190
Fudge Iced Golden Cake	1/8 cake (2.2 oz)	260	2	11	25	37	1	150
Louisiana Crunch	1/8 cake (2.7 oz)	310	3	13	45	47	tr	300
Utlimate Super Cinnamons	1/2 bun (2.5 oz)	280	4	10	25	41	1	180
Vanilla Bean Iced	1/8 cake (2.2 oz)	290	1	17	25	36	0	160
Fiber One								
Toaster Pastry Blueberry	1 (1.8 oz)	180	3	4	0	36	5	130
Toaster Pastry Chocolate Fudge	1 (1.8 oz)	160	3	4	0	35	5	140
Fillo Factory								
Organic Apple Strudel	1 (4.4 oz)	290	3	10	0	47	2	110
Organic Apple Turnovers	1 (3 oz)	180	2	6	0	30	1	90
Foods By George								
Gluten Free Crumb Cake	1/9 cake (2.2 oz)	280	2	14	40	36	tr	80
Gluten Free Pound Cake	1/6 cake (2.7 oz)	290	4	12	130	35	tr	190
French Meadow Bakery								
Gluten Free Cupcake Chocolate	1 (2 oz)	220	24	8	20	35	1	240
Gluten Free Cupcake Yellow	1 (2 oz)	230	20	9	20	35	0	230
Vegan Carrot	1/4 cake (2.6 oz)	130	2	0	65	38	1	150
Glenny's								
Blondie 100 Calorie 75% Organic	1 (1.45 oz)	100	4	3	–	12	7	100
Gourmet Pastries								
Baklava Walnut	1 piece (1.8 oz)	240	3	11	5	30	0	100

FOOD	PORTION	CALS	PROT	FAT	CHOL	CARB	FIBER	SOD
Guiltless Gourmet								
Dessert Bowl Bananas Foster Cake	1 pkg (2 oz)	200	3	2	15	42	tr	250
Dessert Bowl Black Velvet Cake	1 pkg (2 oz)	200	4	3	20	42	3	190
Hostess								
100 Calorie Pack Mini Carrot Cake	1 pkg (1.2 oz)	100	2	3	5	20	4	120
100 Calorie Pack Mini Chocolate Cupcakes	1 pkg (1.3 oz)	100	2	3	10	22	5	140
100 Calorie Pack Mini Coffee Cake Cinnamon Streusel	1 pkg (1.2 oz)	100	2	3	10	21	5	135
100 Calorie Pack Mini Golden Cupcakes	1 pkg (1.2 oz)	100	2	3	5	20	3	150
Cup Cakes Chocolate	1 (1.8 oz)	170	1	6	5	30	1	250
Ho Hos	1	120	1	6	0	18	0	75
Twinkies	1 (1.5 oz)	150	1	5	20	27	0	220
Lance								
Honey Bun	1 (3 oz)	320	4	13	0	47	4	200
Mrs. Freshley's								
Golden Cupcakes Creme Filled	1 pkg (1.3 oz)	100	2	3	10	24	5	135
Mrs. Smith's								
Carrot	1/6 cake (2.9 oz)	300	3	16	30	37	2	320
Cobbler Blackberry	1 serv (4 oz)	260	2	10	0	43	2	250
Singles Heavenly 100 New York Cheesecake	1 (0.9 oz)	100	2	6	25	9	0	75
Neuman's								
Date Nut Bread	1 oz	90	2	2	<5	17	1	154
Pepperidge Farm								
Chocolate Coconut 3 Layer	1/8 cake	240	2	10	20	33	tr	130
Devil's Food 3 Layer	1/8 cake	220	2	9	20	34	tr	170
Golden 3 Layer	1/8 cake	230	2	9	15	34	1	130
Lemon 3 Layer	1/8 cake	240	2	11	25	34	tr	130
Turnover Apple	1	290	4	15	0	36	2	230
Turnover Peach	1	290	4	15	0	35	1	230
Pillsbury								
Caramel Rolls	1 (1.7 oz)	170	2	7	0	24	tr	320

FOOD	PORTION	CALS	PROT	FAT	CHOL	CARB	FIBER	SOD
Cinnamon Rolls w/ Icing	1 (3.5 oz)	310	5	9	0	54	1	640
Cinnamon Rolls w/ Icing Reduced Fat	1 (1.5 oz)	140	2	4	0	24	tr	340
Toaster Strudel	1 (2 oz)	200	3	9	5	28	1	210
Toaster Strudel Blueberry	1 (2 oz)	190	3	9	5	26	tr	190
Toaster Strudel Cream Cheese	1 (2 oz)	200	3	11	10	23	tr	220
Toaster Strudel Raspberry	1 (2 oz)	190	3	9	5	26	tr	190
Toaster Strudel Wildberry	1 (2 oz)	190	3	9	5	25	tr	190
Turnovers Cherry	1 (2 oz)	180	2	8	0	24	0	250
Prosperity								
Limoncello	1 serv (3.5 oz)	300	4	12	55	43	1	240
Tortuga								
Caribbean Rum Golden Original	1 piece (4 oz)	400	4	19	25	54	2	540
TAKE-OUT								
angelfood	1 slice (2 oz)	143	3	tr	0	33	tr	283
apple crisp	1 serv (8.6 oz)	384	4	8	0	76	4	502
apple turnover	1 (6.6 oz)	661	7	34	0	83	3	614
baklava	1 piece (2.7 oz)	334	5	23	35	29	2	253
basbousa namoura	1 piece (1 oz)	60	2	3	0	10	2	144
bean cake	1 cake (1.1 oz)	130	2	7	0	16	1	60
black forest chocolate cherry	1 piece (2.5 oz)	187	2	9	30	27	1	160
boston cream pie	1 slice (3.2 oz)	232	2	8	34	39	1	132
cannoli w/ cannoli cream	1	369	6	21	–	42	–	–
carrot w/ icing	1 slice (4.7 oz)	543	5	28	80	70	2	245
cheesecake	1 slice (4.5 oz)	410	11	25	86	37	tr	484
cheesecake chocolate	1 slice (4.5 oz)	489	8	32	118	49	2	384
chinese moon cake	1 (4.8 oz)	458	9	6	69	92	4	119
cobbler pineapple	1 cup (7.6 oz)	414	4	10	2	80	2	345

FOOD	PORTION	CALS	PROT	FAT	CHOL	CARB	FIBER	SOD
coconut mochiko filipino cake	1 piece (2.7 oz)	252	3	12	0	35	2	76
coffeecake iced	1 piece (1.6 oz)	175	3	8	31	24	1	180
cream puff custard filled chocolate frosted	1 (3.9 oz)	293	7	18	142	27	1	377
eclair	1 (3.5 oz)	262	6	16	127	24	1	337
french apple tart	1 (3.5 oz)	302	4	15	60	37	2	326
fruitcake	1 slice (1.5 oz)	139	1	4	2	26	2	116
funnel cake	1 (3.2 oz)	276	7	14	62	29	1	269
gingerbread	1 piece (2.4 oz)	213	3	7	24	35	1	316
jelly roll	1 slice (1.8 oz)	146	3	2	93	28	tr	92
jelly roll lemon filled	1 slice (3 oz)	210	3	2	35	48	tr	300
napoleon	1 mini (1 oz)	123	2	9	14	9	tr	51
napoleon	1 (3 oz)	348	5	25	39	25	1	144
panettone	1/12 cake (2.9 oz)	300	6	12	90	43	2	120
petit fours	2 (0.9 oz)	120	1	7	0	15	0	15
pineapple upside down	1 piece (4.2 oz)	387	4	15	27	61	1	385
pound	1 slice (1 oz)	120	2	5	32	15	–	96
pound fat free	1 slice (2 oz)	160	3	1	0	35	1	193
pumpkin bread w/ raisins	1 slice (2.1 oz)	178	2	4	26	34	1	151
red velvet cupcake w/ cream cheese frosting	1 sm	272	3	12	63	38	1	178
red velvet w/ cream cheese frosting	1/16 cake	520	6	24	117	70	1	334
sacher torte	1 slice (2.2 oz)	240	4	11	50	30	4	120
sacher torte chocolate + apricot jam	1 serv	430	–	12	–	23	–	–
strawberry shortcake	1 serv (4.1 oz)	211	4	5	109	40	1	112
strudel apple	1 piece (2.2 oz)	175	2	7	4	26	1	172

FOOD	PORTION	CALS	PROT	FAT	CHOL	CARB	FIBER	SOD
strudel cheese	1 piece (2.2 oz)	195	6	8	42	24	tr	111
strudel cherry	1 piece (2.2 oz)	179	3	6	9	29	1	82
strudel pineapple	1 piece (2.2 oz)	159	2	4	10	31	1	88
sweet potato w/ glaze	1 piece (2.7 oz)	275	4	12	40	39	1	285
tiramisu	1 piece (5.1 oz)	409	7	30	171	31	tr	79
tiramisu	1 cake (4.4 lbs)	5732	101	421	2395	439	3	1107
torte chocolate ganache	1 slice (3.5 oz)	400	7	26	90	40	6	120
trifle w/ cream	6 oz	291	4	16	–	34	1	–
white w/ coconut icing	1 slice (3.9 oz)	399	5	12	1	71	1	318
zucchini bread	1 slice (1.4 oz)	150	2	7	26	19	1	115
CAKE ICING								
chocolate	¼ cup	269	1	7	1	53	1	125
vanilla	¼ cup	322	tr	8	0	64	0	152
Betty Crocker								
HomeStyle Mix Fluffy White as prep	6 tbsp	100	tr	0	0	24	–	55
Rich & Creamy Butter Cream	2 tbsp (1.3 oz)	140	0	5	0	15	–	70
Rich & Creamy Chocolate	2 tbsp (1.2 oz)	130	0	5	0	21	tr	95
Rich & Creamy Creamy White	2 tbsp (1.2 oz)	140	0	5	0	23	–	70
Rich & Creamy Lemon	2 tbsp (1.2 oz)	140	0	5	0	23	–	70
Rich & Creamy Vanilla	2 tbsp (1.2 oz)	140	0	5	0	23	–	70
Whipped Fluffy White	2 tbsp (0.8 oz)	100	0	5	–	15	–	25

FOOD	PORTION	CALS	PROT	FAT	CHOL	CARB	FIBER	SOD
Duncan Hines								
Chocolate Butter Cream	2 tbsp (1.2 oz)	140	0	6	0	22	0	90
Chocolate Fudge	2 tbsp (1.2 oz)	130	tr	6	0	21	0	120
Classic Vanilla	2 tbsp	140	0	6	0	23	0	70
Cream Cheese	2 tbsp (1.2 oz)	140	0	6	0	23	0	70
Milk Chocolate	2 tbsp (1.2 oz)	140	0	6	0	22	0	90
Manischewitz								
Dairy Free Chocolate	2 tbsp (1.2 oz)	138	0	5	0	22	0	95
Naturally Nora								
Frosting Mix Chocolate as prep	1/12 pkg	150	1	7	15	24	0	21
Frosting Mix Vanilla as prep	1/12 pkg	170	tr	8	21	25	0	24
CAKE MIX								
Betty Crocker								
Gingerbread as prep	1 piece	220	2	6	27	39	–	360
Pineapple Upside Down as prep	1/6 cake	390	2	13	36	66	–	280
Pound Cake as prep	1/8 cake	260	2	8	54	45	–	190
SuperMoist Carrot as prep	1/12 cake	260	1	12	54	35	–	270
SuperMoist Chocolate as prep	1/12 cake	250	2	11	75	35	1	380
SuperMoist Devil's Food as prep	1/12 cake	260	2	12	54	35	1	370
SuperMoist Lemon as prep	1/12 cake	240	1	9	54	35	–	280
SuperMoist Milk Chocolate as prep	1/12 cake	240	2	9	54	35	tr	280
SuperMoist Spice as prep	1/12 cake	270	2	13	54	34	1	370
SuperMoist Vanilla as prep	1/12 cake	230	2	9	54	35	–	300
SuperMoist White as prep	1/12 cake	220	2	8	0	35	–	300
SuperMoist Yellow as prep	1/12 cake	230	1	9	54	35	–	280
Bisquick								
Heart Smart	1/3 cup	140	3	3	0	27	1	430
Duncan Hines								
Angel Food as prep	1/12 cake	140	31	0	0	31	0	280

FOOD	PORTION	CALS	PROT	FAT	CHOL	CARB	FIBER	SOD
Cupcake Mix Classic Yellow as prep	1	130	2	6	35	17	0	150
Decadent Carrot as prep	1/12 cake	260	4	11	55	37	1	260
Golden Butter Recipe as prep	1/12 cake	270	3	14	75	35	0	240
Lemon Supreme as prep	1/12 cake	270	3	12	55	36	–	310
Red Velvet as prep	1/12 cake	270	4	13	55	35	1	280
Yellow Classic as prep	1/12 cake	270	3	12	55	36	–	310
Naturally Nora								
Cheerful Chocolate as prep	1/12 pkg	300	3	14	39	39	1	168
Sunny Yellow as prep	1/12 pkg	280	2	12	54	39	tr	168
Surprising Stars as prep	1/12 pkg	300	3	12	39	42	tr	168
Uncle Wally's								
Slice 'N Bake Cupcakes Chocolate	1 (2.1 oz)	240	2	11	20	32	1	150

CALZONE (*see* SANDWICHES)

CANADIAN BACON

FOOD	PORTION	CALS	PROT	FAT	CHOL	CARB	FIBER	SOD
grilled	2 slices (1.6 oz)	87	11	4	27	1	0	727
Applegate Farms								
Natural	2 slices (2 oz)	90	12	4	35	1	0	500
Celebrity								
98% Fat Free	3 slices (1.8 oz)	60	10	1	30	1	0	350
Dietz & Watson								
Canadian Style	2 oz	70	11	2	30	1	0	490

CANADIAN BACON SUBSTITUTES

FOOD	PORTION	CALS	PROT	FAT	CHOL	CARB	FIBER	SOD
Yves								
Meatless Canadian Bacon	2 slices (2 oz)	80	17	1	0	2	0	400

CANDY

FOOD	PORTION	CALS	PROT	FAT	CHOL	CARB	FIBER	SOD
butterscotch	1 piece (6 g)	24	0	tr	1	6	–	3
candied cherries	1 (4 g)	12	0	tr	0	3	–	–
candied citron	1 oz	89	tr	tr	0	23	–	82
candied lemon peel	1 oz	90	tr	tr	0	23	–	14
candied orange peel	1 oz	90	tr	tr	0	23	–	14
candied pineapple slice	1 slice (2 oz)	179	tr	tr	0	45	–	–
candy corn	1 oz	105	tr	0	0	27	–	57
caramels	1 piece (8 g)	31	tr	1	1	6	–	20

FOOD	PORTION	CALS	PROT	FAT	CHOL	CARB	FIBER	SOD
caramels chocolate	1 piece (6 g)	22	tr	tr	0	6	–	–
carob bar	1 (3.1 oz)	453	11	28	–	42	–	–
dark chocolate	1 oz	150	1	10	0	16	–	5
fondant	1 piece (0.6 oz)	57	0	0	0	15	–	6
fondant chocolate coated	1 piece (0.4 oz)	40	tr	1	0	9	–	3
fondant mint	1 oz	105	tr	0	0	27	–	57
fruit pastilles	1 tube (1.4 oz)	101	2	0	–	25	–	–
fudge brown sugar w/ nuts	1 piece (0.5 oz)	56	tr	1	1	11	–	14
fudge chocolate marshmallow	1 piece (0.7 oz)	84	1	3	5	14	–	21
fudge chocolate marshmallow w/ nuts	1 piece (0.8 oz)	96	1	4	5	15	–	21
fudge chocolate w/ nuts	1 piece (0.7 oz)	81	1	3	3	14	–	11
fudge peanut butter	1 piece (0.6 oz)	59	1	1	1	13	–	12
fudge vanilla w/ nuts	1 piece (0.5 oz)	62	tr	2	2	11	–	9
gumdrops	10 sm (0.4 oz)	135	0	0	0	35	–	15
gumdrops	10 lg (3.8 oz)	420	0	0	0	108	–	48
hard candy	1 oz	106	0	0	0	28	–	11
jelly beans	10 sm (0.4 oz)	40	0	tr	0	10	–	3
jelly beans	10 lg (1 oz)	104	0	tr	0	26	–	7
lollipop	1 (6 g)	22	0	0	0	6	–	2
marzipan	1 oz	128	3	7	0	15	2	5
milk chocolate	1 bar (1.55 oz)	226	3	14	10	26	–	36
milk chocolate crisp	1 bar (1.45 oz)	203	3	11	8	28	–	59
milk chocolate w/ almonds	1 bar (1.45 oz)	215	4	14	8	22	–	30
nougat nut cream	0.5 oz	49	1	4	–	8	–	–
peanut bar	1 (1.4 oz)	209	6	14	–	19	–	91

FOOD	PORTION	CALS	PROT	FAT	CHOL	CARB	FIBER	SOD
peanut brittle	1 oz	128	2	5	4	20	–	128
peanuts chocolate covered	1 cup (5.2 oz)	773	19	50	13	74	–	61
peanuts chocolate covered	10 (1.4 oz)	208	5	13	4	20	–	16
praline	1 piece (1.4 oz)	177	1	10	0	24	–	24
pretzels chocolate covered	1 (0.4 oz)	50	1	2	–	8	–	10
pretzels chocolate covered	1 oz	130	2	5	–	20	–	–
sesame crunch	20 pieces (1.2 oz)	181	4	12	0	18	–	–
taffy	1 piece (0.5 oz)	56	0	1	1	14	–	13
toffee	1 piece (0.4 oz)	65	tr	4	13	8	–	22
truffles	1 piece (0.4 oz)	59	1	4	6	5	–	8
3 Musketeers								
Bar	1 (2.1 oz)	260	2	8	5	46	1	110
Fun Size	3 bars (1.6 oz)	190	1	6	5	34	1	85
Minis	7 (1.4 oz)	170	1	5	5	32	1	80
Mint	1 bar (1.2 oz)	150	1	5	0	26	1	65
5th Avenue								
Bar	1 (2 oz)	260	4	12	–	37	2	120
Almond Joy								
Bar	1 (1.6 oz)	220	2	13	–	26	2	50
Andes								
Dark Chocolate Covered Cherries	2 (1 oz)	110	1	5	0	19	tr	10
Thins Cherry Jubilee	8 pieces (1.3 oz)	200	2	13	0	22	1	20
Thins Creme De Menthe	8 pieces (1.3 oz)	200	2	13	0	22	tr	20
Annabelle's								
Skinny Hunk Chewy Nougat	1 bar (1 oz)	100	0	1	0	24	0	75
Annie's Homegrown								
Organic Bunny Fruit Summer Strawberry	1 pkg (0.8 oz)	70	0	0	0	18	–	45

FOOD	PORTION	CALS	PROT	FAT	CHOL	CARB	FIBER	SOD
Baby Ruth								
Fun Size	2 bars (1.3 oz)	170	2	8	0	24	tr	85
Snack Bars	2 (1.3 oz)	170	2	8	0	24	tr	85
Bartons								
Cashew Toppers	1 (1 oz)	140	3	9	5	14	1	20
Baskin-Robbins								
Soft Candy Mint Chocolate Chip	2 (0.3 oz)	40	tr	1	0	7	0	15
Sugar Free Hard Candy Cookies 'N Cream	4 (0.6 oz)	40	0	1	0	15	–	10
Benecol								
Smart Chews Caramel	1 piece	20	0	0	0	4	–	15
Benedetto								
Cubetti Mini Caramel Crunch Protein 1st	5 pieces (1.7 oz)	178	19	5	–	17	1	–
Cupola Mini Mint Protein 1st	5 pieces (1.7 oz)	122	11	3	–	15	2	–
Betty Crocker								
Fruit Gushers Rockin' Blue Raspberry	1 pkg (0.9 oz)	90	0	1	0	20	–	45
Blow Pop								
Regular	1 (0.6 oz)	60	0	0	0	16	0	0
Brach's								
Mellowcreme Pumpkins	6 pieces (1.5 oz)	150	0	0	0	38	–	80
Breath Savers								
Peppermint	1 (1.8 g)	5	0	0	0	2	–	–
Bubble Chocolate								
Dark Chocolate	1 bar (1.41 oz)	200	2	15	0	22	3	0
Milk Chocolate	1 bar (1.41 oz)	220	3	15	10	21	tr	30
Cadbury								
Caramello	1 (1.6 oz)	220	3	10	10	29	tr	45
Dairy Milk	7 blocks (1.4 oz)	200	3	11	10	23	tr	40
Milk Chocolate Fruit & Nut	10 blocks (1.4 oz)	200	4	10	5	24	1	30

FOOD	PORTION	CALS	PROT	FAT	CHOL	CARB	FIBER	SOD
Milk Chocolate Roast Almond	7 blocks (1.4 oz)	210	4	13	10	21	1	35
Royal Dark	7 blocks (1.4 oz)	170	2	12	<5	23	3	–
Cella's								
Milk Chocolate Covered Cherries	2 (1 oz)	120	1	5	5	20	1	20
Charleston Chews								
Chocolate	1 bar (1.9 oz)	230	2	6	0	43	1	30
Vanilla	1 bar (1.9 oz)	230	2	8	0	44	0	30
Charms								
Fluffy Stuff Cotton Candy	1 pkg (0.6 oz)	70	0	0	0	17	0	0
Sour Balls	1 (5 g)	20	0	0	0	5	0	0
Squares	2 pieces	20	0	0	0	6	0	0
Chew-ets								
Peanut Chews Original Dark	3 pieces	170	3	9	0	22	2	55
Choward's								
Mints All Flavors	3 (5 g)	20	0	0	0	5	0	0
Chuao Chocolatier								
Choco Pod Banana	1 (0.4 oz)	50	tr	3	–	6	–	10
Choco Pod Passion	1 (0.4 oz)	50	0	4	–	5	–	0
Coombs Family Farms								
Maple Candy	6 pieces (1.5 oz)	160	0	0	0	42	0	5
Crispy Cat								
Roasted Peanut	1 bar (1 oz)	220	4	10	0	29	2	125
Dare								
RealFruit Gummies All Flavors	8 pieces (1.4 oz)	120	2	0	0	28	0	5
Dots								
All Flavors	12 (1.5 oz)	140	0	0	0	35	0	10
Dove								
Dark Chocolate Cranberry Almond	⅓ pkg (1.2 oz)	170	2	10	5	20	2	10
Milk Chocolate Roasted Almond	⅓ bar (1.2 oz)	180	3	12	5	18	1	20

FOOD	PORTION	CALS	PROT	FAT	CHOL	CARB	FIBER	SOD
E. Guittard								
Bar Quevedo Bittersweet 65% Cacao	1 (2 oz)	290	3	23	0	29	5	0
Bar Sur Del Lago Bittersweet 65% Cacao	1 (2 oz)	290	3	23	0	29	5	0
Emily's								
Espresso Beans Dark Chocolate Covered	26 (1.4 oz)	220	2	19	<5	24	3	20
Enjoy Life								
Boom Choco Boom Dark Chocolate Dairy Nut Soy Free	1 bar (1.4 oz)	200	2	15	0	22	3	0
Equal Exchange								
Organic Chocolate Espresso Bean	1 bar (1.4 oz)	216	2	15	0	22	3	2
Organic Milk Chocolate	1 bar (1.4 oz)	230	4	16	12	19	1	40
Organic Very Dark Chocolate	1 bar (1.4 oz)	220	3	17	0	18	5	5
Ferrero								
Rocher	3 pieces (1.3 oz)	220	3	16	0	16	1	15
Rondnoir	3 pieces (1.4 oz)	220	3	14	<5	21	2	25
Frooties								
Chewy Candy Fruit Flavored	12 pieces (1.3 oz)	104	0	3	0	29	0	20
Ghirardelli								
Luxe Milk Chocolate	4 sq (1.5 oz)	220	3	13	10	26	tr	30
Squares Milk Chocolate w/ Caramel Filling	3 (1.6 oz)	220	2	12	10	27	tr	60
Squares Mint Indulgence	3 (1.6 oz)	210	1	11	0	30	2	0
Squares 60% Cacao Dark Chocolate	4 (1.5 oz)	220	2	17	0	23	3	0
Squares 60% Cacao Dark Chocolate w/ Caramel	3 (1.6 oz)	220	2	15	5	25	3	35
Gimme								
Dark Chocolate Omega 3	1 pkg (1 oz)	130	2	7	0	19	2	10
Dark Chocolate Probiotics	1 pkg (1 oz)	130	1	7	0	20	2	5
Milk Chocolate Calcium	1 pkg (1 oz)	120	1	7	0	18	1	30

FOOD	PORTION	CALS	PROT	FAT	CHOL	CARB	FIBER	SOD
Godiva								
Assorted Milk Chocolate	4 pieces (1.4 oz)	190	2	12	5	22	1	40
Truffles Assorted	2 pieces (1.4 oz)	210	3	13	10	20	2	20
Good & Plenty								
Licorice	33 (1.4 oz)	140	tr	0	0	35	–	120
Guylian								
Twists Milk Chocolate Truffle	5 pieces (1.2 oz)	230	2	19	10	15	1	20
Twists Original Praline	4 pieces (1.2 oz)	200	3	13	10	19	1	20
Hammond's								
Root Beer Drops	3 (0.6 oz)	60	0	0	0	14	0	5
Heath								
Bar	1 (1.4 oz)	210	1	13	10	24	tr	135
Hershey's								
Bar Milk Chocolate w/ Almonds	1 (1.4 oz)	210	4	14	10	21	2	25
Bar Special Dark	1 (1.4 oz)	180	2	12	<5	25	3	15
Bliss Dark Chocolate Bar	1 (1.3 oz)	160	2	12	<5	21	3	10
Bliss Milk Chocolate	6 (1.5 oz)	210	3	14	5	24	1	40
Bliss Milk Chocolate Meltaway	6 (1.5 oz)	220	3	15	5	24	1	65
Bliss Milk Chocolate Raspberry Meltaway	6 (1.5 oz)	220	3	14	5	24	tr	55
Cacao Reserve 35% Cacao Milk Chocolate w/ Hazelnuts	3 sq (1.3 oz)	220	3	15	10	18	1	25
Cacao Reserve 65% Cacao Dark	3 blocks (1.3 oz)	180	4	15	<5	18	4	0
Kisses Cherry Cordial	9 (1.5 oz)	180	2	7	5	30	–	25
Kisses Hugs	9 (1.4 oz)	210	3	12	10	23	–	45
Kisses Milk Chocolate	9 (1.4 oz)	200	3	12	10	25	1	35
Kisses Special Dark	9 (1.4 oz)	180	2	12	<5	25	3	15
Milk Chocolate Bar	1 (1.5 oz)	210	3	13	10	26	1	35
Milk Chocolate w/ Almonds Bar	1 (1.5 oz)	210	3	13	5	25	2	50
Miniatures Special Dark	5 (1.4 oz)	190	3	13	<5	24	3	25
Nuggets Milk Chocolate	4 (1.4 oz)	200	3	12	10	25	1	35

FOOD	PORTION	CALS	PROT	FAT	CHOL	CARB	FIBER	SOD
Nuggets Milk Chocolate w/ Almonds	4 (1.3 oz)	200	4	13	10	20	2	25
Pieces All Flavors	51 (1.4 oz)	190	4	9	–	25	1	75
Ice Breakers								
Coolmint	1 (0.8 g)	0	0	0	0	tr	–	–
Jay's								
Cotton Candy	1 pkg (2 oz)	220	3	0	0	56	–	0
Jelly Belly								
Jelly Beans Cocktail Classics	1 pkg (0.75 oz)	80	0	0	0	20	–	10
Jer's								
Balls Peanut Butter Chocolate	1 piece (0.5 oz)	80	2	5	0	8	–	25
Original IncrediBar Peanut Butter	1 (1.8 oz)	210	6	12	0	21	2	65
Jolly Rancher								
Gummies	9 (1.4 oz)	120	2	0	0	28	–	35
Original Assortment	3 (0.5 oz)	50	0	0	0	13	–	20
Junior								
Caramels	1 box (1.4 oz)	170	1	3	0	35	tr	30
Mints	1 box (1.4 oz)	170	1	3	0	35	tr	30
KitKat								
Bar	1 (1.5 oz)	210	3	11	<5	28	tr	30
Kopali								
Organic Dark Chocolate Covered Espresso Beans	½ pkg (1 oz)	120	1	7	0	17	2	0
Lance								
Chewz Strawberry	1 pkg (1.1 oz)	120	0	1	–	28	–	0
Peanut Bar	1 (2.3 oz)	340	13	19	0	29	3	100
Let's Do Organic								
Black Licorice Bars	1 (0.9 oz)	80	1	0	0	20	tr	20
Black Licorice Chews	8 (1.4 oz)	130	2	0	0	30	tr	30
Gummi Bears	1 pkg (0.9 oz)	80	0	0	0	22	0	15
Lindt								
Lindor Truffles 60% Extra Dark	3 pieces (1.3 oz)	210	2	19	<5	15	tr	0

FOOD	PORTION	CALS	PROT	FAT	CHOL	CARB	FIBER	SOD
Lindor Truffles Swiss Dark Chocolate	3 (1.4 oz)	240	2	18	<5	17	2	10
Petits Desserts Assorted	4 (1.3 oz)	210	2	15	10	20	tr	15
Love Candy								
Dark Chocolate	1 bar (1.5 oz)	190	2	11	20	21	1	55
Milk Chocolate	1 bar (1.5 oz)	200	1	11	25	22	tr	65
Yogurt Supreme	1 bar (1.5 oz)	190	1	11	20	23	tr	60
Mama's Goodies								
Butter Nut Crunch Almond	1 piece (1.33 oz)	220	3	15	10	20	1	30
Butter Nut Crunch Sesame Seed	1 piece (1.33 oz)	220	2	14	10	20	1	30
Nut Butter Crunch Macadamia & Coconut	1 piece (1.33 oz)	220	1	17	10	20	1	30
Mamba								
Fruit Flavor	6 (0.9 oz)	170	0	3	0	36	0	0
Sour	6 (0.9 oz)	100	0	2	0	22	0	20
Mike & Ike								
All Flavors	1 pkg (2 oz)	200	0	0	0	50	–	–
Milk Duds								
Chocolate	13 (1.4 oz)	170	1	6	–	28	–	100
Milkfuls								
Candy	6 (1.4 oz)	170	tr	3	5	35	0	10
Milky Way								
Fun Size	2 bars (1.2 oz)	150	1	6	5	24	0	55
Mounds								
Bar	1 (1.7 oz)	230	2	13	–	29	3	55
Mr.Goodbar								
Bar	1 (1.7 oz)	250	5	17	<5	26	2	65
Necco								
Banana Splits	4 (1.4 oz)	150	0	2	0	36	0	55
Clark Junior Bar	1 (0.5 oz)	60	1	3	0	10	0	20
Conversation Hearts Tiny	40 (1.4 oz)	160	0	0	0	39	0	0
Double Dipped Peanuts	15 (1.4 oz)	200	3	11	0	25	1	25
Junior Assorted Wafers	1 roll (0.5 oz)	50	0	0	0	13	–	0
Mary Janes	5 (1.4 oz)	160	1	4	0	32	0	65

FOOD	PORTION	CALS	PROT	FAT	CHOL	CARB	FIBER	SOD
Mint Juleps	4 (1.4 oz)	150	0	2	0	36	0	55
Nonpareils	10 (1.4 oz)	190	1	9	0	29	0	0
Squirrel Nut Caramel	5 (1.6 oz)	170	1	3	0	37	0	70
Nestle								
Crunch Stix	1 (0.6 oz)	90	tr	5	0	12	0	30
NibMor								
Organic Vegan Dark Chocolate w/ Crispy Brown Rice	½ bar (1 oz)	110	1	7	0	13	2	45
Organic Vegan Dark Chocolate	½ bar (1.1 oz)	120	1	7	0	13	2	20
Organic Vegan Dark Chocolate w/ Almonds	½ bar (1.1 oz)	130	2	8	0	12	3	45
Organic Vegan Dark Chocolate w/ Cacao Nibs	½ bar (1.1 oz)	120	2	7	0	14	3	45
Panda								
Licorice Cherry	1 bar (1.1 oz)	100	1	0	0	24	0	65
PayDay								
Peanut Caramel	1 (1.8 oz)	240	7	13	–	27	2	120
Pot Of Gold								
Nut Assortment	4 (1.4 oz)	210	3	13	<5	23	2	40
Pecan Caramel Clusters	4 (1.4 oz)	200	2	12	<5	23	1	60
Truffle Assortment	3 (1.5 oz)	200	2	9	5	27	1	20
Pure Fun								
Organic Vegan Barrels Of Fun Root Beer Float	2 (0.5 oz)	60	0	0	0	13	0	10
Organic Vegan Candy Canes	1 (0.5 oz)	62	0	0	0	14	1	0
Organic Vegan Chocolate Meltdowns All Flavors	3 (0.6 oz)	70	0	0	0	16	0	10
Organic Vegan Citrus Slices All Flavors	3 (0.6 oz)	60	0	0	0	15	0	10
Organic Vegan Cotton Candy All Flavors	¼ pkg (0.5 oz)	60	0	0	0	15	0	0
Organic Vegan Jaw Boulders All Flavors	2 (0.5 oz)	58	0	0	0	13	0	8
Organic Vegan Pure Pops All Flavors	3 (0.6 oz)	60	0	0	0	15	0	10

FOOD	PORTION	CALS	PROT	FAT	CHOL	CARB	FIBER	SOD
Raisinets								
Candy	3 pkg (1.7 oz)	200	2	8	5	34	1	15
Reese's								
Crispy Crunchy Bar	1 (1.7 oz)	250	5	14	<5	29	2	85
FastBreak	1 (2 oz)	260	5	12	–	35	2	190
NutRageous	1 (1.8 oz)	260	6	16	–	28	2	100
Peanut Butter Cups Miniatures Dark Chocolate	5 (1.5 oz)	220	4	14	<5	24	2	120
Pieces Peanut Butter	1 pkg (1.5 oz)	210	5	10	–	26	1	85
ReeseSticks								
Wafer Bar Chocolate & Peanut Butter	1 (1.5 oz)	210	4	13	–	23	1	130
Ricochet								
Coffee Shots Sugar Free	5 (3 g)	10	0	0	0	2	–	0
Riesen								
Candy	4 (1.3 oz)	170	1	4	0	28	0	15
Ritter Sport								
Bar Cappuccino	1 (3.5 oz)	574	6	39	18	50	2	77
Bar Chocolate Marzipan	1 (3.5 oz)	484	6	27	tr	53	5	16
Bar Chocolate & Cornflakes	1 (3.5 oz)	525	6	29	9	59	2	184
Bar Chocolate Butter Biscuit	1 (3.5 oz)	556	7	35	15	53	2	148
Bar Dark Chocolate	1 (3.5 oz)	525	5	33	tr	51	7	20
Bar Milk Chocolate	1 (3.5 oz)	533	7	31	11	57	3	99
Bar Mousse Au Chocolat	1 (3.5 oz)	544	5	36	9	48	7	15
Bar White Chocolate Whole Hazelnuts	1 (3.5 oz)	562	7	38	20	48	2	114
Rolo								
Chewy Caramels In Milk Chocolate	3 pkg (1.7 oz)	220	2	10	5	33	–	80
Russell Stover								
Assorted Chocolates	4 pieces (2 oz)	280	2	13	5	39	1	90
Private Reserve Triple Chocolate Mousse	3 pieces (1.3 oz)	220	2	17	<5	19	2	15
Private Reserve Vanilla Bean Brulee	3 pieces (1.3 oz)	180	3	13	<5	19	3	25

FOOD	PORTION	CALS	PROT	FAT	CHOL	CARB	FIBER	SOD
See's								
Assorted Chocolates	2 (1.2 oz)	160	2	9	10	20	tr	40
Nuts & Chews	3 (1.6 oz)	240	4	16	10	25	2	50
Soft Centers	2 (1.4 oz)	170	1	9	10	25	tr	40
Sencha Naturals								
Green Tea Mints All Flavors	3	5	0	0	0	1	0	–
Shaman Chocolates								
Organic Extra Dark Chocolate 82% Cacao	½ bar (1 oz)	158	2	14	0	7	4	0
Organic Milk Chocolate w/ Macadamia Nuts & Hawaiian Pink Sea Salt	½ bar (1 oz)	91	1	1	0	13	2	773
Skittles								
Original Fruit	1 pkg (2.2 oz)	250	0	3	0	56	0	10
Sour	1 pkg (1.8 oz)	200	0	0	0	44	0	5
Skor								
Toffee & Milk Chocolate	1 (1.4 oz)	200	1	12	20	25	tr	130
Slim-Fast								
Protein Snack Chews Peanut Butter	1 pkg (0.9 oz)	100	6	4	0	12	0	90
Smile Chocolatiers								
Choclatea Ginger Tea Milk Chocolate 37% Cacao	½ bar (1.5 oz)	230	3	15	10	23	1	30
Choclatea Herbal Chai Tea Dark Chocolate 64% Cacao	½ bar (1.5 oz)	220	2	17	0	22	5	0
Choclatea Pistachio Green Tea White Chocolate	½ bar (1.5 oz)	240	5	16	10	22	1	0
Choclatea Pomegranate White Tea Very Dark Chocolate 72% Cacao	½ bar (1.5 oz)	220	3	16	0	16	2	5
Choclatea White Tea Very Dark Chocolate 72% Cacao	½ bar (1.5 oz)	220	2	17	0	22	5	0
Sour Patch								
Kids Soft & Chewy	1 pkg (1 oz)	100	0	0	0	25	–	20
Starbucks								
Truffles Caffe Mocha	3 (1.3 oz)	200	3	14	10	19	1	35

FOOD	PORTION	CALS	PROT	FAT	CHOL	CARB	FIBER	SOD
Sugar Babies								
Candy	30 pieces (1.5 oz)	180	0	2	0	41	0	40
Chocolate	19 pieces (1.4 oz)	180	1	5	5	33	0	35
Sugar Daddy								
Pop	1 lg (1.7 oz)	200	1	3	0	43	0	65
Surf Sweets								
Gummy Bears	16 (1.4 oz)	130	3	0	0	30	0	15
Gummy Worms	4 (1.4 oz)	130	3	0	0	30	0	15
Jelly Beans	31 (1.4 oz)	140	0	0	0	34	0	35
Sour Worms	8 (1.4 oz)	130	0	0	0	32	1	140
Symphony								
Almonds & Toffee	1 (1.5 oz)	220	4	14	10	23	tr	65
Take 5								
Original	1 pkg (1.5 oz)	200	4	11	–	25	1	180
Terra Nostra								
Organic Bar Creamy Milk Raisins & Pecans	4 sections (1.2 oz)	180	2	11	5	18	1	20
Organic Bar Vegan Intense Dark	4 sections (1.2 oz)	180	2	12	0	15	4	0
Organic Bar Vegan Ricemilk Choco	4 sections (1.2 oz)	190	tr	14	0	18	0	30
Organic Bar Vegan Robust Dark Raisins & Pecans	4 sections (1.2 oz)	170	2	11	0	16	3	0
Thorntons								
Chocolates Summer Collection	1	65	1	4	–	7	–	–
Toblerone								
Bittersweet w/ Honey & Almond Nougat	⅓ bar (1.2 oz)	170	1	9	5	20	2	5
Milk Chocolate w/ Honey & Almond Nougat	⅓ bar (1.2 oz)	170	2	9	10	21	1	15
White w/ Honey & Almond Nougat	⅓ bar (1.2 oz)	180	2	10	5	20	1	30
Toffifay								
Candy	5 (1.4 oz)	200	2	11	<5	25	1	50
Tootsie Roll								
Midgees	6	140	0	3	0	28	0	10

FOOD	PORTION	CALS	PROT	FAT	CHOL	CARB	FIBER	SOD
Mini Chews	30 pieces (1.4 oz)	170	2	7	5	27	1	20
Pops	1 (0.6 oz)	60	0	0	0	15	0	0
Pops Caramel Apple	1 (0.6 oz)	60	0	1	0	15	0	15
Truffulls								
Chocolate Caramel Gluten Free	1 (1.13 oz)	120	8	4	0	17	5	80
Chocolate Mint Gluten Free	1 (1.13 oz)	120	8	4	10	17	5	70
Twix								
Fun Size	1 (0.6 oz)	80	1	4	0	10	0	70
Twizzlers								
Licorice	4 (1.6 oz)	150	1	1	–	35	–	210
Strawberry	4 (1.6 oz)	160	1	1	–	36	–	95
Werther's								
Caramel Milk Chocolate	6 (1.3 oz)	230	2	16	10	18	0	50
Original	3 (0.5 oz)	60	0	1	<5	13	0	60
Original Sugar Free	5 (0.5 oz)	40	0	1	<5	14	0	55
Whitman's								
Assorted Chocolates	4 pieces (1.5 oz)	210	2	10	5	29	1	55
Whoppers								
Malted Milk Balls	18 (1.4 oz)	190	1	7	–	31	–	115
Wolfgang								
Blueberries Dipped In Dark Chocolate	2 (0.7 oz)	80	0	4	0	13	tr	10
Cranberries Dipped In Dark Chocolate	2 (1 oz)	130	1	6	0	18	1	10
Raspberries Dipped In Dark Chocolate	2 (1.1 oz)	130	1	6	0	21	1	5
Wonka Exceptionals								
Bar Chocolate Waterfall	4 sq (1.4 oz)	210	2	13	5	23	tr	30
Bar Domed Dark Chocolate	4 sq (1.4 oz)	200	2	13	5	24	3	0
Fruit Jellies All Flavors	14 (1.5 oz)	130	0	0	0	34	–	0
Fruit Marvels All Flavors	10 (1.4 oz)	140	0	0	0	34	–	0
York								
Peppermint Patty	1 (1.4 oz)	140	tr	3	–	31	tr	10
Young & Smylie								
Licorice Black	11 (1.5 oz)	140	tr	2	–	32	–	190
Licorice Strawberry	11 (1.5 oz)	150	1	2	–	33	–	30

FOOD	PORTION	CALS	PROT	FAT	CHOL	CARB	FIBER	SOD
Zagnut								
Peanut Butter & Coconut	3 (1.5 oz)	200	3	8	–	31	1	90
Zero								
Bar	1 (1.8 oz)	230	3	8	–	37	–	115
CANTALOUPE								
dried	3.5 pieces (1.4 oz)	140	0	0	0	34	1	110
fresh cubed	1 cup	57	1	tr	0	13	1	14
fresh half	½	94	2	1	0	22	2	23
Chiquita								
Fresh Cup Up	1 cup (6.2 oz)	60	1	0	0	16	2	28
CAPERS								
capers	1 tbsp	2	tr	tr	0	tr	tr	255
CARAWAY								
seed	1 tbsp	22	1	1	0	3	3	1
CARDAMOM								
ground	1 tsp	6	tr	tr	0	1	1	0
CARDOON								
fresh cooked w/o salt	1 serv (3.5 oz)	22	1	tr	0	5	2	176
fresh shredded	1 cup (6.2 oz)	30	1	tr	0	7	3	303
Ocean Mist								
Cardone Fresh Shredded	1 cup (6.2 oz)	36	1	tr	0	9	3	303
CARIBOU								
roasted	3 oz	142	25	4	93	0	0	51
CARISSA								
fresh	1	12	tr	tr	0	3	–	1
CAROB								
carob mix	3 tsp	45	tr	0	0	11	–	12
carob mix as prep w/ whole milk	9 oz	195	8	8	33	23	–	132
flour	1 cup	185	5	1	0	92	–	36
flour	1 tbsp	14	tr	tr	0	7	–	3

FOOD	PORTION	CALS	PROT	FAT	CHOL	CARB	FIBER	SOD
Bob's Red Mill								
Powder Toasted	2 tsp	25	1	0	0	11	2	5
Tree Of Life								
Chips Malt Sweetened	50 (0.5 oz)	70	1	4	0	9	1	5
CARP								
fresh cooked	3 oz	138	19	6	72	0	0	54
fresh cooked	1 fillet (6 oz)	276	39	12	143	0	0	107
fresh raw	3 oz	108	15	5	56	0	0	42
roe raw	1 oz	37	7	tr	103	tr	–	–
roe salted in olive oil	2 tbsp (1 oz)	40	–	–	100	6	0	1400
CARROT JUICE								
canned	6 oz	73	2	tr	0	17	–	54
Hollywood								
100% Juice	1 can (12 oz)	120	2	1	0	27	1	250
Lakewood								
Organic	6 oz	73	2	0	0	17	2	45
Odwalla								
100% Juice	8 oz	70	2	0	0	15	1	160
CARROTS								
CANNED								
slices	½ cup	17	tr	tr	0	4	1	176
slices low sodium	½ cup	17	tr	tr	0	4	1	31
Allens								
Tiny Sliced	½ cup	35	0	0	0	8	3	40
Del Monte								
Savory Sides Honey Glazed	½ cup	70	1	0	0	18	tr	440
S&W								
Julienne	½ cup (4.3 oz)	35	0	0	0	8	3	300
FRESH								
baby raw	1 (0.5 oz)	6	tr	tr	0	1	–	5
raw	1 (2.5 oz)	31	1	tr	0	7	2	25
raw shredded	½ cup	24	1	tr	0	6	2	19
slices cooked	½ cup	35	1	tr	0	8	–	52
Chiquita								
Carrot Bites w/ Ranch Dressing	1 pkg (2.5 oz)	50	1	3	5	7	2	150

FOOD	PORTION	CALS	PROT	FAT	CHOL	CARB	FIBER	SOD
Earthbound Farms								
Organic Tops On	1 (2.7 oz)	35	1	0	0	8	2	40
Organic w/ Organic Ranch Dip	1 pkg (2.2 oz)	90	1	8	5	5	1	180
Ready Pac								
Baby Carrots	7 (3 oz)	40	1	0	0	9	2	45
FROZEN								
slices cooked	½ cup	26	1	tr	0	6	–	43
Birds Eye								
Steam & Serve Carrots & Cranberries	1 cup	130	1	5	10	20	3	230
C&W								
Whole Baby	⅔ cup	35	tr	0	0	7	2	60
Green Giant								
Honey Glazed	1 cup	90	1	3	0	15	3	190
Joy Of Cooking								
Bite Size	½ cup (3.3 oz)	70	1	3	5	12	2	115

CASABA

cubed	1 cup (6 oz)	46	2	tr	0	11	2	15
melon fresh	¼ (14 oz)	115	5	tr	0	27	4	37

CASHEW JUICE

O.N.E.								
Cashew Fruit	1 bottle (11 oz)	140	tr	0	0	34	1	20

CASHEWS

cashew butter w/o salt	1 tbsp	94	3	8	0	4	–	2
dry roasted w/ salt	18 nuts (1 oz)	160	4	13	0	9	1	180
dry roasted w/ salt	1 oz	163	4	13	0	9	–	213
oil roasted w/ salt	1 oz	163	5	14	0	8	–	209
oil roasted w/o salt	1 oz	163	5	14	0	8	–	5
Arrowhead Mills								
Organic Cashew Butter	2 tbsp	160	4	13	0	9	tr	0
Back To Nature								
Jumbo Sea Salt Roasted	1 oz	160	5	13	0	9	1	100

FOOD	PORTION	CALS	PROT	FAT	CHOL	CARB	FIBER	SOD
Lance								
Cashews	1 pkg (1.5 oz)	270	8	22	0	11	3	230
Navitas Naturals								
Cashews	1 oz	160	5	12	0	9	1	0
Peeled Snacks								
Nut Picks Cashew Later	1 pkg (1 oz)	180	4	14	0	9	tr	120
Planters								
Chocolate Lovers Milk Chocolate	10 pieces (1.5 oz)	230	5	16	5	20	tr	25
Dry Roasted	19 pieces (1 oz)	160	5	12	0	9	tr	140
Organic	23 pieces (1 oz)	170	5	13	0	8	1	115
Sunfood								
Organic	1 oz	164	5	12	0	9	1	3
Tree Of Life								
Cashew Butter Creamy	2 tbsp	180	4	15	–	9	1	0
Yumnuts								
Chili Lime	¼ cup (1 oz)	170	6	13	0	7	3	110
Chocolate	¼ cup (1 oz)	160	4	11	0	12	2	10
Honey	¼ cup (1 oz)	170	5	12	0	10	1	0
Toasted Coconut	½ cup (1 oz)	170	5	13	0	9	2	0
CASSAVA								
diced cooked w/o fat	1 cup (4.6 oz)	213	2	tr	0	51	2	257
root raw	1 (14.3 oz)	653	6	1	0	155	7	57
TAKE-OUT								
fritter crab meat stuffed	1 (4.4 oz)	341	12	16	45	38	2	680
CATFISH								
channel breaded & fried	3 oz	194	15	11	69	7	–	238
wolffish atlantic baked	3 oz	105	19	3	50	0	0	93
Simmons								
Farm Raised	4 oz	140	17	6	50	0	0	40
CAULIFLOWER								
flowerets fresh	1 (0.5 oz)	3	tr	tr	0	1	tr	4
flowerets fresh cooked w/o salt	3 (2 oz)	12	1	tr	0	2	1	8

FOOD	PORTION	CALS	PROT	FAT	CHOL	CARB	FIBER	SOD
fresh	1 cup	25	2	tr	0	5	3	30
fresh cooked w/o salt	1 cup	29	2	1	0	5	3	19
fresh head small	1 (9.2 oz)	66	5	tr	0	14	7	80
frzn cooked w/o salt	1 cup	34	3	tr	0	7	5	32
green fresh	1 cup	20	2	tr	0	4	2	15
green fresh small head	1 (11.4 oz)	101	10	1	0	20	10	75
pickled	¼ cup	14	tr	tr	0	3	1	60
pickled chow chow	¼ cup	74	1	1	0	16	1	323
Birds Eye								
Steamfresh Garlic Cauliflower	1 cup (2.4 oz)	40	1	2	0	5	1	330
Jake & Amos								
Sweet Pickled Hot Cauliflower	1 tbsp	40	0	0	0	10	0	70
Mann's								
Cauliettes Fresh	1 serv (3 oz)	20	2	0	0	4	2	25
TAKE-OUT								
batter dipped fried	1 piece (0.9 oz)	55	1	4	4	4	1	48
batter dipped fried	1 cup	178	3	13	14	12	2	156
w/ cheese sauce	1 cup	249	12	18	36	12	3	440
CAVIAR								
black or red	2 tbsp	81	8	6	188	1	0	480
CELERY								
fresh	1 lg stalk (2.2 oz)	9	tr	tr	0	2	1	51
pickled	½ cup	10	tr	tr	0	2	1	192
raw diced	½ cup	8	tr	tr	0	2	1	48
seed	1 tsp	1	tr	tr	0	tr	tr	0
strips	1 cup	17	1	tr	0	4	2	99
Dole								
Stalks	2 med (3 oz)	20	1	0	0	5	2	100
Earthbound Farms								
Organic Hearts	2 stalks (3.9 oz)	20	1	0	0	5	2	100
Ready Pac								
Sticks	5 (3 oz)	10	1	0	0	3	1	70
TAKE-OUT								
creamed	½ cup	87	3	6	3	7	1	383

FOOD	PORTION	CALS	PROT	FAT	CHOL	CARB	FIBER	SOD
stir fried	½ cup	30	1	2	0	3	1	238
stuffed w/ cheese	1 (5 inch)	38	1	3	10	1	tr	84
CELERY JUICE								
juice	1 cup	42	2	tr	0	9	4	215
CELERY ROOT								
fresh cooked w/o salt	1 cup (5.4 oz)	42	1	tr	0	9	2	95
fresh cut up	1 cup (5.5 oz)	66	2	tr	0	14	3	156
CELTUCE								
raw	3.5 oz	22	1	tr	0	4	–	11
CEREAL								
bran flakes	¾ cup	90	4	1	0	22	–	264
corn flakes	1¼ cups	110	2	tr	0	24	–	351
farina as prep w/ water	¾ cup	88	2	tr	0	19	2	0
granola	½ cup	285	9	15	0	32	6	15
oatmeal instant as prep w/ water	1 cup (8.2 oz)	138	6	2	0	24	4	377
oatmeal regular & quick as prep w/ water	¾ cup (6.1 oz)	149	5	2	0	19	3	2
oatmeal regular & quick not prep	⅓ cup (0.9 oz)	104	4	2	0	18	3	1
puffed rice	1 cup	56	1	tr	0	13	tr	0
puffed wheat	1 cup	44	2	tr	0	10	1	0
shredded mini wheats	1 cup	107	3	1	0	24	3	3
shredded wheat rectangular	1 biscuit (0.8 oz)	85	3	tr	0	19	2	0
Alpen								
High Fibre	1 serv (1.6 oz)	154	4	3	–	28	tr	tr
No Sugar Added	1 serv (1.6 oz)	158	5	2	–	29	4	tr
Alti Plano Gold								
Instant Quinoa Hot Cereal Spiced Apple Raisin	1 pkg	160	3	2	0	35	5	110
Instant Quinoa Organic Hot Cereal Oaxacan Chocolate	1 pkg	170	6	3	0	30	5	120

FOOD	PORTION	CALS	PROT	FAT	CHOL	CARB	FIBER	SOD
Amy's								
Bowls Organic Cream Of Rice	1 pkg (8.9 oz)	170	2	1	0	39	2	220
Bowls Organic Multigrain	1 pkg (8.9 oz)	190	4	2	0	40	5	300
Arrowhead Mills								
Organic Amaranth Flakes	1 cup	140	4	2	0	26	3	0
Organic Kamut Flakes	1 cup	120	4	1	0	25	2	70
Organic Multigrain Flakes	1 cup	170	5	2	0	33	3	180
Organic Nature O's	1 cup	130	4	2	0	25	2	0
Organic Puffed Corn	1 cup	60	2	1	0	12	2	5
Organic Puffed Millet	1 cup	60	2	1	0	11	1	0
Organic Puffed Wheat	1 cup	60	3	0	0	12	2	0
Organic Rice Flakes Sweetened	1 cup	180	3	1	0	40	1	190
Organic Shredded Wheat	1 cup	190	7	1	0	38	6	5
Organic Spelt Flakes	1 cup	120	4	1	0	24	3	100
Back To Nature								
Granola Apple Blueberry	½ cup (1.8 oz)	200	6	3	0	39	4	10
Granola Chocolate Delight	½ cup (1.75 oz)	220	5	6	0	37	4	5
Granola Classic	½ cup (1.8 oz)	200	6	3	0	39	4	0
Granola Sunflower & Pumpkin Seed	½ cup (1.6 oz)	290	6	7	0	31	4	140
Granola To Go Ginger Roasted Almonds w/ Flax Seed	1 serv (1.5 oz)	190	5	7	0	29	4	20
Granola To Go Wild Blueberry Walnut w/ Flax Seed	1 serv (1.5 oz)	190	5	6	0	30	4	20
Bakery On Main								
Granola Apple Cinnamon Walnut	½ cup (2 oz)	240	6	12	0	29	4	20
Granola Fiber Power Cinnamon Raisin	½ cup (2 oz)	230	7	6	0	40	9	50
Granola Maple Raisin Almond	½ cup (2 oz)	240	6	12	0	30	4	20
Granola Super Fruit & Nut	½ cup (2 oz)	250	6	13	0	29	4	20

FOOD	PORTION	CALS	PROT	FAT	CHOL	CARB	FIBER	SOD
Barbara's Bakery								
Alpen No Sugar Added	⅔ cup	200	7	3	0	40	4	30
Organic Breakfast O's Fruit Juice Sweetened	1 cup	120	4	2	0	22	3	125
Organic Brown Rice Crisps Fruit Juice Sweetened	1 cup	120	2	1	0	25	1	125
Organic Corn Flakes Fruit Juice Sweetened	1 cup	110	2	1	0	25	1	140
Organic Ultima High Fiber	½ cup	90	3	1	0	24	8	130
Organic Ultima Pomegranate	½ cup	100	3	1	0	24	5	85
Organic Wild Puffs	1 cup	100	2	1	0	23	tr	40
Organic Wild Puffs Fruity Punch	1 cup	110	2	1	0	26	1	55
Puffins Cinnamon	⅔ cup	100	2	1	0	26	6	150
Puffins Originals	¾ cup (0.9 oz)	90	2	1	0	23	5	190
Shredded Oats Bite Size	1¼ cups (2 oz)	220	6	3	0	46	5	260
Shredded Wheat	2 biscuits (1.4 oz)	140	4	1	0	31	5	0
Basic 4								
Whole Grain	1 cup (1.9 oz)	200	4	2	0	43	3	320
Bear Naked								
Cranberry Raisin	⅔ cup (2 oz)	210	5	5	0	41	4	140
Fit Vanilla Almond Crunch	¼ cup (1.1 oz)	120	4	3	0	22	2	10
Granola Fruit And Nut	¼ cup (1.1 oz)	140	3	7	0	17	2	0
Granola Heavenly Chocolate	¼ cup (1.1 oz)	130	3	4	0	21	2	10
Peak Flax Oats And Honey w/ Blueberries	¼ cup (1.1 oz)	130	3	4	0	22	2	0
Better Balance								
Protein Cereal All Flavors Gluten Free	1 oz	100	9	2	0	15	3	140
Bob's Red Mill								
Farina Creamy Brown Rice not prep	¼ cup	150	3	1	0	32	2	5

FOOD	PORTION	CALS	PROT	FAT	CHOL	CARB	FIBER	SOD
Muesli Old Country	¼ cup	110	4	3	0	21	4	0
Natural Granola No Fat	½ cup	180	5	3	0	35	4	10
Organic Right Stuff Hot Cereal 6 Grain not prep	¼ cup	140	6	2	0	27	4	0
Rolled Oats Gluten Free not prep	½ cup	160	7	3	0	27	4	0
Boo Berry								
Cereal	3 cups (1.2 oz)	130	1	1	0	28	1	190
Bready Brek								
Original	1 serv (1 oz)	108	4	3	–	18	2	tr
Cascadian Farm								
Organic Clifford Crunch	1 cup	100	2	1	0	25	5	160
Organic Granola Oats & Honey	⅔ cup (1.9 oz)	230	5	6	0	42	3	110
Chappaqua Crunch								
Original Granola	⅓ cup	115	4	2	0	20	3	0
Simply Granola w/ Raisins	⅓ cup	120	4	2	0	22	3	15
Simply Granola w/ Raspberries	⅓ cup	110	4	2	0	21	3	0
Cheerios								
Apple Cinnamon	¾ cup (1 oz)	120	2	2	0	24	2	135
Banana Nut	¾ cup (1 oz)	120	1	1	0	26	0	180
Crunch Oat Clusters	¾ cup	100	2	1	0	22	2	140
Honey Nut	¾ cup (1 oz)	110	2	2	0	22	2	190
Whole Grain Oat	1 cup (1 oz)	100	3	2	0	20	3	160
Yogurt Burst Strawberry	¾ cup (1 oz)	120	2	2	0	24	2	180
Chex								
Chocolate	¾ cup (1.1 oz)	130	1	3	0	26	tr	240
Corn Gluten Free	1 cup (1.2 oz)	120	2	1	0	26	1	290
Multi-Bran	¾ cup (1.6 oz)	160	3	2	0	39	6	310
Rice Gluten Free	1 cup (0.9 oz)	100	2	0	0	23	tr	240
Wheat	¾ cup (1.6 oz)	160	5	2	0	38	5	340
Chia Goodness								
Apple Almond Cinnamon	2 tbsp (1 oz)	130	4	6	0	16	4	125

FOOD	PORTION	CALS	PROT	FAT	CHOL	CARB	FIBER	SOD
Cranberry Ginger	2 tbsp (1 oz)	130	4	7	0	16	4	120
Original	2 tbsp (1 oz)	140	6	8	0	14	5	125
Cinnamon Toast Crunch								
Cinnamon Sugar	¾ cup (1.1 oz)	130	1	3	0	25	1	220
Cocoa Puffs								
Cereal	¾ cup (1 oz)	100	1	2	0	23	2	150
Cookie Crisp								
Cereal	¾ cup (0.9 oz)	100	1	1	0	22	1	150
Count Chocula								
Cereal	¾ cup (0.9 oz)	110	1	1	0	23	1	160
Country Choice Organic								
Multigrain Hot Cereal not prep	½ cup	130	5	1	0	29	5	0
Oats Old Fashioned not prep	½ cup	150	5	3	0	27	4	0
Oats Quick not prep	½ cup	150	5	3	0	27	4	0
Dorset Cereals								
Berries & Cherries	½ cup	150	4	1	<5	40	3	5
Simply Delicious Muesli	½ cup	200	6	5	<5	37	4	15
Super Cranberry Cherry & Almond	½ cup	200	5	5	<5	39	4	90
Earthbound Farms								
Organic Granola Maple Almond	½ cup	260	6	14	0	31	4	0
Enjoy Life								
Allergen Gluten Free Granola Cinnamon	½ cup	160	3	3	0	31	5	10
Erewhon								
Aztec Crunchy Corn & Amaranth	1 cup (1 oz)	110	2	0	0	26	1	70
Barley Plus not prep	¼ cup (1.6 oz)	170	5	1	0	37	4	0
Brown Rice Cream not prep	¼ cup (1.6 oz)	170	5	1	0	36	1	30
Cocoa Crispy Brown Rice	1 cup (1.8 oz)	200	3	2	0	44	1	190

FOOD	PORTION	CALS	PROT	FAT	CHOL	CARB	FIBER	SOD
Crispy Brown Rice No Salt Added	1 cup (1 oz)	110	2	0	0	25	1	10
Crispy Brown Rice Original	1 cup (1 oz)	110	2	0	0	25	1	180
Organic Instant Oatmeal Apple Cinnamon not prep	1 pkg (1.2 oz)	130	5	2	0	24	3	100
Organic Instant Oatmeal w/ Oat Bran	1 pkg (1.8 oz)	130	6	3	0	25	4	0
Rice Twice	¾ cup (1 oz)	120	2	0	0	26	0	60
Erin Baker's								
Granola Fruit & Nut	½ cup (1.6 oz)	190	5	8	0	25	4	0
Granola Oatmeal Raisin	½ cup (1.6 oz)	180	4	6	0	30	4	0
Granola Ultra Protein Power Crunch	½ cup (1.6 oz)	200	8	6	0	25	4	75
Farina								
Original as prep	1 cup	120	3	0	0	22	tr	0
Feed								
Granola Apple A Day	¼ cup (1 oz)	130	3	3	0	23	3	40
Granola Bittersweet'ness	¼ cup (1 oz)	130	3	4	0	22	3	40
Granola Raisin Nut	¼ cup (1 oz)	130	3	4	0	20	2	35
Sweet Mango	¼ cup (1 oz)	120	3	3	0	23	3	15
Fiber One								
Caramel Delight	1 cup (1.8 oz)	180	3	3	0	41	9	230
Frosted Shredded Wheat	1 cup (2.1 oz)	200	5	1	0	50	9	0
Honey Clusters	1 cup (1.8 oz)	160	3	2	0	44	13	230
Original	½ cup (1 oz)	60	2	1	0	25	14	105
Raisin Bran Clusters	1 cup (2 oz)	170	4	1	0	45	11	260
Glucerna								
Crunchy Flakes 'N Raisins	1 bowl (1.6 oz)	140	4	1	0	36	6	270
Crunchy Flakes 'N Strawberries	1 bowl (1.5 oz)	150	4	1	0	37	7	320
Glutenfreeda								
Granola Apple Almond Honey	¼ cup (1 oz)	150	3	11	0	10	2	45

FOOD	PORTION	CALS	PROT	FAT	CHOL	CARB	FIBER	SOD
Oatmeal Instant as prep	1 pkg (1.8 oz)	190	8	3	0	34	5	0
Glutino								
Gluten Free Apple Cinnamon	½ cup	120	1	2	0	24	1	180
Gluten Free Honey Nut	½ cup	130	2	3	0	24	1	150
Golden Grahams								
Cereal	¾ cup (1.1 oz)	120	2	1	0	26	1	270
Health Valley								
Empower	1 cup	200	6	3	0	42	6	170
Granola Low Fat Tropical Fruit	⅔ cup	180	5	1	0	43	6	90
Heart Wise	1 cup	200	11	3	0	37	5	140
Organic Cherry Lemon Blast Ems	¾ cup	120	2	1	0	25	2	90
Organic Golden Flax	¾ cup	190	6	3	0	38	6	80
Organic Multigrain Apple Cinnamon Square Ems	1¼ cups	210	5	3	0	44	8	125
Organic Oat Bran O's	¾ cup	100	3	0	0	23	3	90
Rice Crunch-Ems	1 cup	110	4	0	0	26	2	150
Honest Foods								
Granola Planks Maple Almond Crunch	½ bar (2 oz)	250	6	10	0	37	5	150
Kashi								
7 Whole Grain Flakes	1 cup	180	6	1	0	41	6	150
7 Whole Grain Honey Puffs	1 cup	120	3	1	0	25	2	6
7 Whole Grain Nuggets	½ cup	210	7	2	0	47	7	260
7 Whole Grain Pilaf as prep	½ cup	170	6	3	0	30	6	15
GoLean	1 cup	140	13	1	0	30	10	85
GoLean Crunch!	1 cup	190	9	3	0	36	8	95
GoLean Crunch Honey Almond Flax	1 cup	200	9	5	0	34	8	140
GoLean Instant Hot Cereal Creamy Truly Vanilla	1 pkg	150	9	2	0	25	7	100
GoLean Instant Hot Cereal Hearty Honey & Cinnamon	1 pkg	150	8	2	0	26	5	100
Good Friends	1 cup	170	5	2	0	43	12	130
Granola Mountain Medley	½ cup	220	6	7	0	37	6	10

FOOD	PORTION	CALS	PROT	FAT	CHOL	CARB	FIBER	SOD
Heart To Heart Instant Oatmeal Golden Brown Maple	1 pkg	160	4	2	0	33	5	100
Heart To Heart Instant Oatmeal Raisin Spice	1 pkg	150	3	2	0	33	4	100
Heart To Heart Oat Flakes & Blueberry Clusters	1¼ cups	200	6	3	0	42	4	130
Heart To Heart Toasted Oat	¾ cup	110	4	2	0	25	5	90
Honey Sunshine	¾ cup (1.1 oz)	100	2	2	0	25	6	135
Mighty Bites All Flavors	1 cup	110	5	2	0	23	3	160
Organic Promise Autumn Wheat	1 cup	190	5	1	0	45	6	0
Organic Promise Cinnamon Harvest	1 cup	190	4	1	0	44	5	0
Organic Promise Strawberry Fields	1 cup	120	2	0	0	28	1	200
Vive Probiotic Digestive Wellness	1¼ cups	170	4	3	0	43	12	60
Kellogg's								
Corn Pops	1 box (1 oz)	110	1	0	0	24	3	105
Raisin Bran	1 cup (2.1 oz)	190	5	1	0	46	7	250
Special K	1 box (0.8 oz)	90	5	0	0	17	tr	170
Kix								
Corn Puffs	1¼ cups (1 oz)	110	2	1	0	25	3	190
Honey	1¼ cups (1.1 oz)	120	2	1	0	28	3	190
Kozy Shack								
Ready Grains Apple Cinnamon	1 pkg (7 oz)	210	7	2	15	39	7	200
Ready Grains Maple Brown Sugar	1 pkg (7 oz)	190	7	2	15	33	7	180
Ready Grains Original	1 pkg (7 oz)	180	8	2	20	30	7	200
Ready Grains Strawberry	1 pkg (7 oz)	210	7	2	15	38	7	190
Lucky Charms								
Swirled	¾ cup (1 oz)	110	2	1	0	22	1	190

FOOD	PORTION	CALS	PROT	FAT	CHOL	CARB	FIBER	SOD
Lundberg								
Purely Organic Hot'n Creamy Rice	⅓ cup	190	4	2	0	43	3	0
Malt-O-Meal								
Balance	¾ cup	120	3	1	0	26	3	220
Cinnamon Toasters	¾ cup	130	1	4	0	24	1	104
Colossal Crunch	¾ cup	120	1	2	0	26	0	230
Creamy Hot Wheat not prep	3 tbsp	130	4	0	0	27	1	0
Crispy Rice	1¼ cups	130	2	0	0	29	0	300
Frosted Flakes	¾ cup	120	2	0	0	28	1	180
Frosted Mini Spooners	1 cup	190	5	1	0	45	6	10
Honey & Oat Blenders	¾ cup	120	2	2	0	25	1	150
Honey Buzzers	1⅓ cups	110	1	1	0	26	1	220
Instant Oatmeal Apple & Cinnamon	1 pkg	130	3	2	0	27	3	170
Instant Oatmeal Cinnamon & Spice	1 pkg	170	4	2	0	36	3	240
Instant Oatmeal Maple & Brown Sugar	1 pkg	160	4	2	0	33	3	240
Original Hot Wheat not prep	3 tbsp	130	5	1	0	27	1	0
Puffed Rice	1 cup	60	1	0	0	13	0	0
Raisin Bran	1 cup	220	5	1	0	47	7	350
McCann's								
Irish Oatmeal Instant Apples & Cinnamon not prep	1 pkg (1.2 oz)	130	3	2	0	27	3	170
Irish Oatmeal Instant Maple & Brown Sugar not prep	1 pkg (1.5 oz)	160	4	2	0	32	3	240
Irish Oatmeal Instant Regular not prep	1 pkg (1 oz)	100	4	2	0	18	3	80
Irish Oatmeal Quick Cooking not prep	½ cup (1.4 oz)	150	4	2	0	26	4	0
Irish Oatmeal Steel Cut not prep	¼ cup (1.4 oz)	150	4	2	0	26	4	0
Mom's Best Naturals								
Oatmeal Instant	1 pkg	160	4	2	0	33	3	240
Raisin Bran	1 cup	230	5	2	0	49	6	340

FOOD	PORTION	CALS	PROT	FAT	CHOL	CARB	FIBER	SOD
Toasted Wheat-fuls	1 cup	200	8	1	0	44	7	10
Toasty O's	1 cup	120	4	2	0	23	3	200
Naked Granola								
Taste Of Seattle Nights	½ pkg (1.2 oz)	110	4	6	0	12	5	–
Natural Ovens								
Great Granola	½ cup	250	6	9	0	38	3	10
Nature's Path								
Organic Flax Plus Granola Pumpkin	¾ cup (1.9 oz)	260	6	10	0	37	5	45
Organic Granola Pomegran Plus	½ cup	140	2	5	0	21	2	35
Organic Smart Bran	⅔ cup	90	3	1	0	24	13	130
Nature's Plus								
Organic Oatmeal Hemp Plus	1 pkg	160	5	3	0	30	4	105
New Morning								
Cocoa Crispy Rice	¾ cup (1 oz)	120	2	1	0	26	1	100
Oatios Original	1 cup (1 oz)	110	5	2	0	22	3	125
Newman's Own								
Sweet Enough Honey Flax Flakes	¾ cup	100	3	1	0	24	4	80
Sweet Enough Honey Nut O's	¾ cup	110	3	2	0	22	2	170
Sweet Enough Wheat Puffs	¾ cup	100	3	1	0	22	1	45
Oatmeal Crisp								
Crunchy Almond	1 cup (2.1 oz)	240	6	5	0	47	4	130
Post								
100% Bran	½ cup (0.8 oz)	80	4	1	0	22	9	0
Bran Flakes	1 cup	100	3	1	0	24	5	220
Cocoa Pebbles	¾ cup (1 oz)	110	1	2	0	26	3	180
Golden Crisp	¾ cup (1 oz)	110	1	0	0	25	1	25
Grape-Nuts	½ cup (2 oz)	200	6	1	0	48	7	290
Grape-Nuts O's	1 cup (1 oz)	120	2	0	0	28	2	140
Grape-Nuts Trail Mix Crunch	1 cup (1.7 oz)	170	4	2	0	37	5	210
Great Grains Raisins Dates & Pecans	¾ cup (2 oz)	210	4	5	0	40	4	130

FOOD	PORTION	CALS	PROT	FAT	CHOL	CARB	FIBER	SOD
Honey Bunches Of Oats	¾ cup	130	2	2	0	25	2	150
Honey Bunches Of Oats Peaches	1 cup	120	2	2	0	26	2	135
Honeycomb	1⅓ cups (1 oz)	120	2	1	0	28	3	170
LiveActive Mixed Berry Crunch	1 cup	190	4	2	0	43	7	250
LiveActive Nut Harvest Crunch	1 cup	220	5	6	0	39	8	270
Oreo O's	1 cup	110	1	2	0	22	1	90
Raisin Bran	1 cup (2 oz)	190	4	1	0	46	8	300
Selects Blueberry Morning	2 oz	220	3	3	0	45	2	280
Selects Cranberry Almond Crunch	¾ cup (1.8 oz)	200	4	3	0	40	3	115
Shredded Wheat Frosted	2 oz	180	4	1	0	43	5	0
Shredded Wheat 'N Bran	2 oz	200	6	1	0	49	8	0
Shredded Wheat Original	2 biscuits (1.6 oz)	160	5	1	0	37	6	0
Shredded Wheat Spoon Size	1 cup (1.7 oz)	170	6	1	0	40	6	0
Toasties Corn Flakes	1 cup (1 oz)	100	2	0	0	24	1	260
Quaker								
Instant Oatmeal Apples & Cinnamon	1 pkg (1.2 oz)	130	3	2	0	27	3	160
Instant Oatmeal Cinnamon & Spice	1 pkg	170	4	2	0	35	3	250
Instant Oatmeal Cinnamon Roll	1 pkg	160	4	2	0	33	3	240
Instant Oatmeal Crunch Mixed Berry	1 pkg	190	4	3	0	39	3	250
Instant Oatmeal Express Baked Apple	1 pkg	200	4	3	0	42	4	320
Instant Oatmeal For Kids Dinosaur Eggs	1 pkg	190	4	4	0	37	3	260
Instant Oatmeal Lower Sugar Maple & Brown Sugar	1 pkg	120	4	2	0	24	3	290
Instant Oatmeal Maple Brown Sugar w/ Pecans	1 pkg	160	4	4	0	30	4	75

FOOD	PORTION	CALS	PROT	FAT	CHOL	CARB	FIBER	SOD
Instant Oatmeal Nutrition For Women Golden Brown Sugar	1 pkg	170	5	2	0	32	3	330
Instant Oatmeal Organic Regular	1 pkg	100	4	2	0	19	3	0
Instant Oatmeal Regular	1 pkg	100	4	2	0	19	3	80
Instant Oatmeal Simple Harvest Multigrain Maple Brown Sugar w/ Pecans	1 pkg (1.48 oz)	160	4	4	0	30	4	75
Instant Oatmeal Strawberries & Cream	1 pkg	130	3	3	0	27	2	190
Instant Oatmeal Supreme Apple Raisin	1 pkg	150	4	2	0	32	3	290
Instant Oatmeal Supreme Cinnamon Pecan	1 pkg	180	4	4	0	33	3	290
Instant Oatmeal Take Heart Golden Maple	1 pkg	160	4	3	0	33	5	110
Instant Oatmeal Weight Control Banana Bread	1 pkg	160	7	3	0	29	6	260
Oat Bran Hot Cereal not prep	½ cup	150	7	3	0	25	6	0
Oatmeal Squares	1 cup (2 oz)	210	6	3	0	44	5	190
Ralston								
Corn Flakes	1 cup (1 oz)	100	2	0	0	24	tr	200
Raisin Bran	1 cup (2 oz)	190	4	1	0	46	7	350
Ready Brek								
Chocolate	1 serv (1 oz)	108	3	2	–	19	2	tr
Rice Krispies								
Roasted Rice	1¼ cups (1.2 oz)	130	2	0	0	29	tr	220
Roman Meal								
Cream Of Rye not prep	⅓ cup (1.4 oz)	130	6	0	0	27	6	0
Elements Cranberry Passion	1 cup (1.6 oz)	160	5	3	0	33	5	120
Hot Cereal not prep	⅓ cup (1.3 oz)	120	6	2	0	26	6	0
Silhouette Solution								
Oatmeal Cinnamon Apple	1 pkg. (1.39 oz)	150	15	2	15	17	4	310

FOOD	PORTION	CALS	PROT	FAT	CHOL	CARB	FIBER	SOD
Skinner's								
Raisin Bran	1 cup (1.9 oz)	170	6	1	0	41	7	85
South Beach								
Crunch Strawberry Harvest	1 cup	170	7	2	0	37	8	290
Crunch Vanilla Almond	1 cup	180	8	4	0	35	8	280
Granola Clusters Cherry Almond	1 pkg (1 oz)	130	6	4	0	18	6	55
Granola Clusters Mixed Berry	1 pkg (1 oz)	130	6	4	0	18	6	55
Stark Sisters								
Granola Lo-Fat Raspberry Blueberry	½ cup	230	4	7	0	38	4	0
Granola Nutty Maple	½ cup	250	6	11	0	32	4	5
Granola Original Maple Almond	½ cup	240	6	10	0	33	5	0
Sunbelt								
Granola Low Fat Cinnamon & Raisins	½ cup	250	4	3	0	52	3	90
Total								
Cinnamon Crunch	1 cup (1.8 oz)	190	4	3	0	40	4	200
Raisin Bran	1 cup (1.9 oz)	160	3	1	0	40	5	230
Whole Grain	¾ cup (1 oz)	100	2	1	0	23	3	190
Trix								
Swirls	1 cup (1.1 oz)	120	1	2	0	28	1	190
Udi's								
Gluten Free Granola Au Naturel	¼ cup (1.1 oz)	120	3	4	0	19	3	0
Uncle Sam								
Mixed Berries	1 cup (1.9 oz)	190	7	4	0	39	10	130
Original	¾ cup (1.9 oz)	190	7	5	0	38	10	135

FOOD	PORTION	CALS	PROT	FAT	CHOL	CARB	FIBER	SOD
Weetabix								
Crunchy Bran	1 serv (1.4 oz)	122	5	1	–	23	8	tr
Multigrain	1 serv (1.3 oz)	127	4	1	–	26	4	tr
Oatibix Bites	1 serv (1.4 oz)	148	4	3	–	27	4	tr
Oatibix Flakes	1 serv (1 oz)	114	3	2	–	22	2	tr
Organic	2 biscuits (1.2 oz)	120	4	1	0	28	4	130
Organic Crispy Flakes	¾ cup	110	3	1	0	24	4	180
Wheatena								
Toasted Wheat	⅓ cup	160	5	1	0	33	5	0
Wheaties								
Cereal	¾ cup (1 oz)	100	3	1	0	22	3	190
YogActive								
Probiotic High Fibre Wheat Strawberry Raspberry	⅔ cup	160	5	3	0	29	6	115
Probiotic Kiwi	⅔ cup	120	3	2	25	23	1	150
Probiotic Strawberry	⅔ cup	130	3	2	30	25	1	170
Probiotic Strawberry Dark Chocolate	⅔ cup	130	3	3	0	26	2	170
Yogi								
Granola Crisps Baked Cinnamon Raisin	½ cup	120	3	3	0	21	2	50
Granola Crisps Fresh Strawberry Crunch	½ cup	120	3	3	0	21	2	50
Granola Crisps Mountain Blueberry Flax	½ cup	110	3	3	0	21	2	50

CEREAL BARS (*see also* ENERGY BARS)

FOOD	PORTION	CALS	PROT	FAT	CHOL	CARB	FIBER	SOD
Alpen								
Fruit & Nut	1	109	2	2	–	20	1	tr
Light Chocolate & Fudge	1	63	1	1	–	11	5	tr
Raspberry & Yogurt	1	120	2	3	–	22	1	tr
Aristo								
Acai Blueberry Lime	1 (1.3 oz)	130	3	4	5	22	3	40
Pomegranate & Cranberry	1 (1.3 oz)	140	3	5	5	21	3	40

FOOD	PORTION	CALS	PROT	FAT	CHOL	CARB	FIBER	SOD
Attune								
Wellness Yogurt & Granola Lemon Creme	1 (1.4 oz)	180	5	7	0	24	2	60
Wellness Yogurt & Granola Strawberry Bliss	1 (1.4 oz)	180	5	7	0	24	5	60
Bakery On Main								
Granola Gluten Free Extreme Trail Mix	1 (1.3 oz)	140	3	5	0	23	1	120
Granola Gluten Free Peanut Butter Chocolate Chip	1 (1.2 oz)	140	2	5	0	24	1	85
Barbara's Bakery								
Fruit & Yogurt Cherry Apple	1	150	3	3	0	29	1	125
Nature's Choice Blueberry	1 (1.3 oz)	150	2	2	0	29	2	85
Organic Crunchy Granola Cinnamon Crisp	2 (1.5 oz)	190	4	8	0	27	3	10
Bear Naked								
Grainola Tropical Fruit	1 (2 oz)	220	3	7	0	38	4	60
Cascadian Farm								
Organic Chewy Granola Fruit & Nut	1 (1.2 oz)	140	2	4	0	24	1	110
Cheerios								
Chocolate	¾ cup (1 oz)	100	1	1	0	23	1	170
Honey Nut	1 (1.4 oz)	160	3	4	0	28	1	120
Cinnamon Toast Crunch								
Milk 'N Cereal	1 (1.6 oz)	180	3	4	0	33	1	150
Corazonas								
Oatmeal Squares Banana Walnut	1 (1.8 oz)	190	6	6	0	27	5	105
Oatmeal Squares Chocolate Chip	1 (1.8 oz)	190	6	6	0	28	5	110
Oatmeal Squares Cranberry Flax	1 (1.8 oz)	180	6	5	0	28	6	110
Country Choice Organic								
Oatmeal Squares Apple Cinnamon	1 (2 oz)	210	4	3	0	41	1	190
Oatmeal Squares Maple	1 (2 oz)	210	4	3	0	41	4	180
Enjoy Life								
Allergen Gluten Free Caramel Apple	1 (1 oz)	110	2	3	0	21	2	95

FOOD	PORTION	CALS	PROT	FAT	CHOL	CARB	FIBER	SOD
Fullbar								
Cocoa Chip	1 (1.59 oz)	160	4	3	0	31	4	95
Fit Chewy Brownie	1 (1.76 oz)	180	15	4	0	24	5	170
Fit Toffee Crunch	1 (1.76 oz)	180	15	5	0	24	5	250
Peanut Butter Crunch	1 (1.59 oz)	170	6	5	0	27	4	95
Glenny's								
Organic Muesli Chocolate Chip	1 (1.6 oz)	170	3	3	0	34	3	50
Organic Muesli Raisins & Dates	1 (1.6 oz)	170	3	3	0	34	3	50
Slim Carb Bars Brownie Cheesecake	1 (1.3 oz)	130	12	3	–	19	1	180
Slim-1 w/ Acai Very Berry Blast	1 (1.1 oz)	100	2	3	–	21	2	40
Slim-1 w/ GreenTea Double Fudge	1 (1.1 oz)	100	3	3	–	20	2	90
Glutino								
Gluten Free Breakfast Bar Apple	1 (1.4 oz)	120	2	1	0	25	3	10
Gluten Free Breakfast Bar Chocolate	1 (¼ oz)	110	2	1	0	25	4	10
Gluten Free Organic Chocolate & Peanut	1 (1 oz)	110	2	3	0	19	1	50
Gluten Free Organic Wildberry	1 (1 oz)	100	1	1	0	21	1	65
Health Valley								
Cafe Creations Cinnamon Danish	1 (1.4 oz)	130	2	3	0	27	2	80
Date Almond Low Fat	1 (1.5 oz)	150	1	3	0	32	tr	25
Granola Chocolate Chip Low Fat	1 (1.5 oz)	160	2	3	0	32	1	20
Granola Moist & Chewy Dutch Apple	1 (1 oz)	100	1	2	0	20	tr	10
Granola Trail Mix Cranberries Nuts & Yogurt Chips	1 (1.2 oz)	140	3	4	0	23	1	100
Organic Fig Cobbler	1 (1.4 oz)	130	2	3	0	26	2	80
Organic Raspberry Tarts	1 (1.4 oz)	150	2	3	0	30	tr	95
Organic Strawberry Cobbler	1 (1.3 oz)	130	2	3	0	26	1	85

FOOD	PORTION	CALS	PROT	FAT	CHOL	CARB	FIBER	SOD
Peanut Butter & Grape	1 (1.3 oz)	130	2	3	0	26	1	140
Hershey's								
Sweet & Salty Granola Bar Reese's w/ Chocolate	1 (1.2 oz)	160	4	9	–	18	1	170
Sweet & Salty Granola Bar w/ Pretzels	1 (1.2 oz)	140	3	5	–	22	1	240
Honest Foods								
Cran Lemon Zest	1 (2.2 oz)	240	6	9	0	35	4	150
Farmer's Trail Mix	1 (2.2 oz)	240	6	9	0	35	4	150
Jungle Grub								
Berry Bamboozle w/ Vanilla Icing Gluten Free	1 (0.9 oz)	100	4	4	0	14	1	55
Chocolate Chip Cookie Dough w/ Chocolate Coating Gluten Free	1 (0.9 oz)	100	4	4	0	13	4	60
Peanut Butter Groove w/ Vanilla Icing Gluten Free	1 (0.9 oz)	100	4	4	0	13	1	140
Kardea								
Lemon Ginger	1 (1.34 oz)	140	7	5	0	20	7	75
Kashi								
TLC Chewy Granola Dark Mocha Almond	1 (1.2 oz)	130	6	4	0	21	4	90
TLC Chewy Granola Honey Almond Flax	1 (1.2 oz)	140	5	5	0	19	4	115
TLC Soft Baked Apple Spice	1 (1.2 oz)	110	2	3	0	21	3	105
TLC Soft Baked Blackberry Graham	1 (1.2 oz)	110	2	1	0	21	3	125
TLC Soft Baked Ripe Strawberry	1 (1.2 oz)	110	2	3	0	21	3	105
Kellogg's								
FiberPlus Antioxidants Berry Yogurt Crunch	1 box (1.4 oz)	130	3	1	0	32	8	150
FiberPlus Antioxidants Chocolate Chip	1 (1.2 oz)	120	2	4	0	26	9	55
FiberPlus Antioxidants Chocolatey Peanut Butter	1 (1.2 oz)	130	3	5	0	24	9	95
FiberPlus Antioxidants Dark Chocolate Almond	1 (1.2 oz)	130	2	5	0	24	9	50

FOOD	PORTION	CALS	PROT	FAT	CHOL	CARB	FIBER	SOD
KeriBar								
Vegan Apple Peanut Butter	1 (1.4 oz)	140	6	6	0	21	5	115
Vegan Cherry Almond	1 (1.4 oz)	140	8	6	0	21	5	75
Vegan Strawberry Chocolate Chip	1 (1.4 oz)	130	6	5	0	23	5	85
Kind								
Peanut Butter Dark Chocolate + Protein	1 (1.4 oz)	180	7	12	0	17	2	65
Kudos								
Granola Chocolate Chip	1 (1 oz)	120	1	4	0	20	1	70
Lean Body								
Hi-Protein Granola Peanuts 'N Chocolate	1 (2.8 oz)	340	20	11	0	39	4	580
Natural Ovens								
Great Granola Mixed Fruit	1 (1.4 oz)	150	4	3	0	27	2	140
Nature Valley								
Chewy Trail Mix Fruit & Nut	1 (1.2 oz)	140	3	4	0	25	2	65
Post								
Honey Bunches Of Oats Banana Nut	1 (1.2 oz)	140	2	4	0	24	1	115
Honey Bunches Of Oats Oatmeal Raisin	1 (1.2 oz)	130	2	3	0	25	2	105
ProBar								
Cran-Lemon Twister Organic Vegan	1 (3 oz)	360	9	16	0	49	7	55
Fruition Vegan Blueberry	1 (1.7 oz)	160	3	2	0	34	4	20
Fruition Vegan Cran-Raspberry	1 (1.7 oz)	160	3	2	0	34	4	20
Fruition Vegan Peach	1 (1.7 oz)	160	3	2	0	34	4	20
Fruition Vegan Strawberry	1 (1.7 oz)	160	3	2	0	34	4	20
Quaker								
Breakfast Bar Apple Crisp	1 (1.3 oz)	130	1	3	0	27	1	90
Breakfast Bar Iced Raspberry	1 (1.3 oz)	130	1	3	0	26	1	100
Breakfast Bites Iced Raspberry	1 pkg (1.3 oz)	130	1	3	0	28	3	75
Breakfast Bites Strawberry	1 pkg (1.3 oz)	130	1	3	0	27	2	90
Chewy Chocolate Chip	1 (0.8 oz)	100	1	3	0	18	1	75
Chewy Cookies & Cream	1 (0.8 oz)	90	1	3	0	18	2	85

FOOD	PORTION	CALS	PROT	FAT	CHOL	CARB	FIBER	SOD
Chewy 90 Calorie Cinnamon Sugar	1 (1 oz)	90	1	2	0	19	1	80
Chewy 90 Calorie Honey Nut	1 (0.8 oz)	90	1	2	0	19	1	80
Chewy Dipps Peanut Butter	1 (1 oz)	150	3	7	0	18	1	105
Chewy Granola w/ Protein Peanut Butter & Chocolate	1 (1 oz)	110	5	3	0	18	1	140
Chewy Low Fat S'mores	1 (1 oz)	110	1	2	0	22	1	70
Crunchy Granola Oats & Berries	1 (1 oz)	130	2	4	0	23	1	125
Oatmeal To Go Oatmeal Raisin	1 (2.1 oz)	220	4	4	15	43	5	240
Oatmeal To Go Raspberry Streusel	1 (2.1 oz)	220	4	4	15	43	5	220
Q-Smart Cranberry Vanilla Almond	1 (1 oz)	120	10	6	0	9	2	106
Trail Mix Cranberry Raisin & Almond	1 (1.2 oz)	150	2	5	0	24	1	50
Reese's								
SnackBarz Peanut Butter	1 (0.9 oz)	120	2	5	–	16	tr	95
Revolution Foods								
Jammy Sammy Apple Cinnamon & Oatmeal	1 (1 oz)	100	1	2	0	21	1	50
Organic Jammy Sammy PB & Grape	1 (1 oz)	110	2	3	0	19	1	55
Organic Jammy Sammy PB & Strawberry	1 (1 oz)	110	2	3	0	19	1	55
Roman Meal								
Whole Grain & Fruit	1 (2 oz)	190	4	2	0	43	6	240
Silhouette Solution								
Blueberry Pomegranate	1 (1.3 oz)	130	15	3	5	14	3	180
Peanut Passion	1 (1.3 oz)	130	15	4	5	14	3	180
South Beach								
Fiber Fit Granola Mocha	1 (1.2 oz)	120	2	4	0	25	9	125
Fiber Fit Granola S'Mores	1 (1.2 oz)	120	2	4	0	25	9	125
Weetabix								
Oaty Chocolate	1	67	2	2	–	12	6	tr
Weetos	1	88	1	3	–	14	tr	tr

FOOD	PORTION	CALS	PROT	FAT	CHOL	CARB	FIBER	SOD
Wings Of Nature								
Organic Almond Raisin	1 (1.4 oz)	170	5	11	0	17	3	15
Organic Cafe Mocha Coffee	1 (1.2 oz)	153	3	9	0	18	3	26
Organic Cranberry Crunch	1 (1.4 oz)	170	5	10	0	18	2	20
Organic Espresso Coffee	1 (1.4 oz)	180	3	10	0	21	2	25
Yotta								
Apple Cinnamon	1 (1.2 oz)	120	2	1	0	25	2	40
Cherry	1 (1.2 oz)	120	2	1	0	26	1	40
Orange	1 (1.2 oz)	120	2	1	0	26	2	45
CHAMPAGNE								
champagne	1 serv (3.5 oz)	84	tr	0	0	3	0	5
mimosa	1 serv	117	1	tr	0	12	tr	1
punch	1 serv (4 oz)	73	tr	tr	0	8	0	6
sekt german champagne	1 serv (3.5 oz)	84	tr	0	0	5	–	–
CHAYOTE								
fresh cooked	1 cup	38	1	1	0	8	–	1
raw	1 (7 oz)	49	2	1	0	11	–	8
raw cut up	1 cup	32	1	tr	0	7	–	198
CHEESE (*see also* CHEESE DISHES, CHEESE SUBSTITUTES, COTTAGE CHEESE, CREAM CHEESE, CREAM CHEESE SUBSTITUTES, NEUFCHATEL)								
american	1 oz	93	6	7	18	2	–	337
american cheese spread	1 oz	82	5	6	16	2	–	381
beaufort	1 oz	115	8	9	34	tr	0	128
bel paese	1 oz	112	7	9	–	0	0	–
blue	1 oz	100	6	8	21	1	–	396
blue crumbled	1 cup (4.7 oz)	477	29	39	102	3	–	1884
bocconcini smoked	1 oz	90	6	6	25	1	0	90
brick	1 oz	105	7	8	27	1	–	159
brie	1 oz	95	8	8	28	tr	–	178
cacio di roma sheep's milk cheese	1 oz	130	8	10	30	0	0	170
caerphilly	1.4 oz	150	9	13	–	0	0	–
camembert	1 oz	85	6	7	20	tr	–	239
cantal	1 oz	105	7	9	26	tr	0	269
caraway	1 oz	107	7	8	–	1	–	196

FOOD	PORTION	CALS	PROT	FAT	CHOL	CARB	FIBER	SOD
chabichou	1 oz	95	6	8	23	tr	0	189
chaource	1 oz	83	5	7	20	tr	0	230
cheddar	1 oz	114	7	9	30	tr	–	176
cheddar low sodium	1 oz	113	7	9	28	1	–	6
cheddar lowfat	1 oz	49	9	2	6	1	–	174
cheddar reduced fat	1.4 oz	104	13	6	–	0	0	–
cheddar shredded	1 cup	455	28	37	119	1	–	701
cheshire	1 oz	110	7	9	29	1	–	198
cheshire reduced fat	1.4 oz	108	13	6	–	tr	0	–
colby	1 oz	112	7	9	27	1	–	171
colby low sodium	1 oz	113	7	9	28	1	–	6
colby lowfat	1 oz	49	9	2	6	1	–	174
comte	1 oz	114	8	9	34	tr	0	105
coulommiers	1 oz	88	6	7	23	tr	0	195
crottin	1 oz	105	6	9	23	tr	0	133
derby	1.4 oz	161	10	14	–	0	0	–
edam reduced fat	1.4 oz	92	13	4	–	tr	0	–
emmentaler	1 oz	115	8	9	26	tr	–	129
feta	1 oz	75	4	6	25	1	–	316
fontina	1 oz	110	7	9	33	tr	–	–
frais	1.6 oz	51	3	3	–	3	0	–
gjetost	1 oz	132	3	8	–	12	–	170
gloucester double	1.4 oz	162	10	14	–	0	0	–
goat fresh	1 oz	23	1	2	5	tr	0	18
goat hard	1 oz	128	9	10	30	1	–	98
gorgonzola	1 oz	107	5	9	–	tr	–	–
gouda	1 oz	101	7	8	32	1	–	232
grana padano parmesan shaved	1 tbsp	20	2	2	5	0	0	45
gruyere	1 oz	117	8	9	31	tr	–	95
lancashire	1.4 oz	149	9	12	–	0	0	–
leicester	1.4 oz	160	10	14	–	0	0	–
limburger	1 oz	93	8	8	26	tr	–	227
lymeswold	1.4 oz	170	6	16	–	tr	0	–
maroilles	1 oz	97	6	8	26	tr	0	300
monterey	1 oz	106	7	9	–	tr	–	152
morbier	1 oz	99	7	8	23	tr	0	283
mozzarella	1 oz	80	6	6	22	1	–	106
mozzarella fresh	1 oz	80	6	6	20	tr	0	160
mozzarella part skim	1 oz	72	7	5	16	1	–	132

FOOD	PORTION	CALS	PROT	FAT	CHOL	CARB	FIBER	SOD
muenster	1 oz	104	7	9	27	tr	–	178
parmesan grated	1 tbsp	23	2	2	4	tr	–	93
parmesan hard	1 oz	111	10	7	19	1	–	454
picodon	1 oz	99	6	8	23	tr	0	–
pimento	1 oz	106	6	9	27	tr	–	405
pont l'eveque	1 oz	86	6	7	20	tr	0	191
port du salut	1 oz	100	7	8	35	tr	–	151
provolone	1 oz	100	7	8	20	1	–	248
pyrenees	1 oz	101	6	8	26	tr	0	235
quark 20% fat	1 oz	33	4	1	5	1	–	10
quark 40% fat	1 oz	48	3	3	11	1	–	10
quark made w/ skim milk	1 oz	22	4	tr	tr	1	–	11
queso anejo	1 oz	106	6	9	30	1	–	321
queso asadero	1 oz	101	6	8	30	1	–	186
queso chihuahua	1 oz	106	6	8	30	2	–	175
queso fresco	1 oz	41	4	2	–	1	0	–
queso manchego	1 oz	107	8	8	27	tr	0	341
queso panela	1 oz	74	6	5	–	1	0	–
raclette	1 oz	102	7	8	26	tr	0	217
reblochon	1 oz	88	6	7	23	tr	0	240
ricotta part skim	½ cup (4.4 oz)	171	14	10	38	6	–	155
ricotta whole milk	½ cup (4.4 oz)	216	14	16	63	4	–	104
romadur 40% fat	1 oz	83	7	6	–	tr	–	–
romano	1 oz	110	9	8	29	1	–	340
roquefort	1 oz	105	6	9	26	1	–	513
rouy	1 oz	95	7	8	23	tr	0	138
saint marcellin	1 oz	94	5	8	23	tr	0	171
saint nectaire	1 oz	97	6	8	23	tr	0	169
saint paulin	1 oz	85	7	6	20	tr	0	174
sainte maure	1 oz	99	6	8	23	tr	0	411
selles sur cher	1 oz	93	5	8	20	tr	0	181
stilton blue	1.4 oz	164	9	14	–	0	0	–
stilton white	1.4 oz	145	8	13	–	0	0	–
swiss	1 oz	107	8	8	26	1	–	74
swiss processed	1 oz	95	7	7	24	1	–	388
tilsit	1 oz	96	7	7	29	1	–	213
tome	1 oz	92	6	7	23	tr	0	231
triple creme	1 oz	113	3	11	34	tr	0	86

FOOD	PORTION	CALS	PROT	FAT	CHOL	CARB	FIBER	SOD
vacherin	1 oz	92	5	8	23	tr	0	129
wensleydale	1.4 oz	151	9	13	–	0	0	–
whey cheese	1 oz	126	4	8	–	9	0	146
yogurt cheese	1 oz	80	6	7	15	0	0	60
Alpine Lace								
Reduced Fat Provolone	1 slice (0.8 oz)	70	6	5	10	1	0	135
Reduced Fat Swiss	1 slice (0.8 oz)	70	7	5	15	1	0	95
Reduced Fat White American	1 slice (0.8 oz)	70	5	5	15	1	0	310
Reduced Sodium Muenster	1 slice (0.8 oz)	90	6	7	15	0	0	110
Applegate Farms								
Organic Cheddar Milk	1 slice (0.7 oz)	85	5	6	20	0	0	130
Organic Muenster Kase	1 slice (0.8 oz)	85	5	7	20	0	0	130
Yogurt Cheese w/ Probiotics	1 slice (0.7 oz)	80	5	6	15	tr	–	105
Athenos								
Traditional	¼ cup	90	7	7	25	2	tr	390
Traditional Reduced Fat	¼ cup	70	7	5	10	1	tr	470
Bel Gioioso								
Mozzarella Fresh	1 in cube (1 oz)	80	5	6	20	0	0	85
Boar's Head								
Imported Swiss	1 oz	110	8	8	20	tr	0	70
Cabot								
Cheddar Extra Sharp	1 oz	110	7	9	30	tr	0	180
Cheddar Horseradish	1 oz	110	7	9	30	tr	0	180
Cheddar Light 50% Reduced Fat	1 oz	70	8	5	15	tr	0	170
Cheddar Light 50% Reduced Fat Omega-3	1 oz	70	8	5	15	tr	0	170
Cheddar Light 75% Reduced Fat	1 oz	60	9	3	10	tr	0	200
Cheddar Shake	2 tsp	25	1	2	5	1	0	220
Cheddar Tomato Basil	1 oz	110	7	9	30	tr	0	180
Monterey Jack	1 oz	110	7	9	30	tr	0	170

FOOD	PORTION	CALS	PROT	FAT	CHOL	CARB	FIBER	SOD
Pepper Jack 50% Reduced Fat	1 oz	70	8	5	15	tr	0	170
Swiss Slices	1 (1 oz)	110	8	8	25	1	0	60
Connoisseur								
Asiago Spread	1 tbsp	90	5	7	20	2	0	240
Brie Spread	2 tbsp	90	4	7	25	2	0	250
Gorgonzola Spread	1 tbsp	90	5	7	20	2	0	340
Wheel Asiago Pesto	2 tbsp	90	5	6	20	4	0	240
Wheel Swiss Bacon	2 tbsp	90	5	7	25	2	0	260
Cracker Barrel								
Fontina	1 slice (0.7 oz)	80	6	7	15	tr	0	230
Sharp Cheddar 2% Milk	1 oz	90	7	6	20	tr	0	240
Dietz & Watson								
Aalsbruk Edam	1 oz	90	6	7	25	1	0	180
American Yellow	1 slice (1 oz)	110	6	8	10	0	0	370
Cheddar Sharp	1 oz	110	6	9	28	1	0	270
Danish Blue	1 oz	100	6	12	15	0	0	310
Danish Havarti	1 oz	110	6	9	28	1	0	270
Gorgonzola	1 oz	100	6	8	20	0	0	390
Muenster	1 slice (0.7 oz)	75	5	6	19	0	0	203
DiGiorno								
Shredded Three Cheese Parmesan Romano & Asiago	¼ cup (1 oz)	110	9	8	25	1	0	270
Dragone								
Mozzarella Whole Milk	1 oz	90	6	7	20	tr	0	170
Parmesan Wedge	1 oz	100	9	7	20	tr	0	390
Ricotta Part Skim	¼ cup (2.2 oz)	90	6	6	30	4	0	85
Easy Cheese								
American	2 tbsp (1.1 oz)	90	5	6	20	2	0	410
Cheddar	2 tbsp (1.1 oz)	90	5	6	20	2	0	410
Finlandia								
Swiss Thin Sliced	1 slice (0.5 oz)	55	4	4	10	0	0	39

FOOD	PORTION	CALS	PROT	FAT	CHOL	CARB	FIBER	SOD
Fresh Made								
Farmers Cheese Nonfat	2 tbsp	15	5	0	3	1	0	10
Friendship								
Farmer	2 tbsp (1 oz)	50	5	3	10	0	0	120
Farmer No Salt Added	2 tbsp (1 oz)	50	5	3	10	0	0	10
Frigo								
Mozzarella Part Skim	1 oz	80	7	6	15	tr	0	210
Parmesan Shredded	¼ cup (1 oz)	100	9	7	20	1	tr	430
Ricotta Whole Milk	¼ cup (2.2 oz)	110	7	8	35	2	0	150
Romano Shredded	¼ cup (1 oz)	100	8	7	20	1	tr	460
Hans All Natural								
Spread Cheddar & Jalapeno	2 tbsp (1 oz)	90	5	7	20	3	0	240
Spread Swiss Cheese & Almonds	2 tbsp (1 oz)	90	5	7	20	3	0	200
Haolam								
Cheddar Sliced	1 slice (1 oz)	114	7	9	28	1	0	181
Horizon Organic								
American	1 slice (0.7 oz)	60	4	5	15	1	0	250
Cheddar	1 oz	110	7	9	30	tr	0	180
Monterey Jack	1 oz	100	7	8	30	0	0	170
Shred Mexican	¼ cup	110	7	9	30	tr	0	180
Shred Parmesan	1 tbsp	20	2	2	5	0	0	70
Slice Provolone	1 slice (0.7 oz)	70	5	6	15	0	0	140
Sticks Colby	1 (1 oz)	110	7	9	30	tr	0	180
String Mozzarella	1 stick (1 oz)	80	8	5	15	tr	0	170
J.L. Kraft								
Spreadable Feta & Spinach	2 tbsp	80	3	7	25	1	0	160
Kraft								
Cheddar Sharp Shredded 2% Milk	¼ cup	80	7	6	20	tr	0	230
Crumbles Three Cheese	¼ cup (1 oz)	110	6	9	25	tr	0	190
LiveActive 1% Milk Cheddar Cubes	7 (1 oz)	90	8	6	20	tr	0	260
LiveActive 2% Milk Marbled Colby & Monterey Jack	1 stick (1 oz)	90	8	6	20	tr	0	240

FOOD	PORTION	CALS	PROT	FAT	CHOL	CARB	FIBER	SOD
LiveActive Cheddar Cheese Sticks	1 (1 oz)	120	6	10	30	0	0	180
LiveActive Colby & Monterey Jack Cubes	7 (1 oz)	110	7	9	30	tr	0	200
LiveActive Mozzarella Sticks	1 (1 oz)	80	8	5	15	tr	0	200
Shredded Mexican Style Cheddar & Monterey Jack	¼ cup	110	6	9	25	1	0	190
Swiss Extra Thin Slices	1 (0.6 oz)	60	4	5	15	0	0	25
Land O Lakes								
American	1 slice (0.7 oz)	70	4	5	15	2	0	280
Chedarella	1 oz	110	7	9	25	0	0	190
Cheddar	1 oz	110	7	9	30	0	0	190
Snack 'N Cheese To Go Cheddar Mild	1 serv (0.7 oz)	80	7	7	20	0	0	140
Snack 'N Cheese To Go Cheddar Mild Reduced Fat	1 serv (0.5 oz)	60	5	5	15	0	0	115
Snack 'N Cheese To Go Co-Jack	1 serv (0.7 oz)	80	5	7	20	0	0	140
Snack 'N Cheese To Go Co-Jack Reduced Fat	1 serv (0.7 oz)	60	5	5	15	0	0	120
Swiss	1 oz	110	8	8	25	1	0	115
Laughing Cow								
Blue Light	1 wedge (0.7 oz)	35	2	2	5	2	0	230
Creamy Swiss Light	1 wedge (0.7 oz)	35	2	2	<5	1	0	210
Creamy Swiss Original	1 wedge (0.7 oz)	50	2	4	10	1	0	210
French Onion Light	1 wedge (0.7 oz)	35	2	2	<5	1	0	210
Garlic & Herb Light	1 wedge (0.7 oz)	35	2	2	<5	1	0	210
Mozzarella Sun-Dried Tomato & Basil Light	1 wedge (0.7 oz)	35	2	2	5	2	0	220
Queso Fresco & Chipotle	1 wedge (0.7 oz)	35	2	2	5	2	0	240

FOOD	PORTION	CALS	PROT	FAT	CHOL	CARB	FIBER	SOD
Lifeway								
Farmer	2 tbsp (1.1 oz)	40	3	2	6	4	–	10
Farmer Lite	2 tbsp (1.1 oz)	25	3	1	<5	2	–	10
Sweet Kiss Spread Peach	1 oz	50	3	2	<5	6	–	10
Sweet Kiss Spread Raisins	1 oz	45	3	1	<5	6	–	10
Molly McButter								
Natural Cheese	1 tsp (2 g)	5	0	0	0	1	0	125
Organic Valley								
Blue Crumbles	1 oz	100	6	8	25	1	0	380
Cheddar Mild	1 oz	110	7	9	30	0	0	170
Feta	1 oz	60	5	4	10	tr	0	430
Monterey Jack Shredded	¼ cup	80	8	5	15	1	0	180
Muenster	1 slice (0.7 oz)	80	5	6	20	0	0	160
Provolone	1 slice (0.7 oz)	70	5	6	15	0	0	190
Swiss	1 oz	110	7	9	25	0	0	125
Pizza Zing								
Spicy Hot Cheese Shake	2 tsp	15	2	1	5	0	0	86
Rosenborg								
Danish Camembert	1 oz	80	5	7	23	0	0	168
Rouge Et Noir								
Breakfast	1 oz	90	6	7	25	0	0	210
Brie Garlic	1 oz	90	6	7	30	0	0	210
Brie Pesto	1 oz	90	6	7	30	0	0	210
Brie Tomato Basil	1 oz	90	6	7	30	0	0	210
Brie Triple Creme	1 oz	110	4	10	30	0	0	160
Camembert	1 oz	90	6	7	30	0	0	210
Le Petit Bleu	1 oz	110	4	10	30	0	0	160
Le Petit Chevre	1 oz	90	5	6	20	0	0	210
Marin French Blue	1 oz	110	4	10	30	0	0	160
Marin French Gold	1 oz	110	4	10	30	0	0	160
Schlosskranz	1 oz	85	5	7	30	0	0	390
Saladena								
Goat Crumbles	¼ cup	80	5	7	30	tr	0	110
Sap Sago								
Fat Free Cheese Grated	1 tsp	10	2	0	0	0	0	136

FOOD	PORTION	CALS	PROT	FAT	CHOL	CARB	FIBER	SOD
Sargento								
4 Cheese Italian Shredded	¼ cup	80	8	5	15	1	0	220
4 Cheese Mexican Reduced Fat Shredded	¼ cup (1 oz)	80	8	6	15	1	0	190
American Burger	1 slice (0.7 oz)	70	4	6	20	tr	0	240
Bistro Blends Shredded Italian Pasta Cheese	¼ cup (1 oz)	90	7	6	15	2	0	310
Blue Crumbled	¼ cup (1 oz)	100	6	8	25	1	0	380
Cheddar Chipotle Shredded	¼ cup	100	6	8	15	1	0	190
Cheddar Chipotle Sticks	1 (0.7 oz)	80	5	6	0	1	0	150
Cheddar Mild Cubes	7 (1 oz)	120	7	10	30	tr	0	190
Cheddar Mild Shredded Reduced Sodium	¼ cup (1 oz)	110	7	9	25	1	0	135
Cheddar White Vermont Sharp	1 slice (0.7 oz)	80	5	7	20	0	0	125
Cheddar White Vermont Sharp Shredded	¼ cup (1 oz)	110	7	9	25	1	0	190
Cheese Dips Cheddar & Buttery Pretzels	1 pkg (3.8 oz)	360	9	16	15	47	2	1430
Cheese Dips Cheddar & Tortilla Chips	1 pkg (3 oz)	320	7	21	15	26	1	880
Colby-Jack Sticks Reduced Sodium	1 (0.7 oz)	80	5	7	20	tr	0	105
Jarlsberg	1 slice (0.8 oz)	80	6	6	15	tr	0	110
Monterey Jack Shredded	¼ cup (1 oz)	110	7	9	30	1	0	190
Mozzarella Reduced Fat Shredded	¼ cup (1 oz)	80	8	5	10	tr	0	200
Mozzarella Shredded	¼ cup (1 oz)	80	7	6	15	1	0	190
Muenster	1 slice (0.7 oz)	80	5	6	20	tr	0	135
Nacho & Taco Shredded	¼ cup (1 oz)	110	7	9	30	1	0	200
Parmesan Grated	2 tsp (5 g)	25	2	2	5	0	0	80
Parmesan Shredded	2 tsp	20	2	2	<5	0	0	55
Pepper Jack Reduced Sodium	1 slice (0.7 oz)	70	4	6	15	0	0	90
Provolone	1 slice (0.7 oz)	70	5	5	15	0	0	125

FOOD	PORTION	CALS	PROT	FAT	CHOL	CARB	FIBER	SOD
Provolone Reduced Sodium	1 slice (0.7 oz)	70	5	5	15	0	0	100
Ricotta Fat Free	¼ cup	50	5	0	10	5	0	65
Ricotta Light	¼ cup	60	5	3	15	3	0	55
Ricotta Whole Milk	¼ cup	90	7	8	25	3	0	75
String Light	1 piece (0.7 oz)	50	6	3	10	1	0	160
String Reduced Sodium	1 (0.7 oz)	60	6	4	10	tr	0	110
Swiss Reduced Fat	1 slice (0.7 oz)	60	7	4	15	1	0	30
Swiss Shredded	¼ cup (1 oz)	110	8	8	25	tr	0	60
Swiss Thick Slice	1 slice (1 oz)	110	8	8	25	1	0	60
Swiss Thin Sliced	1 slice (0.6 oz)	70	5	5	20	0	0	40
Smart Balance								
Creamy Cheddar Slices	1 (0.7 oz)	40	4	2	<5	2	0	290
Fat Free Lactose Free Slices	1 (0.7 oz)	40	4	2	<5	2	0	290
Sorrento								
Mozzarella Fresh	1 oz	90	5	6	30	0	0	130
Stella								
3 Cheese Italian Shredded	¼ cup	100	8	7	25	1	tr	410
Asiago Wedge	1 oz	110	6	9	30	tr	0	280
Gorgonzola Wedge	1 oz	100	6	9	25	tr	0	390
Kasseri Wedge	1 oz	110	6	9	30	tr	0	280
The Greek Gods								
Kefir Cheese	2 tbsp (1 oz)	80	2	5	20	2	0	25
Treasure Cave								
Blue Cheese Crumbled	¼ cup (1 oz)	100	6	8	20	tr	–	400
Feta Crumbled	¼ cup (1 oz)	80	5	6	20	1	tr	320
Gorgonzola Crumbled	¼ cup (1 oz)	100	6	8	20	tr	–	310
Weight Watchers								
String Light	1 stick (0.8 oz)	50	6	3	5	tr	0	150
Wholesome Valley								
Organic American	1 slice (0.7 oz)	50	3	4	10	tr	0	210

CHEESE DISHES

FOOD	PORTION	CALS	PROT	FAT	CHOL	CARB	FIBER	SOD
Banquet								
Mozzarella Nuggets	7	270	10	16	35	21	tr	570

FOOD	PORTION	CALS	PROT	FAT	CHOL	CARB	FIBER	SOD
Farm Rich								
Cheese Sticks Breaded	2 (2.1 oz)	210	9	12	15	17	tr	290
Mozzarella Bites Breaded	4 (2.2 oz)	150	8	7	10	13	1	270
Original Cheese Bites Breaded	7 (2.1 oz)	180	9	11	15	13	tr	440
Fillo Factory								
Tyropita Cheese Fillo Appetizers	3 (3 oz)	230	7	14	40	19	0	310
Stouffer's								
Welsh Rarebit	¼ pkg (2.5 oz)	140	6	10	20	6	0	270
TAKE-OUT								
fondue	½ cup (3.8 oz)	247	15	15	49	4	–	142
fried mozzarella sticks	3 (4.6 oz)	503	33	32	107	20	1	759
souffle	1 serv (7 oz)	504	23	38	370	18	1	848
welsh rarebit	1 slice	228	8	16	–	14	1	–

CHEESE SUBSTITUTES

FOOD	PORTION	CALS	PROT	FAT	CHOL	CARB	FIBER	SOD
mozzarella	1 oz	70	3	3	0	7	–	194
soya cheese	1.4 oz	128	7	11	–	tr	0	–
Daiya								
Cheddar Style Shreds	¼ cup (1 oz)	90	1	6	0	7	1	250
Mozzarella Style Shreds	¼ cup (1 oz)	90	1	6	0	7	1	280
Playfood								
Cheesey Cheese	1 oz	60	2	5	0	4	1	190
Rice								
American Flavor	1 slice (0.7 oz)	50	4	3	0	tr	0	230
American Flavor Vegan	1 slice (0.7 oz)	45	1	3	0	0	0	130
Shreds Mozzarella Flavor	⅓ cup (1 oz)	70	6	4	0	3	0	370
Sheese								
Blue Style	1 oz	100	4	8	0	3	0	340
Cheddar Style Medium	1 oz	100	4	8	0	3	0	340
Creamy Mexican	2 tbsp	80	2	7	0	2	0	140
Creamy Original	2 tbsp	80	2	7	0	2	0	140
Super Stix								
Mozzarella Flavor	1 (1 oz)	70	6	5	0	0	0	370

FOOD	PORTION	CALS	PROT	FAT	CHOL	CARB	FIBER	SOD
Vegan Gourmet								
Cheese Alternative Cheddar	1 oz	50	2	4	0	2	2	200
Cheese Alternative Monterey Jack	1 oz	70	1	7	0	2	2	150
Cheese Alternative Mozzarella	1 oz	70	1	8	0	1	1	120
Cheese Alternative Nacho	1 oz	45	2	4	0	2	2	210
Veggie								
American Flavor	1 slice (0.6 oz)	40	3	3	0	tr	0	220
Grated Parmesan Flavor	2 tsp	15	2	1	0	0	0	90
Pepper Jack Flavor	1 oz	60	6	4	0	2	0	390
Shreds Cheddar Flavor	1 oz	70	6	4	0	0	0	260
Veggy								
Mozzarella Flavor	1 slice (0.7 oz)	40	4	3	0	tr	0	230
CHERIMOYA								
fresh	1	515	7	2	0	131	–	–
CHERRIES								
CANNED								
maraschino	¼ cup (1.4 oz)	66	tr	tr	0	17	1	2
maraschino	1 (4 g)	7	tr	tr	0	2	tr	0
sour in heavy syrup	½ cup	116	1	tr	0	30	1	9
sour in light syrup	½ cup	94	1	tr	0	24	1	9
sour water packed	½ cup	44	1	tr	0	11	1	9
sweet juice pack	½ cup	68	1	tr	0	17	2	4
sweet pitted in heavy syrup	½ cup	105	1	tr	0	27	2	4
sweet water pack	½ cup	57	1	tr	0	15	2	1
Chukar Cherries								
Cherry Jubilee Dessert Sauce	1 tbsp	40	0	0	0	10	tr	0
Del Monte								
Sweet Dark Pitted In Heavy Syrup	½ cup (4.2 oz)	100	tr	0	0	24	tr	10
Jake & Amos								
Brandied Sweet	½ cup (4.4 oz)	90	1	0	0	22	2	9

FOOD	PORTION	CALS	PROT	FAT	CHOL	CARB	FIBER	SOD
S&W								
Sliced	½ cup (4.7 oz)	140	1	0	0	34	1	10
The Gracious Gourmet								
Spiced Sour Cherry Spread	1 tbsp (0.5 oz)	15	0	0	0	4	0	25
DRIED								
bing unsulfured	¼ cup	130	0	0	0	31	2	10
montmorency tart pitted	⅓ cup	160	2	1	0	36	2	0
tart	½ cup	200	2	1	0	49	2	0
yogurt covered	¼ cup	170	1	6	0	29	5	20
Bob's Red Mill								
Tart	⅓ cup	140	1	0	0	33	11	0
Chukar Cherries								
Bing	3 tbsp	130	1	1	0	33	3	10
Bing Chocolate Covered	3 tbsp (1.4 oz)	180	2	9	0	24	2	20
Cabernet Dark Chocolate Covered	2 tbsp (1.5 oz)	180	2	9	<5	26	3	10
Columbia River Tart	⅓ cup	120	2	1	0	36	2	0
Rainier	3 tbsp	130	tr	1	0	33	3	10
Totally Tart	⅓ cup	140	1	1	0	33	3	0
De-Lite								
Tart	1 oz	95	1	tr	0	23	1	14
Emily's								
Dark Chocolate Covered	11 (1.4 oz)	180	1	9	0	27	2	0
Peeled Snacks								
Fruit Picks Cherry-Go-Round	1 pkg (1.5 oz)	130	2	0	0	30	4	0
Raisinets								
Dark & Milk Chocolate	¼ cup (1.6 oz)	200	1	8	5	32	2	5
Stoneridge Orchards								
Bing	⅓ cup (1.4 oz)	130	1	0	0	32	1	10
Organic Montmorency Whole	⅓ cup (1.4 oz)	135	0	1	0	33	2	12
Sunsweet								
Cherries	¼ cup (1.4 oz)	100	1	0	0	30	2	5

FOOD	PORTION	CALS	PROT	FAT	CHOL	CARB	FIBER	SOD
FRESH								
sour	1 cup	52	1	tr	0	13	2	3
sour pitted	1 cup	78	2	tr	0	19	3	5
sweet	20	86	1	1	0	22	3	0
Chiquita								
Cherries	1 cup (4.8 oz)	87	1	0	0	22	3	0
FROZEN								
sour unsweetened	½ cup	36	1	tr	0	9	1	1
sweet sweetened	½ cup	115	2	tr	0	29	3	1
CHERRY JUICE								
tart cherry concentrate	1 cup	140	1	0	0	34	0	25
Cheribundi								
Skinny Cherry	8 oz	90	0	0	0	23	–	5
Tru Cherry 100% Juice	8 oz	130	1	0	0	32	–	5
Whey Cherry	8 oz	160	8	0	0	30	–	20
Froose								
Cheerful Cherry	1 box (4.2 oz)	80	0	0	0	19	3	15
HP								
Tart Montmorency Concentrate	1 oz	80	tr	0	0	19	0	15
Old Orchard								
100% Pure Tart Cherry	8 oz	140	0	0	0	34	–	25
Santa Cruz								
Organic 100% Juice Red Tart	8 oz	120	0	0	0	30	0	25
Smart Juice								
Organic 100% Juice Tart Cherry	8 oz	140	1	0	0	32	1	20
Tart Is Smart								
Tart Cherry Concentrate	1 oz	80	1	0	0	19	0	15
CHERVIL								
seed	1 tsp	1	tr	tr	0	tr	–	tr
CHESTNUTS								
chinese steamed	3 (1 oz)	43	1	tr	0	10	–	1
creme de marrons	1 oz	73	1	tr	0	18	1	1
japanese roasted	1 oz	57	1	tr	0	13	–	5

FOOD	PORTION	CALS	PROT	FAT	CHOL	CARB	FIBER	SOD
ready-to-eat vacuum packed	5 (1 oz)	40	tr	0	0	8	0	10
roasted	3 (1 oz)	70	1	1	0	15	1	1
Gefen								
Whole Roasted & Peeled	¼ cup (1.4 oz)	52	1	0	0	11	1	1
CHEWING GUM								
bubble gum	1 block	20	0	tr	0	5	tr	0
stick	1 piece	7	0	tr	0	2	tr	0
sugarless	1 piece	5	0	tr	0	2	0	0
Bubble Yum								
Original	1 piece (8 g)	25	0	0	0	6	–	–
Sugarless	1 piece (5 g)	10	0	0	0	3	–	–
Choward's								
Scented Gum	3 pieces	10	0	0	0	3	0	0
Dubble Bubble								
Gumball	1 piece	10	0	0	0	2	0	0
Extra								
Sugar Free All Flavors	1 piece	5	0	0	0	2	–	0
Flare								
Warming Cinnamon	1 piece	5	0	0	0	2	–	0
Orbit								
Sugarfree Citrusmint	1 piece	<5	0	0	0	1	–	0
White Melon Breeze	2 pieces	5	0	0	0	2	0	0
Stride								
All Flavors	1 piece (1.9 g)	<5	0	0	0	1	–	0
Spark	1 piece (1.9 g)	5	0	0	0	1	–	0
Trident								
Extra Care	1 piece	<5	0	0	0	1	–	0
Splash Strawberry Lime	1 piece	<5	0	0	0	2	–	0
Winterfresh								
Gum	1 stick	10	0	0	0	2	–	0
CHIA SEEDS								
dried	1 oz	134	5	7	0	14	–	–
CHICKEN (*see also* CHICKEN DISHES, CHICKEN SUBSTITUTES, DINNER, HOT DOG, MEATBALLS)								
CANNED								
chicken spread	1 serv (2 oz)	88	10	10	31	2	tr	404

FOOD	PORTION	CALS	PROT	FAT	CHOL	CARB	FIBER	SOD
meat drained	1 can (5 oz)	230	32	10	62	1	0	169
w/ broth	½ can (2.5 oz)	117	15	6	–	0	0	357
Hormel								
Chunk White & Dark	2 oz	70	10	3	45	0	0	250
Premium Chunk Breast	2 oz	60	12	2	40	0	0	250
Swanson								
Chunk Breast In Water	2 oz	50	9	1	25	1	0	300
Tyson								
Premium Chunk	½ can (2 oz)	60	10	3	30	0	0	200
Premium Chunk Breast	½ can (2 oz)	60	13	1	30	0	0	200
FRESH								
back w/ skin roasted bones removed	1 (3.7 oz)	318	28	22	93	0	0	92
back w/o skin roasted bones removed	1 (2.8 oz)	191	23	11	72	0	0	77
breast roasted diced	1 cup (5 oz)	231	43	5	119	0	0	104
breast w/ skin battered fried bones removed	½ breast (4.9 oz)	364	35	18	119	13	tr	385
breast w/ skin floured fried bones removed	1 (3.4 oz)	218	31	9	87	2	tr	74
breast w/ skin roasted bones removed	½ breast (3.4 oz)	193	29	8	82	0	0	70
breast w/ skin stewed bones removed	½ breast (3.9 oz)	202	30	8	82	0	0	68
breast w/o skin fried bones removed	½ breast (3 oz)	161	29	4	78	tr	0	68
breast w/o skin roasted bones removed	½ breast (3 oz)	142	27	3	73	0	0	64
breast w/o skin stewed bones removed	1 (3.3 oz)	143	28	3	73	0	0	60
broiler/fryer w/ skin roasted bones removed	½ (10.5 oz)	715	82	41	263	0	0	245
capon meat & skin roasted bones removed	½ (1.4 lbs)	1459	184	74	548	0	0	312
cornish hen w/ skin roasted	1 (9 oz)	668	57	47	337	0	0	164
cornish hen w/ skin roasted	½ (4.5 oz)	335	29	23	169	0	0	83
cornish hen w/o skin roasted	1 (7.7 oz)	295	51	9	233	0	0	139

FOOD	PORTION	CALS	PROT	FAT	CHOL	CARB	FIBER	SOD
cornish hen w/o skin roasted	½ (4 oz)	147	26	4	117	0	0	69
dark meat w/o skin roasted diced	1 cup (5 oz)	287	38	14	130	0	0	130
drumstick w/ skin battered floured & fried bones removed	1 (1.7 oz)	120	13	7	44	1	0	44
drumstick w/ skin battered fried bones removed	1 (2.5 oz)	193	16	11	62	6	tr	194
drumstick w/ skin roasted bones removed	1 (1.8 oz)	112	14	6	47	0	0	47
drumstick w/ skin stewed bones removed	1 (2 oz)	116	14	6	47	0	0	43
drumstick w/o skin fried bones removed	1 (1.5 oz)	82	12	3	39	0	0	40
drumstick w/o skin roasted bones removed	1 (1.5 oz)	76	12	2	41	0	0	42
drumstick w/o skin stewed bones removed	1 (1.6 oz)	78	13	3	40	0	0	37
feet cooked	1 (1.2 oz)	73	7	5	29	tr	0	23
ground crumbled fried	3 oz	161	20	9	91	0	0	64
ground patty cooked	1 med (2.1 oz)	142	16	8	52	0	0	242
ground patty cooked	1 lg (2.8 oz)	190	22	11	70	0	0	323
ground patty cooked	1 sm (1.7 oz)	114	13	6	42	0	0	194
meat & skin stewed bones removed	¼ chicken (4.6 oz)	372	35	25	103	0	0	95
neck w/ skin battered fried	1 (1.8 oz)	172	10	12	47	5	–	144
neck w/ skin fried	1 (1.3 oz)	120	9	9	34	2	–	30
neck w/ skin simmered	1 (1.3 oz)	94	7	7	27	0	0	20
roaster meat & skin roasted bones removed	¼ chicken (8.4 oz)	535	58	32	182	0	0	175
skin battered fried from ½ chicken	6.7 oz	749	20	55	141	44	–	1104
skin floured fried from ½ chicken	2 oz	281	11	24	41	5	–	30
skin roasted from ½ chicken	2 oz	254	11	23	46	0	0	36
skin stewed from ½ chicken	2.5 oz	261	11	24	45	0	0	40

FOOD	PORTION	CALS	PROT	FAT	CHOL	CARB	FIBER	SOD
tail cooked	1 (1 oz)	84	7	5	25	3	tr	85
thigh w/ skin battered & fried bones removed	1 (3 oz)	238	19	14	80	8	tr	248
thigh w/ skin floured fried bones removed	1 (2.2 oz)	162	17	9	60	2	tr	55
thigh w/ skin roasted bones removed	1 (2.2 oz)	153	16	10	58	0	0	52
thigh w/ skin stewed bones removed	1 (2.4 oz)	158	16	10	57	0	0	48
thigh w/o skin fried bones removed	1 (1.8 oz)	113	15	5	53	1	0	49
thigh w/o skin roasted bones removed	1 (1.8 oz)	109	13	6	49	0	0	46
thigh w/o skin stewed bones removed	1 (1.9 oz)	107	14	5	50	0	0	41
wing w/ skin battered fried bones removed	1 (1.7 oz)	159	10	11	39	5	tr	157
wing w/ skin floured fried bones removed	1 (1.1 oz)	103	8	7	26	1	0	25
wing w/ skin roasted bones removed	1 (1.4 oz)	100	9	7	28	0	0	27
wing w/o skin fried bones removed	1 (0.7 oz)	42	6	2	17	0	0	18
wing w/o skin roasted bones removed	1 (0.7 oz)	43	6	2	18	0	0	19
wing w/o skin stewed bones removed	1 (0.8 oz)	43	7	2	18	0	0	18
Coleman								
Organic Breast Boneless Skinless	4 oz	120	26	2	65	0	0	75
Organic Drumsticks	4 oz	180	22	10	90	0	0	95
Perdue								
Boneless Skinless Breasts cooked	3 oz	110	25	1	70	0	0	30
Breast Boneless Herb & Pepper	1 piece (4.8 oz)	140	29	2	80	0	0	330
Breast Boneless Roasted Garlic w/ White Wine	1 piece (4.8 oz)	110	29	2	80	1	–	520
Breast Boneless Skinless cooked	3 oz	100	23	1	65	0	0	25

FOOD	PORTION	CALS	PROT	FAT	CHOL	CARB	FIBER	SOD
Breast Perfect Portions Boneless Skinless	1 (4.8 oz)	130	19	2	80	0	–	350
Ground cooked	3 oz	170	18	11	125	0	0	50
Ground Breast cooked	3 oz	80	19	1	55	0	0	60
Oven Ready Cornish Hen Seasoned	4 oz	160	16	10	75	1	–	420
Oven Ready Roaster Bone-In Breast	4 oz	140	20	7	75	1	0	410
Oven Ready Roaster Seasoned	4 oz	210	17	15	70	1	–	430
Oven Stuffer Drumstick	1 (3.6 oz)	190	25	11	125	0	0	85
Patties cooked	1 (3 oz)	170	19	11	130	0	0	75
Thigh Filets Boneless Skinless	4 oz	150	22	8	110	0	0	85
Thighs Tender & Tasty Boneless Skinless cooked	3 oz	150	17	9	90	0	0	380
Whole Chicken Tender & Tasty cooked	3 oz	150	20	8	110	0	0	280
Whole Dark Meat cooked	3 oz	210	18	15	100	0	0	60
Whole White Meat cooked	3 oz	170	21	9	80	0	0	50
Wingettes cooked	3 oz	170	20	10	135	0	0	250
Wings cooked	3 oz	170	20	10	135	0	0	250
Rocky								
The Range Chicken Whole	4 oz	240	21	17	100	0	0	80
Rosie								
Organic Breast Boneless Skinless	4 oz	120	26	2	65	0	0	75
Tyson								
Breasts Boneless Skinless	4 oz	110	23	3	65	0	0	180
Cornish Hen	1 serv (4 oz)	200	19	14	130	0	0	65
Drumsticks	4 oz	150	18	9	95	0	0	180
Thigh Cutlets Boneless Skinless	4 oz	130	18	7	90	0	0	160
Whole Cut Up	4 oz	220	19	16	80	0	0	170
Wings	4 oz	220	17	17	105	0	0	190
FROZEN								
breast roll roasted	2 oz	75	8	4	22	1	0	494
fajita strips	1 (0.3 oz)	13	2	1	8	tr	0	75
patty cooked	1 (3.5 oz)	287	15	20	43	13	tr	532

FOOD	PORTION	CALS	PROT	FAT	CHOL	CARB	FIBER	SOD
Banquet								
Wings Hot & Spicy	1/4 pkg (3 oz)	260	19	17	55	8	5	320
Barber								
Buffalo Fingers	1 (3.3 oz)	160	15	4	35	18	tr	380
Nuggets 4 Cheese Stuffed	3 (3 oz)	230	14	16	45	9	tr	570
Nuggets Cheddar & Bacon Stuffed	3 (3 oz)	240	14	17	45	8	tr	520
Potato Chip Sticks	2 pieces (4.5 oz)	350	18	24	60	16	tr	950
Bell & Evans								
Breaded Breast Nuggets	1 serv (4 oz)	220	21	9	45	13	1	380
Breasts Grilled	1 (2.75 oz)	90	21	1	50	1	0	320
Breasts Grilled Buffalo Style	1 (3 oz)	110	24	1	65	0	0	340
Burgers	1 (4 oz)	160	31	6	95	3	0	140
Chicken Tenders Gluten Free	1 serv (4 oz)	180	19	6	45	12	1	440
Wings Honey Barbeque	3 (4.6 oz)	160	17	8	80	6	0	27
Coleman								
Breast Nuggets Gluten Free	6 (2.7 oz)	130	12	6	30	10	0	380
Breast Strips	6 (2.7 oz)	130	13	3	30	14	1	250
Health Is Wealth								
Nuggets	4 (3 oz)	130	13	4	35	11	0	230
Organic Prairie								
Breast Boneless Skinless	4 oz	150	32	2	90	1	tr	160
Ground	4 oz	200	21	12	95	1	–	90
Perdue								
Breast Chunks Breaded BBQ Glazed	3 oz	190	11	8	25	17	–	630
Breast Chunks Breaded General Tso's Glazed	3 oz	190	12	8	25	16	–	610
Breast Chunks Breaded Honey BBQ Glazed	3 oz	180	12	8	55	17	–	520
Breast Chunks Breaded Honey Dijon Glazed	3 oz	200	12	11	30	16	–	600
Tyson								
Any'tizers Barbeque Style Wings	3 (3.2 oz)	200	19	13	110	7	0	380
Any'tizers Homestyle Chicken Fries	7 (3.2 oz)	230	13	11	25	19	1	590
Any'tizers Popcorn Chicken	6 (2.8 oz)	220	12	10	25	19	1	670

FOOD	PORTION	CALS	PROT	FAT	CHOL	CARB	FIBER	SOD
Breast Pattie	1 (2.6 oz)	180	10	11	25	12	1	300
Cordon Bleu	1 piece (5.9 oz)	380	22	24	80	20	1	790
Diced Strips	1 serv (3 oz)	90	20	1	45	0	0	250
Kiev	1 piece (5.9 oz)	480	17	37	150	19	1	420
READY-TO-EAT								
Applegate Farms								
Organic Roasted	2 oz	60	10	2	30	1	0	580
Butterball								
Breast Oven Roasted Thin Sliced	4 slices (2 oz)	50	11	1	20	1	0	480
Breast Strips Oven Roasted	½ pkg (3 oz)	90	18	2	60	1	–	760
Carl Buddig								
Chicken Sliced	2 oz	85	10	5	–	1	–	–
Dietz & Watson								
Breast Southern Fried	3 slices (1.9 oz)	70	11	2	30	1	0	390
Healthy Ones								
Oven Roasted 97% Fat Free	4 slices (2 oz)	60	9	2	25	2	0	410
Hormel								
Natural Choice Carved Breast Grilled	½ pkg (2 oz)	60	12	1	35	0	0	230
Oscar Mayer								
Breast Oven Roasted Thin Sliced	⅓ pkg (2 oz)	60	10	2	30	1	0	710
Breast Strips Breaded	½ pkg (3 oz)	170	15	6	30	14	–	800
Breast Strips Grilled	½ pkg (3 oz)	110	19	3	55	1	–	770
Perdue								
Breast Bites Popcorn Breaded	12 (3 oz)	190	10	12	30	14	–	580
Breast Strips Breaded Original	2 (2.6 oz)	160	9	10	25	12	–	500
Cutlets Breaded Original	1 (3 oz)	200	10	13	45	13	–	450
Nuggets Original	5 (2.9 oz)	200	10	13	45	13	–	450
Nuggets w/ Whole Grain Breading	4 (2.8 oz)	160	11	8	30	13	–	450
Short Cuts Carved Chicken Breast Original Roasted	½ cup (2.5 oz)	90	16	2	60	1	–	460

FOOD	PORTION	CALS	PROT	FAT	CHOL	CARB	FIBER	SOD
Short Cuts Chicken Breast Grilled	½ cup (2.5 oz)	90	16	2	60	1	–	460
Sara Lee								
Breast Oven Roasted	4 slices (2 oz)	45	10	1	25	0	0	430
Tyson								
Chicken Strips Fajita	1 serv (3 oz)	110	19	2	60	3	0	450
Honey Roasted Breast	2 slices (1.6 oz)	50	8	1	15	3	0	530
Hot Wings Buffalo Style	4	220	20	15	110	1	0	560
Roasted Whole Chicken Lemon Pepper	1 serv (3 oz)	120	17	6	75	1	0	510
Salad Kit Chunk Chicken	1 pkg (3.4 oz)	210	18	9	50	15	1	640
TAKE-OUT								
chicken tenders	4 (2.2 oz)	180	11	10	31	11	tr	445

CHICKEN DISHES

FOOD	PORTION	CALS	PROT	FAT	CHOL	CARB	FIBER	SOD
FROZEN								
Banquet								
Boneless Popcorn Chicken	11 pieces	180	8	9	20	18	tr	510
Wings Honey BBQ	¼ pkg (3 oz)	270	17	17	65	12	5	520
Barber								
Broccoli & Cheese Reduced Fat	1 piece (5.5 oz)	250	25	13	55	11	tr	610
Cordon Bleu	1 piece (6 oz)	370	28	23	95	14	0	840
Cordon Bleu Reduced Fat	1 piece (5.5 oz)	260	27	13	75	11	0	700
Creme Brie & Apple	1 piece (6 oz)	350	25	21	90	18	tr	830
Kiev	1 piece (6 oz)	430	27	29	110	15	tr	720
Mashed Potato Stuffed	1 piece (6 oz)	340	21	18	85	21	tr	630
Skinless Breast Stuffed	1 piece (6 oz)	280	21	11	45	24	tr	860
MIX								
Chicken Helper								
Asian Chicken Fried Rice as prep	1 cup	250	3	8	117	22	1	552

FOOD	PORTION	CALS	PROT	FAT	CHOL	CARB	FIBER	SOD
Classic Creamy Chicken & Noodles as prep	1 cup	280	3	8	60	24	tr	744
Jambalaya as prep	1 cup	280	3	8	57	15	1	816
REFRIGERATED								
Tyson								
Chicken Breast Medallions In White Wine & Garlic Sauce	1 serv (5 oz)	140	19	6	45	3	1	500
Ventera								
Rollatini w/ Rice Stuffing & Marsala Wine Sauce	1 serv + sauce (6 oz)	230	24	10	70	9	0	590
TAKE-OUT								
arroz con pollo	1 serv (16 oz)	579	48	14	126	62	2	1433
barbecued pulled chicken	1 serv (9 oz)	312	36	2	147	37	2	794
boneless breast w/ apple stuffing	1 serv (5 oz)	260	32	9	80	10	1	250
breast & wing breaded & fried	2 pieces (5.7 oz)	494	36	30	148	20	–	975
buffalo wing + sauce	2 (1.7 oz)	147	12	10	39	tr	0	97
cacciatore breast + sauce	1 serv (5.9 oz)	323	29	18	88	9	1	422
cacciatore drumstick + sauce	1 serv (3.2 oz)	172	15	9	47	5	1	225
cacciatore thigh + sauce	1 serv (3.8 oz)	204	18	11	56	6	1	268
cacciatore wing + sauce	1 serv (2.1 oz)	113	10	6	31	3	tr	148
chicharrones de pollo	3 (2.6 oz)	289	16	18	58	14	1	898
chicken & dumplings	1 cup (8.6 oz)	368	26	19	88	22	1	920
chicken & noodles in cream sauce	1 cup (8 oz)	323	22	11	76	32	1	706
chicken a la king	1 cup (8.5 oz)	465	24	34	190	16	1	880
chicken breast parmigiana	1 serv (5.8 oz)	278	25	14	119	13	1	684
chicken cordon bleu + sauce	1 roll (8 oz)	504	44	29	188	11	1	598
chicken creole w/o rice	1 cup (8.6 oz)	187	29	4	69	8	2	598

FOOD	PORTION	CALS	PROT	FAT	CHOL	CARB	FIBER	SOD
chicken kiev breast meat	1 serv (9 oz)	653	72	34	276	11	1	975
chicken meatloaf	1 lg slice (5 oz)	243	29	9	122	11	1	658
chicken paprikash	1½ cups	296	–	10	90	–	–	–
chicken pie w/ top crust	1 slice (5.6 oz)	472	19	31	–	32	1	–
chicken satay + peanut sauce	2 skewers	239	27	12	64	6	1	439
creamed chicken	1 cup (8.5 oz)	388	30	23	87	14	tr	641
croquette	1 (2.2 oz)	159	10	9	28	8	tr	239
curry	1 cup (8.3 oz)	288	27	16	83	9	2	1187
curry breast half + sauce	1 (7 oz)	244	23	14	70	8	2	1006
curry drumstick + sauce	1 (3.7 oz)	129	12	7	37	4	1	533
curry thigh + sauce	1 (4.4 oz)	154	14	9	44	5	1	634
curry wing + sauce	1 (2.4 oz)	84	8	5	24	3	1	347
drumstick & thigh breaded & fried	2 pieces (5.2 oz)	431	30	27	166	16	–	755
fricassee	1 cup (8.6 oz)	322	29	18	85	8	tr	695
groundnut stew hkatenkwan	1 serv (15.7 oz)	576	38	40	116	18	4	1009
jamaican jerk wings	4 wings (9.9 oz)	709	57	51	172	3	tr	1045
jambalaya w/ sausage & rice	1 cup (8.6 oz)	393	26	21	98	23	1	488
kobete turkish chicken w/ pastry	1 serv	513	–	13	71	–	–	551
rotisserie seasoned breast w/ skin	1 serv (3.5 oz)	184	27	8	96	0	0	347
rotisserie seasoned breast w/o skin	1 serv (3.5 oz)	148	29	3	89	0	0	314
rotisserie seasoned thigh w/ skin	1 serv (3.5 oz)	233	23	16	132	0	0	345
rotisserie seasoned thigh w/o skin	1 serv (3.5 oz)	196	24	11	130	0	0	337
sancocho de pollo dominican chicken stew	1 serv	702	71	30	195	34	1	653

FOOD	PORTION	CALS	PROT	FAT	CHOL	CARB	FIBER	SOD
stew	1 cup (8.8 oz)	176	15	5	43	19	3	496
tandoori chicken breast	1 serv	260	–	13	–	5	–	–
tandoori chicken leg & thigh	1 serv	300	–	17	–	6	–	–
tetrazzini	1 cup (8.6 oz)	369	20	18	49	29	2	669
CHICKEN SUBSTITUTES								
Chicken Free Chicken								
Country Smoked	2 oz	80	11	2	0	5	0	245
Gardein								
Buffalo Wings	1 serv (3.5 oz)	120	16	3	0	8	2	630
Chick'n Filets	1 (3.5 oz)	120	20	2	0	7	2	470
Chick'n Scallopini	1 piece (2.5 oz)	90	14	2	0	4	2	330
Crispy Fingers	2 (3.2 oz)	160	16	5	0	12	2	430
Crispy Tenders	1 (1.8 oz)	90	9	2	0	9	1	260
Tuscan Breasts	1 (5.3 oz)	150	22	3	0	11	3	550
Gardenburger								
Chik'n Grill	1 (2.5 oz)	100	13	3	0	5	5	360
Health Is Wealth								
Chicken-Free Nuggets	3 pieces (2.9 oz)	120	14	2	0	14	2	450
Loma Linda								
Fried Chik'n w/ Gravy	2 pieces (2.8 oz)	150	12	10	0	5	2	430
Morningstar Farms								
Chik'n Roasted Herb	1 pattie (2.2 oz)	110	13	3	0	9	2	380
Meal Starters Chik'n Strips	12 pieces (3 oz)	140	23	4	0	6	1	510
Veat								
Chick'n Free Nuggets	1 serv (2.5 oz)	140	21	5	0	5	2	690
Vegetarian Breast	1 (1.8 oz)	90	11	3	0	5	tr	280
Veggie Patch								
Chick'n Nuggets	4 (2.7 oz)	170	9	7	0	20	2	440
Vjana								
Chickin Fillets	1 (3.5 oz)	270	25	15	0	10	2	790
Chickin Nuggets	3 (2.6 oz)	200	16	12	0	8	2	590

FOOD	PORTION	CALS	PROT	FAT	CHOL	CARB	FIBER	SOD
Worthington								
FriChik Original	2 pieces (3.2 oz)	140	12	8	0	3	1	430
Meatless Chicken Style	1 slice (2 oz)	90	9	5	0	2	1	240
Yves								
Meatless Chicken Burger	1 (2.6 oz)	100	15	3	0	5	2	420
Meatless Smoked Chicken Slices	4 (2.2 oz)	100	14	2	0	5	0	460
CHICKPEAS								
CANNED								
chickpeas	1 cup	285	12	3	0	54	–	718
Allens								
Garbanzo Beans	½ cup	120	5	3	0	19	8	330
Green Giant								
Garbanzo Beans	½ cup	100	5	2	0	17	4	430
Progresso								
Chick Peas	½ cup (4.6 oz)	120	5	3	0	20	5	280
DRIED								
cooked	1 cup	269	15	4	0	45	–	11
Arrowhead Mills								
Organic Dried Chickpeas not prep	¼ cup	160	9	3	0	27	8	10
CHICORY								
endive fresh chopped	½ cup	4	tr	tr	0	1	–	6
greens raw chopped	½ cup	21	2	tr	0	4	–	41
root raw	1 (2.1 oz)	44	1	tr	0	11	–	30
roots raw cut up	½ cup (1.6 oz)	33	1	tr	0	8	–	23
witloof head raw	1 (1.9 oz)	9	tr	tr	0	2	–	1
witloof raw	½ cup (1.6 oz)	8	tr	tr	0	2	–	1
CHILI								
powder	1 tbsp	24	1	1	0	4	3	76
Ahh!Gourmet								
Wriggly Sambal Chili Sauce Paste	4 tbsp	170	7	9	32	15	4	391
Allergaroo								
Gluten Free Chili Mac	1 pkg (8 oz)	240	5	4	0	50	3	700

FOOD	PORTION	CALS	PROT	FAT	CHOL	CARB	FIBER	SOD
Amy's								
Organic Black Bean Medium	1 cup	200	13	2	0	31	15	680
Whole Meals Chili & Cornbread	1 pkg	340	11	6	10	59	10	680
Comfort Care								
Vegetarian White	1 cup (8 oz)	150	11	2	0	26	5	310
Dennison's								
Con Carne	1 cup	350	22	15	40	31	11	970
Fat Free w/ Beans	1 cup	210	20	2	60	29	8	1020
Turkey	1 cup	210	16	3	45	29	7	850
Vegetarian	1 cup	190	9	2	0	34	9	800
Dynasty								
Thai Chili Garlic Paste	1 tsp (5 g)	0	0	0	0	0	0	40
Health Valley								
Chunky Spicy Vegetarian No Salt Added	1 cup	150	9	1	0	31	10	75
Vegetarian Spicy	1 cup	150	9	1	0	31	10	480
Heinz								
Chili Sauce	1 tbsp (0.6 oz)	20	0	0	0	5	0	230
High Plains Bison								
Campfire Chili	1 cup (8 oz)	190	15	6	100	18	6	720
Hormel								
Chili Mac	1 pkg (9.9 oz)	270	17	7	30	34	6	980
Chili No Beans	1 pkg (7.3 oz)	190	14	8	35	16	2	860
Chili No Beans Less Sodium	1 serv (8.3 oz)	220	16	9	40	18	3	710
Chili w/ Beans	1 serv (8.7 oz)	260	16	7	30	33	7	1200
Chili w/ Beans Less Sodium	1 serv (8.7 oz)	260	16	7	30	33	7	880
Turkey Chili w/ Beans	1 serv (8.7 oz)	210	17	3	45	28	6	1250
Vegetarian Chili w/ Beans	1 serv (8.7 oz)	190	11	1	0	35	10	780

FOOD	PORTION	CALS	PROT	FAT	CHOL	CARB	FIBER	SOD
Master Chili								
Chipotle Chicken No Bean	1 serv (8.3 oz)	230	18	10	95	18	3	990
Roasted Tomato w/ Bean	1 serv (8.7 oz)	210	14	6	25	25	7	990
McIlhenny								
Original Recipe	½ cup	50	2	1	0	10	3	610
Meals To Live								
White Chicken Chili Relleno w/ Ranchero Sauce	1 pkg (9 oz)	210	15	5	25	20	4	480
Mimi's Gourmet								
Organic Vegan Gluten Free 3 Bean w/ Rice	1 pkg (11.5 oz)	270	10	6	0	46	10	670
Organic Vegan Gluten Free Black Bean & Corn	1 pkg (10.5 oz)	250	10	6	0	40	11	680
Organic Vegan Gluten Free White Bean	1 pkg (10.5 oz)	230	10	6	0	35	9	660
Spice Hunter								
Powder Blend Salt Free	¼ tsp	0	0	0	0	0	0	0
Thai Kitchen								
Roasted Red Chili Paste	1 tbsp (0.5 oz)	50	1	3	5	6	0	180
Truitt Brothers								
Beef Natural Shredded	1 cup (9.4 oz)	240	16	5	25	32	7	1110
Vegetarian	1 cup (9.4 oz)	220	11	2	0	42	10	920
Worthington								
Vegetarian	1 cup	280	24	10	0	25	8	1130
TAKE-OUT								
chiles rellenos cheese filled	1 (5 oz)	365	17	30	167	8	1	496
chili con carne w/ beans	1 cup	264	21	11	53	22	7	1275
chili con carne w/ beans & chicken	1 cup (8.9 oz)	218	19	7	53	19	6	945
con carne w/ beans & rice	1 cup	298	11	9	28	45	7	1172
vegetarian con carne	1 cup	272	19	7	0	35	11	1090

CHILI PEPPER (*see* PEPPERS)

CHINESE FOOD (*see* ASIAN FOOD)

FOOD	PORTION	CALS	PROT	FAT	CHOL	CARB	FIBER	SOD
CHINESE PRESERVING MELON								
cooked	½ cup	11	tr	tr	0	3	–	93
CHIPS (*see also* SNACKS)								
apple chips	10 (0.8 oz)	101	tr	5	0	16	2	22
banana	1 oz	147	1	10	0	17	2	2
carrot	28 (1 oz)	95	2	tr	0	22	7	77
corn	1 oz	147	2	8	0	18	2	175
plantain	1 oz	158	tr	10	–	16	1	111
potato salted	1 oz	155	2	11	0	14	1	149
potato sticks	½ cup (0.6 oz)	94	1	6	0	10	1	45
potato sticks	1 pkg (1 oz)	148	2	10	0	15	1	45
potato unsalted	1 oz	152	2	10	0	15	1	2
potato unsalted reduced fat	1 oz	138	2	6	0	19	2	2
shrimp	4 sm (0.4 oz)	56	1	4	8	5	tr	142
shrimp	4 med (0.9 oz)	141	2	9	21	13	tr	355
shrimp	4 lg (1.4 oz)	219	3	14	33	20	tr	551
soy	1 oz	107	8	2	0	15	1	239
sweet potato	1 oz	141	1	7	0	18	1	10
taro	10 (0.8 oz)	115	1	6	0	16	2	79
tortilla lowfat baked	1 oz	118	3	2	0	23	2	119
tortilla lowfat unsalted	1 oz	118	3	2	0	23	2	4
tortilla white corn	1 oz	139	2	7	0	19	2	119
tortilla yellow corn	1 oz	139	2	6	0	19	1	80
Athenos								
Pita Chips Original	11 (1 oz)	120	3	4	0	19	0	270
Beanitos								
Pinto Bean & Flax	10 (1 oz)	150	4	8	0	14	5	190
Better Balance								
Protein Chips Gluten Free All Flavors	1 oz	110	10	4	0	14	3	230
Betty Crocker								
Potato Kettle Cooked Lightly Salted	1 oz	120	2	5	0	15	1	105
Boulder Canyon								
Potato 50% Reduced Salt	14 (1 oz)	150	2	8	0	17	2	68
Potato Sour Cream & Chive	14 (1 oz)	150	2	8	0	15	2	205
Potato Spinach & Artichoke	14 (1 oz)	150	2	8	0	17	2	334

FOOD	PORTION	CALS	PROT	FAT	CHOL	CARB	FIBER	SOD
Brothers-All-Natural								
Potato Crisps Fresh Onion & Fresh Garlic	1 pkg	45	1	0	0	10	1	250
Potato Crisps Original w/ Sea Salt	1 pkg	45	1	0	0	10	1	280
Burger King								
Potato Flame Broiled	16 (1 oz)	150	1	8	0	19	1	170
Potato Ketchup & Fries	16 (1 oz)	150	1	8	0	19	1	240
Butterfield								
Potato Sticks Shoestring	1 pkg (1.7 oz)	250	3	15	0	26	3	150
Corazonas								
Potato Lightly Salted	1 oz	130	3	6	0	18	2	90
Potato Parmesan Peppercorn	1 oz	140	2	6	0	18	2	160
Potato Spicy Rio Habanero	1 oz	130	2	6	0	18	2	120
Tortilla Lightly Salted	14 (1 oz)	140	2	7	0	18	3	75
Tortilla Squeeze Of Lime	14 (1 oz)	140	2	7	0	17	3	170
Deep River Snacks								
Potato Baked Fries Sweet Maui Onion	1 oz	135	3	5	0	19	1	235
Potato Kettle Cooked Asian Sweet & Spicy	1 oz	150	2	8	0	15	1	160
Potato Kettle Cooked Original Salted	1 oz	150	2	8	0	16	1	110
Potato Kettle Cooked Rosemary & Olive Oil	1 oz	150	2	8	0	16	1	180
Potato Kettle Cooked Salt & Vinegar	1 oz	150	2	8	0	15	1	240
Potato Zesty Jalapeno	1 oz	150	2	8	0	15	1	240
Flat Earth								
Baked Fruit Crisps Apple Cinnamon Grove	14 (1 oz)	130	1	5	0	21	2	35
Baked Fruit Crisps Peach Mango Paradise	14 (1 oz)	130	1	5	0	21	1	35
Baked Fruit Crisps Wild Berry Patch	14 (1 oz)	130	1	5	0	21	1	40
Baked Veggie Crisps Farmland Cheddar	14 (1 oz)	130	2	5	0	19	2	190

FOOD	PORTION	CALS	PROT	FAT	CHOL	CARB	FIBER	SOD
Baked Veggie Crisps Garlic & Herb Field	14 (1 oz)	130	2	5	0	19	2	190
Baked Veggie Crisps Tangy Tomato Ranch	14 (1 oz)	130	2	5	0	19	2	210
FoodShouldTasteGood								
Tortilla Buffalo	10 (1 oz)	130	2	6	0	18	3	270
Tortilla Chocolate Gluten Free	1 pkg (1 oz)	140	2	7	0	19	3	80
Tortilla Multigrain Gluten Free	1 pkg (1 oz)	140	3	7	0	18	3	80
Tortilla Sweet Potato Gluten Free	10 (1 oz)	130	2	6	0	18	3	80
French's								
Potato Sticks Barbecue	¾ cup	160	2	10	0	16	1	190
Potato Sticks Original	¾ cup	190	2	12	0	16	1	190
Fritos								
Original	32 (1 oz)	160	2	10	0	16	1	160
Glenny's								
Organic Soy Barbeque	1 oz	110	8	3	–	13	3	350
Organic Soy Creamy Ranch	1 oz	110	9	3	–	12	3	300
Soy Crisps Apple Cinnamon	½ pkg (0.6 oz)	70	5	2	–	10	2	90
Soy Crisps Caramel	½ pkg (1.3 oz)	70	5	2	0	9	1	125
Soy Crisps Low Fat Lightly Salted	½ pkg (0.6 oz)	70	5	1	–	9	2	170
Soy Crisps No Salt	½ pkg (0.6 oz)	70	5	1	–	9	2	100
Soy Crisps Salt & Pepper	½ pkg (0.6 oz)	70	5	1	–	9	2	190
Soy Crisps White Cheddar	½ pkg (0.6 oz)	70	5	2	–	9	2	180
Spud Delites Sea Salt	1 pkg (1.1 oz)	100	2	1	–	21	1	270
Veggie Fries	½ pkg (0.6 oz)	70	1	1	0	13	0	120
Zen Health Tortilla Crisps Original	1 oz	110	9	3	0	12	tr	250
Guiltless Gourmet								
Tortilla Blue Corn	18 (1 oz)	120	3	3	0	23	2	250

OOD	PORTION	CALS	PROT	FAT	CHOL	CARB	FIBER	SOD
otato Original	1 oz	150	2	7	0	19	3	90
weet Potato Baked	1 oz	110	1	2	0	23	1	310
ortilla Gluten Free MultiGrain	10 (1 oz)	150	2	7	0	19	3	80
Tortilla White Corn	1 oz	140	2	5	0	23	2	110
Stacy's								
Pita Chips Multigrain	1 pkg	140	3	6	0	17	2	240
Pita Chips Parmesan Garlic & Herb	1 oz	140	4	5	0	19	2	200
Pita Chips Texarkana Hot	1 oz	130	3	5	0	19	2	260
Soy Thin Chips Sticky Bun	18 (1 oz)	130	6	5	0	15	3	180
Soy Thin Crisps Simply Cheese	18 (1 oz)	130	7	6	0	13	3	230
SunChips								
Original	16 (1 oz)	140	2	6	0	18	2	120
T.G.I. Friday's								
Potato Cheese Pizza	16 (1 oz)	160	2	9	0	17	1	190
Tater Skins								
Cheddar Bacon	16 (1 oz)	150	1	8	0	19	1	170
Original	16 (1 oz)	150	1	8	0	19	1	170
Terra								
Exotic Vegetable Original	14 (1 oz)	150	7	9	0	16	3	150
Exotic Vegetable Zesty Tomato	14 (1 oz)	150	1	9	0	16	3	190
ettles Potato Sea Salt & Pepper	15 (1 oz)	140	2	6	0	18	tr	65
snip Chips	12 (1 oz)	150	2	10	0	13	5	50
to Au Natural	18 (1 oz)	150	2	9	0	15	2	0
o Blues	1 oz	130	2	6	0	19	3	115
Frites Sea Salt egar	1 oz	150	2	8	0	18	3	200
olds Original	1 oz	130	2	5	0	19	0	80
pourri	1 oz	140	2	7	0	17	4	110
Bliss	1 oz	140	1	7	0	18	2	110
Exotic	1 oz	150	1	9	0	16	3	110
	17 (1 oz)	160	1	11	0	15	3	10
	16 (1 oz)	150	2	9	0	15	1	5
	1 oz	140	1	6	0	19	4	110

FOOD	PORTION	CALS	PROT	FAT	CHOL	CARB	FIBER	SOD
Tortilla Chili Lime	18 (1 oz)	120	2	3	0	19	2	150
Tortilla Chipotle	18 (1 oz)	123	2	3	0	22	2	250
Tortilla Yellow Corn	18 (1 oz)	120	2	3	0	22	2	250
Tortilla Yellow Corn Unsalted	18 (1 oz)	120	3	2	0	22	2	26
Hippie Chips								
Baked Potato Chive-Talkin' Sour Cream	1 pkg (0.7 oz)	90	2	3	0	14	tr	300
Baked Potato Haight AshBerry Jalapeno	1 pkg (0.7 oz)	90	1	3	0	15	tr	310
Baked Potato Memphis Blues Barbecue	1 pkg (0.7 oz)	90	1	3	0	15	tr	310
Baked Potato Sea Of Love Salt	1 pkg (1 oz)	125	2	4	0	21	1	280
Baked Potato Woodstock Ranch	1 pkg (0.7 oz)	90	2	3	0	14	tr	300
Jay's								
Potato	1 oz	150	2	10	0	14	1	190
Late July								
Organic Multigrain Dude Ranch	13 (1 oz)	120	2	5	0	17	2	190
Organic Multigrain Mild Green Mojo	13 (1 oz)	110	2	5	0	17	2	210
Little Wings								
Multi Grain Hot Buffalo Wing w/ Bleu Cheese Drizzle	1 pkg (0.5 oz)	60	1	3	0	10	2	200
Lundberg								
Rice Chips Original Sea Salt	1 oz	140	2	7	0	18	tr	110
Rice Chips Sesame Seaweed	1 oz	140	2	7	0	18	tr	90
Rice Chips Wasabi	1 oz	140	2	6	0	18	1	210
Madhouse Munchies								
Potato Sea Salt	16	150	2	9	0	16	1	80
Potato Sea Salt & Vinegar	16	150	2	9	0	16	2	130
Tortilla White	9	140	2	6	0	19	1	110
Mexi-Snax								
Tortilla Multi-Grain Blue	15 (1 oz)	140	2	7	0	17	2	110
Tortilla Pico De Gallo	15 (1 oz)	140	2	7	0	18	2	185

FOOD	PORTION	CALS	PROT	FAT	CHOL	CARB	FIBER	SOD
Tortilla Salted	15 (1 oz)	140	2	7	0	18	2	70
Tortilla Tamari	15 (1 oz)	130	2	6	0	17	2	170
Michael Season's								
Potato Crisps Thin Baked Low Fat	14	120	2	2	0	23	2	180
Potato Kettle Style Reduced Fat	18	130	2	6	0	18	1	240
Potato Reduced Fat	20	140	2	7	0	17	1	130
Potato Reduced Fat Unsalted	20	140	2	7	0	17	1	10
Poore Brothers								
Original	14 (1 oz)	140	2	9	0	15	1	180
Salt & Vinegar	15 (1 oz)	150	2	9	0	15	1	470
Sweet Maui Onion	14 (1 oz)	140	2	9	0	15	1	247
Popchips								
Potato Barbeque	19 (1 oz)	120	1	4	0	20	1	250
Potato Cheddar	20 (1 oz)	120	2	4	0	20	1	290
Potato Original	22 (1 oz)	120	1	4	0	20	1	280
Potato Parmesan Garlic	20 (1 oz)	120	2	4	0	20	1	310
Potato Salt & Pepper	11 (0.4 oz)	50	1	2	0	8	1	120
Potato Sea Salt & Vinegar	20 (1 oz)	120	1	4	0	20	1	290
Potato Sour Cream & Onion	20 (1 oz)	120	2	4	0	20	1	290
Pringles								
Jalapeno	15 (1 oz)	150	1	10	0	14	tr	190
Loaded Baked Potato	15 (1 oz)	150	1	10	0	14	tr	170
Minis Cheddar Cheese	1 pkg	120	1	7	0	12	tr	220
Minis Original	1 pkg	120	1	7	0	13	tr	140
Original	14 (1 oz)	160	1	11	0	14	tr	170
Pizza	15 (1 oz)	150	1	10	0	14	tr	190
Select Cinnamon Sweet Potato	28 (1 oz)	150	1	9	0	16	1	15
Select Parmesan Garlic	28 (1 oz)	140	1	9	0	15	tr	180
Snack Stacks Original	1 pkg	140	1	10	0	12	tr	150
Revolution Foods								
Organic Popalongs Whole Grains Cheesy Cheese	16 (0.7 oz)	90	2	3	5	14	1	210
Organic Popalongs Whole Grains Original	16 (0.7 oz)	100	2	3	0	15	1	200

FOOD	PORTION	CALS	PROT	FAT	CHOL	CARB	F	
Organic Popalongs Whole Grains Simply Cinnamon	16 (0.7 oz)	100	1	3	0	16		
Rhythm								
Crispy Kale Kool Ranch	½ pkg (1 oz)	100	6	5	0	10		
Crispy Kale Zesty Nacho	½ pkg (1 oz)	106	5	5	0	12	2	
Crispy Kate Bombay Curry	½ pkg (1 oz)	101	4	2	0	11	2	
Robert's American Gourmet								
Soy Crisps Country Barbecue	1 oz	130	7	4	0	15	3	
Salba Smart								
Organic Blue Corn Omega-3 Enriched	1 oz	104	2	6	0	19	4	
Seneca								
Crispy Apple Apple Pie Ala Mode	12 (1 oz)	140	0	7	0	20	2	4[illegible]
Crispy Apple Caramel	12 (1 oz)	140	0	7	0	20	2	15
Crispy Apple Cinnamon	14 (1 oz)	150	1	7	0	18	4	30
Crispy Apple Original	12 (1 oz)	140	0	7	0	20	2	15
Crispy Apple Sour Apple	12 (1 oz)	150	0	9	0	18	3	10
Sensible Portions								
Garden Veggie Sea Salt	1 pkg (0.5 oz)	70	1	4	0	8	tr	
Snikiddy								
Fries Potato Bold Buffalo Gluten Free	1 oz	130	2	5	0	20	1	
Fries Potato Classic Ketchup Gluten Free	1 oz	130	2	5	0	21		
Fries Potato Original Gluten Free	1 oz	130	2	5	0			
Fries Potato Southwest Cheddar Gluten Free	1 oz	130	2	5				
Snyder's Of Hanover								
Kosher Dill	1 oz	140	2					
MultiGrain Sunflower	1 oz	140	2					
MultiGrain Sunflower Southwestern Cheddar	1 oz	140						
MultiGrain Tortilla Lightly Salted	1 oz	1[illegible]						
MultiGrain Tortilla Strips Flaxseed Gold	1 oz							
Organic Veggie Crisps	1 oz	140						

Pa
Pota
Potat
Potato
& Vin
Potato G
Potato Po
Potato Red
Stix Original
Vegetable
Sweet Potato
Sweets & Beets
Taro

FOOD	PORTION	CALS	PROT	FAT	CHOL	CARB	FIBER	SOD
The Whole Earth								
Tortilla Really Seedy Multigrain	9 (1 oz)	140	2	9	0	14	2	150
Thunder								
Potato Buffalo Wing w/ Blue Cheese	22 (1 oz)	150	1	8	0	16	tr	280
Sour Cream & Onion	22 (1 oz)	150	2	9	0	15	tr	280
Utz								
Pita Natural w/ Sea Salt	1 oz	120	3	5	0	18	tr	140
Potato	20 (1 oz)	150	2	9	0	14	1	95
Potato Baked	1 oz	110	2	2	0	23	2	170
Potato BBQ	20 (1 oz)	150	2	10	0	14	1	200
Potato Grandma Kettle	1 oz	140	2	8	5	14	1	120
Potato Homestyle Kettle	1 oz	140	2	8	0	14	1	120
Potato Kettle Classics	20 (1 oz)	150	2	9	0	15	1	120
Potato Mystic Kettle	1 oz	150	2	9	0	15	1	120
Potato Mystic Kettle Reduced Fat	1 oz	130	2	6	0	18	1	120
Potato Natural Lightly Salted Kettle	1 oz	140	2	8	0	15	1	95
Potato No Salt Added	20 (1 oz)	150	2	9	0	14	1	5
Potato Onion & Garlic	1 oz	150	2	9	0	14	1	180
Potato Ripple	20 (1 oz)	150	2	10	0	14	1	95
Sweet Potato Kettle Classics	20 (1 oz)	150	1	9	0	16	2	65
Tortilla Baked	10	120	2	2	0	23	1	125
Tortilla Organic Yellow Corn	1 oz	140	2	6	0	19	2	100
Vegetable Natural Exotic Medley	1 oz	160	2	10	0	15	2	110
Yogachips								
Organic Apple Chips Peach	1 pkg (0.35 oz)	35	0	0	0	9	tr	7
Zapp's								
Potato Cajun Dill	1 oz	150	2	8	0	17	1	180
Potato No Salt	1 oz	150	2	9	0	18	1	0
Potato Original	1 oz	150	2	8	0	17	1	50
Potato Sizzlin Steak	1 oz	150	2	8	0	17	1	270
Sweet Potato Lightly Salted	1 oz	150	1	8	0	17	1	30

FOOD	PORTION	CALS	PROT	FAT	CHOL	CARB	FIBER	SOD
CHITTERLINGS								
pork cooked	3 oz	258	9	24	122	0	0	33
CHIVES								
freeze-dried	1 tbsp	1	tr	tr	0	tr	–	–
fresh chopped	1 tsp	0	tr	tr	0	tr	–	0
fresh chopped	1 tbsp	1	tr	tr	0	tr	–	0
CHOCOLATE (*see also* CANDY, CHOCOLATE SPREAD, CHOCOLATE SYRUP, COCOA, HOT CHOCOLATE, ICE CREAM TOPPINGS, MILK DRINKS)								
BAKING								
baking	1 oz	145	3	15	0	8	–	1
grated unsweetened	¼ cup	165	4	17	0	10	6	8
liquid unsweetened	1 oz	134	3	14	0	10	5	3
mexican baking	1 sq (0.7 oz)	85	1	3	0	15	1	1
squares unsweetened	1 sq (1 oz)	145	4	15	0	9	5	7
Hershey's								
Unsweetened Block	1 (0.5 oz)	70	2	7	–	4	2	–
CHIPS								
milk chocolate	1 cup (6 oz)	862	12	52	38	100	–	138
semisweet	1 cup (6 oz)	804	7	50	0	106	–	19
semisweet	60 pieces (1 oz)	136	1	9	0	18	–	3
E. Guittard								
Cappuccino	30 (0.5 oz)	80	tr	5	0	9	0	15
Milk Chocolate	12 (0.5 oz)	80	1	5	5	9	0	10
Semisweet	30 (0.5 oz)	70	tr	4	0	10	tr	0
Ghirardelli								
Semi-Sweet	32 (0.5 oz)	70	1	5	0	10	tr	0
Hershey's								
Milk Chocolate	1 tbsp (0.5 oz)	70	1	5	<5	9	1	10
Premier White	1 tbsp (0.5 oz)	80	1	4	–	9	–	30
Semi-Sweet	1 tbsp (0.5 oz)	70	tr	4	–	10	tr	–
Special Dark	1 tbsp (0.5 oz)	70	tr	5	–	9	1	5
Sugar Free	1 tbsp (0.5 oz)	70	tr	5	–	9	1	–

FOOD	PORTION	CALS	PROT	FAT	CHOL	CARB	FIBER	SOD
MIX								
drink mix powder	2–3 heaping tsp	75	1	1	0	20	–	45
drink mix powder as prep w/ whole milk	9 oz	226	9	9	33	31	–	165
Nesquik								
Chocolate Powder	2 tbsp (0.6 oz)	60	tr	1	0	14	tr	30
Chocolate Powder No Sugar Added	2 tbsp (0.4 oz)	35	1	1	0	7	1	70
Sunfood								
Organic Powder	2 tbsp (1 oz)	120	6	4	0	15	9	6

CHOCOLATE MILK (*see* MILK DRINKS)

CHOCOLATE SPREAD

FOOD	PORTION	CALS	PROT	FAT	CHOL	CARB	FIBER	SOD
Love'n Bake								
Chocolate Schmear	2 tbsp	140	4	8	0	14	2	0

CHOCOLATE SYRUP

FOOD	PORTION	CALS	PROT	FAT	CHOL	CARB	FIBER	SOD
chocolate fudge	1 tbsp (0.7 oz)	73	1	3	–	12	–	27
chocolate fudge	1 cup (11.9 oz)	1176	15	46	–	200	–	442
syrup	2 tbsp	82	1	tr	0	22	–	36
syrup	1 cup	653	6	3	0	177	–	287
syrup as prep w/ whole milk	1 cup (9.9 oz)	254	9	8	25	36	1	133
Hershey's								
Lite	2 tbsp (1.2 oz)	45	0	0	0	11	tr	70
Sugar Free	2 tbsp (1.1 oz)	15	tr	0	0	5	tr	120
Sundae Syrup Double Chocolate	2 tbsp (1.3 oz)	100	tr	0	0	24	1	15
Syrup	2 tbsp (1.4 oz)	100	tr	0	0	24	1	15
Nesquik								
Calcium Fortified	2 tbsp (1.3 oz)	100	0	0	0	25	tr	55
Santa Cruz								
Organic	2 tbsp	110	1	0	0	27	tr	0

FOOD	PORTION	CALS	PROT	FAT	CHOL	CARB	FIBER	SOD
Steel's								
No Sugar Added Fat Free	2 tbsp (1 oz)	50	1	0	0	17	0	10
U-Bet								
Original	2 tbsp (1.4 oz)	128	1	0	0	29	–	35
CHUTNEY								
apple	1.2 oz	68	tr	0	–	18	1	–
coconut	2 oz	87	1	9	0	1	3	217
fresh mint	2 oz	18	1	0	0	3	1	432
mango	¼ cup (2 oz)	227	2	5	0	43	10	–
tomato	1 oz	90	1	7	6	6	2	269
Beth's Farm Kitchen								
Blazing Tomato	2 tbsp (1 oz)	25	0	0	0	6	0	10
Chukar Cherries								
Curried Cherry	1 tbsp	30	0	0	0	8	tr	85
Patak's								
Major Grey	1 tbsp	60	0	0	0	14	0	290
Mango Hot	1 tbsp	60	0	0	0	14	0	300
Mango Sweet	1 tbsp	60	0	1	0	14	0	310
Robert Rothchild Farm								
Hot Peach & Apple	2 tbsp	45	0	0	0	12	tr	35
School House Kitchen								
Bardshar	1 oz	80	0	0	0	20	1	240
The Gracious Gourmet								
Mango Pineapple	2 tbsp (1 oz)	45	0	1	0	9	0	5
Wild Thymes Farm								
Apricot Cranberry Walnut	1 tbsp	16	tr	0	0	4	tr	0
Plum Currant Ginger	1 tsp	20	tr	0	0	5	tr	1
CILANTRO								
fresh	¼ cup	1	tr	tr	0	tr	tr	2
fresh sprigs	5 (5 g)	1	tr	tr	0	tr	tr	3
CINNAMON								
cinnamon sugar	1 tsp	16	tr	tr	0	4	tr	0
ground	1 tsp	6	tr	tr	0	2	1	0
sticks	0.5 oz	39	1	tr	–	8	3	4
McCormick								
Grinder Cinnamon Sugar	1 tsp (3.5 g)	10	0	0	0	2	0	0

FOOD	PORTION	CALS	PROT	FAT	CHOL	CARB	FIBER	SOD
CISCO								
raw	3 oz	84	16	2	–	0	0	47
smoked	1 oz	50	5	3	9	0	0	135
CLAMS								
CANNED								
liquid only	1 cup	6	1	tr	–	tr	–	516
liquid only	3 oz	2	tr	tr	–	tr	–	183
meat only	3 oz	126	22	2	57	4	–	95
meat only	1 cup	236	41	3	107	8	–	179
Polar								
Baby	¼ cup	30	5	0	20	3	0	280
FRESH								
cooked	20 sm	133	23	2	60	5	–	100
cooked	3 oz	126	22	2	57	4	–	95
raw	20 sm (6.3 oz)	133	23	2	60	5	–	100
raw	9 lg (6.3 oz)	133	23	2	60	5	–	100
raw	3 oz	63	11	1	29	2	–	47
FROZEN								
Mrs. Paul's								
Fried	18 (3 oz)	270	9	13	20	29	1	690
SeaPak								
Oven Crunchy Strips	1 serv (3 oz)	250	7	14	15	24	0	420
TAKE-OUT								
breaded & fried	20 sm	379	27	21	115	19	–	684
CLEMENTINE JUICE								
Izze								
Sparkling Clementine	1 bottle (12 oz)	120	0	0	0	30	–	25
CLEMENTINES								
Cuties								
Fresh	2 (6 oz)	80	1	1	0	17	4	0
Disney Garden								
Clementines	1	35	1	0	0	9	1	1
CLOVES								
ground	1 tsp	7	tr	tr	0	1	1	5

FOOD	PORTION	CALS	PROT	FAT	CHOL	CARB	FIBER	SOD
COCOA (*see also* HOT CHOCOLATE)								
cocoa butter	1 tbsp	120	0	14	0	0	0	0
powder unsweetened	1 tbsp	12	1	1	0	3	2	1
CocoaVia								
Beverage Mix Dark Chocolate	1 pkg (0.28 oz)	30	1	1	–	5	1	90
Hershey's								
Cocoa	1 tbsp (5 g)	10	tr	1	–	3	2	–
COCONUT								
dried sweetened shredded	¼ cup	116	1	8	0	11	1	61
dried toasted	1 oz	168	2	13	0	13	–	10
dried unsweetened	1 oz	187	2	18	0	7	5	10
fresh from 1 coconut	14 oz	1405	13	133	0	60	36	79
fresh shredded	¼ cup	71	1	7	0	3	2	4
Bob's Red Mill								
Shredded	3 tbsp	120	1	11	0	4	2	5
Let's Do Organic								
Organic Reduced Fat Shredded	1 can (0.5 oz)	70	1	6	0	4	2	0
Shredded	3 tbsp (0.5 oz)	110	1	10	0	4	2	5
Mounds								
Sweetened Flakes	2 tbsp (0.5 oz)	70	tr	5	–	6	1	35
Prosperity								
Organic Coconut Flax Butter Garlic & Onion	1 tbsp	140	0	15	0	0	0	0
COCONUT JUICE								
coconut water fresh	½ cup	23	1	tr	0	4	1	126
creamed sweetened canned	½ cup	264	1	12	0	39	tr	27
milk canned	½ cup	276	3	29	0	7	3	18
Coco King								
Roasted w/ Pulp	1 can (11.75 oz)	130	1	0	0	29	1	80
W/ Pulp	1 can (11.85 oz)	130	0	2	0	30	–	60

FOOD	PORTION	CALS	PROT	FAT	CHOL	CARB	FIBER	SOD
Goya								
Coconut Water	1 can (11.8 oz)	120	0	1	0	29	tr	130
Let's Do Organic								
Creamed	1 oz	220	4	19	0	8	6	10
Milk	¼ cup	100	1	11	0	2	0	5
O.N.E.								
Natural Coconut Water	1 box (11 oz)	60	1	0	0	15	0	60
Thai Kitchen								
Lite Coconut Milk	2 oz	45	0	4	0	1	0	0
Zico								
Coconut Water All Flavors	1 pkg (11 oz)	60	1	0	0	15	0	60
COD								
atlantic canned	3 oz	89	19	1	47	0	0	185
atlantic canned	1 can (11 oz)	327	71	3	171	0	0	680
atlantic dried	3 oz	246	53	2	129	0	0	5973
atlantic fresh cooked	3 oz	89	19	1	47	0	0	66
atlantic fresh cooked	1 fillet (6.3 oz)	189	41	2	99	0	0	141
atlantic fresh raw	3 oz	70	15	1	37	0	0	46
pacific fresh baked	3 oz	95	21	1	43	0	0	82
roe canned	1 oz	34	6	1	–	tr	–	–
roe tarama	3.5 oz	547	8	55	–	6	–	600
Mrs. Paul's								
Filets Lightly Breaded	1 (4 oz)	220	12	11	40	17	1	430
TAKE-OUT								
roe baked w/ butter & lemon juice	1 oz	36	6	1	–	tr	–	21
COFFEE (*see also* COFFEE BEVERAGES, COFFEE SUBSTITUTES)								
INSTANT								
decaffeinated as prep	8 oz	2	tr	0	0	0	0	5
decaffeinated powder	1 rounded tsp	4	tr	0	0	1	0	0
regular powder	1 rounded tsp	4	tr	tr	0	1	0	64
REGULAR								
brewed	8 oz	2	tr	tr	0	0	0	5
roasted beans	1 oz	64	4	4	–	18	2	–
Spava								
Calm Decaffeinated	1 cup	0	0	0	0	0	0	0

FOOD	PORTION	CALS	PROT	FAT	CHOL	CARB	FIBER	SOD
COFFEE BEVERAGES								
Click								
Espresso Protein Drink as prep	2 scoops (1.1 oz)	120	15	2	<5	12	tr	115
Coffee Spoons								
Flavored	1 (0.6 oz)	90	1	5	0	11	1	15
Emmi								
Caffe Latte Light	1 pkg (7.7 oz)	80	8	0	10	12	1	170
General Foods								
International Coffees Vanilla Bean Latte	1 serv	60	0	2	–	12	–	50
Health Is Wealth								
Nutriccino Vitamin Infused All Flavors	1 bottle (9.5 oz)	190	4	3	10	37	0	260
Vitamin Coffee Ener-G Infused Vanilla Latte	1 bottle (9.5 oz)	190	4	3	10	37	0	260
Iced 'Spresso								
Ultra Light American Vanilla	1 bottle (9.5 oz)	90	6	3	10	11	0	180
Ultra Light Espresso Latte	1 bottle (9.5 oz)	70	6	0	0	11	0	190
N.O. Brew								
Iced Coffee not prep	1 serv (2.6 oz)	10	0	0	0	1	0	0
O.N.E.								
Coffee Fruit	1 bottle (11 oz)	107	tr	1	0	26	1	10
POMx								
Iced Cafe Au Lait	1 bottle (10.5 oz)	170	7	3	15	29	0	130
Iced Cafe Vanilla	1 bottle (10.5 oz)	180	11	0	0	43	0	130
Wolfgang Puck								
Culinary Iced All Flavors	1 bottle (8.5 oz)	120	3	3	10	23	–	150
TAKE-OUT								
cafe amaretto w/ alcohol	1 serv	192	1	9	33	15	0	14
cafe au lait	1 cup (8 oz)	77	4	4	17	6	–	62
cafe brulot	1 cup	48	tr	0	0	3	–	2
cafe brulot w/ alcohol	1 serv	130	1	tr	0	16	3	4

FOOD	PORTION	CALS	PROT	FAT	CHOL	CARB	FIBER	SOD
cappuccino	1 cup (8 oz)	77	4	4	17	6	–	62
coffee con leche	1 cup (6 oz)	104	3	4	10	16	0	36
cuban coffee w/ rum & creme de cacao	1 (9 oz)	112	3	2	–	6	0	–
dutch coffee w/ gin	1 (7 oz)	181	1	10	29	6	0	19
espresso	1 cup (4 oz)	2	tr	tr	0	0	0	17
french coffee w/ orange liqueur & kahlua	1 (8 oz)	232	1	10	29	24	0	–
irish coffee	1 serv (8 oz)	209	1	11	38	5	0	13
italian coffee w/ strega	1 (7 oz)	163	1	10	–	12	0	19
latte w/ skim milk	1 serv (13 oz)	88	8	tr	4	12	0	128
latte w/ whole milk	1 serv (14 oz)	143	9	6	20	15	0	126
mocha	1 serv (17 oz)	403	11	9	29	69	2	199
puerto rican coffee w/ rum & kahlua	1 (8 oz)	166	1	10	29	9	0	–
turkish	1 cup (4 oz)	50	tr	1	0	12	0	1

COFFEE SUBSTITUTES

Pixie								
Mate Latte Chai	½ cup (4 oz)	80	0	0	0	18	tr	5
Mate Latte Dark Roast	½ cup (4 oz)	70	0	0	0	16	tr	0
Mate Latte Mocha	½ cup (4 oz)	70	0	0	0	18	0	0
Mate Latte Original	½ cup (4 oz)	70	0	0	0	17	0	0

COFFEE WHITENERS

Baileys								
Caramel	1 tbsp (0.5 oz)	40	0	2	0	6	0	0
French Vanilla	1 tbsp (0.5 oz)	40	0	2	5	6	0	0
Hazelnut	1 tbsp (0.5 oz)	35	0	2	5	5	0	5
Original Irish Cream	1 tbsp (0.5 oz)	40	0	2	5	5	0	5
Farmland								
Nondairy Creamer	2 tbsp	40	1	3	15	2	0	15
International Delight								
Amaretto	1 tbsp (0.5 oz)	40	0	2	0	7	0	5

FOOD	PORTION	CALS	PROT	FAT	CHOL	CARB	FIBER	SOD
Caramel Macchiato	1 tbsp (0.5 oz)	40	0	2	0	7	0	5
Caribbean Cinnamon Creme	1 tbsp (0.5 oz)	45	0	2	0	6	0	5
Dark Chocolate Cream	1 tbsp (0.5 oz)	35	0	2	5	6	0	0
English Almond Toffee	1 tbsp (0.5 oz)	45	0	2	0	6	0	5
French Vanilla	1 tbsp (0.5 oz)	45	0	2	0	6	0	5
French Vanilla Fat Free	1 tbsp (0.5 oz)	30	0	0	0	7	0	0
French Vanilla Sugar Free	1 tbsp (0.5 oz)	20	0	2	0	1	0	0
Irish Creme	1 tbsp (0.5 oz)	40	0	2	0	7	0	5
Vanilla Caramel Cream	1 tbsp (0.5 oz)	35	0	2	5	6	0	0
Vanilla Latte	1 tbsp (0.5 oz)	40	0	2	0	7	0	5
Silk								
French Vanilla	1 tbsp (0.5 oz)	20	0	1	0	3	0	10
Original	1 tbsp (0.5 oz)	15	0	1	0	1	0	10
WildWood								
Soymilk Creamer Plain	1 tbsp	15	0	2	0	1	0	0
COLESLAW								
Fresh Express								
3 Color Deli	1½ cups	20	1	0	0	5	2	15
Kit w/ Sweet & Creamy Dressing as prep	1 cup	120	1	8	5	12	2	135
Old Fashioned	2 cups	25	1	0	0	5	2	15
Mann's								
Broccoli Cole Slaw w/o Dressing	1 serv (3 oz)	25	2	0	0	5	3	25
Ready Pac								
Coleslaw	1½ cups (3 oz)	20	1	0	0	5	2	20

FOOD	PORTION	CALS	PROT	FAT	CHOL	CARB	FIBER	SOD
Coleslaw Mix as prep	1 cup (3.5 oz)	130	1	9	5	13	2	160
TAKE-OUT								
coleslaw w/ dressing	¾ cup	147	1	11	5	13	–	267
vinegar & oil coleslaw	3.5 oz	150	1	9	0	16	–	480
COLLARDS								
fresh cooked	½ cup	17	1	tr	0	4	–	10
frzn chopped cooked	½ cup	31	3	tr	0	6	–	42
raw chopped	½ cup	6	tr	tr	0	1	–	4
Allens								
Seasoned Southern Style	½ cup (4.1 oz)	35	2	0	0	6	2	930
Glory								
Green Fresh	2 cups	25	2	0	0	5	3	15
Seasoned canned	½ cup	35	2	0	0	5	2	490
Sensibly Seasoned canned	½ cup	20	2	0	0	4	2	240
Seabrook Farms								
Chopped Greens frzn	½ cup (3.1 oz)	30	2	0	0	2	2	20
COOKIES								
MIX								
chocolate chip	1 (0.56 oz)	79	1	4	7	10	–	47
oatmeal	1 (0.6 oz)	74	1	3	7	10	tr	75
oatmeal raisin	1 (0.6 oz)	74	1	3	7	10	tr	75
Betty Crocker								
Caramelita Bars as prep	1	190	2	8	9	28	1	115
Chocolate Chip as prep	2	170	1	8	27	21	tr	105
Oatmeal as prep	2	160	2	7	27	22	tr	105
Peanut Butter as prep	2	150	2	7	12	20	–	140
Reese's Dessert Bar Mix No Bake as prep	1	180	2	10	12	20	1	125
Sugar as prep	2	160	1	8	27	21	0	80
Sunkist Lemon Bars as prep	1	140	tr	4	39	24	–	80
Turtle Cookie Bars as prep	1	180	2	8	9	27	tr	140
Duncan Hines								
Chocolate Chip as prep	2 (1.1 oz)	180	1	9	10	23	0	85
READY-TO-EAT								
animal crackers	1 (2.5 g)	11	tr	tr	–	2	–	10

FOOD	PORTION	CALS	PROT	FAT	CHOL	CARB	FIBER	SOD
animal crackers	1 box (2.4 oz)	299	4	9	11	51	–	274
animal crackers	11 (1 oz)	126	2	4	–	21	–	112
australian anzac biscuit	1	98	1	3	0	17	1	59
butter	1 (5 g)	23	tr	1	–	3	tr	18
chocolate chip	1 (0.4 oz)	48	1	2	–	7	tr	32
chocolate chip	1 box (1.9 oz)	233	3	12	12	36	–	188
chocolate chip low sugar low sodium	1 (0.24 oz)	31	tr	1	0	5	–	1
chocolate chip lowfat	1 (0.25 oz)	45	1	2	0	7	–	38
chocolate chip soft-type	1 (0.5 oz)	69	1	4	0	9	tr	49
chocolate w/ creme filling	1 (0.35 oz)	47	1	2	–	7	tr	36
chocolate w/ creme filling chocolate coated	1 (0.60 oz)	82	1	5	–	11	–	55
chocolate w/ creme filling sugar free low sodium	1 (0.35 oz)	46	1	2	–	7	–	24
chocolate w/ extra creme filling	1 (0.46 oz)	65	1	3	–	9	–	64
chocolate wafer	1 (0.2 oz)	26	tr	1	0	4	–	35
cream cheese	1 (1.1 oz)	141	2	9	25	14	tr	53
digestive biscuits plain	2	141	2	7	–	21	1	–
fig bars	1 (0.56 oz)	56	1	1	–	11	1	56
fortune	1 (0.28 oz)	30	tr	tr	–	7	tr	22
fudge	1 (0.73 oz)	73	1	1	–	17	tr	40
gingersnaps	1 (0.24 oz)	29	tr	1	0	5	–	48
graham	1 sq (0.24 oz)	30	1	1	0	5	–	42
graham chocolate covered	1 (0.49 oz)	68	1	3	0	9	–	41
graham honey	1 (0.24 oz)	30	1	1	0	5	tr	42
hermits	1 (1 oz)	117	2	5	23	18	1	54
jumbles coconut	1 (1 oz)	121	1	7	26	13	1	19
ladyfingers	1 (0.38 oz)	40	1	1	40	7	–	16
macaroons	1 (0.8 oz)	97	1	3	0	17	–	59
madeleines	1 (0.8 oz)	86	2	5	46	10	tr	34
marshmallow chocolate coated	1 (0.46 oz)	55	1	2	–	9	–	22
marshmallow pie chocolate coated	1 (1.4 oz)	165	2	7	–	26	–	66
molasses	1 (0.5 oz)	65	1	2	0	11	–	69
neapolitan tri-color cookie	1 (0.6 oz)	79	1	5	17	8	tr	10

FOOD	PORTION	CALS	PROT	FAT	CHOL	CARB	FIBER	SOD
oatmeal	1 (0.6 oz)	81	1	3	0	12	1	69
oatmeal soft-type	1 (0.5 oz)	61	1	2	–	10	tr	52
oatmeal raisin	1 (0.6 oz)	81	1	3	0	12	1	69
oatmeal raisin low sugar no sodium	1 (0.24 oz)	31	tr	1	0	5	–	1
oatmeal raisin soft-type	1 (0.5 oz)	61	1	2	–	10	tr	52
peanut butter sandwich	1 (0.5 oz)	67	1	3	0	9	–	52
peanut butter sandwich sugar free low sodium	1 (0.35 oz)	54	1	3	–	5	–	41
peanut butter soft-type	1 (0.5 oz)	69	1	4	0	9	tr	50
pinenut cookies	1 (1.1 oz)	134	4	9	0	11	1	11
raisin soft-type	1 (0.5 oz)	60	1	2	0	10	–	51
reginette queen's biscuit	1 (0.8 oz)	86	2	3	tr	13	tr	83
shortbread	1 (0.28 oz)	40	1	2	2	5	–	36
shortbread pecan	1 (0.49 oz)	79	1	5	5	8	tr	39
spritz	1 (0.4 oz)	42	1	2	6	6	tr	9
sugar	1 (0.52 oz)	72	1	3	8	10	–	53
sugar low sugar sodium free	1 (0.24 oz)	30	1	1	0	5	–	0
sugar wafers w/ creme filling	1 (0.12 oz)	18	tr	1	0	3	–	5
sugar wafers w/ creme filling sugar free sodium free	1 (0.14 oz)	20	tr	1	0	3	–	0
toll house original	1 (0.8 oz)	105	2	6	15	13	tr	57
vanilla sandwich	1 (0.35 oz)	48	tr	2	0	7	tr	35
vanilla wafers	1 (0.21 oz)	28	tr	1	–	4	–	18
zeppole	1 (0.8 oz)	78	1	6	24	6	tr	14
6 Hour Energy								
Almond Cranberry Chocolate Chunk	½ (1.25 oz)	100	4	6	0	12	5	–
ABC								
Vegan Colossal Chocolate Chip	1 (2.1 oz)	240	3	7	0	41	1	190
Vegan Double Chocolate Decadence	1 (2.1 oz)	240	3	8	0	39	2	120
Vegan Luscious Lemon Poppyseed	1 (2.1 oz)	240	3	7	0	40	0	125
Vegan Mac The Chip	1 (2.1 oz)	250	4	10	0	35	3	200

FOOD	PORTION	CALS	PROT	FAT	CHOL	CARB	FIBER	SOD
Vegan Peanut Butter Chocolate Chip	1 (2.1 oz)	240	4	8	0	39	1	160
Vegan Phenomenal Pumpkin Spice	1 (2.1 oz)	220	4	7	0	39	3	115
Almond Joy								
Cookies	2 (1 oz)	140	2	8	–	17	tr	60
Almondina								
BranTreats w/ Cinnamon	4 (1 oz)	127	3	3	0	22	2	11
Gingerspice	4 (1 oz)	137	3	4	0	22	1	10
Sesame	4 (1 oz)	138	3	5	0	21	2	10
The Original	4 (1 oz)	133	3	4	0	22	1	9
The Original Chocolate Dipped	2	130	3	5	0	16	4	15
Anna's Swedish Thins								
Almond Cinnamon	6 (1 oz)	140	2	7	0	18	1	150
Cappuccino	6 (1 oz)	140	2	7	0	18	2	150
Chocolate Mint	6 (1 oz)	150	2	8	5	17	2	100
Orange	6 (1 oz)	140	2	7	0	19	3	150
Archway								
Coconut Macaroon	2 (1.3 oz)	160	1	8	0	22	2	85
Frosty Lemon	1 (0.9 oz)	110	1	5	0	18	0	105
Fruit Filled Raspberry	1 (0.8 oz)	90	1	3	0	15	0	75
Arico								
Gluten Free Casein Free Almond Cranberry	1 bar (1.4 oz)	140	3	6	25	22	4	120
Gluten Free Casein Free Double Chocolate	1 (0.9 oz)	100	2	5	15	15	3	70
Gluten Free Casein Free Lemon Ginger	1 (0.9 oz)	90	2	4	15	15	3	85
Gluten Free Casein Free Peanut Butter	1 bar (1.4 oz)	160	5	7	25	19	4	140
Arrowroot								
Biscuit	1 (5 g)	20	0	1	0	4	0	15
Aunt Gussie's								
Biscotti Almond	1 (0.8 oz)	110	2	6	15	13	1	10
Biscotti Almond Sugar Free	2 (1 oz)	150	2	10	20	14	1	40
Biscotti Cinnamon Raisin No Sugar Added	1 (0.8 oz)	110	2	6	15	14	1	10
Biscotti Italian w/ Olive Oil	2 (1.2 oz)	160	3	5	25	25	1	30
Coconut Crisp	2 (1.1 oz)	170	2	9	20	18	1	65

FOOD	PORTION	CALS	PROT	FAT	CHOL	CARB	FIBER	SOD
Latte Sugar Free	1 (0.9 oz)	110	2	6	15	18	0	15
Lemon Sugar Free	3 (1.2 oz)	160	2	9	30	22	1	55
Mexican Wedding Cakes	3 (1.2 oz)	160	2	10	20	19	1	45
Snickerdoodle	2 (1.1 oz)	180	2	12	25	16	1	45
Vanilla Spritz Sugar Free Gluten Free	2 (0.9 oz)	110	0	5	25	17	0	15
Back To Nature								
Granola Cranberry Pecan	1 (1.1 oz)	130	2	6	0	20	2	105
Granola Honey Nut	1 (1.1 oz)	140	3	7	0	18	2	105
Bahlsen								
Delice	6 (1.1 oz)	150	2	8	0	19	tr	135
Hannover Waffeln	6 (1.1 oz)	180	1	11	0	19	1	30
Hit Minis Chocolate Filled	5 (1.2 oz)	170	2	8	0	23	tr	75
Waffeletten	4 (1 oz)	160	2	9	5	18	1	55
Barbara's Bakery								
Fig Bars Traditional	1	60	0	1	0	14	–	20
Fig Bars Wheat Free	1	60	0	0	0	13	1	25
Organic 100 Calorie Mini Ginger	1 pkg (0.9 oz)	100	1	2	5	19	–	150
Snackimals Chocolate Chip	10	120	1	4	0	19	–	80
Snackimals Wheat Free Oatmeal	10	120	1	5	0	17	1	130
Barnum's								
Animal Crackers	10 (1 oz)	120	2	4	0	22	1	140
Barry's Bakery								
French Twists Wild Raspberry	2 (0.5 oz)	60	0	2	0	9	0	25
Bear Naked								
Granola Soft Baked Fruit & Nut	1 (1 oz)	130	2	6	0	18	2	40
Breaktime								
Ginger	4 (1 oz)	130	2	4	0	23	0	100
Oatmeal	4 (1 oz)	130	2	4	0	22	tr	190
Brown & Haley								
Almond Roca	6 (1 oz)	110	1	4	5	19	0	105
Brown Butter Cookie								
Brown Butter Sea Salt	1 (0.7 oz)	94	1	5	14	11	0	41
Buzz Strong's								
Real Coffee	1 (1.2 oz)	150	2	7	10	22	1	125

FOOD	PORTION	CALS	PROT	FAT	CHOL	CARB	FIBER	SOD
Cameo								
Sandwich Creme	2 (1 oz)	130	1	5	0	21	0	105
Chips Ahoy!								
Chocolate Chip	1 pkg (1.4 oz)	190	2	9	0	27	1	140
Mini	1 pkg (1.2 oz)	170	2	8	0	24	1	115
Reduced Fat	1 pkg (1.1 oz)	140	2	5	0	23	1	150
Comfort Care								
Cabin Hearth Chocolate Chip	1 (2 oz)	250	3	11	15	38	1	230
Cabin Hearth Oatmeal Peach	1 (2 oz)	200	3	7	15	31	3	220
Cabin Hearth Oatmeal Raisin	1 (2 oz)	200	3	7	15	31	3	220
Country Choice Organic								
Fit Kids Snackin' Grahams Chocolate	18 (1 oz)	110	2	3	0	20	2	115
Oatmeal Chocolate Chip	1 (0.8 oz)	100	1	4	5	15	1	60
Oatmeal Raisin	1 (0.8 oz)	100	1	3	5	16	1	65
Dare								
Lemon Creme	1 (0.7 oz)	100	tr	4	0	14	0	70
Maple Leaf Creme	1 (0.6 oz)	80	tr	4	0	12	0	60
Delacre								
Royal Moments Milk Chocolate Biscuits	2 (0.9 oz)	130	2	6	33	18	0	30
DiCamillo								
Biscotti DiPrato	5 (1 oz)	130	3	4	15	21	tr	130
Divvies								
Chocolate Chip Vegan	1	130	1	7	0	17	tr	105
Oatmeal Raisin Vegan	1	120	1	5	0	17	tr	35
Do Goodie								
Gluten Free Chocolate Chip	1	140	1	7	20	18	1	115
Gluten Free Oatmeal Raisin	1	120	1	4	15	21	1	60
Earthbound Farms								
Organic Ginger Snaps	2	120	2	6	20	18	0	70
Emily's								
Fortune Dark Chocolate Covered	2 (1.4 oz)	140	2	6	0	23	2	0

FOOD	PORTION	CALS	PROT	FAT	CHOL	CARB	FIBER	SOD
Graham Cracker Milk Chocolate Covered	1 (1 oz)	150	2	9	<5	17	tr	45
Enjoy Life								
Allergen Gluten Free Gingerbread Spice	2 (1 oz)	100	1	4	0	19	2	120
Allergen Gluten Free No Oats Oatmeal	2 (1 oz)	120	1	4	0	21	1	50
Allergen Gluten Free Snickerdoodle	2 (1 oz)	130	1	5	0	21	2	110
Snack Bar Sunbutter Crunch	1 (1 oz)	140	3	5	0	20	3	110
Entenmann's								
Original Chocolate Chip	3 (1 oz)	140	1	7	<5	20	tr	90
Erin Baker's								
Breakfast Banana Toasted Flax	1 (3 oz)	300	6	5	0	55	6	250
Breakfast Banana Walnut	1 (3 oz)	300	7	8	0	52	5	240
Breakfast Caramel Apple	1 (3 oz)	280	6	4	0	55	5	240
Breakfast Double Chocolate Chunk	1 (3 oz)	300	7	6	0	53	6	230
Breakfast Mini Fruit & Nut	1 (1 oz)	100	2	3	0	17	2	75
Breakfast Oatmeal Raisin	1 (3 oz)	290	6	5	0	55	5	230
Breakfast Vegan Chocolate Chip	1 (3 oz)	310	6	6	0	57	6	250
Organic Breakfast Mini Peanut Butter	1 (1 oz)	110	3	3	0	16	2	115
Fauchon								
Assorted Chocolate	4 (2 oz)	330	4	15	55	34	5	165
Foods By George								
Gluten Free Biscotti	1 (0.8 oz)	90	2	5	0	11	1	25
French Meadow Bakery								
Coconutty Macaroons	2 (1.1 oz)	150	2	8	5	17	1	85
Gluten Free Chocolate Chip	1 (2.1 oz)	320	1	16	25	43	1	260
Rhubarb Bar	1 (2.7 oz)	250	3	11	30	34	1	80
Vegan Peanut Butter Bliss	2 (1.2 oz)	150	2	7	0	19	1	260
Gak's Snacks								
Organic Brownie Chip	1 (1 oz)	130	2	5	0	20	1	115
Organic Chocolate Chip	1 (1 oz)	140	1	6	0	21	1	95
Organic Oatmeal	1 (1 oz)	120	2	4	0	19	2	75

FOOD	PORTION	CALS	PROT	FAT	CHOL	CARB	FIBER	SOD
Ginger Snaps								
Cookies	4 (1 oz)	120	1	3	0	23	0	190
Girl Scout								
Lemon Chalet Cremes	3 (1.3 oz)	170	1	7	0	26	tr	95
Gluten-Free Pantry								
Gluten Free Buckwheat Raisin	1 (1 oz)	140	1	6	5	21	1	135
Gluten Free Chocolate Chunk	1 (1 oz)	140	1	8	5	19	1	120
Glutenfreeda								
Kookies Sugar	1	142	1	7	33	19	0	97
Glutino								
Gluten Free Wafers Chocolate	4	160	1	8	5	19	3	25
Gluten Free Wafers Lemon	3	150	0	6	0	24	0	25
Gottena								
Exquisit	5	170	2	10	0	19	1	25
Gourmet Pastries								
Kourabiethes Butter Almond	1 (1.1 oz)	150	2	9	25	15	1	110
Phoenicia Honey & Spice	1 (1.3 oz)	140	2	5	0	20	0	60
Health Valley								
Mini Mint Chocolate Chip	4 (1 oz)	120	1	6	5	16	1	125
Oatmeal Raisin	1 (0.8 oz)	90	2	4	0	14	1	50
Raisin Oatmeal Low Fat	3	110	2	2	0	23	1	105
White Chocolate Chunk	1 (1 oz)	140	1	7	10	17	0	150
Home Free								
Organic Chocolate Chip	1 (1 oz)	140	1	6	0	21	1	95
Organic Oatmeal	1 (1 oz)	120	2	4	0	19	2	75
Honey Maid								
Grahams Honey	1 (1.1 oz)	130	2	4	0	24	1	180
Grahams Honey Low Fat	1 (1.1 oz)	120	2	2	0	25	1	190
Jules Destrooper								
Butter Crisp	2 (0.9 oz)	120	2	4	15	19	tr	75
Kashi								
TLC Happy Trail Mix	1 (1 oz)	130	2	5	0	21	4	80
TLC Oatmeal Dark Chocolate	1 (1 oz)	130	2	5	0	21	3	70
TLC Oatmeal Raisin Flax	1 (1 oz)	130	2	5	0	20	4	75

FOOD	PORTION	CALS	PROT	FAT	CHOL	CARB	FIBER	SOD
Kay's Naturals								
Protein + Cookie Bites All Flavors Gluten Free	1 oz	110	10	3	0	15	3	336
Kedem								
Tea Biscuits Chocolate	2 (0.3 oz)	32	1	1	0	6	tr	29
Tea Biscuits Vanilla	2 (0.3 oz)	32	1	1	0	6	tr	29
Keebler								
100 Calorie RightBites Fudge Shoppe Fudge Grahams	1 pkg (0.7 oz)	100	1	4	0	15	tr	70
100 Calorie RightBites Sandies Shortbread	1 pkg (0.7 oz)	100	1	3	0	17	tr	90
Animal Crackers Frosted	8	150	1	7	0	22	tr	80
Chips Deluxe Chocolate Lovers	1	90	tr	5	0	10	0	65
Chips Deluxe Coconut	2	150	2	9	0	18	1	90
Chips Deluxe Fudge Stripes	1	100	1	6	0	13	tr	60
Chips Deluxe Original	1 pkg (2 oz)	300	3	16	0	37	1	180
Chocolate Dip & Cookie Sticks	1 pkg (1 oz)	130	1	6	0	18	tr	65
Danish Wedding	4	130	1	6	0	18	tr	70
Dipping Delights Cheesecake	1	90	<2	4	0	13	0	50
E.L. Fudge Original	1	90	1	4	<5	13	tr	50
Fudge Shoppe Fudge Stripes	3	150	1	7	0	21	tr	110
Fudge Shoppe Grasshoppers	4	140	1	7	0	19	tr	75
Fudge Shoppe Mint Creme Filled	2	160	tr	9	0	20	tr	65
Graham Honey	8 (1 oz)	110	2	2	0	22	tr	150
Graham Original	8 (1 oz)	130	2	4	0	22	tr	160
Oatmeal Country Style	2	130	2	6	0	18	1	115
Sandies Drops Butter Pecan	4	140	1	7	0	18	tr	60
Sandies Fudge Drops	4 (1 oz)	140	1	7	0	18	tr	60
Sandies Pecan Shortbread Reduced Fat	1	80	tr	4	0	11	0	65
Scooby-Doo Graham Sticks	9	130	2	4	0	21	tr	120

FOOD	PORTION	CALS	PROT	FAT	CHOL	CARB	FIBER	SOD
S'mores Snack	1 pkg (0.8 oz)	110	1	6	0	14	0	40
Soft Batch Chocolate Chip	1	80	tr	4	0	11	tr	55
Vanilla Wafers	8	140	1	6	0	21	tr	120
Vienna Fingers	2 (1.1 oz)	150	1	6	0	23	tr	95
Vienna Fingers Reduced Fat	2 (1.1 oz)	140	1	5	0	24	tr	115
Khaya								
Krunchi Orange & Chocolate	5 (1.53 oz)	240	3	12	21	29	2	14
Shortbread Grapeseed	13 (1.15 oz)	193	tr	10	26	27	tr	64
Shortbread Orange Rooibos	13 (1.15 oz)	259	tr	14	36	36	tr	88
La Choy								
Fortune	4 (1 oz)	110	2	0	0	25	0	10
Lance								
Oatmeal Creme	1 (2.5 oz)	300	3	12	0	45	2	300
Van-O-Lunch	1 pkg (1.6 oz)	230	3	10	0	34	0	140
Late July								
Organic Mini Sandwich Milk Chocolate	10 (1 oz)	130	2	6	0	19	1	85
Organic Mini Sandwich White Chocolate	10 (1 oz)	140	2	7	0	18	1	85
Lean Body								
Cookie Bar Hi-Protein S'Mores	1 (3.2 oz)	360	30	13	60	30	2	310
Liz Lovely								
Vegan Cowboy	½ cookie (1.3 oz)	190	3	9	0	24	2	90
Vegan Cowgirl	½ cookie (1.5 oz)	210	2	9	0	30	0	130
Vegan Ginger Snapdragons	½ cookie (1.5 oz)	190	2	7	0	29	0	230
Loacker								
Quadratini Dark Chocolate	9 (1.1 oz)	160	2	8	0	20	2	25
Lorna Doone								
Shortbread	4 (1 oz)	140	1	7	0	20	0	150
LU								
Le Chocolatier	3 (1 oz)	150	1	9	0	17	1	5
Le Fondant	4 (1.1 oz)	170	2	10	0	19	1	5

FOOD	PORTION	CALS	PROT	FAT	CHOL	CARB	FIBER	SOD
Le Petit Beurre	4 (1.2 oz)	140	3	4	5	24	tr	230
Petit Ecolier Dark Chocolate	2 (0.9 oz)	130	1	6	5	17	1	50
Petit Ecolier Milk Chocolate	2 (0.9 oz)	130	2	6	5	17	tr	55
Shortbread	2 (1 oz)	140	1	8	25	16	tr	95
Lucy's								
Chocolate Chip Gluten Free Vegan	3	130	2	5	0	20	2	170
Cinnamon Thin Gluten Free Vegan	3	130	2	5	0	21	1	180
Oatmeal Gluten Free Vegan	3	120	2	5	0	18	1	170
Sugar Gluten Free Vegan	3	130	2	5	0	21	1	180
Luna								
Berry Pomegranate	1 (1.4 oz)	140	3	3	0	27	4	100
Peanut Butter Chocolate	1 (1.4 oz)	150	4	6	0	23	3	170
M&M's								
Milk Chocolate	1 pkg (1.15 oz)	150	2	5	5	22	1	110
Mallomars								
Cookies	2 (0.9 oz)	120	1	5	0	18	1	40
Market Day								
Chocolate Chip Peanut Free	1 (1 oz)	150	1	9	10	17	0	65
Mauna Loa								
Macadamia Nut Chocolate Chip	4 (1 oz)	150	1	9	–	17	<1	80
Montana Monster Munchies								
Original	½ (1.4 oz)	177	4	9	22	21	2	33
Raisin	½ (1.4 oz)	172	3	9	21	22	2	32
MoonPie								
Mini All Flavors	1 pkg (1.2 oz)	130	2	4	0	23	2	110
Mrs. Fields								
Cookie Dough Snacks Brownie Chocolate Chip	7 (1 oz)	120	tr	3	5	18	0	80
Cookie Dough Snacks Chocolate Chip	7 (1 oz)	120	1	4	<5	19	tr	55
Murray's								
Sugar Free Chocolate Sandwich	3 (1 oz)	130	1	7	0	19	1	55

FOOD	PORTION	CALS	PROT	FAT	CHOL	CARB	FIBER	SOD
Sugar Free Chocolate Chip	3 (1.1 oz)	160	2	9	<5	20	1	130
Sugar Free Fudge Dipped Grahams	4 (1 oz)	150	2	8	0	19	1	80
Sugar Free Ginger Snap	7 (1.1 oz)	130	2	5	0	23	2	115
Sugar Free Oatmeal	3 (1.1 oz)	140	2	7	0	21	3	130
Sugar Free Shortbread	8 (1 oz)	130	2	5	0	21	2	140
Nabisco								
100 Calorie Pack Alpha-Bits Mini	1 pkg	100	1	3	0	16	0	120
100 Calorie Pack Barnum's Animal Choco	1 pkg	100	1	3	0	17	tr	115
100 Calorie Pack Lorna Doone	1 pkg	100	1	3	0	16	0	120
100 Calorie Pack Teddy Grahams Mini Cinnamon	1 pkg	100	1	3	0	16	1	115
Grahams Original	8 (1.1 oz)	130	2	3	0	24	1	190
Nairn's								
Oat Fruit & Cinnamon	2 (0.7 oz)	85	2	3	0	15	2	50
Oat Stem Ginger	2 (0.7 oz)	87	2	3	0	14	1	60
Nana's								
No Gluten Berry Vanilla	1 bar (1.2 oz)	130	1	4	0	22	tr	135
No Gluten Chocolate	1 (3.5 oz)	360	4	12	0	62	2	380
No Gluten Ginger	1 (3.5 oz)	360	4	10	0	64	2	170
No Gluten Nana Banana	1 bar (1.2 oz)	130	1	5	0	23	0	130
No Wheat Oatmeal Raisin	1 (3.5 oz)	280	6	10	0	46	6	150
Vegan Chocolate Chip	1 (4 oz)	320	6	14	0	48	6	210
Vegan Peanut Butter	1 (4 oz)	360	8	16	0	46	4	220
Vegan Sunflower	1 (3.5 oz)	380	8	14	0	60	6	360
Napolitanke								
Lemon Orange	4 (0.7 oz)	108	1	6	–	13	–	12
Mocca	4 (0.7 oz)	101	1	5	–	13	–	27
Natural Ovens								
Oatmeal Raisin	1 (1.3 oz)	120	2	4	0	20	2	50
New Morning								
Honey Grahams	2 (1 oz)	130	3	3	0	24	1	180
New York Style								
Biscotti Almond	3 (1 oz)	130	3	5	25	20	1	35

FOOD	PORTION	CALS	PROT	FAT	CHOL	CARB	FIBER	SOD
Newtons								
Fig	2 (1.1 oz)	110	1	2	0	22	1	125
Fig 100% Whole Grain	2 (1.3 oz)	130	1	3	0	26	3	135
Fig Fat Free	2 (1 oz)	90	1	0	0	22	1	130
Raspberry	2 (1 oz)	100	1	2	0	21	0	110
Nilla Wafers								
Cookies	1 oz	140	1	6	0	21	0	115
Reduced Fat	1 oz	110	1	2	0	24	0	110
Nonni's								
Biscotti Cioccolati	1 (0.8 oz)	110	2	5	20	17	1	70
Biscotti Limone	1 (0.8 oz)	110	2	5	20	17	0	75
Biscotti Original	1 (0.7 oz)	90	2	3	20	14	0	65
NutraBalance								
High Fibre	1 (0.7 oz)	90	1	4	0	13	3	85
Nutter Butter								
Bites	1 pkg (1.2 oz)	170	3	7	0	24	1	135
Sandwich Cookie	1 (1 oz)	130	2	6	0	19	1	110
Oreo								
Cakesters Mini Golden 100 Calorie Pack	1 pkg (0.8 oz)	100	1	5	0	15	0	65
Double Stuff	1 (1 oz)	140	1	7	0	21	1	120
Golden Chocolate Creme	3 (1.2 oz)	170	2	7	0	25	tr	135
Reduced Fat	3 (1.2 oz)	150	1	5	0	27	1	160
Sandwich Cookie	2 (1.2 oz)	160	2	7	0	25	1	190
Orion								
Choco Pie	1 (1 oz)	120	1	5	<5	19	tr	65
Pepperidge Farm								
Bordeaux	4 (1 oz)	130	2	5	10	19	tr	95
Chantilly Raspberry	2	120	1	3	0	23	tr	115
Chessmen	3 (0.9 oz)	120	2	5	20	18	tr	80
Dark Chocolate Mint Chocolate Chunk	1	140	2	7	10	16	0	80
Gingerman	4	130	2	4	10	21	tr	100
Lemon	4 (1.1 oz)	160	2	8	5	21	0	105
Medallion Milk Chocolate	5	160	2	8	10	20	0	40
Milano	3 (1.2 oz)	180	2	10	10	21	tr	80
Milano French Vanilla	2	130	1	5	<5	18	tr	65
Milano Mint Chocolate Covered	4	130	2	6	<5	18	1	40

FOOD	PORTION	CALS	PROT	FAT	CHOL	CARB	FIBER	SOD
Milano Sugar Free	3	170	2	9	5	21	tr	65
Nantucket Chocolate Dipped	1	150	2	8	10	20	tr	100
Nantucket Dark Chocolate Chunk	1	140	2	7	10	16	0	80
Pirouettes Cappuccino	2	120	1	5	<5	18	0	40
Pirouettes Chocolate Mint	2	120	1	5	<5	18	tr	40
Sausalito Milk Chocolate Macadamia Nut	1	140	2	8	10	16	0	80
Shortbread	2	140	2	7	10	16	tr	105
Soft Baked Milk Chocolate	1	150	1	7	5	21	tr	70
Soft Baked Oatmeal Cranberry	1	130	2	4	5	22	tr	110
Soft Baked Sugar	1	140	2	5	10	22	0	90
Tahiti	2	170	2	10	5	17	2	40
Verona Apricot Raspberry	3	140	2	5	10	22	tr	100
Pirouette								
Sandwich Vanilla Creamed	3 (1.1 oz)	133	1	4	0	22	0	34
Polar								
Fortune	2	56	2	0	0	12	0	47
Q.bel								
Wafer Rolls Dark Chocolate	1 pkg (0.9 oz)	120	1	6	0	18	1	25
Wafer Rolls Milk Chocolate	1 pkg (0.9 oz)	130	2	6	0	18	tr	35
Quaker								
Breakfast Cookie Oatmeal Raisin	1	180	3	5	0	33	5	200
Ruger								
Wafers Vanilla	3 (1 oz)	160	1	9	5	20	0	25
Simply Shari's								
Gluten Free Almond Shortbread	2 (1 oz)	120	1	6	15	15	0	75
Gluten Free Chocolate Chip	2 (1 oz)	120	1	6	10	17	1	55
Gluten Free Fudge Brownies	2 (1 oz)	130	1	7	10	16	1	70
Gluten Free Shortbread	2 (1 oz)	130	1	6	15	17	0	85
SnackWell's								
Cookie Cakes Chocolate Mint	1 (0.6 oz)	50	1	1	0	12	0	40

FOOD	PORTION	CALS	PROT	FAT	CHOL	CARB	FIBER	SOD
Devil's Food Fat Free	1 (0.5 oz)	50	1	0	0	12	0	25
Sugar Free Lemon Creme	2 (1.1 oz)	130	1	6	0	23	2	135
Sugar Free Shortbread	2 (1 oz)	130	2	6	5	21	2	140
Snikiddy								
Cherry Oaties	1 pkg (0.8 oz)	110	2	4	0	17	1	115
South Beach								
Fiber Fit Double Chocolate Chunk	1 pkg (0.8 oz)	100	1	5	0	17	5	85
Fiber Fit Oatmeal Chocolate Chunk	1 pkg (0.8 oz)	100	1	5	0	17	5	80
Wafer Sticke Dark Chocolate Hazelnut Creme	1 pkg	100	5	6	0	10	3	70
Wafer Sticke Dark Chocolate Peanut Butter	1 pkg	100	5	6	0	10	3	75
Starbucks								
Almond Roca Buttercrunch Toffee	6 (1 oz)	110	1	4	5	19	0	105
Biscotti Chocolate Hazelnut	1 (0.9 oz)	100	2	5	20	14	1	70
Madeleines Petite French Cakes	3 (1.8 oz)	230	19	11	70	32	tr	100
White Chocolate & Raspberry	2 (0.9 oz)	120	1	6	0	15	tr	85
Stella D'oro								
100 Calorie Pack Breakfast Treats Original	1 pkg (0.8 oz)	100	2	2	15	19	1	96
Almond Delight	1 (1 oz)	150	2	8	10	18	tr	85
Angelica Goodies	1 (0.7 oz)	90	1	3	10	15	0	45
Anginetti	4 (1.1 oz)	130	1	3	25	25	0	5
Biscotti Almond	1 (0.7 oz)	90	2	4	5	15	1	40
Biscotti French Vanilla	1 (0.7 oz)	90	1	3	5	15	0	50
Breakfast Treats Chocolate	1 (0.9 oz)	110	1	4	20	19	tr	70
Breakfast Treats Original	1 (0.7 oz)	90	1	3	20	14	0	65
Coffee Treats Almond Toast	2 (0.9 oz)	100	2	2	25	20	tr	90
Coffee Treats Angel Wings	3 (1 oz)	160	2	10	0	16	0	90
Coffee Treats Anisette Sponge	2 (0.9 oz)	90	2	1	40	18	0	80
Coffee Treats Anisette Toast	3 (1.2 oz)	130	2	1	35	27	tr	110
Coffee Treats Roman Egg Biscuits	1 (1.1 oz)	130	3	5	15	19	0	125

FOOD	PORTION	CALS	PROT	FAT	CHOL	CARB	FIBER	SOD
Egg Jumbo	3 (1.2 oz)	120	2	2	50	25	0	85
Lady Stella	3 (1 oz)	130	1	5	<5	19	tr	60
Margherite	2 (1 oz)	130	2	5	20	20	0	85
Swiss Fudge	3 (1.2 oz)	170	2	9	<5	22	tr	80
Teddy Grahams								
Chocolate	24 (1.1 oz)	130	2	5	0	22	2	160
Honey	24 (1 oz)	130	2	4	0	23	1	150
Temptations								
Chocolate Alps	1 bar (1.6 oz)	170	2	7	0	28	1	130
Chocolate Mocha	1 bar (1.6 oz)	170	2	6	0	27	1	130
No Gluten Chocolate Rush	1 bar (1.6 oz)	170	1	9	0	25	1	90
Voortman								
Chinese Almond	1 (0.9 oz)	130	1	7	0	16	0	–
Coconut Delight	1 (0.6 oz)	90	1	6	0	10	tr	tr
Dutch Creme	1 (0.8 oz)	110	1	4	0	16	0	60
Fudge Swirl	1 (0.6 oz)	80	1	4	0	10	0	30
Gingerboy	1 (0.7 oz)	100	1	4	0	15	0	90
Maple Leaf	1 (0.6 oz)	90	1	4	0	13	0	tr
Molasses	1 (1 oz)	110	2	3	0	20	tr	80
Oatmeal Apple	1 (0.7 oz)	90	2	4	0	13	1	100
Peanut Delight	1 (0.9 oz)	130	2	7	0	15	tr	90
Shortbread	1 (0.6 oz)	90	1	5	0	11	tr	40
Sugar Free Chocolate Chip	1 (0.7 oz)	80	1	5	0	13	0	50
Sugar Free Lemon Wafers	3 (1 oz)	130	0	8	0	17	0	40
Sugar Free Vanilla Creme	2 (0.7 oz)	100	1	6	0	13	0	40
Sugar Free Wafers Peanut Butter	4 (1 oz)	150	2	8	0	17	0	50
Sugar Free Wafers Vanilla	3 (1 oz)	130	0	8	0	17	0	40
Turnover Blueberry	1 (0.9 oz)	110	1	4	0	18	tr	60
Turnover Cherry	1 (0.9 oz)	110	1	4	0	18	tr	50
Turnover Strawberry	1 (0.9 oz)	110	1	4	0	18	tr	60
Wafer Chocolate Covered	1 (0.7 oz)	100	tr	5	0	13	0	15
Wafer Vanilla	3 (1 oz)	140	1	7	0	20	0	25
Wafers Mini Chocolate	5 (1 oz)	130	tr	6	0	19	0	20
Walkers								
Shortbread Chocolate Chip	2 (1 oz)	140	1	8	20	17	tr	80
Shortbread Rounds	2 (1.2 oz)	180	2	10	30	20	tr	115
Whippet								
Original	2 (1.2 oz)	150	1	5	0	24	1	50

FOOD	PORTION	CALS	PROT	FAT	CHOL	CARB	FIBER	SOD
World Of Grains								
Apple Cinnamon	1 pkg	130	3	4	5	21	3	85
Cranberry	1 pkg	130	3	4	5	21	3	85
Multigrain	1 pkg	130	3	5	5	21	3	100
Zwieback								
Toast	1 (8 g)	35	1	1	0	6	0	10
REFRIGERATED								
chocolate chip	1 (0.42 oz)	59	1	3	3	8	–	28
chocolate chip dough	1 oz	126	1	6	7	17	–	59
oatmeal	1 (0.4 oz)	56	1	3	3	8	–	39
oatmeal raisin	1 (0.4 oz)	56	1	3	3	8	–	39
peanut butter	1 (0.4 oz)	60	1	3	4	7	–	52
peanut butter dough	1 oz	130	2	7	8	15	–	112
sugar	1 (0.42 oz)	58	1	3	4	8	–	56
sugar dough	1 oz	124	1	6	8	17	–	120
Pillsbury								
Chocolate Chip	2 (1.3 oz)	170	2	9	10	22	tr	125
Gingerbread	2 (1.1 oz)	170	1	7	10	18	0	105
Oatmeal Chocolate Chip	2 (1.3 oz)	170	2	8	10	23	1	95
Peanut Butter	2 (1 oz)	130	2	6	5	16	0	135
S'Mores	2 (1.3 oz)	160	1	7	5	23	tr	120
Sugar	2 (1.3 oz)	170	2	9	10	22	0	100
TAKE-OUT								
biscotti w/ nuts chocolate dipped	1 (1.3 oz)	117	2	6	18	16	1	33
black & white	1 lg (3 oz)	302	4	9	58	52	1	72
finikia	1 (1.2 oz)	171	2	5	27	16	1	26
koulourakia butter cookie twist	1 (0.9 oz)	113	2	6	32	14	tr	59
linzer tart	1 (2.4 oz)	280	2	14	40	34	0	130
CORIANDER								
cilantro fresh	1 tsp (2 g)	tr	tr	tr	0	tr	tr	1
leaf dried	1 tsp	2	tr	tr	0	tr	tr	1
leaf fresh	¼ cup	1	tr	tr	0	tr	–	1
seed	1 tsp	5	tr	tr	0	1	1	1
CORN								
CANNED								
cream style	½ cup	93	2	1	0	23	–	365
w/ red & green peppers	½ cup	86	3	1	0	21	–	396

FOOD	PORTION	CALS	PROT	FAT	CHOL	CARB	FIBER	SOD
white	½ cup	66	2	1	0	15	–	–
yellow	½ cup	66	2	1	0	15	1	–
Del Monte								
Cream Style Sweet Corn	½ cup (4.4 oz)	70	1	1	0	14	4	300
Savory Sides In Butter Sauce	½ cup	90	2	3	5	14	tr	530
Savory Sides Santa Fe	½ cup	70	3	1	0	16	1	510
Green Giant								
Mexicorn	⅓ cup	70	2	1	0	14	1	250
Super Sweet Yellow & White	⅓ cup (2.6 oz)	60	2	1	0	12	1	200
Jake & Amos								
Pickled Dill Baby Corn	2 tbsp	5	0	0	0	1	0	217
Orchids								
Whole Young Spears	½ cup (4.6 oz)	25	2	0	0	4	2	280
DRIED								
Crunchies								
Freeze Dried Corn Snack	⅓ cup (1 oz)	130	2	7	0	19	4	85
Freeze Dried Sweet Buttered	½ cup (1 oz)	100	3	2	0	21	3	210
FRESH								
white cooked	½ cup	89	3	1	0	21	–	14
white raw	½ cup	66	2	1	0	15	–	12
yellow cooked	1 ear (2.7 oz)	83	3	1	0	19	–	13
yellow cooked	½ cup	89	3	1	0	21	–	14
yellow raw	½ cup	66	2	1	0	15	–	12
yellow raw	1 ear (3 oz)	77	3	1	0	17	–	14
FROZEN								
cooked	½ cup	67	2	tr	0	17	–	4
on the cob cooked	1 ear (2.2 oz)	59	2	tr	0	14	–	3
Birds Eye								
Steamfresh Singles Super Sweet	1 pkg (3.2 oz)	80	3	1	0	14	2	0
Steamfresh Southwestern	⅔ cup (2.9 oz)	90	2	2	0	16	1	260

FOOD	PORTION	CALS	PROT	FAT	CHOL	CARB	FIBER	SOD
Steamfresh Sweet Mini Corn On The Cob	1 (3 oz)	90	3	1	0	19	1	0
C&W								
Cheddar Bacon	½ cup	130	4	5	10	18	3	210
Early Harvest Supersweet Petite	⅔ cup	70	3	1	0	14	2	0
Salsa Corn	1 cup	90	3	1	0	17	3	250
Glory								
Savory Accents Fried Corn	½ cup	110	3	2	0	24	2	470
Green Giant								
Cream Style	½ cup	110	2	1	0	24	2	320
Nibblers On-The-Cob	1 (2.1 oz)	70	2	1	0	14	1	5
Health Is Wealth								
Creamed	½ pkg (4.5 oz)	110	4	2	5	23	1	40
Stouffer's								
Souffle	½ pkg (6 oz)	150	5	5	65	22	2	490
TAKE-OUT								
fritters	1 (1 oz)	62	2	2	12	9	1	126
on the cob w/ butter cooked	1 ear	155	4	3	6	32	–	30
scalloped	1 cup	257	10	11	152	34	3	666

CORN CHIPS (see CHIPS)

CORNISH HEN (see CHICKEN)

CORNMEAL

FOOD	PORTION	CALS	PROT	FAT	CHOL	CARB	FIBER	SOD
cornmeal mush as prep w/ water	1 cup	223	5	1	0	47	5	523
cornmeal yellow	½ cup (2.2 oz)	236	4	1	0	52	1	1
whole grain blue	½ cup (1.9 oz)	201	5	3	0	41	5	3
yellow self-rising	½ cup (3 oz)	296	7	2	0	62	5	1121
Indian Head								
Stone Ground	¼ cup	100	3	1	0	20	2	0
Martha White								
White Self Rising	3 tbsp (1.1 oz)	100	2	1	0	22	2	440

FOOD	PORTION	CALS	PROT	FAT	CHOL	CARB	FIBER	SOD
White Enriched	3 tbsp (1.2 oz)	120	3	1	0	24	2	0
Yellow Self Rising	3 tbsp (1.1 oz)	110	2	1	0	22	2	460
Quaker								
Quick Grits not prep	¼ cup (1.3 oz)	130	3	1	0	29	2	0
TAKE-OUT								
corn pone	1 piece (2.1 oz)	128	2	3	0	23	2	275
fritter puerto rican style	1 (1.4 oz)	109	3	7	8	8	1	223
harina de maize con coco	½ cup	383	4	27	0	36	4	287
harina de maize con leche	1 cup	295	8	7	25	51	7	300
hush puppies	1 (0.8 oz)	74	2	3	10	10	1	147
johnnycake	1 piece (1.7 oz)	134	4	4	35	21	2	432

CORNSTARCH

FOOD	PORTION	CALS	PROT	FAT	CHOL	CARB	FIBER	SOD
cornstarch	¼ cup (1.1 oz)	122	tr	tr	0	29	tr	3
cornstarch	1 tbsp (0.3 oz)	34	tr	0	0	8	tr	1
Argo								
Cornstarch	1 tbsp (0.3 oz)	30	0	0	0	7	–	0
Bob's Red Mill								
Cornstarch	1 tbsp	30	0	0	0	7	0	0
Clabber Girl								
Cornstarch Calcium Fortified	1 tbsp (0.4 oz)	35	0	0	0	8	–	0
Rumford								
Cornstarch Calcium Fortified	1 tbsp (0.4 oz)	35	0	0	0	8	–	0

COTTAGE CHEESE

FOOD	PORTION	CALS	PROT	FAT	CHOL	CARB	FIBER	SOD
creamed large curd	½ cup (4 oz)	110	13	5	19	4	0	410
creamed small curd	½ cup (3.7 oz)	103	12	5	18	4	0	382
dry curd	½ cup (2.5 oz)	52	8	tr	5	5	0	239

FOOD	PORTION	CALS	PROT	FAT	CHOL	CARB	FIBER	SOD
lowfat 1%	½ cup (4 oz)	81	14	1	5	3	0	459
lowfat 1% lactose reduced	½ cup (4 oz)	84	14	1	5	4	1	250
Axelrod								
Lowfat 1%	½ cup (4 oz)	90	14	2	15	6	0	480
Breakstone's								
2% Low Fat Small Curd	½ cup (4.4 oz)	100	12	3	15	6	0	370
LiveActive	1 pkg (4 oz)	90	10	2	15	8	3	380
LiveActive Mixed Berries	1 pkg (4 oz)	120	8	2	10	18	3	310
Cabot								
Cottage Cheese	½ cup	100	13	5	15	4	0	400
No Fat	½ cup	70	13	0	5	5	0	410
Friendship								
1% Lowfat	½ cup	90	16	1	5	3	0	360
1% Lowfat No Salt Added	½ cup	90	16	1	0	4	1	50
1% Lowfat Whipped	½ cup	90	16	1	5	3	0	360
2% Digestive Health	½ cup	90	14	3	10	5	3	360
2% Pot Style	½ cup	90	15	3	10	3	0	400
4% California Style	½ cup	110	15	5	20	3	1	380
Nonfat	½ cup	80	15	0	0	4	0	380
Horizon Organic								
Lowfat	½ cup	100	13	3	15	4	0	390
Regular	½ cup	120	13	5	20	4	0	390
Knudsen								
LiveActive Pineapple	1 pkg (4 oz)	110	8	2	10	17	3	310
Land O Lakes								
1% Lowfat	½ cup (4 oz)	90	13	2	10	5	0	460
2% Lowfat	½ cup (3.7 oz)	100	13	3	15	5	0	480
Cottage Cheese	½ cup (3.7 oz)	110	11	5	20	5	0	410
Fat Free	½ cup (4 oz)	80	14	0	0	6	0	380
Nancy's								
Organic Lowfat	½ cup	80	14	1	5	3	0	304
Organic Valley								
Low Fat	½ cup	100	15	2	10	4	0	450
COTTONSEED								
kernels roasted	1 tbsp	51	3	4	0	2	–	3

FOOD	PORTION	CALS	PROT	FAT	CHOL	CARB	FIBER	SOD
COUSCOUS								
cooked	1 cup (5.5 oz)	176	6	tr	0	36	2	8
dry	1 cup (6.1 oz)	650	22	1	0	134	9	17
Marrakesh Express								
Mango Salsa as prep	1 cup	190	7	0	0	38	1	380
Mushroom as prep	1 cup	190	8	1	0	39	1	600
Plain as prep	1 cup	270	10	0	0	57	2	10
Near East								
Mediterranean Curry as prep	1 cup	220	8	4	0	40	3	552
Original Plain as prep	1 cup	190	7	2	0	37	3	0
Parmesan as prep	1 cup	220	8	4	9	39	2	600
Toasted Pine Nut as prep	1 cup	230	8	5	0	39	2	510
Wild Mushroom & Herb as prep	1 cup	230	8	4	9	40	3	624
CRAB								
CANNED								
blue	½ cup	67	14	1	60	0	0	225
blue drained	1 can (6.5 oz)	124	26	2	111	0	0	416
Ace Of Diamonds								
Fancy w/ Leg Meat	¼ cup (2 oz)	40	7	0	50	2	0	400
Polar								
Claw Meat	¼ cup (2 oz)	37	10	0	53	1	0	393
Jumbo Lump Meat	¼ cup (2 oz)	39	8	1	52	0	0	304
Wild Planet								
Dungeness	2 oz	62	12	1	142	tr	–	321
FRESH								
alaska king meat only steamed	3 oz	82	16	1	45	0	0	911
blue cooked flaked	1 cup (4 oz)	120	24	2	118	0	0	329
dungeness steamed	3 oz	94	19	1	65	1	0	321
queen steamed	3 oz	98	20	1	60	0	0	587
Dockside Classics								
Crabcakes	1 (2.5 oz)	150	7	11	25	7	0	380
FROZEN								
Mama Belle's								
Crab Cakes Maryland Style	1 (2 oz)	100	9	5	70	4	0	340

FOOD	PORTION	CALS	PROT	FAT	CHOL	CARB	FIBER	SOD
Mrs. Paul's								
Deviled Crab Cakes	1 (3 oz)	220	20	12	60	12	3	320
SeaPak								
Maryland Style Crab Cakes + Sauce	1 (4 oz)	240	11	13	55	19	1	830
TAKE-OUT								
alaska king leg steamed	1 leg (4.7 oz)	130	26	2	71	0	0	1436
baked	1 (3.8 oz)	160	29	2	184	4	–	550
cakes	2 (4.2 oz)	186	24	9	180	1	0	396
crab imperial	1 crab (6.8 oz)	289	30	15	242	6	0	782
crab salad	1 serv (5.5 oz)	285	21	21	109	3	1	736
crab thermidor	1 serv (6.4 oz)	456	22	37	313	8	tr	664
deviled	1 serv (4.5 oz)	254	17	13	126	17	1	825
dungeness steamed	1 crab (4.5 oz)	140	28	2	97	1	0	480
empanada de jueyes	1 (4.4 oz)	341	12	16	45	38	2	680
fried crab puffs	4 (3.2 oz)	323	10	18	85	30	1	792
kenagi korean crab cooked	1 serv (3 oz)	71	16	tr	–	0	0	204
salmorejo de jueyes (in tomato sauce)	1 serv (4.5 oz)	215	20	14	99	3	tr	785
soft-shell breaded & fried	1 med (2.3 oz)	216	13	13	79	11	1	353
taco de jueyes	1 (4.2 oz)	266	16	14	79	18	2	800

CRACKER CRUMBS

FOOD	PORTION	CALS	PROT	FAT	CHOL	CARB	FIBER	SOD
cracker meal	1 cup	440	11	2	0	93	3	32
graham cracker crumbs	1 cup	355	6	8	0	65	2	508
Honey Maid								
Graham Cracker Crumbs	2½ tbsp (0.6 oz)	70	1	2	0	13	0	95
Keebler								
Graham	¼ cup	93	1	2	0	17	1	187

CRACKERS

FOOD	PORTION	CALS	PROT	FAT	CHOL	CARB	FIBER	SOD
melba toast round	1	12	tr	tr	0	2	tr	25
oyster cracker	¼ cup	48	1	1	0	8	tr	121

FOOD	PORTION	CALS	PROT	FAT	CHOL	CARB	FIBER	SOD
saltines	1	13	tr	tr	0	2	tr	32
water biscuits	3	92	2	3	–	16	1	–
zwieback	1 oz	107	3	1	–	21	1	75
34 Degrees								
Crispbread Sesame	19 (1.1 oz)	140	5	3	0	26	1	360
Whole Grain	9 (0.5 oz)	35	1	0	0	7	1	110
Athenos								
Pita Chips Whole Wheat	11 (1 oz)	120	4	4	0	18	2	270
Aunt Gussie's								
Cracker Flats Spelt Cinnamon Raisin	1 (1 oz)	100	3	2	0	19	1	40
Cracker Flats Spelt Everything	1 (0.8 oz)	60	2	2	0	12	2	80
Back To Nature								
Poppy Thyme	17 (1 oz)	130	2	4	0	21	1	270
Rice Thin Sesame Ginger	16	120	2	3	0	23	0	180
Sesame Tarragon	17 (1 oz)	130	2	5	0	21	1	270
Barbara's Bakery								
Rite Rounds Lite Original	5 (0.5 oz)	60	1	2	0	11	–	200
Wheatines Original	4	60	1	1	0	11	tr	80
Better Cheddars								
Original	1.1 oz	160	3	8	5	18	1	360
Blue Diamond								
Nut-Thins Almond Country Ranch	16 (1 oz)	130	3	4	0	22	tr	220
Bran Crispbread								
GG Scandinavian	1 (0.4 oz)	12	1	0	0	7	5	30
Bremner Wafers								
Cracked Wheat	7 (0.5 oz)	70	2	2	0	11	0	100
Original	7 (0.5 oz)	70	2	2	0	11	0	105
Soup & Chili Crackers	50 (0.5 oz)	60	2	2	0	11	0	110
Breton								
Garden Vegetable	4 (0.7 oz)	100	1	4	0	13	1	160
Minis Cheddar Cheese	20 (0.7 oz)	100	3	5	5	13	1	240
Brown Rice Snaps								
Cheddar	6	60	1	1	0	12	tr	40
Original Tamari Seaweed	9	60	1	0	0	12	tr	120
Unsalted Plain	8	60	1	0	0	13	tr	0

FOOD	PORTION	CALS	PROT	FAT	CHOL	CARB	FIBER	SOD
Cheese Nips								
Cheddar	1 pkg (1.2 oz)	170	3	7	0	22	1	400
Chicken Biskit								
Original	1.1 oz	160	2	8	0	19	1	300
Daelia's								
Biscuits For Cheese Almond w/ Raisins	4 (1 oz)	133	3	4	0	22	1	9
Biscuits For Cheese Hazelnut w/ Figs	4 (1 oz)	133	3	5	0	20	1	10
Dare								
Crackers	3 (0.5 oz)	70	1	4	0	9	0	70
Original	4 (0.7 oz)	90	2	4	0	13	1	170
Reduced Fat & Salt	5 (0.7 oz)	80	3	2	0	16	1	105
Dr. Kracker								
Flatbread Klassic Seed	1 (1 oz)	120	6	5	0	13	4	220
Flatbread Pumpkin Seed Cheddar	1 (1 oz)	120	5	5	<5	12	4	220
Flatbread Seeded Spelt	1 (1 oz)	120	5	6	0	12	4	200
Flatbread Seedlander	1 (1 oz)	120	5	5	0	15	3	220
Flatbread Spelt Sunflower Cheddar	1 (1 oz)	120	5	6	<5	12	4	220
Krispy Grahams	5 (1 oz)	110	2	3	4	17	2	120
Flatout								
Edge On Baked Flatbread Four Cheese	15 (1 oz)	130	6	5	0	15	5	290
Edge On Baked Flatbread Garlic Herb	15 (1 oz)	120	6	4	0	16	5	330
Glutino								
Gluten Free	4 (0.5 oz)	70	tr	2	5	12	0	120
Gluten Free Rusks	2 (0.7 oz)	80	0	2	0	15	2	140
GrainsFirst								
Autumn Harvest	7 (1.1 oz)	140	3	7	0	16	3	410
Grissol								
Crispy Baguettes Garden Herb	8 (1 oz)	110	3	2	0	19	1	210
Health Valley								
Organic Bruschetta Vegetable	4	70	1	3	0	10	0	210
Organic Cracked Pepper	4	70	1	3	0	10	0	190

FOOD	PORTION	CALS	PROT	FAT	CHOL	CARB	FIBER	SOD
Organic Cracker Stix Garlic Herb	8	70	1	3	0	9	tr	210
Organic Whole Wheat	4	70	2	3	0	9	1	170
Kashi								
Heart To Heart Whole Grain	7 (1 oz)	120	3	4	0	22	4	85
TLC Natural Ranch	15 (1 oz)	130	4	3	0	22	2	200
TLC Original 7 Grain	15 (1 oz)	130	3	3	0	22	2	160
TLC Party Mediterranean Bruschetta	4	120	3	4	0	18	3	140
TLC Snack Fire Roasted Vegetable	5	130	3	4	0	21	2	210
TLC Toasted Asiago	15 (1.1 oz)	130	3	4	0	21	2	200
Keebler								
Club Multi-Grain	4	70	1	3	0	10	tr	150
Club Original	4 (0.5 oz)	70	1	3	0	9	tr	125
Club Reduced Fat	5	70	1	3	0	12	tr	190
Club Snack Sticks	12	130	1	6	0	19	tr	320
Puffed Original	24	140	2	6	0	20	1	310
Sandwich Cheese & Peanut Butter	1 pkg (1.4 oz)	200	4	10	0	23	1	400
Sandwich Toast & Peanut Butter	1 pkg (1.4 oz)	200	4	10	0	23	1	410
Sandwich Wheat & Cheddar	1 pkg (1.3 oz)	190	2	10	<5	23	tr	370
Toasteds Harvest Wheat	16	130	2	6	0	20	1	260
Toasteds Sesame	5	80	1	4	0	10	tr	140
Toasteds Wheat	5	80	1	4	0	10	tr	160
Town House Bistro	2	80	1	3	0	11	tr	130
Town House FlipSides Original	5	70	1	4	0	10	tr	200
Town House Original	5 (0.5 oz)	80	tr	5	0	10	tr	130
Town House Reduced Fat	6	60	tr	2	0	11	tr	160
Town House Reduced Sodium	5	80	tr	5	0	10	tr	80
Town House Toppers	3	70	1	3	0	9	0	135
Wheatables 33% Less Fat	19	140	2	4	0	22	1	320
Wheatables Original	17	140	2	6	0	20	1	340
Zesta Saltine Fat Free	5	60	1	0	0	13	tr	280
Zesta Saltine Original	5	60	1	2	0	11	tr	200

FOOD	PORTION	CALS	PROT	FAT	CHOL	CARB	FIBER	SOD
Kellogg's								
All Bran Garlic Herb	18 (1 oz)	120	3	6	0	19	5	330
Kitchen Table Bakers								
Aged Parmesan	3	80	7	6	15	tr	0	150
Everything	3	80	7	6	15	tr	0	150
Garlic	3	80	6	6	15	tr	0	150
Jalapeno	3	80	6	6	15	2	1	150
Lance								
Captain Wafers	4	70	1	3	0	9	0	105
Nekot	1 pkg (1.7 oz)	240	7	11	0	30	1	150
Nipchee	1 pkg (1.4 oz)	190	4	11	<5	22	1	340
Peanut Butter On Wheat	1 pkg (1.4 oz)	200	4	9	0	21	1	250
Toastchee	1 pkg (1.5 oz)	220	5	11	<5	23	2	430
Toastchee Reduced Fat	1 pkg (1.4 oz)	180	6	7	0	23	2	230
Larzaroni								
Bruschette w/ Olives	9 (1.1 oz)	140	4	5	0	21	1	350
Mary's Gone Crackers								
Wheat Free Gluten Free Black Pepper	13 (1 oz)	140	3	5	0	21	3	180
Wheat Free Gluten Free Onion	13 (1 oz)	140	3	5	0	21	3	190
Wheat Free Gluten Free Original Seed	13 (1 oz)	140	3	5	0	21	3	190
Nabisco								
Garden Harvest Apple Cinnamon	16 (1 oz)	120	2	3	0	22	3	65
Garden Harvest Banana	16 (1 oz)	120	2	3	0	22	3	60
Garden Harvest Tomato Basil	16 (1 oz)	120	2	4	0	20	3	220
Garden Harvest Vegetable Medley	16 (1 oz)	120	2	4	0	20	3	240
Vegetable Thins	21 (1 oz)	150	2	7	0	20	tr	330
Nairn's								
Oatcake Fine	2 (0.5 oz)	70	2	3	0	10	1	110
Oatcake Rough	2 (0.8 oz)	91	2	4	0	14	2	160

FOOD	PORTION	CALS	PROT	FAT	CHOL	CARB	FIBER	SOD
New York Style								
Crispini Seeds & Spice	6	120	4	4	0	19	tr	190
Panetini Original	2	80	2	4	0	10	0	90
Panetini Three Cheese	2	80	2	5	0	9	0	150
Pita Chips Garlic	7	130	3	5	0	17	1	440
Pita Chips Natural Whole Wheat	7	120	3	5	0	17	3	350
Nonni's								
Panetini Roasted Garlic	5 (1 oz)	120	4	4	0	19	tr	300
Panetini Sun Dried Tomato Basil	5 (1 oz)	120	4	4	0	17	tr	170
Orkney								
Oatcakes Thin	4 (1.8 oz)	227	6	12	–	25	3	600
Pepperidge Farm								
100 Calorie Pack Goldfish Cheddar	1 pkg	100	3	4	<5	14	1	170
100 Calorie Pack Goldfish Pretzel	1 pkg	100	2	2	0	18	tr	200
Goldfish Cinnamon Graham	1 pkg	210	3	8	5	32	1	220
Goldfish Pizza	55	140	3	5	0	20	tr	230
Goldfish Reduced Sodium Cheddar	60	140	4	5	<5	20	tr	170
Goldfish w/ Whole Grain Cheddar	55 (1.1 oz)	140	4	5	<5	19	2	250
Snack Sticks Pumpernickel	15	120	3	2	0	24	2	410
Water Crackers	4	60	0	1	0	12	tr	90
Wheat Crisps Spicy Salsa	16	140	2	6	0	21	2	270
Premium								
Saltines Fat Free	5 (0.5 oz)	60	1	0	0	12	0	170
Saltines Low Sodium	5 (0.5 oz)	80	1	2	0	11	0	25
Saltines Multigrain	5 (0.5 oz)	60	1	2	0	10	tr	170
Saltines Original	5 (0.5 oz)	60	1	2	0	11	0	190
Ritz								
Bites Cheese	13 (1 oz)	150	2	9	0	17	0	250
Hint Of Salt	0.5 oz	80	1	4	0	10	0	35
Original	0.5 oz	80	1	5	0	10	0	135
Reduced Fat	5 (0.5 oz)	70	1	2	0	11	0	160
Roasted Vegetable	5 (0.5 oz)	80	1	4	0	10	0	150

FOOD	PORTION	CALS	PROT	FAT	CHOL	CARB	FIBER	SOD
Sociables								
Original	0.5 oz	70	1	4	0	9	0	140
SunRidge Farms								
Japanese Rice	¼ cup (1 oz)	110	2	0	0	26	0	220
Suzie's								
Flatbreads Garlic Salt	1 oz	70	2	1	0	15	0	190
Triscuit								
Cracked Pepper & Olive Oil	6 (1 oz)	120	3	4	0	20	3	140
Deli-Style Rye	1 oz	120	3	5	0	19	3	150
Original	1 oz	120	3	5	0	19	3	180
Reduced Fat	1 oz	120	3	3	0	21	3	160
True North								
Peanut Crunches	¼ cup (1 oz)	150	5	8	0	13	4	130
Pistachio Crisps	12 (1 oz)	140	5	7	0	15	2	240
Utz								
Cheese Peanut Butter	6	200	4	10	<5	21	2	390
Vegetable Thins								
Original	21 (1.1 oz)	150	2	7	0	19	1	320
Vinta								
Original	3 (0.7 oz)	100	2	5	0	12	1	180
Wasa								
Hearty	1 (0.5 oz)	45	1	0	0	11	2	70
Light Rye	2 (0.6 oz)	60	2	0	0	14	3	70
Multi Grain	1 (0.5 oz)	45	2	0	0	10	2	80
Sourdough	1 (0.4 oz)	35	1	0	0	9	2	45
Whole Grain	1 (0.4 oz)	40	1	0	0	10	2	50
Whole Wheat	1 (0.5 oz)	50	2	1	0	10	1	70
Water Crackers								
Original	6 (0.5 oz)	60	2	2	0	11	0	120
Westminster								
Oyster	1 pkg (0.5 oz)	66	1	2	0	11	0	60
Wheat Thins								
100% Whole Grain	1 oz	140	2	6	0	21	2	290
Low Sodium	1.1 oz	150	2	6	0	22	1	80
Original	16 (1.1 oz)	140	2	5	0	22	2	230
Reduced Fat	1 oz	130	3	4	0	21	1	260
Wheatsworth								
Crackers	5 (0.5 oz)	80	2	4	0	10	1	180

FOOD	PORTION	CALS	PROT	FAT	CHOL	CARB	FIBER	SOD
CRANBERRIES								
cranberry orange relish	¼ cup	118	tr	tr	0	31	2	1
dried	½ cup	85	tr	tr	0	23	2	1
fresh chopped	1 cup	13	tr	tr	0	3	1	1
fresh whole	1 cup	11	tr	tr	0	3	1	1
sauce	1 slice (2 oz)	86	tr	tr	0	22	1	17
sauce	¼ cup	109	tr	tr	0	27	1	20
Chukar Cherries								
North Cove Dried	¼ cup	100	0	0	0	24	2	0
Craisins								
Blueberry	⅓ cup	140	0	0	0	34	–	0
Cherry	⅓ cup	130	0	0	0	33	–	0
Dried Cranberries	⅓ cup	130	0	0	0	33	–	0
Orange	⅓ cup	130	0	0	0	33	–	0
De-Lite								
Dried Sweetened	1 oz	92	tr	tr	0	23	1	3
Earthbound Farms								
Organic Dried	⅓ cup	130	0	0	0	34	2	2
Emily's								
Milk Chocolate Covered	¼ cup (1.4 oz)	180	tr	10	<5	24	2	0
Fool								
Cranberry Spread	1 tbsp	30	0	0	0	7	1	0
Fruitaceuticals								
OmegaCrans Dried	¼ cup	91	0	1	0	22	1	0
Mariani								
Dried Sweetened	⅓ cup	130	0	0	0	35	2	0
Ocean Spray								
Fresh	2 oz	30	–	0	0	6	–	0
Jellied Sauce	¼ cup (2.5 oz)	110	0	0	0	25	tr	10
Whole Berry Sauce	¼ cup (2.5 oz)	110	0	0	0	25	1	10
S&W								
Sauce Jellied	¼ cup (2.5 oz)	100	0	0	0	26	1	35
Sauce Whole Berry	¼ cup (2.5 oz)	100	0	0	0	26	1	35

FOOD	PORTION	CALS	PROT	FAT	CHOL	CARB	FIBER	SOD
Sarabeth's								
Relish	1 tbsp (0.7 oz)	45	0	0	0	36	3	0
Stoneridge Orchards								
Dried	⅓ cup (¼ oz)	140	0	0	0	33	2	10
Sun-Maid								
Dried Cape Cod	⅓ cup (1.4 oz)	130	0	0	0	33	2	0
Sunsweet								
Dried	⅓ cup (1.4 oz)	140	0	0	0	35	2	0
Tree Of Life								
Organic Jellied	¼ cup (2.5 oz)	100	0	0	0	26	1	35
Truitt Brothers								
Sauce Orchard Medley	⅓ cup (2.7 oz)	90	0	0	0	24	2	25
Wild Thymes Farm								
Cranberry Fig Sauce	1 tsp	19	tr	0	0	5	tr	0
Original Cranberry Sauce	1 tbsp	21	0	0	0	5	tr	0
CRANBERRY BEANS								
canned	½ cup	108	7	tr	0	20	8	432
dried cooked w/o salt	½ cup	120	8	tr	0	22	9	1
Goya								
Roman Beans Dried not prep	¼ cup (1.4 oz)	80	8	0	0	24	13	15
CRANBERRY JUICE								
cranberry juice cocktail low calorie w/ vitamin C	8 oz	46	tr	tr	0	11	0	7
cranberry juice cocktail w/ vitamin C	8 oz	137	0	tr	0	34	0	5
unsweetened	8 oz	116	1	tr	0	31	tr	5
Apple & Eve								
100% Juice	8 oz	130	0	0	0	32	–	25
Lakewood								
Organic	6 oz	50	1	0	0	12	1	4
Organic Light	6 oz	45	1	0	0	18	1	3

FOOD	PORTION	CALS	PROT	FAT	CHOL	CARB	FIBER	SOD
Nantucket Nectars								
Cranberry Cocktail	8 oz	130	0	0	0	33	0	25
Northland								
100% Juice No Sugar Added	8 oz	130	0	0	0	33	–	35
Ocean Spray								
100% Juice Cranberry Blend	8 oz	140	0	0	0	36	–	35
Cocktail	8 oz	120	0	0	0	30	–	35
Cocktail Light	8 oz	40	0	0	0	10	–	75
Diet	8 oz	5	0	0	0	2	–	50
White Cocktail Light	8 oz	40	0	0	0	10	–	75
White Cranberry	8 oz	110	0	0	0	27	–	50
White Cranberry Strawberry	8 oz	110	0	0	0	27	–	50
Old Orchard								
Cocktail	8 oz	140	0	0	0	34	–	30
Santa Cruz								
Organic Nectar	8 oz	110	tr	0	0	27	0	25
SSips								
Cocktail	1 box (7 oz)	110	0	0	0	28	–	0
CRAYFISH								
cooked	3 oz	97	20	1	151	0	0	58
raw	3 oz	76	16	1	118	0	0	45
raw	8	24	5	tr	37	0	0	14
CREAM (*see also* WHIPPED TOPPINGS)								
clotted cream	2 tbsp (1 oz)	164	tr	18	48	1	0	18
creme fraiche	2 tbsp (1 oz)	100	1	11	40	1	0	10
half & half	1 tbsp (0.5 oz)	20	tr	2	6	1	–	6
half & half	1 cup (8.5 oz)	315	7	28	89	10	–	98
heavy whipping	1 tbsp (0.5 oz)	52	tr	6	21	tr	–	6
heavy whipping whipped	1 cup (4.1 oz)	411	5	44	163	7	–	89
light coffee	1 cup (8.4 oz)	496	6	46	159	9	–	95

FOOD	PORTION	CALS	PROT	FAT	CHOL	CARB	FIBER	SOD
light coffee	1 tbsp (0.5 oz)	29	tr	3	10	1	–	6
light whipping	1 tbsp (0.5 oz)	44	tr	5	17	tr	–	5
light whipping whipped	1 cup (4.2 oz)	345	5	37	132	7	–	82
Cabot								
Whipped	2 tbsp	15	0	2	<5	1	0	0
Horizon Organic								
Half & Half	2 tbsp	35	1	3	10	1	0	15
Heavy Whipping	1 tbsp	50	0	5	20	0	0	10
Land O Lakes								
Aerosol Whipped Light Cream	2 tbsp (0.2 oz)	20	0	2	5	1	0	0
Half & Half	2 tbsp (1.1 oz)	35	tr	4	10	1	0	15
Half & Half Fat Free	2 tbsp (1.1 oz)	20	1	0	0	3	0	30
Heavy Whipping	1 tbsp (0.5 oz)	50	0	5	20	0	0	5
Organic Valley								
Half & Half	2 tbsp (1 oz)	40	tr	4	10	1	0	10
Straus								
Organic Whipping Cream	1 tbsp (0.5 oz)	52	0	6	25	0	0	0

CREAM CHEESE

FOOD	PORTION	CALS	PROT	FAT	CHOL	CARB	FIBER	SOD
cream cheese	1 pkg (3 oz)	297	6	30	93	2	–	251
cream cheese	1 oz	99	2	10	31	1	–	84
Connoisseur								
Wheel Mango Peach	2 tbsp	110	1	7	20	10	0	110
Wheel Wild Blueberry	2 tbsp	100	1	7	20	9	0	120
Earth Balance								
Brick	2 tbsp	80	3	6	0	2	0	105
Tub	2 tbsp	80	3	6	15	2	0	105
Horizon Organic								
Reduced Fat	2 tbsp	70	2	7	25	2	0	100
Lifeway								
Whipped	2 tbsp	80	2	8	25	1	0	75

FOOD	PORTION	CALS	PROT	FAT	CHOL	CARB	FIBER	SOD
Nancy's								
Organic	2 tbsp	95	1	9	35	2	0	35
Organic Valley								
Cream Cheese	1 oz	100	2	10	35	1	0	105
Soft	2 tbsp	90	1	9	25	2	0	140
Philadelphia								
⅓ Less Fat	1 oz	70	2	6	20	tr	0	120
Original	1 oz	100	2	9	35	1	0	105
Whipped	2 tbsp	60	1	6	20	1	0	90
CREAM CHEESE SUBSTITUTES								
Vegan Gourmet								
Alternative Cream Cheese	2 tbsp (1 oz)	90	2	8	0	3	2	130
CREAM OF TARTAR								
cream of tartar	1 tsp	8	0	0	0	2	0	2
CREPES								
basic crepe unfilled	1 (7 in)	112	4	6	78	11	tr	142
Ekizian								
Chickpea Crepe	1 (7 in) (1.5 oz)	212	7	13	2	16	3	514
CROAKER								
atlantic breaded & fried	3 oz	188	15	11	71	6	–	296
atlantic raw	3 oz	89	15	3	52	0	0	47
CROCODILE								
cooked	3 oz	78	17	1	–	0	0	–
CROISSANT								
apple	1 (2 oz)	145	4	5	18	21	1	156
butter	1 lg (2.4 oz)	272	5	14	45	31	2	498
butter mini	1 (1 oz)	114	2	6	19	13	1	208
cheese	1 (1.5 oz)	174	4	9	24	20	1	233
chocolate	1 (2 oz)	237	5	14	34	25	2	383
TAKE-OUT								
w/ egg & cheese	1 (4.5 oz)	368	13	25	216	24	–	551
w/ egg & sausage	1 (5 oz)	497	16	34	237	31	2	878
w/ egg cheese & bacon	1 (4.1 oz)	385	16	24	253	25	1	806
w/ egg cheese & ham	1 (5.1 oz)	402	21	24	264	25	1	1092
w/ egg cheese & sausage	1 (5.6 oz)	539	20	39	280	26	1	1045
w/ ham & cheese	1 (4 oz)	338	15	20	64	25	1	836

FOOD	PORTION	CALS	PROT	FAT	CHOL	CARB	FIBER	SOD
CROUTONS								
plain	1 cup (1 oz)	122	4	2	0	22	2	209
seasoned	1 cup (1.4 oz)	186	4	7	–	25	2	495
Edward & Sons								
Organic Lightly Salted	2 tbsp	30	tr	1	0	5	0	25
Fresh Gourmet								
Butter & Garlic	7 (7 g)	35	1	2	0	4	0	80
Cheese & Garlic	12 (0.5 oz)	70	1	3	0	9	0	115
Classic Caesar	6 (7 g)	35	1	2	0	4	0	75
Cornbread Sweet Butter	½ cup (1 oz)	110	3	1	0	22	1	260
Country Ranch	6 (7 g)	35	1	2	0	4	–	75
Fat Free Garlic Caesar	12 (7 g)	30	1	0	0	5	0	45
Italian Seasoned	6 (7 g)	35	1	2	0	4	0	70
Organic Seasoned	5 (7 g)	30	1	2	0	4	0	70
Pepperidge Farm								
Whole Grain Seasoned	6	30	1	1	0	5	tr	70
Zesty Italian	6	30	tr	1	0	5	0	55
CUCUMBER								
fresh peeled	1 med (7 oz)	24	1	tr	0	4	1	4
fresh sliced	1 cup	14	1	tr	0	3	1	2
fresh w/ peel sliced	½ cup	34	tr	tr	0	2	tr	1
TAKE-OUT								
cucumber & onion salad w/ vinegar	1 cup	52	1	tr	0	12	1	375
cucumber raita	1 serv (3.3 oz)	40	2	3	6	3	1	233
cucumber salad w/ oil & vinegar	1 cup	183	1	15	0	11	1	329
cucumber salad w/ sour cream dressing	1 cup	68	1	6	12	3	1	16
kimchee	½ cup (1.8 oz)	36	tr	2	0	4	tr	173
tzatziki	½ cup (3.4 oz)	72	2	6	5	4	1	197
CUMIN								
seed	1 tsp (2 g)	8	tr	tr	0	1	tr	4
seed	1 tbsp (6 g)	22	1	1	0	3	1	10

FOOD	PORTION	CALS	PROT	FAT	CHOL	CARB	FIBER	SOD
CURRANT JUICE								
black currant nectar	7 oz	110	tr	0	–	26	–	10
red currant nectar	7 oz	108	tr	tr	–	26	–	tr
Fructal								
Black Currant	1 bottle (6.75 oz)	102	0	0	0	25	1	1
GoodBelly								
Black Currant Probiotic Drink	8 oz	120	tr	0	0	31	0	30
CURRANTS								
black fresh	½ cup	36	1	tr	0	9	–	1
zante dried	½ cup	204	3	tr	0	53	–	6
Sun-Maid								
Zante	¼ cup (1.4 oz)	120	1	0	0	30	2	10
CURRY								
curry powder	1 tsp	7	tr	tr	0	1	1	1
curry sauce mix as prep	1 cup	120	3	6	0	14	–	1142
curry sauce mix as prep w/ milk	1 cup	270	11	15	35	26	–	1276
paste	1 tube (6 oz)	465	7	36	16	30	12	4394
Ethnic Gourmet								
Gujarati Vegetable Curry	1 pkg (10 oz)	380	8	11	0	63	4	540
Malay Chicken Curry	1 pkg (10 oz)	410	18	11	35	59	2	530
Simmer Sauce Bombay Curry	4 oz	70	2	3	0	10	2	540
Fortun's								
Finishing Sauce Mulligatawny Curry	¼ cup (2 oz)	60	1	2	5	10	1	370
French Meadow Bakery								
Fragrant Chicken Curry	1 pkg (12 oz)	280	28	5	65	36	3	590
Helen's Kitchen								
Indian Curry w/ Tofu Steaks & Rice	1 pkg (9 oz)	300	14	8	0	63	5	300

FOOD	PORTION	CALS	PROT	FAT	CHOL	CARB	FIBER	SOD
Kikkoman								
Sauce Thai Red Curry	¼ cup (2.2 oz)	90	1	6	0	7	0	500
Sauce Thai Yellow Curry	¼ cup (2.2 oz)	90	1	6	0	6	0	510
Knorr								
Curry Sauce Indian Madras	1 oz	30	tr	2	5	2	–	140
Curry Sauce Thai	1 oz	35	tr	3	0	3	–	90
Patak's								
Curry Paste Biryani	2 tbsp	180	1	16	0	6	3	890
Garam Masala Paste	2 tsp	130	1	12	0	4	0	1080
Tandoori Paste	2 tbsp	30	1	1	0	5	1	800
Vegetable Curry w/ Rice Rich Creamy Coconut	1 pkg	400	6	18	10	54	5	990
Vegetable Curry w/ Rice Rich Tomato & Onion	1 pkg (10.5 oz)	290	6	6	0	53	5	900
Vegetable Curry w/ Rice Tangy Lemon & Cilantro	1 pkg	300	5	7	0	54	5	1020
Vindaloo Paste	2 tbsp	160	1	16	0	4	0	1020
So-Yah!								
Creamy Coconut Curry	1 pkg (10 oz)	190	4	10	0	21	5	850
Red Vindaloo Curry	1 pkg (10 oz)	150	3	4	0	24	8	710
Spice Hunter								
Curry Seasoning Salt Free	¼ tsp	0	0	0	0	0	0	0
TastyBite								
Green Curry Vegetables & Jasmine Rice	1 pkg (12 oz)	320	6	10	0	52	2	530
Yellow Curry Vegetables & Jasmine Rice	1 pkg (12 oz)	380	7	13	0	61	3	440
Thai Kitchen								
Green Curry Paste	1 tbsp (0.5 oz)	15	0	0	0	3	0	510
TAKE-OUT								
beef curry	1 cup	432	27	31	68	14	3	1293
beef kurma	1 serv (10 oz)	611	41	47	114	6	6	589
chicken curry ½ breast	1 serv	160	15	9	45	6	1	624
chicken curry boneless	1 serv (6.2 oz)	219	20	12	62	8	2	857
chicken curry leg & thigh	1 serv	180	17	10	51	7	1	702

FOOD	PORTION	CALS	PROT	FAT	CHOL	CARB	FIBER	SOD
chickpea curry	1 serv (8.3 oz)	305	18	15	12	23	15	1206
eggplant curry	1 serv (8 oz)	241	4	19	0	12	5	1009
lamb curry	1 cup	257	28	14	90	4	1	496
mixed vegetable curry	1 serv (7.7 oz)	398	4	33	–	22	–	–
pea & potato curry	1 serv (7 oz)	284	5	22	–	19	6	–
pork vindaloo curry	1 serv	620	–	47	–	3	–	–
potato curry	1 serv (5.5 oz)	791	29	60	12	35	14	668
sambhar dhal curry	1 serv (10 oz)	177	8	7	0	21	8	1314
shrimp curry	1 cup (8.3 oz)	276	25	14	250	13	1	1239
CUSK								
fillet baked	3 oz	106	23	1	50	0	0	38
CUSTARD								
MIX								
egg custard as prep w/ 2% milk	1 serv (3.5 oz)	112	4	3	49	18	0	87
egg custard as prep w/ whole milk	1 serv (3.5 oz)	122	4	4	51	18	0	84
flan as prep w/ 2% milk	1 serv (3.5 oz)	103	3	2	7	19	0	113
flan as prep w/ whole milk	1 serv (3.5 oz)	113	3	3	12	19	0	112
READY-TO-EAT								
Kozy Shack								
Custard	1 pkg (4 oz)	130	7	3	15	19	0	90
Signature								
Flan Coffee	1 pkg (4.5 oz)	340	11	12	175	48	0	140
Flan Vanilla	1 pkg (4.5 oz)	350	11	13	185	49	0	150
TAKE-OUT								
baked	½ cup (5 oz)	147	7	6	118	16	0	86
flan	½ cup (5.4 oz)	222	7	6	138	35	0	81

FOOD	PORTION	CALS	PROT	FAT	CHOL	CARB	FIBER	SOD
flan de calabaza	1 serv (3.5 oz)	225	5	10	112	30	tr	342
flan de coco	½ cup (4.3 oz)	345	10	13	145	49	tr	163
flan de pina	1 serv (4.2 oz)	186	7	5	222	28	tr	74
flan de pini	½ cup (4.6 oz)	202	7	6	240	31	tr	81
puerto rican corn custard	½ cup (4.9 oz)	553	5	34	0	65	5	882
tocino del cielo heaven's delight	1 cup	856	14	21	967	156	0	48
zabaione	½ cup (2 oz)	135	3	5	213	13	0	9
CUTTLEFISH								
steamed	3 oz	134	28	1	190	1	–	632
DANDELION GREENS								
fresh cooked	½ cup	17	1	tr	0	3	–	23
raw chopped	½ cup	13	1	tr	0	3	–	21
DANISH PASTRY								
TAKE-OUT								
cheese	1 (2.5 oz)	266	6	16	11	26	1	320
cinnamon	1 (5 oz)	572	10	32	30	63	2	527
fruit	1 (5 oz)	527	8	27	162	68	3	503
lemon	1 (2.5 oz)	263	4	13	28	34	1	251
raisin nut	1 (2.3 oz)	280	5	16	30	30	1	236
DATES								
deglet noor chopped	¼ cup (1.3 oz)	104	1	tr	0	28	3	1
deglet noor dried	1 (7 g)	20	tr	tr	0	5	1	0
jujube dried	1 oz	75	1	tr	–	19	2	2
jujube fresh	1 oz	30	tr	tr	0	7	–	1
jujube preserved in sugar	1 oz	91	tr	tr	–	22	–	2
medjool	1 (0.8 oz)	66	tr	tr	0	18	2	0
Bard Valley Growers								
Medjool	1	63	1	0	0	17	2	0
Bob's Red Mill								
Dried Crumbles	⅓ cup	130	1	0	0	33	4	15

FOOD	PORTION	CALS	PROT	FAT	CHOL	CARB	FIBER	SOD
Earthbound Farms								
Organic Dried	6 (1.4 oz)	120	1	0	0	31	3	0
SunDate								
Fancy Medjool	3 (1.4 oz)	120	1	0	0	31	3	0
Sun-Maid								
Pitted	¼ cup (1.4 oz)	110	1	0	0	30	4	0
Tree Of Life								
Deglet Noor Pitted	5 (1.5 oz)	120	1	0	0	31	3	0
Organic Medjool	5 (1.5 oz)	120	1	0	0	31	3	0

DEER (*see* JERKY, VENISON)

DELI MEATS/COLD CUTS (*see also* BEEF, CHICKEN, HAM, MEAT SUBSTITUTES, TURKEY)

FOOD	PORTION	CALS	PROT	FAT	CHOL	CARB	FIBER	SOD
barbecue loaf pork & beef	1 slice (0.8 oz)	40	4	2	9	1	0	307
beerwurst beef	2 oz	155	8	13	35	2	1	410
berliner pork & beef	1 slice (0.8 oz)	53	4	4	11	1	0	298
blood sausage	1 slice (0.9 oz)	95	4	9	30	tr	0	170
bologna beef	1 slice (1 oz)	88	3	8	16	1	0	302
bologna beef & pork	1 slice (1 oz)	87	4	7	17	2	0	209
bologna beef & pork low fat	1 slice (1 oz)	64	3	5	11	1	0	310
bologna beef lowfat	1 slice (1 oz)	57	3	4	12	1	0	330
bologna beef reduced sodium	1 slice (1 oz)	88	3	8	16	1	0	191
braunschweiger pork	1 slice (1 oz)	92	4	8	50	1	0	325
corned beef brisket	2 oz	90	11	5	35	0	0	370
dutch brand loaf pork & beef	1 slice (1.3 oz)	104	5	9	23	1	tr	401
headcheese pork	1 slice (1.6 oz)	71	6	5	31	0	0	374
honey loaf pork & beef	1 slice (1 oz)	35	4	1	10	1	0	370
lebanon bologna beef	2 slices (1 oz)	105	11	6	31	tr	0	783
mortadella beef & pork	1 slice (0.5 oz)	47	2	4	8	tr	0	187
olive loaf pork	2 slices (2 oz)	134	7	9	22	5	0	846
pastrami beef	1 slice (1 oz)	41	6	2	19	tr	tr	248

FOOD	PORTION	CALS	PROT	FAT	CHOL	CARB	FIBER	SOD
peppered loaf pork & beef	1 slice (1 oz)	41	5	2	13	1	0	426
pepperoni pork & beef	15 slices (1 oz)	135	6	12	34	1	tr	519
picnic loaf pork & beef	1 slice (1 oz)	65	4	5	11	1	0	326
salami cooked beef & pork	1 slice (0.8 oz)	58	3	5	15	1	0	245
salami hard pork	3 slices (0.9 oz)	14	6	8	27	1	0	543
salami hard pork & beef less sodium	1 slice (1 oz)	113	4	9	26	2	tr	177
sandwich spread pork & beef	¼ cup	141	5	10	23	7	tr	608
summer sausage thuringer cervelat	2 oz	203	10	17	41	2	0	728
Applegate Farms								
Organic Genoa Salami Sliced	1 oz	100	7	7	25	0	0	400
Butterball								
Turkey Bologna	1 slice (1 oz)	60	3	5	15	3	–	300
Turkey Ham	1 slice (1 oz)	35	4	2	10	1	–	340
Carl Buddig								
Beef	2 oz	90	10	5	–	1	–	–
Corned Beef	2 oz	90	10	5	–	1	–	–
Dietz & Watson								
Bologna Beef	3 slices (1.9 oz)	170	7	14	35	3	0	490
Mortadella	2 oz	150	19	14	30	2	0	560
Sopressata	1 oz	90	8	7	24	1	0	500
Healthy Ones								
Pastrami 97% Fat Free	4 slices (2 oz)	60	10	2	25	3	0	450
High Plains Bison								
Pastrami	3 oz	80	14	2	25	0	0	1280
Oscar Mayer								
Salami Beef	3 slices (1.8 oz)	150	8	13	40	1	0	640
DILL								
seed	1 tsp	6	tr	tr	0	1	tr	0
sprigs fresh	5 (0.3 oz)	0	tr	tr	0	tr	–	1
weed dry	1 tbsp	8	1	tr	0	2	tr	6

FOOD	PORTION	CALS	PROT	FAT	CHOL	CARB	FIBER	SOD
DINNER (*see also* ASIAN FOOD, CURRY, PASTA DINNERS, POT PIE, SPANISH FOOD)								
A La Carte								
Stuffed Zucchini w/ Barley Risotto Chicken Stuffing in Tomato Sauce	1 serv (5 oz)	140	6	7	25	14	2	280
Amy's								
Country Dinner Vegetable Salisbury Steak	1 pkg (10.9 oz)	380	12	16	30	50	7	680
Banquet								
Boneless Pork Ribs	1 pkg	370	6	17	30	47	4	710
Chicken Fingers	1 pkg	460	13	15	20	69	11	730
Corn Dog Meal	1 pkg	470	11	18	35	68	8	730
Crock Pot Classics Chicken & Dumplings	⅔ cup	200	10	8	35	21	6	940
Crock Pot Classics Hearty Beef & Vegetables	⅔ cup	140	12	6	35	15	4	620
Crock Pot Classics Meatballs In Stroganoff Sauce	⅔ cup	300	14	14	45	29	5	800
Fish Sticks	1 pkg	360	13	13	25	46	3	600
Fried Beef Steak	1 pkg	390	14	19	35	41	3	1040
Meatloaf	1 pkg	300	14	15	35	28	5	820
Original Fried Chicken	1 pkg	380	14	20	30	35	5	930
Salisbury Steak	1 pkg	300	14	16	25	25	5	1090
Swedish Meatballs	1 pkg	430	20	23	90	35	5	950
Turkey	1 pkg	200	14	8	30	27	5	980
Betty Crocker								
Complete Meals Chicken & Buttermilk Biscuits	⅕ pkg (5.4 oz)	280	9	11	15	37	2	950
Complete Meals Stroganoff	⅕ pkg (5 oz)	200	10	5	15	30	1	760
Birds Eye								
Steamfresh Meals For Two Asian Chicken Vegetable Medley	½ pkg (11.9 oz)	290	20	6	50	36	10	1290
Steamfresh Meals For Two Grilled Chicken Marinara	½ pkg (11.9 oz)	360	21	10	30	45	4	1030
Steamfresh Meals For Two Sweet & Spicy Chicken	½ pkg (11.9 oz)	370	20	10	35	53	4	930
Voila! Pasta Primavera w/ Chicken	1⅔ cups	250	14	3	10	42	7	1130

FOOD	PORTION	CALS	PROT	FAT	CHOL	CARB	FIBER	SOD
Voila! Shrimp Scampi	1¾ cups	190	11	3	60	31	3	540
Voila! Southwestern Chicken	2 cups	250	14	6	30	32	2	640
C&W								
Stir Fry Feast Pot Sticker + Sauce	2 cups	200	10	4	15	30	4	1200
Stir Fry Feast Ultimate + Sauce	1½ cups	190	11	5	30	25	3	1350
Campbell's								
Supper Bakes Cheesy Chicken w/ Pasta	⅙ pkg	170	6	4	5	28	1	840
Supper Bakes Garlic Chicken w/ Pasta	⅙ pkg	220	9	2	<5	42	2	760
Supper Bakes Savory Pork Chops w/ Herb Stuffing	⅙ box	160	5	2	<5	30	1	780
Supper Bakes Traditional Roast Chicken w/ Stuffing	⅙ pkg	160	5	3	<5	29	2	740
Contessa								
Beef Goulash not prep	1¾ cups	210	12	5	50	32	3	850
Chicken Cacciatore not prep	1¾ cups	230	14	7	35	24	6	810
Chicken Alfredo not prep	1¾ cups	330	15	18	70	28	2	660
Fillo Factory								
Organic Fillo Pie Eggplant & Red Pepper	1 serv (5 oz)	230	4	9	0	35	3	310
French Meadow Bakery								
Garlic Ginger Chicken	1 pkg (12 oz)	310	24	5	60	42	3	880
Gardein								
Burgundy Trio	1 pkg	230	22	4	0	26	4	700
Thai Trio	1 pkg	250	19	8	0	25	3	750
Glory								
Savory Singles Chicken & Dumplings	1 pkg	290	16	8	75	40	6	1400
Savory Singles Chicken Smoked Sausage & Rice Casserole	1 pkg	440	18	18	60	49	1	1390
Savory Singles Ham & Sausage Jambalaya	1 pkg	400	17	18	50	42	2	1320

FOOD	PORTION	CALS	PROT	FAT	CHOL	CARB	FIBER	SOD
Savory Singles Turkey & Gravy w/ Cornbread Stuffing	1 pkg	440	18	18	30	49	2	1380
Gluten Free Cafe								
Lemon Basil Chicken	1 pkg (9.2 oz)	340	18	11	55	42	3	720
Glutino								
Gluten Free Chicken Pomodoro w/ Brown Rice & Vegetables	1 pkg (9.1 oz)	190	11	3	15	33	3	910
Gluten Free Chicken Ranchero w/ Brown Rice	1 pkg (9.1 oz)	180	14	2	20	30	4	790
Green Giant								
Create A Meal Stir Fry Sweet & Sour as prep	1 cup	280	2	7	54	36	3	528
Skillet Meal Chicken Teriyaki as prep	1½ cups	240	13	1	20	46	3	780
Healthy Choice								
Beef Pot Roast w/ Gravy	1 pkg (11 oz)	310	15	7	45	45	5	500
Beef Tips Portabello	1 pkg (11.25 oz)	270	18	6	45	34	6	520
Cafe Steamers Beef Merlot	1 pkg (10 oz)	220	17	6	25	22	5	580
Cafe Steamers Cajun Style Chicken & Shrimp	1 pkg (10.4 oz)	250	18	3	40	36	3	600
Cafe Steamers Chicken Margherita	1 pkg (10 oz)	340	23	8	30	43	4	550
Cafe Steamers Creamy Dill Salmon	1 pkg (9.8 oz)	240	19	6	15	26	5	600
Cafe Steamers Grilled Basil Chicken	1 (10.6 oz)	290	20	6	25	37	5	580
Cafe Steamers Grilled Whiskey Steak	1 pkg (9.4 oz)	250	18	4	30	34	6	580
Chicken Parmigiana	1 pkg (11.6 oz)	350	16	10	25	49	7	580
Country Herb Chicken	1 pkg (11.35 oz)	240	15	5	30	34	5	600
Fire Roasted Tomato Chicken	1 pkg (11.7 oz)	310	19	5	35	46	6	500

FOOD	PORTION	CALS	PROT	FAT	CHOL	CARB	FIBER	SOD
Fresh Mixers Southwestern Chicken	1 pkg (7.9 oz)	310	13	3	15	60	5	550
Golden Roasted Turkey Breast	1 pkg (10.5 oz)	290	17	5	30	44	8	460
Lemon Pepper Fish	1 pkg (10.7 oz)	310	14	5	25	50	5	450
Mandarin Chicken	1 pkg (9.1 oz)	240	13	3	15	39	5	510
Pineapple Chicken	1 pkg (9 oz)	380	9	7	10	68	5	210
Salisbury Steak	1 pkg (12.5 oz)	360	20	9	40	46	7	600
Slow Roasted Turkey Medallions	1 pkg (8.5 oz)	220	14	5	35	28	5	500
Sweet & Sour Chicken	1 pkg (12 oz)	430	16	9	20	69	5	600
Traditional Turkey Breast	1 pkg	300	21	4	25	42	6	550
Hormel								
Compleats Microwave Meals Beef Steak & Peppers w/ Noodles	1 pkg (9.9 oz)	210	20	5	50	22	2	580
Compleats Microwave Meals Chicken Breast & Dressing	1 pkg (9.9 oz)	270	23	7	45	29	2	800
Compleats Microwave Meals Chicken Breast & Gravy w/ Mashed Potatoes	1 pkg (9.9 oz)	200	19	3	35	24	2	950
Compleats Microwave Meals Homestyle Beef w/ Potatoes & Gravy	1 pkg (9.9 oz)	220	11	6	15	30	3	600
Compleats Microwave Meals Meatloaf w/ Potatoes & Gravy	1 pkg (9.9 oz)	310	18	11	40	34	3	940
Compleats Microwave Meals Salisbury Steak w/ Slice Potato & Gravy	1 pkg (9.9 oz)	280	16	11	50	30	2	980
Compleats Microwave Meals Santa Fe Chicken w/ Rice & Beans	1 pkg (9.9 oz)	280	20	4	40	41	4	550

FOOD	PORTION	CALS	PROT	FAT	CHOL	CARB	FIBER	SOD
Compleats Microwave Meals Swedish Meatballs	1 pkg (9.9 oz)	350	15	18	70	32	1	980
Compleats Microwave Meals Sweet & Sour Chicken w/ Rice	1 pkg (9.9 oz)	290	13	2	35	54	2	960
Compleats Microwave Meals Teriyaki Chicken w/ Rice	1 pkg (9.9 oz)	270	13	2	20	50	2	930
Compleats Microwave Meals Tuna Casserole	1 pkg (9.9 oz)	240	17	7	35	26	2	880
Compleats Microwave Meals Turkey & Dressing w/ Gravy	1 pkg (9.9 oz)	290	20	9	45	31	2	960
Compleats Microwave Meals Turkey & Hearty Vegetables	1 pkg (9.9 oz)	180	14	4	25	24	4	1200
Joy Of Cooking								
Braised Beef Tips & Egg Noodles	1 cup (7.7 oz)	220	17	7	75	24	1	650
Roasted Herb Chicken	1 cup (7.7 oz)	170	11	3	25	27	3	640
Kashi								
Black Bean Mango	1 pkg (10 oz)	340	8	8	0	58	7	430
Lemon Rosemary Chicken	1 pkg (10 oz)	330	17	9	15	45	5	640
Lime Cilantro Shrimp	1 pkg (10 oz)	250	12	8	0	33	6	690
Southwest Style Chicken	1 pkg (10 oz)	240	16	5	30	32	6	680
Sweet & Sour Chicken	1 pkg (10 oz)	320	18	4	35	55	6	380
Lean Cuisine								
Cafe Classics Sweet & Sour Chicken	1 pkg (10 oz)	300	18	3	30	51	2	560
Dinnertime Selects Lemon Garlic Shrimp	1 pkg (12 oz)	350	18	7	75	54	5	830
Marie Callender's								
Chicken Fried Beef	1 meal	540	19	28	45	51	6	1510
Chicken Teriyaki	1 meal	430	19	4	45	78	5	1230

FOOD	PORTION	CALS	PROT	FAT	CHOL	CARB	FIBER	SOD
Golden Battered Filet Dinner	1 meal	450	22	16	35	53	4	1170
Herb Roasted Chicken	1 meal	460	30	25	65	26	5	1030
Meat Loaf w/ Gravy	1 meal	480	31	22	60	39	3	1080
Old Fashioned Beef Pot Roast	1 meal	330	27	10	45	32	9	970
Salisbury Steak	1 meal	400	27	16	50	38	7	820
Slow Roasted Beef	1 meal	370	25	13	40	37	7	1370
Sweet & Sour Chicken	1 meal	600	22	20	25	88	10	860
Turkey w/ Stuffing	1 meal	400	32	9	65	45	4	1230
Meals To Live								
Grilled White Chicken w/ Brown Rice & Vegetables Gluten Free	1 pkg (9 oz)	260	17	5	30	30	5	470
Grilled White Chicken w/ Red Roasted Potatoes & Green Beans	1 pkg (8 oz)	200	14	3	30	30	3	470
Shrimp Jambalaya Gluten Free	1 pkg (9 oz)	220	13	4	90	31	4	480
Sliced Turkey w/ Balsamic Sauce & Butternut Squash Gluten Free	1 pkg (7 oz)	230	17	5	40	28	4	450
Stacked Eggplant w/ Seasoned White Chicken	1 pkg (9 oz)	200	14	5	20	28	3	480
White Chicken Fajita w/ Santa Fe Rice Gluten Free	1 pkg (9 oz)	240	17	5	30	34	5	480
Mon Cuisine								
Vegan Moroccan Couscous	1 pkg (10 oz)	280	20	4	0	46	10	440
Vegan Veal Schnitzel In Sauce	1 pkg (10 oz)	300	24	8	0	38	7	440
Vegetarian Stuffed Cabbage In Tomato Sauce	1 pkg (10 oz)	220	13	5	0	36	5	260
Moosewood								
Organic Vegetarian Moroccan Stew	1 pkg (10 oz)	150	5	3	0	29	5	400

FOOD	PORTION	CALS	PROT	FAT	CHOL	CARB	FIBER	SOD
Organic Bistro								
Alaskan Salmon Cakes	1 pkg (10 oz)	410	28	16	70	39	8	250
Chicken Citron	1 pkg (13.5 oz)	490	31	17	60	53	6	400
Ginger Chicken	1 pkg (13.25 oz)	490	31	17	60	53	6	400
Jamaican Shrimp Cakes	1 pkg (12 oz)	380	23	8	130	55	7	140
Savory Turkey	1 pkg (12 oz)	430	35	14	65	43	8	290
Spiced Chicken Morocco	1 pkg (12.2 oz)	390	26	11	50	46	7	330
Wild Salmon	1 pkg (13.1 oz)	500	35	23	95	41	8	80
Organic Classics								
Chicken Marsala w/ Mashed Potatoes	1 pkg (9.5 oz)	330	14	16	60	31	3	530
Jamaican Style Jerk Chicken w/ Wehani Rice	1 pkg (9.5 oz)	270	16	7	40	37	4	620
Lemon Chicken w/ Wehani Rice	1 pkg (9.5 oz)	320	14	8	35	49	3	320
South Beach								
Chicken Santa Fe Style Rice & Beans	1 pkg (8.9 oz)	340	22	12	80	35	4	750
Meatloaf w/ Gravy	1 pkg (8.9 oz)	210	16	9	50	17	4	910
Roasted Turkey	1 pkg (9.4 oz)	240	17	9	50	27	4	920
Stouffer's								
Beef Stew	1 pkg (11 oz)	280	21	9	40	28	4	1000
Beef Stroganoff	1 pkg (9.75 oz)	380	22	17	70	34	2	990
Chicken A La King	1 pkg (11.5 oz)	360	18	12	35	44	0	800
Corner Bistro Bourbon Steak Tips	1 pkg (12 oz)	520	25	22	50	56	3	1000
Corner Bistro Sesame Chicken	1 pkg (12.63 oz)	510	22	15	75	72	5	1380

FOOD	PORTION	CALS	PROT	FAT	CHOL	CARB	FIBER	SOD
Country Fried Beef Steak	1 pkg (16 oz)	610	22	33	40	55	6	1330
Creamed Chipped Beef	½ pkg (5.5 oz)	140	9	7	35	9	0	590
Fish Filet	1 pkg (9 oz)	400	27	16	55	36	4	1050
Fried Chicken Breast	1 pkg (8.88 oz)	360	20	18	45	30	2	880
Green Pepper Steak	1 pkg (10.5 oz)	240	18	4	30	32	3	910
Grilled Chicken Teriyaki	1 pkg (9.38 oz)	300	21	4	40	45	3	880
Grilled Lemon Pepper Chicken	1 pkg (9 oz)	240	19	8	40	24	4	670
Meatloaf	1 pkg (6 oz)	560	34	29	110	40	8	1180
Pork Cutlet	1 pkg (10 oz)	370	13	21	25	31	3	1110
Roast Pork	1 pkg (9.5 oz)	320	17	11	50	39	4	960
Roast Turkey Breast	1 pkg (16 oz)	390	21	13	40	48	6	1290
Salisbury Steak	1 pkg (16 oz)	470	29	24	65	34	6	1050
Stuffed Pepper	1 pkg (10 oz)	220	11	10	20	22	2	1000
Swedish Meatballs	1 pkg (11.5 oz)	560	32	27	100	47	3	1250
Sukhis								
Tikka Masala Chicken	1 serv (5 oz)	170	25	6	75	46	0	750
Swanson								
Chicken & Dumplings	1 cup	230	11	10	35	24	2	990
Chicken A La King	1 can	270	14	18	20	12	2	1370
Taste Above								
Meatless Zesty BBQ w/ Veggie Beef & Rice	1 pkg (10 oz)	280	16	6	0	48	7	310
TastyBite								
Beans Marsala & Basmati Rice	1 pkg (12 oz)	426	14	8	0	75	13	600
Spinach Dal & Basmati Rice	1 pkg (12 oz)	372	12	9	0	62	8	640

FOOD	PORTION	CALS	PROT	FAT	CHOL	CARB	FIBER	SOD
Stir Fry Vegetables & Jasmine Rice	1 pkg (12 oz)	450	7	16	0	67	3	480
Vegetable Supreme & Basmati Rice	1 pkg (12 oz)	317	11	6	4	55	11	410
Yves								
Meatless Santa Fe Beef	1 pkg (10.5 oz)	360	15	9	0	57	5	750
Zatarain's								
Blackened Chicken w/ Yellow Rice	1 pkg (10.5 oz)	470	16	13	25	71	3	1310
Jambalaya w/ Sausage	1 pkg (12 oz)	500	13	14	25	79	3	1020
Red Beans & Rice w/ Sausage	1 pkg (12 oz)	510	16	20	30	68	5	1200
Rice Bowl Big Easy	1 pkg (10 oz)	430	22	12	45	56	5	870
Sausage & Chicken Gumbo w/ Rice	1 pkg (12 oz)	300	14	14	30	36	2	1330

DIP

FOOD	PORTION	CALS	PROT	FAT	CHOL	CARB	FIBER	SOD
shrimp cream cheese	¼ cup (2 oz)	152	5	14	74	2	tr	245
spinach sour cream	¼ cup	155	2	15	13	4	1	166
Cabot								
French Onion	2 tbsp	50	1	5	15	1	0	200
Ranch	2 tbsp	50	1	5	15	1	0	140
Cedarlane								
Organic Five Layer Mexican	2 tbsp	60	3	3	10	4	1	100
Emerald Valley								
Organic Black Bean	1 tbsp (1 oz)	45	2	2	0	6	1	120
Guiltless Gourmet								
Black Bean Mild	2 tbsp (1.1 oz)	40	2	0	0	7	2	125
Health Is Wealth								
Vegetarian Spinach & Artichoke	3 tbsp (1 oz)	30	1	2	5	3	0	50
Kraft								
Green Onion	2 tbsp	60	tr	5	0	3	0	170
LiteHouse								
Avocado	2 tbsp	140	1	15	15	2	0	210
Caramel Low Fat	1 tbsp	110	1	0	0	27	0	140

FOOD	PORTION	CALS	PROT	FAT	CHOL	CARB	FIBER	SOD
Caramel Original	2 tbsp	110	1	2	0	25	1	125
Dilly	2 tbsp	150	1	16	15	1	0	200
Fruit Dip Chocolate Yogurt	2 tbsp	110	1	6	0	14	0	95
Fruit Dip Vanilla Yogurt	2 tbsp	60	1	2	0	10	0	50
Lite Ranch Veggie	2 tbsp	70	1	7	10	3	0	125
Organic Ranch	2 tbsp	130	1	13	10	2	0	200
Marie's								
French Onion Roasted	2 tbsp	100	1	10	15	2	0	220
Guacamole	2 tbsp	40	1	3	5	3	1	140
Honey Vanilla Cream Fruit Dip	2 tbsp	60	1	5	15	5	0	20
Spinach Parmesan	2 tbsp	90	2	9	15	2	0	200
Naturally Fresh								
Caramel	2 tbsp	100	0	4	5	15	0	130
Chocolate	2 tbsp	70	1	0	0	17	0	40
Cream Cheese Strawberry	2 tbsp	90	1	4	10	14	0	45
Ranch Lite	2 tbsp	80	1	8	5	2	0	240
Ranch Vegetable	2 tbsp	120	1	12	15	2	0	150
Road's End Organics								
Nacho Cheese Gluten Free	2 tbsp	20	2	0	0	3	tr	110
Robert Rothchild Farm								
Artichoke	2 tbsp	60	2	5	<5	2	tr	65
Snyder's Of Hanover								
Three Bean	2 tbsp	25	1	0	0	5	1	150
Utz								
Jalapeno Cheddar	2 tbsp	260	0	4	0	2	0	260
Sour Cream & Onion	2 tbsp	60	1	5	20	2	0	250
Walden Farms								
Blue Cheese Calorie Free	2 tbsp (1 oz)	0	0	0	0	0	0	210
Ranch No Calorie	2 tbsp (1 oz)	0	0	0	0	0	0	230
Wild Thymes Farm								
Indian Vindaloo Curry	1 tbsp	12	tr	1	0	1	tr	51
Indonesian Peanut Sauce	1 tbsp	32	1	2	0	2	tr	74

DOCK

FOOD	PORTION	CALS	PROT	FAT	CHOL	CARB	FIBER	SOD
fresh cooked	3½ oz	20	2	1	0	3	–	3
raw chopped	½ cup	15	1	tr	0	2	–	3

DOUGHNUTS

FOOD	PORTION	CALS	PROT	FAT	CHOL	CARB	FIBER	SOD
chocolate glazed	1 med (1.5 oz)	175	2	8	24	24	1	143

FOOD	PORTION	CALS	PROT	FAT	CHOL	CARB	FIBER	SOD
chocolate w/ chocolate icing	1 med (2 oz)	218	3	12	4	26	1	243
creme filled	1 (3 oz)	307	5	21	20	26	1	263
custard filled	1 (2.3 oz)	235	4	16	16	20	1	201
french cruller glazed	1 med (1.4 oz)	169	1	8	5	24	1	141
jelly filled	1 (3 oz)	289	5	16	22	33	1	249
old fashioned plain	1 med (2 oz)	226	3	13	5	25	1	301
plain chocolate frosted	1 med (1.5 oz)	194	2	11	8	22	1	187
plain glazed	1 med (1.6 oz)	192	2	10	14	23	1	181
whole wheat sugared	1 med (1.6 oz)	162	3	9	9	19	1	160
TAKE-OUT								
andagi okinawan doughnut	1 (0.7 oz)	84	1	5	7	10	0	109
malasada portuguese ball	1 (1.1 oz)	118	2	5	22	16	0	49

DRINK MIXERS

FOOD	PORTION	CALS	PROT	FAT	CHOL	CARB	FIBER	SOD
whiskey sour mix not prep	1 pkg (0.6 oz)	64	tr	0	0	16	–	46
whiskey sour mix	2 oz	55	0	0	0	14	0	66
Angostura								
Bloody Mary	4 oz	20	0	0	0	4	0	560
Daiquiri	2 oz	72	0	0	0	18	0	5
Grenadine	1 tsp	10	0	0	0	3	0	5
Margarita	4 oz	80	0	0	0	30	0	5
Pina Colada	4 oz	60	0	0	0	16	0	120
Strawberry Daiquiri	8 oz	120	0	0	0	31	0	240
Dave's Gourmet								
Bloody Mary Original	2 oz	25	1	0	0	5	tr	210
Fever-Tree								
Bitter Lemon	1 bottle (6.8 oz)	75	tr	0	0	18	0	2
McIlhenny								
Bloody Mary Mix as prep	1 cup	70	2	0	0	15	2	1930
Modmix								
Mojito	2 oz	50	0	0	0	13	0	10
Organic Citrus Margarita	2 oz	70	0	0	0	19	0	0

FOOD	PORTION	CALS	PROT	FAT	CHOL	CARB	FIBER	SOD
Organic French Martini	2 oz	50	0	0	0	13	0	10
Organic Lavender Lemon Drop	2 oz	55	0	0	0	14	0	0
Organic Pomegranate Cosmopolitan	2 oz	55	0	0	0	14	0	10
Organic Wasabi Bloody Mary	2 oz	20	1	0	0	4	0	150
Monin								
Grenadine	1 oz	90	0	0	0	22	–	0
Mojito Mix	1 oz	84	0	0	0	21	–	0
White Sangria Mix	1 oz	91	0	0	0	22	–	0
DRUM								
freshwater fillet baked	5.4 oz	236	35	10	126	0	0	148
freshwater baked	3 oz	130	19	5	70	0	0	82
DUCK								
boneless roasted	½ duck (7.8 oz)	444	52	25	197	0	0	144
boneless w/o skin roasted	3.5 oz	201	23	11	89	0	0	65
boneless w/o skin roasted diced	1 cup (4.9 oz)	281	33	16	125	0	0	91
chinese pressed	3 oz	162	6	8	28	16	1	188
chinese pressed	1 cup (4.9 oz)	267	10	14	46	26	1	309
pekin breast boneless w/ skin roasted	1 (4.2 oz)	242	29	13	163	0	0	101
pekin breast w/o skin broiled	3 oz	133	26	2	136	0	0	100
pekin leg w/ skin w/o bone roasted	1 (3.2 oz)	200	25	10	105	0	0	101
pekin leg w/o skin & bone roasted	1 (2.6 oz)	134	22	5	79	0	0	81
w/ skin & bone roasted	1 serv (6 oz)	583	33	49	145	0	0	102
w/ skin & bone roasted	½ duck (13 oz)	1287	73	108	321	0	0	225
wing roasted bone removed	1 (1.1 oz)	101	6	8	25	0	0	66
Grimaud Farms								
Muscovy Duck Confit	1 serv (3 oz)	170	20	10	95	tr	–	140

FOOD	PORTION	CALS	PROT	FAT	CHOL	CARB	FIBER	SOD
Muscovy Duck Whole	1 serv (3.7 oz)	200	19	14	130	tr	–	125
TAKE-OUT								
breast battered & fried bone removed	½ (3.2 oz)	199	20	10	94	6	tr	310
leg battered & fried bone removed	1 (2.5 oz)	155	16	8	73	5	tr	242

DUMPLING

FOOD	PORTION	CALS	PROT	FAT	CHOL	CARB	FIBER	SOD
Health Is Wealth								
Potstickers Vegan	2 (1.6 oz)	90	6	3	0	13	2	280
Joyce Chen								
Chinese Style Potstickers Chicken & Vegetable	6	170	8	2	15	30	2	125
Chinese Style Potstickers Pork & Vegetable	6	170	8	3	15	30	2	125
Kahiki								
Potstickers Chicken	5 (3.3 oz)	230	7	11	10	24	1	520
Samosas Coconut Curry Chicken	4 (2.8 oz)	170	8	3	15	26	1	520
Pepperidge Farm								
Apple	1	250	3	11	0	32	1	180
Peach	1	320	3	11	0	50	4	150
Traveling Chef								
Potstickers Chicken + Dipping Sauce	5 pieces + 1 tbsp sauce	285	13	7	20	42	1	840
TAKE-OUT								
apple	1 (6.7 oz)	661	7	34	0	83	3	614
bread dumpling	1 lg	330	–	10	–	28	–	–
cherry	1 (2.7 oz)	238	3	12	0	31	1	216
cornmeal	1 (2.8 oz)	134	5	4	62	20	2	278
fried pork	1 (3.5 oz)	338	13	21	27	25	1	363
fried puerto rican style	1 med (1.1 oz)	117	2	7	0	11	tr	182
gyoza potstickers vegetable	8 (4.9 oz)	210	8	4	0	34	5	500
peach	1 (2.7 oz)	253	3	12	0	33	1	248
piroshki meat filled	1 (3.4 oz)	348	12	22	23	25	1	425
steamed meat	1 (1.3 oz)	41	4	1	18	4	tr	161

DURIAN

FOOD	PORTION	CALS	PROT	FAT	CHOL	CARB	FIBER	SOD
fresh	3.5 oz	141	3	2	0	29	–	1

FOOD	PORTION	CALS	PROT	FAT	CHOL	CARB	FIBER	SOD
EDAMAME (*see* SOYBEANS)								
EEL								
fresh cooked	3 oz	200	20	13	137	0	0	55
fresh cooked	1 fillet (5.6 oz)	375	38	24	257	0	0	104
raw	3 oz	156	16	10	107	0	0	43
smoked	3.5 oz	330	19	28	–	0	0	–
EGG (*see also* EGG DISHES, EGG SUBSTITUTES)								
CHICKEN								
fresh large	1 (1.8 oz)	72	6	5	186	tr	0	71
fresh medium	1 (1.5 oz)	63	6	4	164	tr	0	62
fresh small	1 (1.3 oz)	54	5	4	141	tr	0	54
hard or soft cooked	1	77	6	5	186	1	0	139
pickled	1	72	6	5	198	1	0	131
poached	1	73	6	5	184	tr	0	147
scrambled plain	1 (2 oz)	61	6	7	169	1	0	88
sunny side up	2	155	11	12	365	1	0	414
white raw	1 (1.1 oz)	17	4	tr	0	tr	0	55
yolk raw	1 (0.5 oz)	55	3	4	184	1	0	8
Davidson's								
Pasteurized Shell Eggs	1 lg	75	6	5	213	0	0	60
Egg Innovations								
100% Organic Cage Free Large	1 (1.8 oz)	70	6	5	215	1	0	65
Egg-Land's Best								
Extra Large	1 (2 oz)	80	7	5	200	0	0	75
Hard-Cooked Peeled	1 med (1.5 oz)	60	5	4	160	0	0	55
Large	1 (1.8 oz)	70	6	4	175	0	0	60
Good Earth Organics								
Organic Instant Whites	1 pkg (0.5 oz)	50	12	0	0	1	0	0
Horizon Organic								
Jumbo	1 (2.2 oz)	90	8	5	270	1	0	80
Jake & Amos								
Pickled Red Beet Eggs	2 (5.3 oz)	200	10	8	345	21	0	170
Land O Lakes								
Farm Fresh Brown Extra Large	1 (1.8 oz)	70	6	5	215	1	–	65

FOOD	PORTION	CALS	PROT	FAT	CHOL	CARB	FIBER	SOD
Organic Valley								
Egg Whites Pasteurized	¼ cup	25	5	0	0	1	0	90
Large Omega-3	1	70	7	5	225	tr	–	85
Pete & Gerry's								
Organic Large	1 (1.8 oz)	70	6	5	215	1	–	65
Tree Of Life								
White Large Natural Omega-3	1 (1.8 oz)	70	<6	5	250	tr	0	65
OTHER POULTRY								
duck 100 year old	1 (1 oz)	49	4	3	173	1	–	154
duck cooked	1 (2.5 oz)	129	9	10	616	1	0	210
duck preserved hard core	1 (1.8 oz)	80	6	6	220	1	0	350
duck preserved soft core	1 (1.8 oz)	80	7	6	220	1	0	350
duck salted	1 (1 oz)	54	4	4	184	2	–	769
goose cooked	1 (5 oz)	265	20	19	1223	2	0	420
quail canned	1 (0.3 oz)	14	1	1	75	tr	0	47
quail cooked	1 (0.5 oz)	24	2	2	42	0	0	24
turkey raw	1 (2.8 oz)	135	11	9	737	1	0	119

EGG DISHES

FOOD	PORTION	CALS	PROT	FAT	CHOL	CARB	FIBER	SOD
Aunt Jemima								
Eggs & Sausage	1 pkg (6.2 oz)	370	14	27	335	16	2	750
Omelet Ham & Cheese	1 pkg (5.2 oz)	250	13	15	195	17	2	760
Cedarlane								
Zone Omelette Cheese	1 pkg (10.4 oz)	350	25	14	40	31	2	720
Jimmy Dean								
Breakfast Bowls D-Lights Sausage	1 pkg	230	23	7	20	19	2	730
Breakfast Bowls Eggs Potato & Ham	1 pkg	390	24	23	360	23	3	1170
Breakfast Bowls Eggs Potatoes Sausage & Cheddar Cheese	1 pkg	490	23	34	370	20	3	1210
Breakfast Skillets Bacon as prep	1 serv (4.5 oz)	370	10	24	336	14	2	840
Breakfast Skillets Ham as prep	1 serv (4.5 oz)	270	8	15	336	16	2	792

FOOD	PORTION	CALS	PROT	FAT	CHOL	CARB	FIBER	SOD
Breakfast Skillets Smoked Sausage as prep	1 serv (4.5 oz)	380	8	25	345	20	3	792
Omelets Ham & Cheese	1 (4.2 oz)	280	16	19	295	4	0	770
Omelets Sausage & Cheese	1 (4.3 oz)	270	15	22	295	5	0	570
Meals To Live								
Spinach Omelet w/ Turkey Sausage Gluten Free	1 pkg (7.5 oz)	190	17	6	20	18	2	480
TAKE-OUT								
deviled	1 half	62	4	5	121	tr	0	94
eggs benedict	2	825	35	64	784	26	2	1654
omelet cheese	3 eggs	387	25	29	588	6	0	1134
omelet mushroom	3 eggs	251	18	17	511	6	1	796
omelet mushroom & onion	3 eggs	294	20	20	600	7	1	780
omelet plain	3 eggs	338	24	25	736	4	0	854
omelet spanish	3 eggs	496	23	38	626	17	3	876
omelet spinach	3 eggs	279	20	19	568	6	1	687
omelet western	3 eggs	355	24	23	537	6	tr	1007
salad	½ cup	353	10	34	344	2	0	402
scotch egg	1 (4.2 oz)	301	14	21	–	16	2	–
tortilla de amarillo omelet w/ plantain	3 eggs	536	16	35	467	43	3	1017

EGG ROLLS

FOOD	PORTION	CALS	PROT	FAT	CHOL	CARB	FIBER	SOD
egg roll wrapper fresh	1 (1.1 oz)	93	3	tr	3	19	1	183
Blue Horizon Organic								
Spring Rolls Chinese Shrimp	3 (2.1 oz)	130	3	4	0	16	1	210
Spring Rolls Indian	3 (2.1 oz)	110	3	4	0	15	1	250
Spring Rolls Thai	3 (2.1 oz)	110	3	4	0	16	1	210
Spring Rolls Thai Shrimp	3 (2.1 oz)	130	3	4	0	15	1	250
Health Is Wealth								
Spinach	1 (3 oz)	170	8	8	0	18	3	310
Thai Spring Roll	2 (1.6 oz)	90	3	3	0	13	1	300
Kahiki								
Chicken	1 (3 oz)	160	7	6	10	19	1	730
Chipotle Lime Chicken	1 (3 oz)	170	8	4	10	26	2	380
Lemongrass Chicken Stix	3 (2.6 oz)	100	7	2	20	13	tr	380
Pork & Shrimp	1 (3 oz)	140	8	4	30	20	1	630
Vegetable	1 (3 oz)	90	2	4	0	12	1	410

FOOD	PORTION	CALS	PROT	FAT	CHOL	CARB	FIBER	SOD
TAKE-OUT								
chicken	1 (3 oz)	140	7	4	15	20	4	510
lobster	1 (4.8 oz)	270	8	7	0	43	6	460
lumpia vegetable & shrimp	2 (3 oz)	120	4	0	10	26	2	300
meat & shrimp	1 (4.8 oz)	320	10	12	10	41	4	470
pork & shrimp	1 (5 oz)	300	13	10	15	41	7	890
shrimp	1 (2.2 oz)	156	5	7	11	18	2	320
spicy pork	1 (3 oz)	200	6	9	5	23	3	410
spring roll deep fried	1 (0.8 oz)	70	1	4	3	7	1	141
vegetable	1 (3 oz)	170	5	4	0	28	4	520
EGG SUBSTITUTES								
Bob's Red Mill								
Egg White Dried	2 tsp	15	3	0	0	0	0	45
Vegetarian Egg Replacer	1 tbsp	30	3	1	0	2	1	20
Egg Beaters								
Original	¼ cup (2.1 oz)	30	6	0	0	1	0	115
EggPro								
Powder	1 tbsp	15	4	0	0	tr	0	55
Horizon Organic								
Liquid Egg	¼ cup	35	6	0	0	1	0	100
Quick Eggs								
Fat Free Cholesterol Free	¼ cup	30	6	0	0	1	0	115
EGGNOG								
eggnog	1 cup	342	10	19	149	34	–	138
eggnog	1 qt	1368	39	76	596	138	–	553
eggnog flavor mix as prep w/ milk	9 oz	260	8	8	33	39	–	163
Farmland								
Egg Nog	½ cup	180	4	8	50	23	0	150
Horizon Organic								
Lowfat	½ cup	140	6	3	45	22	0	135
Organic Valley								
Ultra Pasteurized	½ cup	180	5	10	90	18	0	85
Straus								
Organic Cream Top	4 oz	160	5	10	70	13	0	55
TAKE-OUT								
eggnog	1 cup	306	5	22	63	16	0	95

FOOD	PORTION	CALS	PROT	FAT	CHOL	CARB	FIBER	SOD
EGGNOG SUBSTITUTES								
Silk								
Nog	½ cup (4 oz)	90	3	2	0	15	0	75
EGGPLANT								
cubed cooked w/ oil	1 cup	133	2	8	0	17	5	1000
pickled	½ cup	33	1	tr	0	7	2	1138
slices grilled	1 (2 oz)	36	tr	2	0	5	1	268
Cedarlane								
Eggplant Mediterranean	1 pkg (10 oz)	230	13	10	20	22	6	590
Celentano								
Eggplant Parmigiana	1 serv (7 oz)	330	9	22	25	26	5	480
Peloponnese								
Baba Ganoush	2 tbsp	40	1	3	0	2	1	250
Stonewall Kitchen								
Eggplant Spread	1 tbsp	25	0	1	–	4	–	90
TastyBite								
Punjab Eggplant	½ pkg (5 oz)	144	4	9	0	13	2	515
The Gracious Gourmet								
Tapenade Roasted Eggplant	2 tbsp (1 oz)	35	1	4	0	3	tr	135
TAKE-OUT								
baba ghannouj	¼ cup	55	2	4	0	5	–	95
caponata	2 tbsp (1 oz)	30	1	2	0	3	–	115
iman bayildi eggplant w/ onion & tomato	1 serv (15.6 oz)	345	3	28	0	25	2	552
indian eggplant runi	1 serv	180	2	14	0	13	1	228
moussaka	1 serv (9 oz)	372	20	24	54	18	5	415
papoutsaki little shoes	1 serv (15.5 oz)	245	12	16	40	15	1	751
tempura	1 serv (1.5 oz)	118	1	10	0	5	1	13
ELDERBERRIES								
fresh	1 cup	105	1	1	0	27	–	–
ELDERBERRY JUICE								
elderberry	7 oz	76	4	0	0	16	–	2
ELK								
eye of round roasted	3.5 oz	151	31	3	63	1	0	50
ground cooked	3.5 oz	143	29	3	70	0	0	56

FOOD	PORTION	CALS	PROT	FAT	CHOL	CARB	FIBER	SOD
Natural Frontier Foods								
Filet	1 (4 oz)	140	26	3	95	0	0	60
EMU								
cooked	3 oz	130	–	–	111	–	–	97
ENERGY BARS (*see also* CEREAL BARS, NUTRITION SUPPLEMENTS)								
Activex								
Organic All Flavors	1 (1.6 oz)	200	8	12	0	17	2	75
Attune								
Wellness Chocolate Crisp	1 (0.7 oz)	100	2	6	0	11	1	20
Wellness Cool Mint Chocolate	1 (0.7 oz)	100	2	6	0	11	1	20
Balance								
100 Calories Peanut Butter Crisp	1 (1 oz)	100	6	5	<5	14	5	180
100 Calories Vanilla Crisp	1 (1 oz)	100	5	4	<5	15	5	180
Carbwell Chocolate Fudge	1 (1.8 oz)	190	14	6	<5	23	2	190
Gold Chocolate Peanut Butter	1 (1.8 oz)	210	14	6	<5	23	tr	125
Gold S'mores Crunch	1 (1.8 oz)	210	15	6	<5	23	0	140
Organic Apricot Mango Crisp	1 (1.6 oz)	180	10	7	0	23	5	120
Organic Cranberry Pomegranate Crisp	1 (1.6 oz)	180	10	7	0	23	5	100
Original Almond Brownie	1 (1.8 oz)	200	14	6	<5	22	2	75
Original Mocha Crisp	1 (1.8 oz)	200	15	6	0	21	tr	95
Pure Banana Cashew	1 (1.6 oz)	180	9	6	0	23	2	80
Pure Cherry Pecan	1 (1.6 oz)	190	9	7	0	22	2	75
Boomi Bar								
Almond Protein Plus	1	270	12	18	15	20	4	12
Cashew Almond Delicacy	1	260	8	17	0	23	1	55
Cranberry Apple	1	210	4	9	0	28	4	50
Merry Macadamia	1	220	3	14	0	26	3	25
Pistachio Pineapple	1	200	5	9	0	28	3	50
Bora Bora								
Organic Island Brazil Nut Almond	1 (1.4 oz)	200	5	12	0	18	2	5
Organic Peanut Peanut	1 (1.4 oz)	230	6	17	0	10	2	10
Organic Sesame Raisin	1 (1.4 oz)	170	5	11	0	17	3	15

FOOD	PORTION	CALS	PROT	FAT	CHOL	CARB	FIBER	SOD
Clif								
Apricot	1 (2.4 oz)	230	10	3	0	45	5	125
Black Cherry Almond	1 (2.4 oz)	250	10	5	0	44	5	110
Builders Chocolate	1 (2.4 oz)	270	20	8	0	30	4	230
Builders Lemon	1 (2.4 oz)	270	20	8	0	31	1	240
Chocolate Almond Fudge	1 (2.4 oz)	250	10	5	0	44	5	140
Chocolate Chip Peanut Crunch	1 (2.4 oz)	260	11	6	0	42	5	200
Crunchy Peanut Butter	1 (2.4 oz)	250	11	6	0	42	5	230
Mojo Chocolate Peanut	1 (1.6 oz)	210	9	10	0	22	3	190
Mojo Honey Roasted Peanuts	1 (1.6 oz)	200	10	10	0	20	2	200
Mojo Mountain Mix	1 (1.6 oz)	180	9	8	0	21	2	220
Mojo Peanut Butter & Jelly	1 (1.6 oz)	220	9	11	0	21	2	115
Nectar Cherry Pomegranate	1 (1.6 oz)	150	3	5	0	29	7	0
Nectar Dark Chocolate Walnut	1 (1.6 oz)	160	3	6	0	27	6	0
Oatmeal Raisin Walnut	1 (2.4 oz)	240	10	5	0	43	5	130
Spiced Pumpkin Pie	1 (2.4 oz)	240	10	5	0	45	5	140
Vanilla Almond	1 (2.4 oz)	270	20	8	0	30	3	240
ZBar Blueberry	1 (1.3 oz)	120	3	3	0	23	3	90
ZBar Honey Graham	1 (1.3 oz)	130	3	3	0	26	3	95
ZBar Spooky S'mores	1 (1.3 oz)	130	2	4	0	23	3	80
Glenny's								
Fruit & Nut Mixed Nut	1	230	6	16	–	14	3	50
Glucerna								
All Flavors	1 (0.7 oz)	80	4	3	0	12	tr	60
Gnu								
Flavor & Fiber Banana Walnut	1 (1.4 oz)	130	3	3	0	30	12	42
Flavor & Fiber Chocolate Brownie Bar	1 (1.4 oz)	140	3	3	0	32	12	55
Granola Gourmet								
Chocolate Espresso	1 (1.23 oz)	150	4	6	0	20	3	15
Ultimate Berry	1 (1.2 oz)	150	5	6	0	19	3	20
Ultimate Cran-Orange	1 (1.2 oz)	140	5	5	0	19	3	30
Ultimate Fudge Brownie	1 (1.3 oz)	150	5	6	0	19	3	30
Ultimate Mocha Fudge	1 (1.2 oz)	150	5	6	0	19	3	35

FOOD	PORTION	CALS	PROT	FAT	CHOL	CARB	FIBER	SOD
Green SuperFood								
Whole Food	1 (2.1 oz)	220	5	8	0	36	4	25
Whole Food Chocolate	1 (2.1 oz)	230	5	9	0	37	0	25
JojoBar								
Chocolate Cashew	1 (1.8 oz)	220	11	14	10	18	2	55
Peanut Butter & Jelly	1 (1.8 oz)	220	13	13	10	17	3	25
Kashi								
GoLean Chocolate Almond Toffee	1 (2.7 oz)	290	13	6	0	45	6	250
GoLean Cookies 'N Cream	1 (2.7 oz)	290	13	6	0	50	6	200
GoLean Crunchy Chocolate Peanut	1 (1.8 oz)	180	9	5	0	30	6	250
GoLean Malted Chocolate Chip	1 (2.7 oz)	290	13	6	0	49	6	200
GoLean Oatmeal Raisin Cookie	1 (2.7 oz)	280	13	5	0	49	6	140
GoLean Peanut Butter & Chocolate	1 (2.7 oz)	290	13	6	0	48	6	280
GoLean Roll Caramel Peanut	1 (1.9 oz)	200	12	5	0	29	6	210
GoLean Roll Fudge Sundae	1 (1.9 oz)	190	12	5	0	27	6	260
TLC Chewy Granola Cherry Dark Chocolate	1 (1.2 oz)	120	5	2	0	24	4	75
TLC Crunchy Granola Honey Toasted 7 Grain	1 (1.4 oz)	180	7	6	0	26	4	160
TLC Crunchy Granola Pumpkin Spice	1 (1.4 oz)	180	6	6	0	26	4	150
TLC Crunchy Granola Roasted Almond	1 (1.4 oz)	180	7	6	0	26	4	160
LaraBar								
Jocalat Chocolate	1 (1.7 oz)	190	5	10	0	24	5	0
Lean Body								
Gold Caramel Cookie Twist	1 (2.9 oz)	330	30	7	0	36	2	430
Living Harvest								
Organic Hemp Protein Forbidden Fruit	1 (1.6 oz)	170	6	6	0	25	4	100
Luna								
Berry Almond	1 (1.7 oz)	170	9	4	0	29	3	115
Chai Tea	1 (1.7 oz)	190	9	5	0	26	3	95
Dulce De Leche	1 (1.7 oz)	170	9	4	0	28	3	120

FOOD	PORTION	CALS	PROT	FAT	CHOL	CARB	FIBER	SOD
Mini Caramel Nut Brownie	1 (0.7 oz)	70	3	3	0	11	2	50
Mini S'mores	1 (0.7 oz)	80	4	2	0	11	1	60
Sunrise Apple Cinnamon	1 (1.7 oz)	180	8	5	0	27	5	100
Sunrise Strawberry Crunch	1 (1.7 oz)	170	8	5	0	26	5	105
Toasted Nuts 'N Cranberry	1 (1.7 oz)	170	9	5	0	26	3	180
Mrs. May's								
Trio Blueberry	1 (1.2 oz)	170	5	12	0	15	2	45
Trio Tropical	1 (1.2 oz)	170	5	12	0	14	2	45
Muscle Milk								
Light Chocolate Peanut Caramel	1 (1.59 oz)	170	15	6	0	18	4	105
Nature's Path								
Optimum Pomegran Cherry	1 (2 oz)	230	4	5	0	39	4	140
Nutiva								
Organic Flax & Raisin	1 (1.4 oz)	200	7	15	0	15	4	0
Organic Flaxseed Flax Chocolate	1 (1.4 oz)	200	6	12	0	19	5	5
Organic Original Hempseed	1 (1.4 oz)	210	9	14	0	11	5	5
Odwalla								
Berries GoMega	1	220	5	5	0	41	5	230
Carrot	1	220	4	4	0	43	4	115
Choco-walla	1	240	5	6	0	42	5	80
Cranberry C Monster	1	220	4	3	0	44	3	85
Super Protein	1	230	16	5	0	31	4	160
Superfood	1	230	4	4	0	43	3	110
POM								
Pomegranate Dipped In Chocolate	1 (1.8 oz)	210	3	8	0	31	4	5
POMx								
Coconut Dipped In Yogurt	1 (1.8 oz)	230	3	12	0	28	3	15
Pomegranate Dipped In Yogurt	1 (1.8 oz)	210	3	8	0	31	4	15
Prana Bar								
Apricot Goji	1 (1.7 oz)	220	4	13	0	26	3	30
Coconut Acai	1 (1.7 oz)	220	4	13	0	26	3	35
Pear Ginseng	1 (1.7 oz)	220	5	15	0	21	4	30
PureFit								
Almond Crunch	1 (2 oz)	230	18	6	0	25	3	190
Peanut Butter Crunch	1 (2 oz)	240	18	7	0	26	2	200

FOOD	PORTION	CALS	PROT	FAT	CHOL	CARB	FIBER	SOD
Sencha Naturals								
Green Tea Bar Lively Lemongrass	1 (2 oz)	220	9	8	0	29	3	115
Green Tea Bar Original	1 (2 oz)	220	9	9	0	29	3	120
Simply Nutrilite								
Sweet & Salty	1 (1.6 oz)	170	4	6	0	27	4	310
Snickers								
Marathon Chewy Chocolatey Peanut	1 (1.94 oz)	210	13	8	5	26	5	170
South Beach								
Energy Mix	1 pkg (1 oz)	160	6	13	0	8	2	45
SoyJoy								
Soy & Fruit Banana	1 (1.1 oz)	130	4	6	20	16	2	50
Soy & Fruit Blueberry	1 (1.1 oz)	140	4	6	20	17	4	45
Soy & Fruit Mango Coconut	1 (1.1 oz)	140	4	6	20	16	3	45
SunRidge Farms								
Energy Nuggets	2 (1.4 oz)	200	6	11	0	18	4	0
Think5								
Red Berry	1 (2.5 oz)	240	4	4	0	48	3	140
Red Berry Chocolate Covered	1 (2.8 oz)	290	4	8	0	52	3	140
ThinkPink								
Blueberry Dark Chocolate	1 (2.1 oz)	240	20	8	0	26	2	80
Lemon Burst	1 (2.1 oz)	230	20	7	0	27	2	150
Peanut Butter Caramel	1 (2.1 oz)	230	20	8	5	26	1	280
White Chocolate Raspberry	1 (2.1 oz)	240	20	8	0	28	3	100

ENERGY DRINKS

FOOD	PORTION	CALS	PROT	FAT	CHOL	CARB	FIBER	SOD
180								
Blue w/ Acai	1 can (8.2 oz)	120	0	0	0	31	–	–
Blue w/ Acai Low Calorie	1 can (8.2 oz)	15	0	0	0	4	–	–
1In3Trinity								
Energy Drink	1 can (8.4 oz)	10	0	0	0	3	0	0
B52								
Zero Sugar Citrus Berry	8 oz	10	0	0	0	1	–	190
Bai								
Antioxidant Infusion Jamaica Blueberry	8 oz	70	0	0	0	18	–	10

FOOD	PORTION	CALS	PROT	FAT	CHOL	CARB	FIBER	SOD
Antioxidant Infusion Kenya Peach	8 oz	70	0	0	0	17	–	10
Antioxidant Infusion Mango Kauai	8 oz	70	0	0	0	18	–	10
Bawls								
Guarana	8 oz	90	0	0	0	25	–	30
Guaranexx Sugar Free	1 bottle (10 oz)	0	0	0	0	0	0	15
Bing								
Energy Drink	1 can (12 oz)	40	0	0	0	10	–	20
Bloom								
All Flavors	1 can (10.5 oz)	100	tr	0	0	24	–	115
Boost								
Beauty	1 bottle (12 oz)	220	2	0	tr	52	tr	30
Youth	1 bottle (12 oz)	200	2	0	tr	48	tr	30
Boozer								
Hangover Remedy	1 can (8.4 oz)	110	0	0	0	28	–	10
Brain Toniq								
Functional Drink	1 can (8.4 oz)	80	0	0	0	20	–	0
C1.5								
Extreme	1 can (8.4 oz)	120	0	0	0	30	–	50
Celsius								
Ginger Ale	1 bottle (12 oz)	10	–	–	–	–	–	6
Orange	1 bottle (12 oz)	10	–	–	–	–	–	6
Cintron								
Citrus Mango	8 oz	110	tr	0	0	27	0	200
Citrus Mango Sugar Free	8 oz	0	tr	0	0	0	0	200
Clif								
Quench Fruit Punch	8 oz	45	0	0	0	11	0	130
Quench Orange	8 oz	45	0	0	0	11	0	130
Coca-Cola								
Zero	8 oz	1	0	0	0	tr	0	28

FOOD	PORTION	CALS	PROT	FAT	CHOL	CARB	FIBER	SOD
Coolah								
Original	8 oz	120	0	0	0	31	–	40
Cytomax								
Performance Drink Cool Citrus	1 pkg (1.4 oz)	140	0	0	0	35	0	190
DNA Energy								
Low Carb Citrus	8 oz	0	0	0	0	0	–	96
Dr. Tim's								
ISO-5	1 bottle (11.2 oz)	60	0	0	0	15	–	35
Jungle Juice	1 bottle (4 oz)	20	2	0	0	8	0	30
Emu								
Energy Drink	1 bottle (8.4 oz)	170	tr	0	0	41	–	220
EQ Thirst Equalizer								
All Flavors	8 oz	60	0	0	0	15	–	15
EX								
Aqua Vitamins Lemon Lime	1 bottle (16.9 oz)	110	0	0	0	27	–	5
Chillout	1 can (8.4 oz)	80	0	0	0	20	–	0
Pure Energy	1 can (8.4 oz)	70	0	0	0	17	–	5
Slim Energy	1 can (8.4 oz)	20	0	0	0	5	–	10
Fever								
Stimulation Beverage All Flavors	8 oz	130	0	0	0	31	–	10
Fitness Edge								
Tropical Orange	1 bottle (12 oz)	170	20	2	5	17	1	85
Function								
Alternative Energy	8 oz	60	0	0	0	15	–	65
Brainiac Carambola Punch	8 oz	60	0	0	0	15	–	–
Urban Detox Citrus Prickly Pear	8 oz	60	0	0	0	17	–	48
Youth Trip Acai Grape	8 oz	60	0	0	0	15	–	10
Fuze								
Refresh Banana Coconut	8 oz	90	0	0	0	25	–	15
Refresh Peach Mango	8 oz	90	0	0	0	23	–	15
Refresh Strawberry Banana	8 oz	100	0	0	0	25	–	15

FOOD	PORTION	CALS	PROT	FAT	CHOL	CARB	FIBER	SOD
Slenderize Cranberry Raspberry	8 oz	5	0	0	0	2	–	5
Slenderize Low Carb Tropical Punch	8 oz	5	0	0	0	tr	–	5
Slenderize Tangerine Grapefruit	8 oz	10	0	0	0	2	–	10
Vitalize Blackberry Grape	8 oz	100	0	0	0	26	–	10
Vitalize Orange Mango	8 oz	100	0	0	0	25	–	10
Gatorade								
All Flavors	8 oz	50	0	0	0	14	–	110
Ginger Boost								
Ginger Orange	8 oz	110	1	0	0	24	1	15
Gleukos								
Performance All Flavors	8 oz	70	0	0	0	17	0	40
Go Girl								
Bliss	1 can (11.5 oz)	35	0	0	0	8	–	30
Glo	1 can (12 oz)	35	0	0	0	9	0	80
Sugar Free	1 can (12 oz)	<5	0	0	0	tr	–	100
Guayaki								
Organic Raspberry Revolution	8 oz	50	0	0	0	12	tr	11
Organic Unsweetened	8 oz	15	0	0	0	3	tr	11
Healthy Shot								
Double Protein Peach	1 bottle (2.5 oz)	100	24	0	0	1	0	80
High Protein All Flavors	1 bottle (2.5 oz)	110	12	0	0	17	0	40
Orange Citrus Blast	1 can (8.2 oz)	120	0	0	0	33	–	–
Orange Citrus Blast Sugar Free	1 can (8.2 oz)	5	0	0	0	1	–	–
Red w/ Gogi	1 can (8.2 oz)	130	0	0	0	31	–	–
Hiro								
Thermo	1 can (8.33 oz)	10	0	0	0	2	–	83
Vitality	1 can (8.33 oz)	10	0	0	0	2	–	48

FOOD	PORTION	CALS	PROT	FAT	CHOL	CARB	FIBER	SOD
Honeydrop								
Alive Blood Orange & Honey	8 oz	40	0	0	0	11	–	0
Strong Blueberries & Honey	8 oz	40	0	0	0	11	–	0
IChill								
Relaxation Shot Blissful Berry	1 bottle (2 oz)	0	0	0	0	0	0	–
Kidstrong								
All Flavors	8 oz	30	0	0	0	7	1	90
King 888								
Original	8 oz	110	0	0	0	28	–	25
Sugar Free	8 oz	0	0	0	0	0	0	25
Liv Naturals								
All Flavors	8 oz	70	0	0	0	16	0	105
Marquis Platinum								
Vitality Drink	1 can	30	0	0	0	16	1	–
Me								
Curious Blueberry Lime	1 can	70	0	0	0	17	–	10
Vivacious Tangerine Pineapple	1 can	70	0	0	0	17	–	10
Mix1								
All Flavors	1 bottle (11 oz)	200	15	3	–	29	3	125
Mr. Re								
Restorative	1 can (11 oz)	80	0	0	0	22	0	0
Neuro								
Bliss	1 bottle (14.5 oz)	35	0	0	0	9	–	–
Gasm	1 bottle (14.5 oz)	35	0	0	0	9	–	–
Sleep	1 bottle (14.5 oz)	35	0	0	0	9	–	–
Sonic	1 bottle (14.5 oz)	35	0	0	0	9	–	–
Sport	1 bottle (14.5 oz)	35	0	0	0	9	–	72
Trim	1 bottle (14.5 oz)	35	0	0	0	9	1	–

FOOD	PORTION	CALS	PROT	FAT	CHOL	CARB	FIBER	SOD
NOS								
High Performance	1 bottle (11 oz)	150	2	0	0	38	–	160
Ocean Spray								
Cranergy Cranberry Lift	8 oz	35	0	0	0	8	–	50
Cranergy Pomegranate Cranberry Lift	8 oz	35	0	0	0	9	–	50
Cranergy Raspberry Cranberry Lift	8 oz	20	0	0	0	9	–	50
Odwalla								
Berries GoMega	8 oz	160	3	2	0	34	5	15
Mo' Beta	8 oz	150	1	0	0	37	1	15
Super Protein Original	8 oz	190	10	1	0	35	1	180
Superfood	8 oz	130	1	1	0	30	0	10
Wellness	8 oz	150	2	1	0	33	1	35
OOBA								
All Flavors	8 oz	90	0	0	0	22	–	5
Palo								
Mamajuana	7 oz	50	0	0	0	15	–	10
Phase III Recovery								
Chocolate	1 bottle (14.5 oz)	330	35	5	35	36	3	120
Vanilla	1 bottle (14.5 oz)	320	35	5	35	34	1	125
Pimpjuice								
Energy Drink	1 can (8 oz)	140	0	0	0	35	–	5
PJ Tight	1 can (8 oz)	20	0	0	0	3	–	5
POMx								
Shot Antioxidant Supplement	1 bottle (3 oz)	100	–	0	0	25	–	–
Purity Organic								
Acerola Cherry	1 bottle	60	0	0	0	15	–	–
Pomegranate Blueberry	1 bottle	60	0	0	0	15	–	–
Pomegranate Raspberry	1 bottle	60	0	0	0	15	–	–
Quench Aid								
Berry	1 pkg	10	0	0	0	2	–	76
Dragonfruit	1 pkg	10	0	0	0	2	–	90
Recharge								
Lemon as prep	8 oz	10	0	0	0	1	–	30
Tropical as prep	8 oz	10	0	0	0	1	–	30

FOOD	PORTION	CALS	PROT	FAT	CHOL	CARB	FIBER	SOD
Red Bull								
Original	1 can (8.3 oz)	110	0	0	0	28	–	200
Sugar Free	1 can (8.3 oz)	10	tr	0	0	3	–	200
Rehab								
Recovery Supplement	1 can (12 oz)	150	0	0	0	38	–	60
Rockstar								
Energy Drink	8 oz	140	0	0	0	31	–	40
Simply Nutrilite								
Berry Antioxidant	1 can (8.4 oz)	120	1	0	0	29	0	15
Solixir								
Blackberry	1 can	50	0	0	0	12	–	10
Orange	1 can	55	0	0	0	13	–	0
Pomegranate	1 can	60	0	0	0	14	–	0
Source Burn								
2	8 oz	130	1	0	0	31	–	10
Energy Drink	8 oz	140	0	0	0	36	–	20
Sugar Free	8 oz	10	1	0	0	0	0	15
Steaz								
Organic Fuel	8 oz	90	0	0	0	23	–	35
Svelte								
Protein Drink All Flavors	1 bottle (15.9 oz)	260	16	10	0	35	5	190
T-Fusion								
Energy Tea	8 oz	0	0	0	0	1	0	50
Therafizz								
Energy	1 pkg	8	–	–	–	–	–	150
Vitamin C	1 pkg	5	0	0	0	tr	–	–
UnderWay								
Appetite Suppressing All Flavors	8 oz	10	0	0	0	2	1	0
Unwind								
All Flavors	1 can (12 oz)	40	0	0	0	10	–	25
Venga								
Brainstorm	8 oz	130	0	0	0	31	–	50
Calorie Burn	8 oz	10	0	0	0	2	–	5

FOOD	PORTION	CALS	PROT	FAT	CHOL	CARB	FIBER	SOD
Energize	8 oz	100	0	0	0	24	–	–
Health&Zen	8 oz	80	0	0	0	20	–	50
VIB								
Chill-N	1 can (8 oz)	40	0	0	0	10	0	0
XOOD								
Endurance Drink All Flavors as prep	1 serv	135	3	0	0	30	–	105
Youth Juice								
Drink	2 oz	10	tr	0	0	3	1	5
Zenergize								
Chill	1 tablet	2	0	0	0	1	0	300
Energy+	1 tablet	2	0	0	0	1	0	220
Hydrate	1 tablet	2	0	0	0	1	0	390

ENGLISH MUFFIN

FOOD	PORTION	CALS	PROT	FAT	CHOL	CARB	FIBER	SOD
READY-TO-EAT								
crumpets	1 (1.5 oz)	80	3	0	0	16	tr	270
plain	1 (2 oz)	129	5	1	0	25	2	206
whole wheat	1 (2.3 oz)	134	6	1	0	27	4	240
Aunt Gussie's								
Gluten Free Cinnamon Raisin	1 (3 oz)	200	3	3	0	41	4	400
Gluten Free Original	1 (3 oz)	200	3	3	0	41	4	440
Fiber One								
100% Whole Wheat	1 (2 oz)	100	5	0	0	22	6	230
Foods By George								
Gluten Free Multigrain	1 (3.6 oz)	220	5	5	0	39	2	280
Gluten Free No-Rye Rye	1 (3.6 oz)	210	4	4	0	40	2	270
Milton's								
Healthy Multi-Grain	1 (2 oz)	150	4	1	0	33	3	180
Pepperidge Farm								
100% Whole Wheat	1	140	6	2	0	26	3	210
Original	1	130	5	2	0	25	1	170
Roman Meal								
English Muffin	1 (2.3 oz)	140	6	1	0	29	3	320
Rudi's Organic Bakery								
MultiGrain w/ Flax	1 (2 oz)	130	5	1	0	25	2	220
Whole Grain Wheat	1 (2 oz)	120	5	1	0	23	3	220
Sun-Maid								
Raisin	1 (2.5 oz)	170	5	1	0	36	2	180

FOOD	PORTION	CALS	PROT	FAT	CHOL	CARB	FIBER	SOD
Thomas'								
100 Calories	1	100	4	1	0	24	5	220
Griller Multi Grain	1 (3.2 oz)	210	7	2	0	41	3	250
Griller Onion	1 (3.2 oz)	200	7	1	0	40	2	320
Light Multi-Grain	1 (2 oz)	100	5	1	0	25	8	170
Oatmeal & Honey	1	130	5	1	0	25	2	180
Original Whole Grain	1	130	5	1	0	26	2	220
Raisin Cinnamon	1 (2.1 oz)	140	4	1	0	29	1	170
Sandwich Size Original	1	190	7	2	0	38	2	280
TAKE-OUT								
w/ butter	1 (2.2 oz)	189	5	6	13	30	–	386
w/ cheese & sausage	1 (4 oz)	365	14	22	46	27	1	721
w/ egg cheese & canadian bacon	1 (4.9 oz)	307	19	13	234	30	1	773
w/ egg cheese & sausage	1 (5.8 oz)	472	22	30	269	29	tr	776
EPAZOTE								
fresh	1 tbsp (1 g)	tr	0	0	0	tr	tr	tr
fresh sprig	1 (2 g)	1	tr	tr	0	tr	tr	1
EPPAW								
raw	½ cup	75	2	1	0	16	–	6
FALAFEL								
Near East								
Falafel Patties Vegetarian as prep	2.5	220	10	13	0	18	5	552
Veggie Patch								
Falafel	4 (3 oz)	180	5	9	0	21	6	380
TAKE-OUT								
falafel	1 (1.2 oz)	57	2	3	0	5	–	50
FAT (*see also* BUTTER, BUTTER SUBSTITUTES, MARGARINE, OIL)								
bacon grease	1 tbsp	116	0	13	12	0	0	19
beef shortening	1 tbsp	115	0	13	13	0	0	0
beef suet	1 oz	242	tr	27	19	0	0	2
chicken	1 tbsp (0.4 oz)	115	0	13	11	0	0	0
duck	1 tbsp (0.4 oz)	113	0	13	13	0	0	0
goose	1 tbsp	115	0	13	13	0	0	0
goose	1 oz	257	0	29	–	0	0	–

FOOD	PORTION	CALS	PROT	FAT	CHOL	CARB	FIBER	SOD
lamb new zealand	1 oz	182	2	19	25	0	0	6
lard	1 tbsp (0.5 oz)	115	0	13	12	0	0	0
lard	1 cup (7.2 oz)	1849	0	205	195	0	0	tr
meat pan drippings	½ tbsp	124	0	14	14	0	0	76
pork raw	1 oz	230	1	25	16	0	0	3
salt pork	1 cube (1 oz)	215	2	23	26	0	0	383
shortening	1 tbsp	113	0	13	0	0	0	–
shortening	1 cup	1812	0	205	0	0	0	–
turkey	1 tbsp	116	0	13	13	0	0	0
ucuhuba butter	1 tbsp	120	0	14	–	0	0	–
whale blubber	1 oz	248	tr	28	0	0	0	–
Crisco								
Butter Flavor	1 tbsp	110	0	12	0	0	0	0
Shortening	1 tbsp	110	0	12	0	0	0	0
Earth Balance								
Natural Shortening	1 tbsp	130	0	14	0	0	0	0
Nebraska Land								
Pork Fatback	½ oz	110	1	11	5	0	0	280
FAVA BEANS								
canned	½ cup	91	7	tr	0	16	–	580
fava fresh cooked	½ cup	94	6	tr	0	17	5	4
Progresso								
Fava Beans	½ cup (4.6 oz)	110	6	1	0	20	5	250
FEIJOA								
fresh	1 (1.75 oz)	25	1	tr	0	5	–	2
puree	1 cup	119	3	2	0	26	–	7
FENNEL								
fresh bulb	1 (8.2 oz)	73	3	tr	0	17	7	122
fresh sliced	1 cup	27	1	tr	0	6	3	45
leaves	1 oz	7	tr	tr	–	1	1	25
seed	1 tsp	7	tr	tr	0	1	1	2
stir fried	1 cup	85	2	6	0	9	3	669
Ocean Mist								
Fennel Sweet Anise Sliced Fresh	1 cup	27	1	1	0	6	3	45

FOOD	PORTION	CALS	PROT	FAT	CHOL	CARB	FIBER	SOD
FENUGREEK								
seed	1 tsp	12	1	tr	0	2	1	2
FIBER								
Benefiber								
Supplement	1 pkg (4 g)	20	0	0	0	4	3	20
Fiber Supreme								
Fiber	1 round tbsp (0.5 oz)	36	1	tr	0	12	7	tr
ND Labs								
Apple Fiber	1 round tbsp (7 g)	15	0	tr	0	7	4	tr
Liquid Fiber Flow	1 tbsp (0.5 oz)	42	0	0	0	11	7	3
UniFiber								
Natural Fiber	1 pkg (4 g)	4	0	0	0	tr	3	–
Wellements								
Fiber-Psyll	1 scoop (0.5 oz)	55	0	0	0	14	12	0
FIDDLEHEAD FERNS								
fresh	3.5 oz	34	5	tr	0	6	–	1
FIG JUICE								
Smart Juice								
Organic 100% Juice	8 oz	131	1	0	0	35	1	2
FIGS								
calimyrna	3 (5.4 oz)	120	1	0	0	28	4	0
canned in heavy syrup	½ cup	114	tr	tr	0	30	3	1
canned in light syrup	½ cup	87	tr	tr	0	23	2	1
canned water pack	½ cup	66	1	tr	0	17	3	1
dried california	½ cup (3.5 oz)	200	4	1	0	58	17	11
dried cooked	½ cup	139	2	1	0	36	5	5
dried small	1 (1.4 oz)	30	tr	tr	0	8	1	0
dried whole	1 (8 g)	21	tr	tr	0	5	1	1
fresh large	1 (2.2 oz)	47	tr	tr	0	12	2	1
California Fresh								
Fresh	3 (5.4 oz)	120	1	0	0	31	4	0
Hermes								
Organic Adriatic Fig Spread	1 tbsp	60	0	0	0	15	0	0

FOOD	PORTION	CALS	PROT	FAT	CHOL	CARB	FIBER	SOD
Jenny								
Kalamata Crown Natural Sundried	4 (1.5 oz)	120	1	0	0	28	5	5
Nuta Figs								
Mission	¼ cup (1.4 oz)	110	1	0	0	26	5	0
Orchard Choice								
Mission	4-5 (1.4 oz)	110	1	0	0	26	5	0
Sun-Maid								
California Mission	4 (1.5 oz)	110	1	0	0	26	5	0
Calimyrna	3 (1.5 oz)	120	1	0	0	28	5	0
FIREWEED								
leaves chopped	1 cup (0.8 oz)	24	1	1	0	4	2	8
FISH (*see also individual names,* SUSHI)								
FROZEN								
breaded fillet	1 (2 oz)	155	9	7	64	14	–	332
sticks	1 stick (1 oz)	76	4	3	31	7	–	163
Dr. Praeger's								
Fillets Lightly Breaded	1 (2.1 oz)	100	5	4	15	12	0	250
Fish Sticks Potato Crusted	3 (2.3 oz)	120	6	8	25	7	tr	220
Fishies Lightly Breaded	3 (1.5 oz)	90	4	4	10	9	0	210
Gorton's								
Classic Crispy Battered Fillets	2	230	6	10	25	22	5	650
Classic Crunchy Golden Fillets	2	140	9	12	36	23	–	500
Fillets Beer Battered	2 (3.6 oz)	250	8	17	20	17	1	600
Fillets Breaded Lemon Herb	2 (3.6 oz)	240	9	13	25	21	–	720
Fillets Potato Crunch	2 (3.6 oz)	240	9	14	25	20	2	790
Fish Sticks Classic Breaded	6	290	10	18	25	19	1	340
Grilled Fillets Cajun Blackened	1 (3.8 oz)	100	17	3	60	1	0	330
Grilled Fillets Lemon Pepper	1 (3.7 oz)	100	17	3	70	1	0	290
Tenders Original Batter	3 pieces (3.6 oz)	230	8	12	20	23	2	660
SeaPak								
Popcorn	8 (3 oz)	190	9	9	30	18	1	370

FOOD	PORTION	CALS	PROT	FAT	CHOL	CARB	FIBER	SOD
Van de Kamp's								
Battered Tenders	4 (4 oz)	210	9	10	20	22	1	700
Crisp & Healthy Breaded Fish Sticks	6 (3.6 oz)	140	9	1	25	24	1	380
Crunchy Fillets	2 (3.5 oz)	230	8	13	20	21	tr	440
Sticks	6 (4 oz)	260	11	13	30	26	1	410
TAKE-OUT								
amuk bok kum korean stir fried fish cake	1 cup (7.6 oz)	267	18	7	65	31	3	1959
fish cake	1 (4.7 oz)	166	18	7	–	6	–	–
jamaican brown fish stew	1 serv	426	48	22	84	9	2	419
kedgeree	5.6 oz	242	21	11	–	15	1	–
mousse	1 serv (3.5 oz)	185	13	14	–	3	tr	540
stew	1 cup (7.9 oz)	157	19	4	–	10	–	–
taramasalata	2 tbsp	124	1	14	10	1	–	182
FISH OIL								
cod liver	1 tbsp	123	0	14	78	0	0	0
herring	1 tbsp	123	0	14	104	0	0	0
menhaden	1 tbsp	123	0	14	71	0	0	0
salmon	1 tbsp	123	0	14	66	0	0	0
sardine	1 tbsp	123	0	14	97	0	0	0
shark	1 oz	270	0	29	–	0	0	–
whale beluga	1 oz	256	0	29	–	0	0	0
whale bowhead	1 oz	252	0	28	–	0	0	–
Nordic Naturals								
Nordic Omega-3 Gummies Tangerine Treats	2 pieces	20	0	0	0	4	–	10
Omega 3-6-9 Junior	2 pieces	9	0	1	–	0	0	–
Omega-3 Effervescent as prep	1 pkg (9.7 g)	39	0	2	–	3	–	209
FISH PASTE								
fish paste	2 tsp	15	1	1	–	tr	0	–
FLAXSEED								
Arrowhead Mills								
Organic	3 tbsp (1 oz)	140	6	9	0	9	7	0

FOOD	PORTION	CALS	PROT	FAT	CHOL	CARB	FIBER	SOD
Bob's Red Mill								
Flaxseed Meal	2 tbsp	60	3	5	0	4	4	0
Carrington Farms								
Organic Flax Paks	1 pkg (0.4 oz)	50	2	5	0	3	3	5
Flax USA								
Flax Sprinkles	2 tbsp (0.5 oz)	70	2	5	0	4	3	0
Natural Ovens								
Flax Complete Supplement	1 tbsp (0.4 oz)	60	2	4	4	4	2	–
Tree Of Life								
Flax Seed	3 tbsp (1 oz)	140	5	10	0	11	6	0
FLOUNDER								
FRESH								
cooked	1 fillet (4.5 oz)	148	31	2	86	0	0	133
cooked	3 oz	99	21	1	58	0	0	89
FROZEN								
Mrs. Paul's								
Filets Lightly Breaded	1 (2.7 oz)	150	8	7	25	12	1	290
TAKE-OUT								
breaded & fried	3.2 oz	211	13	11	31	15	–	484
stuffed w/ crab	1 piece (7.6 oz)	332	43	11	160	14	1	903
FLOUR								
all-purpose self-rising	½ cup (2.2 oz)	221	6	1	0	46	2	794
all-purpose unbleached	½ cup (2.2 oz)	228	6	1	0	48	2	1
arrowroot	½ cup (2.2 oz)	228	tr	tr	0	56	2	1
bread flour	½ cup (2.4 oz)	247	8	1	0	50	2	1
buckwheat whole groat	½ cup (2.1 oz)	201	8	2	0	42	6	7
cake	½ cup (2.4 oz)	248	6	1	0	53	1	1

FOOD	PORTION	CALS	PROT	FAT	CHOL	CARB	FIBER	SOD
carob	1 tbsp (0.2 oz)	13	tr	tr	0	5	2	2
carob	½ cup (1.8 oz)	114	2	tr	0	46	21	18
chickpea besan	½ cup (1.6 oz)	178	10	3	0	27	5	29
peanut lowfat	½ cup (1.1 oz)	128	10	7	0	9	5	0
potato	½ cup (2.8 oz)	286	6	tr	0	66	5	44
rice brown	½ cup (2.8 oz)	287	6	2	0	60	4	6
rice white	½ cup (2.8 oz)	289	5	1	0	63	2	0
rye dark	½ cup (2.2 oz)	207	9	2	0	44	15	1
rye light	½ cup (1.8 oz)	187	4	1	0	41	7	1
soy lowfat	½ cup (1.5 oz)	165	20	4	0	15	7	4
triticale whole grain	½ cup (2.3 oz)	220	9	1	0	48	10	1
white all-purpose enriched bleached	½ cup (2.2 oz)	228	6	1	0	48	2	1
whole wheat	½ cup (2.1 oz)	203	8	1	0	44	7	3
Arrowhead Mills								
Organic Barley	⅓ cup	95	3	1	0	19	4	0
Organic Brown Rice	⅓ cup	130	3	1	0	27	2	0
Organic Kamut	⅓ cup	130	5	1	0	25	4	0
Organic Oat	⅓ cup	120	4	3	0	21	3	0
Organic Rye	¼ cup	110	3	1	0	24	4	0
Organic Spelt	⅓ cup	130	4	1	0	25	4	0
Organic Unbleached White	¼ cup	120	3	1	0	26	tr	0
Organic White Rice	⅓ cup	120	2	0	0	28	tr	0
Azukar Organics								
Coconut	3.5 oz	413	19	9	0	65	39	80
Bob's Red Mill								
Brown Rice	¼ cup	140	3	1	0	31	1	5
Corn	¼ cup	160	2	1	0	22	4	2

FOOD	PORTION	CALS	PROT	FAT	CHOL	CARB	FIBER	SOD
Graham	¼ cup	120	5	1	0	21	3	1
Kamut Organic	¼ cup	94	3	1	0	21	3	0
Sorghum Sweet White Gluten Free	¼ cup	120	4	1	0	25	3	0
Spelt	¼ cup	120	4	1	0	22	4	1
Whole Wheat	¼ cup	110	4	1	0	23	4	0
Whole Wheat Hard White Organic	¼ cup	120	4	1	0	24	4	0
Ceresota								
100% Whole Wheat	¼ cup (1 oz)	100	4	1	0	21	3	0
All Purpose Unbleached	¼ cup (1 oz)	100	3	0	0	22	tr	0
Domata Living Flour								
Gluten Free Casein Free	¼ cup	110	tr	0	0	26	tr	20
Gold Medal								
All Purpose	¼ cup (1 oz)	100	3	0	0	22	tr	0
Self Rising	¼ cup (1 oz)	100	3	0	0	23	tr	400
Whole Wheat	¼ cup (1 oz)	100	4	1	0	21	3	0
Wondra	¼ cup (1 oz)	100	3	0	0	23	tr	0
Heckers								
100% Whole Wheat	¼ cup (1 oz)	100	4	1	0	21	3	0
All Purpose Unbleached	¼ cup (1 oz)	100	3	0	0	22	tr	0
Lundberg								
Brown Rice	¼ cup	110	2	2	0	26	1	0
Manitoba Harvest								
Hemp Seed Flour	¼ cup	120	10	4	0	14	12	0
FOOD COLORS								
blue	1 tsp	0	0	0	0	0	0	86
orange	1 tsp	0	0	0	0	0	0	91
yellow	1 tsp	tr	tr	0	0	0	0	28
FRENCH BEANS								
dried cooked	1 cup	228	12	1	0	43	17	11
FRENCH FRIES (*see* POTATO)								
FRENCH TOAST								
french toast frzn	1 slice (2 oz)	126	4	4	48	19	2	292
Aunt Jemima								
Cinnamon	2 slices (4 oz)	240	8	6	70	39	2	340

FOOD	PORTION	CALS	PROT	FAT	CHOL	CARB	FIBER	SOD
Whole Grain	2 slices (4 oz)	240	8	6	70	39	3	340
Farm Rich								
Original Sticks	5 (4.2 oz)	330	6	15	0	42	2	490
Jimmy Dean								
French Toast Duos	1 serv (3.2 oz)	210	12	10	105	19	1	440
French Toast Griddlers Sandwich	1 (3.6 oz)	210	8	8	60	27	0	390
TAKE-OUT								
plain	1 slice	151	7	7	75	16	–	311
sticks	5 (4.9 oz)	513	8	29	75	58	3	499
w/ butter	2 slices	356	10	19	116	36	–	513
FROG LEGS								
frog legs	3 oz	175	15	–	1	–	–	–
TAKE-OUT								
as prep w/ seasoned flour & fried	1 (0.8)	70	4	5	12	15	–	–
FRUCTOSE								
liquid	1 oz	84	0	0	0	23	0	1
powder	1 tsp (4.2 g)	15	0	0	0	4	0	1
powder	¼ cup (1.7 oz)	180	0	0	0	49	0	6
Bob's Red Mill								
Fructose	1 tsp	15	0	0	0	4	0	0
Tree Of Life								
Fructose	1 tsp (4 g)	15	0	0	0	4	0	0
FRUIT DRINKS (*see also individual names,* SMOOTHIES, YOGURT DRINKS)								
FROZEN								
Chiquita								
Banana Colada as prep	8 oz	125	0	2	0	25	1	35
Mixed Berry as prep	8 oz	120	0	0	0	28	–	40
Peach Mango as prep	8 oz	120	1	0	0	28	–	40
MIX								
Aquafull								
Pomegranate Orange Dietary Supplement	1 pkg (9 g)	30	–	0	0	8	4	–

FOOD	PORTION	CALS	PROT	FAT	CHOL	CARB	FIBER	SOD
Bio Fruit								
Mix	1 scoop (8 g)	42	–	1	0	5	1	–
Crystal Light								
LiveActive On The Go	1 pkg	10	0	0	0	3	3	20
South Beach								
Tide Me Over Strawberry Banana	1 pkg	30	3	0	0	6	5	20
Tide Me Over Tropical Breeze	1 pkg	30	3	0	0	6	5	25
READY-TO-DRINK								
fruit punch	6 oz	87	tr	tr	0	22	–	41
Apple & Eve								
100% Cranberry Apple Juice	8 oz	100	1	0	0	24	–	15
Mango Mangosteen	8 oz	120	0	0	0	30	–	15
Back To Nature								
100% Juice Berry	1 pkg (6 oz)	90	0	0	0	21	–	20
Bolthouse								
Bom Dia Acai Berry 100% Juice	8 oz	140	0	0	0	33	1	15
Brazsoy								
Fruit Juice w/ Soy	8 oz	94	1	1	0	21	–	13
Ceres								
100% Juice Apple Berry Cherry	8 oz	130	0	0	0	32	0	10
Medley Of Fruits 100% Juice	8 oz	130	0	0	0	31	2	10
Crayons								
Kiwi Strawberry	1 bottle (12 oz)	130	0	0	0	45	4	15
Outrageous Orange Mango	1 bottle (12 oz)	140	0	0	0	45	4	15
Redder Than Ever Fruitpunch	1 bottle (12 oz)	130	0	0	0	45	4	15
Drenchers								
Super Fruit Endurance Grape Apple	8 oz	120	1	0	0	29	1	25
Super Juice Fit N' Lean Heart Healthy Tropical Passion	8 oz	10	0	0	0	2	0	5

FOOD	PORTION	CALS	PROT	FAT	CHOL	CARB	FIBER	SOD
Super Juice Fit N' Lean Power Protein Orange Cream	8 oz	20	2	0	0	2	0	10
Super Juice Immunity Fruit & Veggie Berry	8 oz	110	1	0	0	26	1	35
EarthWise								
Orange Carrot Mango	8 oz	110	0	0	0	30	0	15
Essn								
Sparkling Blood Orange & Cranberry	1 can (8.4 oz)	160	1	0	0	38	tr	15
Fizz Ed.								
Pomegranate Cherry	1 can (8.4 oz)	90	0	0	0	22	–	30
Fizzy Lizzy								
Raspberry Lemon	1 bottle (12 oz)	120	0	0	0	28	–	5
Frutzzo								
Organic 100% Juice Pomegranate Passionfruit	1 bottle (12 oz)	140	0	0	0	34	0	10
Organic 100% Juice Pomegranate Acai	1 bottle (12 oz)	140	0	0	0	35	0	10
GoodBelly								
Blueberry Acai Probiotic Drink	1 bottle (2.7 oz)	50	tr	0	0	12	tr	5
Cranberry Watermelon Probiotic Drink	8 oz	100	tr	0	0	24	1	30
Peach Mango Probiotic Drink	1 bottle (2.7 oz)	50	tr	0	0	13	tr	10
Strawberry Rosehips Probiotic Drink	1 bottle (2.7 oz)	50	tr	0	0	12	tr	10
Honest Kids								
Organic Tropical Tango Punch	1 pkg (6.75 oz)	40	0	0	0	10	–	5
Juicy Juice								
Harvest Surprise Orange Mango	8 oz	130	1	0	0	31	1	70
Lakewood								
Lean Green	6 oz	90	1	0	0	26	2	7
Organic Acai Amazon Berry	6 oz	95	2	3	0	21	3	24
Land O Lakes								
Juice Cranberry Apple	1 cup (8 oz)	120	0	0	0	30	0	15

FOOD	PORTION	CALS	PROT	FAT	CHOL	CARB	FIBER	SOD
Minute Maid								
Pomegranate Blueberry 100% Juice	8 oz	120	0	1	0	31	–	20
Moto Bar								
Strawberry Kiwi	8 oz	110	0	0	0	28	0	10
Mott's								
Apple Blueberry	8 oz	130	0	0	0	15	–	35
Fruit Medley	1 bottle (14 oz)	230	1	0	0	54	0	20
Nantucket Nectars								
100% Juice Peach Orange	8 oz	130	0	0	0	32	0	30
100% Juice Pomegranate Cherry	8 oz	120	0	0	0	29	0	30
Kiwi Berry	8 oz	120	0	0	0	29	0	25
Organic Banana Mango Carrot	8 oz	140	0	0	0	32	0	30
Pineapple Orange Guava	8 oz	120	0	0	0	29	0	25
Noble								
Organic 100% Juice Orange Tangerine	8 oz	120	1	0	0	29	–	0
Northland								
100% Juice Cranberry Pomegranate	8 oz	140	0	0	0	34	–	25
NutraShake								
Fruit Punch Plus Fiber	1 pkg (8 oz)	120	0	0	0	29	10	8
Ocean Spray								
100% Juice Cranberry & Concord Grape	8 oz	150	0	0	0	37	–	35
100% Juice Fruit & Veggie Tropical Citrus	8 oz	130	0	0	0	32	–	70
100% Juice Fruit & Veggie Tropical Citrus Light	8 oz	60	0	0	0	15	–	35
Cran-Apple	8 oz	130	0	0	0	32	–	80
Cran-Apple Light	8 oz	40	0	0	0	10	–	70
Cran-Cherry	8 oz	120	0	0	0	30	–	35
Cran-Grape	8 oz	120	0	0	0	31	–	80
Cran-Grape Light	8 oz	40	0	0	0	10	–	75
Cran-Pomegranate	8 oz	120	0	0	0	30	–	35
Cran-Pomegranate Light	8 oz	40	0	0	0	10	–	35
Cran-Raspberry	8 oz	110	0	0	0	28	0	70

FOOD	PORTION	CALS	PROT	FAT	CHOL	CARB	FIBER	SOD
Cran-Raspberry Light	8 oz	40	0	0	0	10	–	70
Ruby Tangerine	8 oz	110	0	0	0	28	–	65
White Cranberry Peach	8 oz	110	0	0	0	27	–	50
Odwalla								
Quenchers AntioxiDance	8 oz	90	0	0	0	23	0	10
Quenchers B Berrier	8 oz	120	0	0	0	30	0	15
Old Orchard								
100% Juice Pomegranate Black Currant	8 oz	130	0	0	0	30	–	25
100% Juice Pomegranate Cherry	8 oz	140	0	0	0	34	–	15
Cocktail Apple Passion Mango	8 oz	120	0	0	0	29	–	15
Healthy Balance Apple Kiwi Strawberry	8 oz	31	0	0	0	6	–	9
Pacific Chai								
Pomegranate Blueberry	8 oz	100	0	0	0	27	0	10
R.W. Knudsen								
Razzleberry 100% Juice	8 oz	120	0	0	0	28	0	15
Sensible Sippers Organic Fruit Punch	1 box (4.23 oz)	30	0	0	0	7	–	0
Sabor Latino								
Guava Mango Drink	1 box (7 oz)	110	0	0	0	29	–	15
Nectar Strawberry Banana + Calcium	8 oz	150	0	0	0	37	1	10
Pina Colada	8 oz	130	0	0	0	32	–	15
Santa Cruz								
Organic Cranberry Goji	8 oz	120	0	0	0	30	0	15
Smart Juice								
Organic 100% Juice Pomegranate Purple Carrot	8 oz	137	1	0	0	35	0	20
Snapple								
100% Juice Fruit Punch	8 oz	170	0	0	0	42	–	15
Juice Drink Acai Blackberry	8 oz	110	0	0	0	27	–	5
Juice Drink Cranberry Raspberry	8 oz	100	0	0	0	26	–	5
SSips								
Cherry Berry	1 box (7 oz)	110	0	0	0	26	–	10

FOOD	PORTION	CALS	PROT	FAT	CHOL	CARB	FIBER	SOD
Sun Shower								
100% Juice Nectarine Mango	8 oz	93	1	0	0	21	2	15
Sundia								
Tropical Medley	½ cup	70	1	0	0	18	2	10
Tree Ripe								
Organic Fruit Punch	8 oz	150	1	0	0	36	0	15
Tropical Grove								
Fruit Punch	8 oz	110	0	0	0	26	–	40
Tropicana								
Fruit Punch	1 cup	130	0	0	0	32	0	15
Fruit Punch Light	8 oz	10	0	0	0	3	0	5
Orange Tangerine Juice	8 oz	110	2	0	0	25	0	0
Orchard Berry	8 oz	110	1	0	0	27	0	25
Organic Orchard Medley	8 oz	120	0	0	0	29	0	25
Twister Berry Blast	8 oz	120	tr	0	0	29	0	10
Twister Citrus Spark	8 oz	120	0	0	0	30	0	10
Twister Fruit Fury	8 oz	120	tr	0	0	30	0	30
Twister Light Strawberry Spiral	8 oz	40	0	0	0	10	0	70
V8								
Light Peach Mango	8 oz	50	0	0	0	13	0	40
Splash Diet Berry Blend	8 oz	10	0	0	0	3	0	35
Splash Mango Peach	8 oz	80	0	0	0	20	0	40
V-Fusion Acai Mixed Berry	8 oz	110	0	0	0	27	0	70
V-Fusion Cranberry Blackberry	8 oz	110	0	0	0	27	–	70
V-Fusion Light Peach Mango	8 oz	50	0	0	0	13	–	40
Vruit								
Apple Carrot	1 box (8.45 oz)	120	1	0	0	29	–	50
Berry Veggie	1 box (8.45 oz)	110	1	0	0	27	–	25
Orange Veggie	1 box (8.45 oz)	110	1	1	0	26	–	20
Tropical Blend	1 box (8.45 oz)	110	1	0	0	27	–	20

FOOD	PORTION	CALS	PROT	FAT	CHOL	CARB	FIBER	SOD
Wadda Juice								
All Flavors	1 bottle (4 oz)	25	0	0	0	7	–	4
Walnut Acres								
Organic Orange Carrot	8 oz	110	0	0	0	27	–	30
Welch's								
100% Black Cherry Concord Grape	8 oz	160	1	0	0	40	–	20
Light Strawberry Mango	8 oz	50	0	0	0	13	–	80
FRUIT MIXED *(see also individual names)*								
CANNED								
fruit cocktail in heavy syrup	½ cup	93	1	tr	0	24	–	7
fruit cocktail juice pack	½ cup	56	1	tr	0	15	–	4
fruit cocktail water pack	½ cup	40	1	tr	0	10	–	5
fruit salad in heavy syrup	½ cup	94	tr	tr	0	24	–	7
fruit salad in light syrup	½ cup	73	tr	tr	0	19	–	7
fruit salad juice pack	½ cup	62	1	tr	0	16	–	7
fruit salad water pack	½ cup	37	tr	tr	0	10	–	4
mixed fruit in heavy syrup	½ cup	92	tr	tr	0	24	–	5
tropical fruit salad in heavy syrup	½ cup	110	1	tr	0	29	–	3
Buddy Fruits								
100% Fruit Apple & Banana	1 pkg (3.2 oz)	50	0	0	0	13	1	10
Del Monte								
Carb Clever Fruit Cocktail	½ cup (4.2 oz)	40	0	0	0	11	1	10
Chunky Mixed Fruit In 100% Juice	½ cup (4.4 oz)	60	0	0	0	15	1	10
Chunky Mixed Fruit In Heavy Syrup	½ cup (4.5 oz)	100	0	0	0	24	1	10
Fruit Cocktail In 100% Juice	½ cup (4.4 oz)	60	0	0	0	15	1	10
Fruit Cocktail In Heavy Syrup	½ cup (4.5 oz)	100	0	0	0	24	1	10
Fruit Cocktail In Light Syrup	½ cup (4.5 oz)	60	0	0	0	21	1	10
Fruit Cocktail In Pear Juice	½ cup (4.4 oz)	60	0	0	0	15	1	10

FOOD	PORTION	CALS	PROT	FAT	CHOL	CARB	FIBER	SOD
Fruit Cocktail Lite	½ cup (4.4 oz)	60	0	0	0	15	1	10
Fruit Naturals Apples & Oranges	½ cup (4.4 oz)	70	0	0	0	18	<2	10
Fruit Naturals Citrus Salad	½ cup (4.4 oz)	70	0	0	0	20	0	20
Fruit Naturals Tropical Medley	½ cup (4.4 oz)	70	tr	0	0	18	tr	5
Mixed Fruit In Light Syrup	½ cup (4.4 oz)	80	0	0	0	18	1	5
Mixed Fruit In Cherry Gel	1 pkg (4.5 oz)	90	0	0	0	23	0	40
Snack Cups Cherry Mixed Fruit	1 pkg (4 oz)	70	tr	0	0	18	tr	10
Superfruit Mixed Fruit Chunks Mango & Passion	1 pkg (6 oz)	120	2	0	0	29	3	25
Superfruit Peach Chunks Pomegranate & Orange	1 pkg (6 oz)	100	2	0	0	26	3	15
Superfruit Pear Chunks Acai & Blackberry	1 pkg (6 oz)	120	2	0	0	31	3	15
Tropical Fruit Salad	½ cup (4.3 oz)	60	0	0	0	16	1	15
Dole								
Mixed Fruit Light Syrup	½ cup (4.3 oz)	80	0	0	0	21	tr	0
Homemade Harvey's								
Crushed Fruit Apple Pear & Spices	1 pkg (4.5 oz)	60	0	0	0	17	2	0
Crushed Fruit Mango Pineapple Banana & Passion Fruit	1 pkg (4.5 oz)	90	1	0	0	22	2	5
Crushed Fruit Strawberries Bananas & Kiwis	1 pkg (4.5 oz)	100	1	1	0	23	2	10
Mott's								
Healthy Harvest Pomegranate	1 pkg (3.9 oz)	50	0	0	0	13	1	0
Polar								
Mixed Fruit Light Syrup	½ cup (4.9 oz)	50	0	0	0	12	2	20

FOOD	PORTION	CALS	PROT	FAT	CHOL	CARB	FIBER	SOD
S&W								
Chunky Mixed In Sweetened Juice	½ cup (4.3 oz)	80	tr	0	0	19	3	20
Fruit Cocktail	½ cup (4.4 oz)	80	0	0	0	20	2	20
DRIED								
mixed	11 oz pkg	712	7	1	0	188	–	52
Brothers-All-Natural								
Crisps Strawberry Banana	1 pkg (0.42 oz)	45	1	0	0	10	2	0
Crunchies								
Freeze Dried Mixed Fruit	¼ cup (7 g)	25	0	0	0	6	1	0
Elizabeth's Natural								
Fancy Mixed	5 pieces	80	1	0	0	20	2	10
Fruitaceuticals								
PomaCrans	¼ cup	100	0	0	0	24	1	0
FruitziO								
Apples & Strawberries Freeze-Dried	1 pkg (0.9 oz)	100	1	0	0	23	2	0
Fun-Yums								
Fresh Crispy Mixed Fruit	1 serv (0.9 oz)	25	–	5	–	18	1	54
Kind								
Bar Apple Cinnamon Nut	1 (1.4 oz)	180	3	10	0	22	5	20
Bar Blueberry Vanilla & Cashew	1 (1.4 oz)	180	3	9	0	24	2	25
Bar Blueberry Pecan + Fiber	1 (1.4 oz)	180	3	10	0	23	5	25
Bar Mango Macadamia	1 (1.4 oz)	190	2	12	0	20	3	20
Bar Pomegranate Blueberry Pistachio + Antioxidants	1 (1.4 oz)	170	3	8	0	24	4	25
Mini Bar Almond & Apricot	1 (0.8 oz)	110	2	7	0	13	3	10
Mini Bar Almond & Coconut + Omega-3	1 (0.8 oz)	107	2	6	0	12	2	0
Mini Bar Cranberry Almond + Antioxidants	1 (0.8 oz)	115	2	8	0	12	2	10
Mini Bar Fruit & Nut Delight	1 (0.8 oz)	108	3	6	0	12	2	10
Mariani								
Berries 'N Cherries	¼ cup	140	tr	0	0	38	2	0

FOOD	PORTION	CALS	PROT	FAT	CHOL	CARB	FIBER	SOD
Sun-Maid								
Fruit Bits	¼ cup (1.4 oz)	120	1	0	0	29	2	20
Mixed	¼ cup (1.4 oz)	100	1	0	0	26	3	35
Sunsweet								
Antioxidant Blend	¼ cup (1.4 oz)	130	1	0	0	31	1	5
Berry Blend	¼ cup (1.4 oz)	120	1	0	0	32	3	5
FRESH								
Chiquita								
Apple & Grape Bites	1 pkg (2.5 oz)	40	0	0	0	10	1	0
FROZEN								
mixed fruit sweetened	1 cup	245	4	tr	0	61	–	8
FRUIT SNACKS								
fruit leather	1 bar (0.8 oz)	81	tr	1	0	18	–	18
fruit leather pieces	1 pkg (0.9 oz)	92	tr	2	0	21	–	109
fruit leather pieces	1 oz	97	tr	2	0	22	–	114
fruit leather rolls	1 sm (0.5 oz)	49	tr	tr	0	12	–	8
fruit leather rolls	1 lg (0.7 oz)	73	tr	1	0	18	–	13
Bare Fruit								
Bananas & Cherries	1 pkg (0.6 oz)	55	2	1	0	12	2	0
Clif								
Twisted Fruit Grape	1 piece (0.7 oz)	70	0	0	0	16	1	5
Twisted Fruit Pineapple	1 piece (0.7 oz)	70	0	0	0	16	1	5
Twisted Fruit Tropical Twist	1 piece (0.7 oz)	70	0	0	0	16	1	5
Funky Monkey								
Bananamon	1 pkg (1 oz)	110	1	0	0	27	3	2
Carnaval Mix	1 pkg (1 oz)	110	1	0	0	26	2	5
Jivealime	1 pkg (1 oz)	110	1	0	0	27	2	1
Purple Funk	1 pkg (1 oz)	120	1	1	0	26	3	1
Jelly Belly								
Fruit Snacks	1 pkg (2.5 oz)	220	0	0	0	58	1	105

FOOD	PORTION	CALS	PROT	FAT	CHOL	CARB	FIBER	SOD
Peeled Snacks								
Fruit & Nuts FigSated	⅓ cup	150	3	6	0	20	3	60
Fruit & Nuts Plu-what?	⅓ cup	150	3	6	0	22	3	50
Revolution Foods								
Organic Mashups Berry	1 pkg (3.2 oz)	40	0	0	0	10	1	5
Organic Mashups Tropical	1 pkg (3.2 oz)	60	1	0	0	13	1	4
Stretch Island								
Fruit Leather Bountiful Blueberry	1 pkg (0.5 oz)	45	0	0	0	12	1	0
Fruit Leather Harvest Grape	1 pkg (0.5 oz)	45	0	0	0	12	1	0
Fruit Leather Mango Sunrise	1 pkg (0.5 oz)	45	0	0	0	11	1	0
Fruit Leather Truly Tropical	1 pkg (0.5 oz)	45	0	0	0	11	1	0
Organic Smooshed Fruit Apple	1 piece (0.4 oz)	40	0	0	0	10	1	0
Organic Smooshed Fruit Strawberry	1 piece (0.4 oz)	40	0	0	0	10	tr	0
Tahitian Noni								
Soft Chews Raspberry	1 pkg (2 oz)	240	2	3	0	50	0	20
Tropicana								
Fruit Wise Bars All Flavors	1 bar (1.4 oz)	140	0	0	0	36	2	10
Fruit Wise Strips All Flavors	1 strip (0.7 oz)	70	0	0	0	17	1	0
Welch's								
Fruit'N Yogurt Strawberry	1 pkg (0.9 oz)	90	1	2	–	17	–	20
Mixed Fruit	1 pkg (0.9 oz)	80	1	0	0	19	–	10
GARLIC								
clove	1	4	tr	tr	0	1	tr	1
fresh chopped	1 tbsp	18	1	tr	0	4	tr	2
powder	1 tsp	9	tr	tr	0	2	tr	1
Jake & Amos								
Sweet Pickled Garlic	1 oz	36	0	0	0	9	0	70
McSweet								
Pickled	8 pieces (1 oz)	40	0	0	0	5	0	420
Spice World								
Ajo Garlic Clove	1 (3 g)	5	0	0	0	1	–	0

FOOD	PORTION	CALS	PROT	FAT	CHOL	CARB	FIBER	SOD
GEFILTE FISH								
sweet	1 piece (1.5 oz)	35	4	1	12	3	–	220
Mrs. Adler's								
Gefilte Fish	1 piece (1.8 oz)	50	5	2	20	3	1	200
Ungar's								
Gefilte Fish	2 slices (1.8 oz)	83	6	5	41	5	0	263
Lite	2 slices (2.4 oz)	80	7	3	20	5	2	190
No Sugar	2 slices (1.8 oz)	70	6	4	15	3	0	180
GELATIN								
READY-TO-EAT								
Jell-O								
Sugar Free Lemon Lime	1 serv (3.2 oz)	10	1	0	0	0	0	45
Kozy Shack								
Gel Treats Sugar Free Strawberry	1 pkg (3.5 oz)	10	0	0	0	2	0	15
Smart Gels Cherry	1 pkg (3.5 oz)	80	0	0	0	21	0	10
Smart Gels Orange	1 pkg (3.5 oz)	80	0	0	0	24	0	10
Smart Gels Strawberry	1 pkg (3.5 oz)	80	0	0	0	24	0	10
Smart Gels Sugar Free Orange	1 pkg (3.5 oz)	5	0	0	0	1	0	15
Tropical	1 pkg (3.5 oz)	80	0	0	0	21	0	10
Tropical Sugar Free	1 pkg (3.5 oz)	5	0	0	0	1	1	15
GIBLETS								
capon simmered	1 cup (5 oz)	238	38	8	629	0	0	80
chicken fried	1 cup (5 oz)	402	47	20	647	6	0	164
chicken simmered	1 cup (5 oz)	289	30	17	419	1	0	93
turkey simmered	1 cup (5 oz)	243	39	7	606	3	–	85
GINGER								
ground	1 tsp	6	tr	tr	0	1	tr	1
pickled	1 tbsp (0.3 oz)	9	0	0	0	2	0	24
preserved	1.5 oz	34	0	0	0	8	1	8
root fresh	5 slices	9	tr	tr	0	2	tr	1
root fresh sliced	¼ cup	19	tr	tr	0	4	1	3

FOOD	PORTION	CALS	PROT	FAT	CHOL	CARB	FIBER	SOD
Dorot								
Crushed Cubes frzn	1 (3.5 g)	0	0	0	0	tr	–	10
Tree Of Life								
Crystallized Pieces	7 (1.4 oz)	150	0	0	0	37	1	25
GINKGO NUTS								
canned	1 oz	32	1	tr	0	6	–	87
dried	1 oz	99	3	tr	0	21	–	4
raw	1 oz	52	1	tr	0	11	–	1
GINSENG								
dried	1 oz	90	5	tr	–	20	2	16
fresh	1 oz	28	1	tr	–	6	tr	5
GIZZARDS								
chicken simmered	1 cup (5 oz)	212	44	4	536	0	0	81
turkey simmered	1 (3 oz)	103	18	3	171	tr	0	56
Perdue								
Fresh Chicken	3 oz	130	23	3	165	1	–	55
GNOCCHI								
Racconto								
Potato Whole Wheat as prep w/o salt	1 cup (5.8 oz)	248	1	0	0	60	8	450
Vantia								
Gnocchi Whole Wheat	¾ cup	210	5	1	0	46	4	630
GOAT								
roasted	3 oz	122	23	3	64	0	0	73
GOJI BERRIES								
dried	1 oz	106	2	3	0	19	2	–
Kopali								
Organic Dark Chocolate Covered	½ pkg (1 oz)	120	2	6	0	18	2	13
Navitas Naturals								
Dried	1 oz	90	4	0	0	18	1	140
Sunfood								
Organic	1 oz	90	4	0	0	18	3	105
Superfood Snacks								
Organic Chocolate Goji Treats	3 pieces (1.4 oz)	150	4	4	5	24	7	55

FOOD	PORTION	CALS	PROT	FAT	CHOL	CARB	FIBER	SOD
Tree Of Life								
Organic	1 oz	110	<4	0	0	25	<5	130
GOJI JUICE								
Arthur's								
Goji Plus	1 bottle (11 oz)	210	3	tr	0	49	2	160
Gojilania								
Organic	8 oz	110	5	0	0	23	0	110
GOOSE								
boneless roasted	2.7 oz	231	19	17	69	0	0	176
meat only raw	6.5 oz	298	42	13	155	0	0	161
w/ skin & bone roasted	1 serv (6.6 oz)	573	47	41	171	0	0	132
wild boneless roasted diced	1 cup (4.9 oz)	426	35	31	127	0	0	325
GOOSEBERRIES								
canned in light syrup	1 cup	184	2	1	0	47	6	5
fresh	1 cup	66	1	1	0	15	7	2
Kopali								
Organic Goldenberry	1 pkg (1.8 oz)	150	4	0	0	31	18	45
Navitas Naturals								
Cape Gooseberry Dried	1 oz	80	2	0	0	17	3	25
GRAINS								
Kashi								
7 Whole Grain Pilaf Fiery Fiesta	1 cup (4.9 oz)	210	8	5	0	40	7	400
7 Whole Grain Pilaf Moroccan Curry	1 cup (4.9 oz)	220	8	5	0	42	7	400
7 Whole Grain Pilaf Original	1 cup (4.9 oz)	220	8	4	0	45	7	0
GRAPE JUICE								
bottled unsweetened	1 cup	154	1	tr	0	38	tr	8
Apple & Eve								
Vintage Concord	8 oz	150	0	0	0	40	–	15
Cascadian Farm								
Organic frzn as prep	8 oz	150	0	0	0	38	–	5

FOOD	PORTION	CALS	PROT	FAT	CHOL	CARB	FIBER	SOD
First Blush								
All Flavors	8 oz	154	1	0	0	38	0	8
Fizzy Lizzy								
Yakima Grape	1 bottle (12 oz)	120	0	0	0	30	–	10
Juicy Juice								
Harvest Surprise	8 oz	120	1	0	0	28	0	80
Kedem								
100% Juice	8 oz	150	tr	0	0	37	–	20
Lakewood								
Organic Concord	6 oz	105	1	0	0	25	1	5
Mott's								
100% Juice Grape Medley	1 bottle (14 oz)	230	1	0	0	55	0	20
Nantucket Nectars								
Grapeade	8 oz	140	0	0	0	33	0	25
Organic Concord Grape	8 oz	130	0	0	0	31	0	35
Old Orchard								
100% Juice White	8 oz	160	0	0	0	38	–	20
R.W. Knudsen								
100% Juice	8 oz	130	1	0	0	32	tr	15
Santa Cruz								
Organic Concord Grape	8 oz	160	tr	0	0	40	0	15
Snapple								
100% Juice Grape	8 oz	170	0	0	0	43	–	15
Grapeade	8 oz	100	0	0	0	26	–	5
Tree Ripe								
Organic 100% Juice	6 oz	120	1	0	0	28	0	10
Tropicana								
Grape	1 bottle (14 oz)	270	tr	0	0	67	0	25
Walnut Acres								
Organic	8 oz	120	0	0	0	31	0	0
Welch's								
100% White	8 oz	160	0	0	0	39	–	20
GRAPE LEAVES								
canned	1 (4 g)	3	tr	tr	0	tr	–	114
fresh raw	1 (3 g)	3	tr	tr	0	1	tr	0
TAKE-OUT								
dolmas w/ beef & rice	1 (0.7 oz)	50	2	4	5	2	1	14

FOOD	PORTION	CALS	PROT	FAT	CHOL	CARB	FIBER	SOD
dolmas w/ lamb & rice	1 (0.7 oz)	56	2	4	5	3	1	14
dolmas w/ rice	1 (2 oz)	92	1	6	0	8	2	93
GRAPEFRUIT								
CANNED								
sections juice pack	½ cup (4.4 oz)	46	1	tr	0	11	1	9
sections light syrup	½ cup (4.5 oz)	76	1	tr	0	20	1	3
sections water pack	½ cup (4.3 oz)	44	1	tr	0	11	1	2
Del Monte								
Fruit Bowls Grapefruit Duo	½ cup (4.4 oz)	60	1	0	0	16	1	10
Fruit Bowls Red	½ cup (4.4 oz)	60	1	0	0	14	tr	15
SunFresh Red No Sugar Added	½ cup (4.2 oz)	40	tr	0	0	10	1	15
FRESH								
pink or red	½ (4.6 oz)	52	1	tr	0	13	2	0
sections pink or red	1 cup (8.1 oz)	97	2	tr	0	25	4	0
sections white	1 cup (8.1 oz)	76	2	tr	0	19	3	0
white	½ (4.1 oz)	39	1	tr	0	10	1	0
Ocean Spray								
Grapefruit	½ med	60	–	0	0	16	–	35
GRAPEFRUIT JUICE								
canned sweetened	1 cup (8.8 oz)	115	1	tr	0	28	tr	5
canned unsweetened	1 cup (8.7 oz)	94	1	tr	0	22	tr	2
pink fresh	1 cup (8.7 oz)	96	1	tr	0	23	–	2
white fresh	1 cup (8.7 oz)	96	1	tr	0	23	tr	2
Apple & Eve								
Ruby Red	8 oz	130	0	0	0	32	–	10
Fizzy Lizzy								
Grapefruit	1 bottle (12 oz)	100	0	0	0	25	–	0
Izze								
Sparkling Fortified Grapefruit	1 can (8.4 oz)	90	0	0	0	23	–	15

FOOD	PORTION	CALS	PROT	FAT	CHOL	CARB	FIBER	SOD
Ocean Spray								
100% Juice Pink	8 oz	100	1	0	0	23	–	35
100% Juice White	8 oz	90	2	0	0	21	–	35
Ruby Drink Light	8 oz	40	0	0	0	10	–	65
Odwalla								
100% Juice	8 oz	90	2	0	0	20	0	5
Sundia								
Ruby	½ cup	70	1	0	0	18	1	0
Tropicana								
Sweet	8 oz	130	1	0	0	31	0	20
GRAPES								
muscadine	10–12 (3.5 oz)	76	5	0	0	14	3	7
scuppernongs	10–12 (3.5 oz)	68	5	0	0	12	3	5
seedless red or green	1 cup	110	1	tr	0	29	1	3
seedless red or green	20	69	1	tr	0	18	1	2
thompson seedless in heavy syrup	½ cup	93	1	tr	0	25	1	6
thompson seedless water pack	½ cup	49	1	tr	0	13	1	7
with seeds red or green	1 cup	106	1	tr	0	28	1	3
with seeds red or green	20	80	1	tr	0	21	1	2
Chiquita								
Grapes	1 cup (3.2 oz)	62	1	0	0	16	1	2
Earthbound Farms								
Organic Black	1½ cups	190	1	1	0	24	1	0
Revolution Foods								
Organic Mashups Grape	1 pkg (3.2 oz)	60	0	0	0	14	0	5
GRAVY								
CANNED								
beef	1 can (10 oz)	155	11	7	9	14	–	1630
beef	1 cup	124	9	6	7	11	–	1305
chicken	1 cup	189	5	14	5	13	–	1375
mushroom	1 cup	120	3	6	0	13	–	1259
turkey	1 cup	122	6	5	5	12	–	–
Campbell's								
Au Jus	¼ cup	5	1	0	0	0	0	230
Chicken	¼ cup	40	0	3	5	3	0	260

FOOD	PORTION	CALS	PROT	FAT	CHOL	CARB	FIBER	SOD
Fat Free Beef	¼ cup	15	1	0	0	3	0	300
Fat Free Turkey	¼ cup	20	1	0	0	4	0	290
Mushroom	¼ cup	20	0	1	<5	3	0	280
Franco-American								
Fat Free Slow Roast Chicken	¼ cup	20	tr	0	0	4	0	250
Slow Roast Chicken	¼ cup	20	1	1	<5	3	0	240
Heinz								
Classic Chicken Fat Free	¼ cup	15	0	0	0	3	0	320
HomeStyle Classic Chicken	¼ cup	25	0	1	0	4	0	340
HomeStyle Roasted Turkey	¼ cup (2.1 oz)	25	1	1	<5	3	0	290
Roasted Turkey Fat Free	¼ cup (2.1 oz)	20	1	0	0	3	0	260
MIX								
au jus as prep w/ water	1 cup	32	1	1	1	4	–	964
brown as prep w/ water	1 cup	75	2	2	2	13	–	1076
chicken as prep	1 cup	83	3	2	3	14	–	1133
mushroom as prep	1 cup	70	2	1	1	14	–	1402
onion as prep w/ water	1 cup	77	2	1	tr	16	–	1013
pork as prep	1 cup	76	2	2	3	13	–	1235
turkey as prep	1 cup	87	3	2	3	15	–	1498
Bournvita								
Extract	2 heaping tsp	34	1	1	–	7	–	–
Bovril								
Extract	1 heaping tsp	9	2	0	–	tr	0	–
Butterball								
Turkey	¼ cup (2 oz)	30	0	0	–	6	0	510
Knorr								
Au Jus Instant as prep	2 oz	10	tr	0	0	2	–	470
Beef Instant as prep	2 oz	20	1	1	0	3	–	330
Brown Instant as prep	2 oz	25	1	0	0	6	–	410
Brown Low Sodium Instant as prep	2 oz	25	1	tr	0	5	–	115
Chicken Instant as prep	2 oz	25	tr	tr	0	5	–	395
Chicken Low Sodium Instant as prep	2 oz	25	1	1	5	4	–	120
Leahey Gardens								
No Beef Brown Gluten Free	¼ cup	9	tr	tr	0	3	–	114
No Chicken Golden	¼ cup	18	tr	2	0	3	–	275

FOOD	PORTION	CALS	PROT	FAT	CHOL	CARB	FIBER	SOD
Loney's								
Brown as prep	¼ cup (2.1 oz)	15	tr	0	0	3	0	200
Turkey as prep	¼ cup (2.1 oz)	20	tr	0	0	4	0	200
Marmite								
Extract	1 heaping tsp	9	2	0	–	tr	–	–
Road's End Organics								
Savory Herb Cholesterol Free Gluten Free	¼ cup	25	tr	0	0	5	0	210
TAKE-OUT								
au jus	1 cup	62	1	6	6	1	tr	290
giblet gravy	¼ cup	45	3	3	23	3	tr	313
GREAT NORTHERN BEANS								
canned	1 cup	299	19	1	0	55	13	11
dried cooked	1 cup	209	15	1	0	37	12	4
HamBeens								
Great Northerns as prep	½ cup	120	7	1	0	22	11	63
GREEN BEANS								
CANNED								
drained	1 cup	27	2	tr	0	6	3	354
Allens								
No Salt	½ cup	15	0	0	0	3	2	10
Del Monte								
French Style	½ cup (4.2 oz)	20	1	0	0	4	2	390
Fresh Cut Italian	½ cup	30	1	0	0	6	3	390
Gertie's Finest								
Pickled	1 oz	15	1	0	0	3	1	160
Green Giant								
50% Less Sodium Cut	½ cup	20	1	0	0	4	1	200
McSweet								
Dilly Beans Whole	5 (1 oz)	30	0	0	0	7	tr	330
S&W								
Cut	½ cup (4.2 oz)	20	1	0	0	4	2	390
Dilled	1 oz	20	0	0	0	5	1	125
FRESH								
cooked w/o salt	1 cup	44	2	tr	0	10	4	1

FOOD	PORTION	CALS	PROT	FAT	CHOL	CARB	FIBER	SOD
raw	1 cup	34	2	tr	0	8	4	7
raw whole beans	10	17	1	tr	0	4	2	3
Ready Pac								
Fast 'N Fresh as prep	1 cup (3 oz)	30	2	0	0	7	3	0
FROZEN								
cooked	1 cup	38	2	tr	0	9	4	12
Birds Eye								
Steamfresh Whole	1 cup (2.9 oz)	35	1	0	0	5	2	0
C&W								
French Cut	1 cup	30	1	0	0	5	2	0
Cascadian Farm								
Organic Petite Whole	1 cup	25	1	0	0	5	2	90
Green Giant								
Green Bean Casserole	⅔ cup	110	2	8	0	8	1	460
TAKE-OUT								
casserole w/ mushroom sauce	1 cup	108	3	6	2	11	3	525
pickled	½ cup	19	1	tr	0	4	2	160
GREENS								
Allens								
Seasoned Mixed	½ cup	45	4	1	0	6	1	830
GROUNDCHERRIES								
fresh	½ cup	37	1	tr	0	8	–	–
GROUPER								
cooked	3 oz	100	21	1	40	0	0	45
cooked	1 fillet (7.1 oz)	238	50	3	95	0	0	107
raw	3 oz	78	16	1	31	0	0	45
GUAR GUM								
Bob's Red Mill								
Guar Gum	1 tbsp	20	0	0	0	6	6	2
GUAVA								
fresh	1	45	1	1	0	11	–	2
guava sauce	½ cup	43	tr	tr	0	11	–	4
GUAVA JUICE								
Apple & Eve								
Nectar	5 oz	130	0	0	0	32	–	35

FOOD	PORTION	CALS	PROT	FAT	CHOL	CARB	FIBER	SOD
Ceres								
100% Juice	8 oz	120	0	0	0	30	2	10
OKF								
Sparkling Fresh Guava	1 bottle (8.3 oz)	20	0	0	0	13	3	3
Sabor Latino								
Nectar + Calcium	8 oz	160	0	0	0	39	–	20
GUINEA HEN								
boneless w/o skin raw	½ hen (9.3 oz)	290	54	7	166	0	0	182
w/ skin raw	½ hen (12 oz)	545	81	22	255	0	0	231
Grimaud Farms								
Guinea Fowl	1 serv (3.7 oz)	130	25	4	105	tr	–	40
HADDOCK								
fresh broiled	4 oz	127	27	1	84	0	0	99
roe raw	1 oz	37	7	tr	103	tr	–	–
smoked	1 oz	33	7	tr	22	0	0	216
Van de Kamp's								
Battered Fillets	2 (3.6 oz)	210	9	11	20	21	2	580
TAKE-OUT								
breaded & fried	4 oz	229	23	10	88	10	1	528
HAGGIS								
scottish haggis	1 serv (6.4 oz)	473	16	32	77	31	5	456
Caledonian Kitchen								
Highland Beef	3 oz	173	8	10	4	12	2	460
Vegetarian	3 oz	190	7	13	5	12	3	320
House of Kenton								
Vegetarian	1 serv (3.5 oz)	249	3	20	–	14	–	–
MacSween								
Traditional	1 (8 oz)	260	12	16	–	18	–	710
Vegetarian	1 (8 oz)	238	7	12	–	22	–	450
HALIBUT								
atlantic & pacific cooked	½ fillet (5.6 oz)	223	42	5	65	0	0	110

FOOD	PORTION	CALS	PROT	FAT	CHOL	CARB	FIBER	SOD
atlantic & pacific cooked	3 oz	119	23	2	35	0	0	59
atlantic & pacific raw	3 oz	93	18	2	27	0	0	46
greenland baked	5.6 oz	380	29	28	94	0	0	163
greenland baked	3 oz	203	16	15	50	0	0	87
FROZEN								
Van de Kamp's								
Battered Fillets	3 (4 oz)	230	10	11	25	22	0	630

HAM

FOOD	PORTION	CALS	PROT	FAT	CHOL	CARB	FIBER	SOD
boneless extra lean roasted	3 oz	123	18	5	45	1	0	1023
boneless roasted	3 oz	151	19	8	50	0	0	1275
canned extra lean roasted	3 oz	116	18	4	26	tr	0	965
canned lean roasted	3 oz	142	18	7	35	tr	0	908
center slice lean & fat roasted	3 oz	173	17	11	46	tr	0	1179
deviled	¼ cup	188	7	17	35	1	0	724
ham salad spread	2 tbsp	65	3	5	11	3	0	274
patty grilled	1 patty (2 oz)	205	8	19	43	1	0	638
prosciutto	4 slices (1.3 oz)	72	10	3	26	tr	0	992
sliced	3 slices (2.9 oz)	137	14	7	48	3	1	1095
sliced extra lean	3 slices (2.2 oz)	69	11	2	30	2	0	697
westphalian smoked	1 oz	105	5	10	–	0	0	398
whole roasted	3 oz	207	18	14	53	0	0	1009
Applegate Farms								
Organic Uncured	2 oz	70	10	2	35	1	0	530
Carl Buddig								
Ham Sliced	2 oz	85	10	5	–	1	–	–
Honey Ham Sliced	2 oz	90	10	5	–	2	–	–
Dietz & Watson								
Boneless Old Fashioned	3 oz	110	14	5	40	1	0	720
Smoked	2 oz	80	11	3	30	1	0	480
Steak Our Traditional	5 oz	100	18	3	50	2	0	680
Healthy Ones								
Honey 97% Fat Free	7 slices (2 oz)	90	9	2	20	2	–	410
Hormel								
Chunk Ham canned	2 oz	90	9	6	30	0	0	620

FOOD	PORTION	CALS	PROT	FAT	CHOL	CARB	FIBER	SOD
Deli Cooked	4 slices (2 oz)	70	10	2	30	1	0	500
Deli Honey	4 slices (2 oz)	70	9	2	25	3	0	500
Deli Smoked	4 slices (2 oz)	60	9	2	25	1	0	500
Dinner	2 oz	70	10	2	30	2	0	550
Organic Prairie								
Hardwood Smoked Bone In Spiral Cut	3 oz	110	19	3	40	tr	0	940
Oscar Mayer								
Ham Brown Sugar Thin Sliced	⅓ pkg (2 oz)	70	10	2	25	4	–	830
Virginia Shaved	2 oz	50	9	1	25	1	0	570
Sara Lee								
Virginia Baked	4 slices (1.8 oz)	60	10	2	20	2	0	550
Tyson								
Glazed Ham Maple & Brown Sugar	1 serv (5 oz)	180	17	5	60	18	0	780
Honey Ham	2 slices (1.6 oz)	50	9	2	25	1	0	740
TAKE-OUT								
croquette	1 (2.2 oz)	149	9	9	18	8	tr	532
salad	½ cup	287	16	23	237	5	tr	671
spam musubi	1 serv (6 oz)	253	6	6	14	42	1	283
thick slice fried	1 (2.2 oz)	140	13	9	33	tr	0	756
HAMBURGER								
Applegate Farms								
Organic Beef Cooked	1 (3 oz)	195	21	12	70	0	0	85
Organic Turkey Burger	1 (4 oz)	190	22	11	75	0	0	70
Hot Pockets								
Cheeseburger	1 (4.5 oz)	310	11	13	25	37	2	630
Lean Pockets								
Cheeseburger	1 (4.5 oz)	280	12	7	25	40	3	560
Oscar Mayer								
Lunchables All-Star Burgers	1 pkg	420	14	14	35	60	1	980
Quaker Maid								
Pure Beef Patties	1 (4 oz)	240	19	18	50	0	0	40
TAKE-OUT								
cheeseburger + condiments	1 reg (4.5 oz)	347	17	17	46	28	1	644

FOOD	PORTION	CALS	PROT	FAT	CHOL	CARB	FIBER	SOD
double hamburger + condiments	1 reg (5.8 oz)	384	23	19	66	30	2	809
single patty + condiments	1 reg (4 oz)	299	15	11	33	35	2	589
HAMBURGER SUBSTITUTES (*see also* MEAT SUBSTITUTES)								
Amy's								
All American Burger	1 (2.5 oz)	120	10	3	0	15	3	390
Cheddar Veggie Burger	1 (2.5 oz)	160	8	5	5	20	3	430
Texas Burger	1 (2.5 oz)	120	12	3	0	14	3	350
Asherah's Gourmet								
Organic Quinoa Vegan Burgers	1 (4 oz)	180	6	5	0	30	5	190
Dr. Praeger's								
Texmex	1 (4 oz)	170	7	6	0	20	6	370
Veggie Burger Bombay	1 (4 oz)	170	7	6	0	20	6	370
Veggie Burger California	1 (4 oz)	170	7	6	0	21	5	310
Veggie Burger California Slider	1 (1.6 oz)	80	3	4	0	8	2	150
Gardenburger								
Black Bean Chipotle	1 (2.5 oz)	80	5	3	0	13	5	250
Flamed Grilled	1 (2.5 oz)	90	11	4	0	5	4	420
GardenVegan	1 (2.5 oz)	100	10	1	0	12	3	230
Original	1 (2.5 oz)	100	5	4	5	14	5	420
Portabella	1 (2.5 oz)	90	5	3	5	15	5	360
Morningstar Farms								
Classic Burger	1 (2.2 oz)	150	14	7	0	10	3	340
Okara Pattie	1 (2.2 oz)	120	12	5	0	6	3	300
Vegan Burger	1 (2.5 oz)	100	13	2	0	8	5	460
Sunshine								
Organic Garden Burger	1 (2.6 oz)	250	8	13	0	14	3	320
Sunshine Burgers								
Original	1 (2.6 oz)	190	8	13	0	14	3	320
Veggie Bites								
Garlic Portabella	1 (2.5 oz)	120	11	6	0	8	4	320
WildWood								
Organic Original Burgers Tofu-Veggie	1 (3.2 oz)	180	12	13	0	8	1	330
HAZELNUTS								
chocolate hazelnut spread	2 tbsp (1.3 oz)	200	2	11	0	23	2	15

FOOD	PORTION	CALS	PROT	FAT	CHOL	CARB	FIBER	SOD
chopped	¼ cup (1 oz)	181	4	17	0	5	3	0
ground	¼ cup (0.7 oz)	118	3	11	0	3	1	0
whole	¼ cup (1.2 oz)	212	5	21	0	6	3	0
whole nuts	21 (1 oz)	178	4	17	0	5	3	0
Chukar Cherries								
Chocolate Covered Spiced	3 tbsp (1.4 oz)	228	4	17	4	21	2	15
Fisher								
Chopped	¼ cup (1 oz)	180	4	17	0	5	3	0
Fundelina								
Choco-Hazelnut Spread All Flavors	2 tbsp (1.3 oz)	200	3	11	0	23	2	14
Love'n Bake								
Hazelnut Praline	2 tbsp	170	3	12	0	13	2	0
HEART								
beef simmered	3 oz	140	24	4	180	tr	0	50
chicken cooked	1 (3 g)	5	1	tr	6	0	0	11
chicken diced simmered	½ cup	134	19	6	175	tr	0	35
lamb braised	3 oz	157	21	7	212	2	0	54
pork braised	1 (4.5 oz)	191	30	7	285	1	0	45
turkey simmered	½ cup	94	16	3	133	tr	0	65
veal braised	3 oz	158	25	6	150	tr	0	49
Rumba								
Beef	4 oz	130	19	4	155	3	0	70
HEARTS OF PALM								
canned	1 (1.2 oz)	9	1	tr	0	2	1	141
canned	½ cup	20	2	tr	0	3	2	311
Del Monte								
Hearts Of Palm	2–3 pieces (4.4 oz)	20	2	0	0	3	2	450
Native Forest								
Organic	1 oz	15	1	0	0	2	1	125
HEMP								
Living Harvest								
Organic Hemp Nuts	2 tbsp (1 oz)	170	10	12	0	5	0	0

FOOD	PORTION	CALS	PROT	FAT	CHOL	CARB	FIBER	SOD
Organic Protein Powder	2 scoops (1 oz)	110	14	3	0	9	1	0
Manitoba Harvest								
Hemp Seed Butter	2 tbsp	160	11	10	0	7	1	10
Organic Pro Fiber	4 tbsp (1 oz)	127	11	3	0	14	14	10
Organic Protein Dark Chocolate	4 tbsp (1 oz)	120	8	3	0	17	9	10
Shelled Seed	2 tbsp	160	11	10	0	7	1	10
Nutiva								
Organic Protein Powder	2 scoops (1 oz)	120	11	3	0	14	14	15
Shelled Hempseed	2 tbsp	110	6	8	0	2	1	0
HERBAL TEA (*see* TEA/HERBAL TEA)								
HERBS/SPICES (*see also individual names*)								
cajun seasoning	1 tbsp	19	1	1	–	3	1	5
chinese five spice	1 tsp	7	0	tr	–	2	tr	1
garam masala	1 tsp	8	tr	tr	0	1	–	2
poultry seasoning	1 tsp	5	tr	tr	0	1	tr	tr
pumpkin pie spice	1 tsp (1.7 g)	6	tr	tr	0	1	tr	1
Bragg								
Herb & Spice Seasoning	¼ tsp	0	0	0	0	0	0	0
Dave's Gourmet								
Insanity Spice	¼ tsp (1 g)	5	0	0	0	0	0	0
Lawry's								
Spices & Seasonings Chimichurri Burrito Casserole	1 tbsp (7 g)	20	tr	0	0	5	–	460
Spices & Seasonings Tuscan Chicken Marsala	1 tbsp (7 g)	20	tr	0	0	5	–	460
McCormick								
Grill Mates Rub Applewood	2 tsp	15	0	0	0	3	0	350
Meat Tenderizer Seasoned	¼ tsp (1 g)	0	0	0	0	0	0	300
Perfect Pinch Salt Free Original	¼ tsp	0	0	0	0	0	0	0
Mrs. Dash								
Grilling Blend Steak	¼ tsp (0.7 g)	0	0	0	0	0	0	0
Original Blend	¼ tsp (0.7 g)	0	0	0	0	0	0	0
Seasoning Blends Caribbean Citrus	¼ tsp (0.7 g)	0	0	0	0	0	0	0

FOOD	PORTION	CALS	PROT	FAT	CHOL	CARB	FIBER	SOD
Seasoning Blends Garlic & Herb	¼ tsp (0.7 g)	0	0	0	0	0	0	0
Seasoning Blends Italian Medley	¼ tsp (0.7 g)	0	0	0	0	0	0	0
Seasoning Blends Table Blend	¼ tsp (0.7 g)	0	0	0	0	0	0	0
Old Bay								
Seasoning	¼ tsp (0.6 g)	0	0	0	0	0	0	160
Seasoning 30% Less Sodium	¼ tsp (0.6 g)	0	0	0	0	0	0	95
Ribber City								
Rib-A-Dub-Rub Dry Rub Seasoning	¼ tsp (0.8 oz)	3	0	0	0	1	0	57
Spice Hunter								
All Purpose Blend	¼ tsp	0	0	0	0	0	0	0
Greek Seasoning Salt Free	¼ tsp	0	0	0	0	0	0	0
HERRING								
atlantic baked	4 oz	230	26	13	87	0	0	130
dried salted	1 fillet (1.4 oz)	161	18	9	61	0	0	680
pickled	1 oz	74	4	5	4	3	0	247
pickled in cream sauce	1 oz	72	3	5	5	2	0	200
roe	1 tbsp	39	6	2	105	tr	0	25
smoked kippered	1 oz	62	7	4	23	0	0	260
TAKE-OUT								
breaded fried	1 serv (4 oz)	225	15	14	67	9	1	432
HIBISCUS								
flowers dried sweetened	⅓ cup	100	0	0	0	23	2	15
Santa Cruz								
Organic Hibiscus Cooler	8 oz	100	tr	0	0	24	0	40
HICKORY NUTS								
dried	1 oz	187	4	18	0	5	–	0
HOMINY								
white canned	1 cup	119	2	1	0	24	4	246
yellow canned	½ cup	115	2	1	0	23	4	336
Allens								
White	½ cup	100	2	1	0	22	4	340

FOOD	PORTION	CALS	PROT	FAT	CHOL	CARB	FIBER	SOD
Bush's								
Golden	½ cup	60	1	0	0	13	3	550
HONEY								
honey	1 tbsp (0.7 oz)	64	tr	0	0	17	–	1
honey	¼ cup (3 oz)	258	tr	0	0	70	tr	3
orange blossom	1 tbsp	60	0	0	0	17	0	0
wild honey	1 tbsp	60	0	0	0	17	–	0
Comfort Care								
Raw Clover	1 tbsp (0.7 oz)	60	0	0	0	17	–	0
Dutch Gold								
Clover	1 tbsp	60	0	0	0	17	0	0
Steel's								
Sugar Free	1 tbsp (0.5 oz)	24	0	0	0	11	0	0
SueBee								
Honey	1 tbsp (0.7 oz)	60	0	0	0	17	–	0
Tastes Like Honey								
Sugar Free	1 tbsp (0.7 oz)	21	0	0	0	0	0	0
Tree Of Life								
Alfalfa Honey Raw Unfiltered	1 tbsp	60	0	0	0	17	–	0
Avocado Honey Raw Unfiltered	1 tbsp (0.7 oz)	60	0	0	0	17	0	0
Buckwheat Honey Raw Unfiltered	1 tbsp	60	0	0	0	17	–	0
Tupelo Honey Raw Unfiltered	1 tbsp	60	0	0	0	17	–	0
Wholesome Sweeteners								
Organic Fair Trade Amber	1 tbsp	60	0	0	0	17	0	0
Organic Fair Trade Raw	1 tbsp (0.7 oz)	60	0	0	0	17	0	0
HONEYDEW								
balls frzn	1 cup (8 oz)	83	1	tr	0	21	2	41
fresh cut up	1 cup	61	1	tr	0	15	1	31

FOOD	PORTION	CALS	PROT	FAT	CHOL	CARB	FIBER	SOD
fresh wedge	⅛ melon (4.5 oz)	45	1	tr	0	11	1	22
whole fresh	1 (35 oz)	360	5	1	0	91	8	180
Chiquita								
Fresh Cut Up	1 cup (6.2 oz)	64	1	0	0	16	1	32
HORSE								
roasted	3 oz	149	24	5	58	0	0	47
HORSERADISH								
japanese wasabi	¼ tsp	1	–	–	0	tr	0	0
sauce	1 tbsp	7	tr	tr	0	2	1	47
wasabi root raw	1 (5.9 oz)	184	8	1	0	40	13	29
wasabi root raw sliced	½ cup (2.3 oz)	71	3	tr	0	15	5	11
Dietz & Watson								
Cranberry Horseradish Sauce	1 tsp (5 g)	10	0	1	0	1	0	5
Gold's								
Horse Radish	1 tsp (5 g)	0	0	0	0	0	0	30
Robert Rothchild Farm								
Sauce	1 tsp	20	0	2	<5	1	0	30
Zatarain's								
Prepared	1 tbsp (0.5 oz)	15	0	0	0	2	0	90
HOT CHOCOLATE								
mix not prep	1 pkg (1 oz)	111	2	1	0	23	1	141
mix w/ no calorie sweetener as prep w/ water	8 oz	72	3	1	0	14	2	180
mix w/ sugar as prep w/ nonfat milk	8 oz	209	9	1	5	30	1	128
mix w/ sugar as prep w/ water	8 oz	138	2	1	0	29	1	182
Hershey's								
Goodnight Hugs	1 pkg (1.2 oz)	140	3	3	<5	27	–	190
Nestle								
Hot Cocoa Carb Select Fat Free	1 pkg	25	1	0	0	5	tr	150

FOOD	PORTION	CALS	PROT	FAT	CHOL	CARB	FIBER	SOD
Hot Cocoa Milk Chocolate	1 pkg (1 oz)	80	tr	3	0	15	tr	180
Hot Cocoa Rich Milk Chocolate as prep w/ water	1 pkg (0.7 oz)	80	tr	3	0	14	tr	180
Silhouette Solution								
Down East not prep	1 pkg (0.88 oz)	90	15	2	0	5	1	300
Starbucks								
Hot Cocoa Mix	1 pkg	130	4	2	0	28	2	170
Swiss Miss								
Cocoa Caramel as prep	1 pkg	120	1	3	0	22	tr	160
Cocoa No Sugar Added as prep	1 pkg	60	2	1	0	10	1	170
Cocoa Rich Creamy as prep	1 pkg	110	2	2	<5	22	tr	170
Cocoa w/ Marshmallows as prep	1 pkg	120	1	2	0	24	1	150
Cocoa w/ Marshmallows Fat Free as prep	1 pkg	140	1	3	0	29	1	160
French Vanilla as prep	1 pkg	110	2	2	0	24	tr	160
Milk Chocolate as prep	1 pkg	120	1	3	0	23	1	170
TAKE-OUT								
chocolate caliente w/ lowfat milk	1 serv (8.4 oz)	221	11	9	12	27	1	158
chocolate caliente w/ whole milk	1 serv (8.4 oz)	276	10	17	38	25	1	149
hot chocolate	1 cup (8.7 oz)	192	9	6	20	30	3	110
mexican hot chocolate	1 cup	173	10	6	18	20	1	150

HOT DOG (*see also* HOT DOG SUBSTITUTES)

FOOD	PORTION	CALS	PROT	FAT	CHOL	CARB	FIBER	SOD
beef	1 (1.5 oz)	149	5	13	24	2	0	513
beef & pork	1 (1.5 oz)	137	5	12	23	1	1	504
beef lowfat	1 (2 oz)	133	7	11	23	1	0	593
chicken	1 (1.5 oz)	116	6	9	45	3	0	617
fat free	1 (2 oz)	62	7	1	23	6	0	455
lowfat	1 (2 oz)	88	6	6	25	3	0	716
low sodium	1 (2 oz)	180	7	16	35	1	0	177
pork and beef cheese smokie	1 (1.5 oz)	141	6	12	29	1	0	465
turkey	1 (1.5 oz)	102	6	8	48	1	0	642

FOOD	PORTION	CALS	PROT	FAT	CHOL	CARB	FIBER	SOD
Applegate Farms								
Natural Beef	1 (1.5 oz)	80	5	6	20	0	0	380
Organic Chicken	1 (1.5 oz)	70	7	5	30	0	0	430
Dietz & Watson								
Beef Foot Long	1 (4 oz)	310	14	26	60	4	0	980
Black Forest Wieners	1 (2 oz)	180	8	16	30	0	0	480
Gourmet Lite	1 (2 oz)	60	7	2	15	5	0	390
Super Franks	1 (3.2 oz)	270	11	24	40	3	0	780
Healthy Ones								
Beef	1 (1.8 oz)	70	6	3	20	7	0	430
Franks	1 (1.8 oz)	70	6	3	20	6	0	430
Johnsonville								
Stadium Beef	1 (2.7 oz)	240	9	22	50	2	–	760
Organic Prairie								
Beef Uncured	1 (1.5 oz)	120	5	11	25	0	0	360
Oscar Mayer								
Beef	1 (1.6 oz)	140	5	13	30	1	0	460
Beef Light	1 (1.6 oz)	90	5	6	20	2	–	500
Cheese Dogs	1 (1.6 oz)	140	5	13	35	1	0	540
Corn Dogs	1	210	6	12	25	21	1	590
Smokies	1 (1.8 oz)	150	6	13	30	1	0	500
TAKE-OUT								
corndog	1	460	17	19	79	56	–	972
w/ bun chili	1	297	14	13	51	31	–	480
w/ bun plain	1	242	10	15	44	18	–	671
HOT DOG SUBSTITUTES								
Health Is Wealth								
Vegetarian Cocktail Franks	3 (2.4 oz)	220	8	16	0	16	3	200
Loma Linda								
Big Franks	1 (1.8 oz)	110	11	6	0	3	2	220
Big Franks Low Fat Vegan	1 (1.8 oz)	80	12	3	0	3	2	240
Morningstar Farms								
Corn Dog Veggie	1 (2.5 oz)	170	8	6	0	22	3	530
Yves								
Meatless Hot Dog	1	50	10	1	0	2	0	400
Tofu Dogs	1	45	8	1	0	2	0	300
HUMMUS								
Athenos								
Original	2 tbsp	80	2	5	0	5	1	180

FOOD	PORTION	CALS	PROT	FAT	CHOL	CARB	FIBER	SOD
Roasted Garlic	2 tbsp	80	2	5	0	5	1	200
Roasted Red Pepper	2 tbsp	80	2	6	0	5	1	130
Cedar's								
Artichoke Spinach	2 tbsp (1 oz)	70	2	4	0	5	1	105
Emerald Valley								
Organic Greek Olive & Roasted Garlic	2 tbsp (1 oz)	60	2	3	0	6	2	190
Organic Original	2 tbsp (1 oz)	50	2	2	0	7	2	200
Organic Spinach Feta	2 tbsp (1 oz)	50	2	2	0	6	2	190
Guiltless Gourmet								
Original	2 tbsp (1.1 oz)	50	2	2	0	8	2	110
Tribe								
40 Spices	2 tbsp	50	1	4	0	3	1	140
French Onion	2 tbsp	50	1	4	0	4	1	120
Organic Classic	2 tbsp	50	2	4	0	4	1	100
Organic Roasted Red Peppers	2 tbsp	40	1	3	0	3	1	95
Roasted Eggplant	2 tbsp	35	1	3	0	3	1	150
Scallion	2 tbsp	50	1	4	0	4	1	125
Zesty Lemon	2 tbsp	50	1	3	0	4	1	130
Wholesome Valley								
Organic Classic	2 tbsp (1 oz)	60	2	4	0	5	1	115
Wild Garden								
Hummus Dip	2 tbsp	35	2	2	0	4	1	70
WildWood								
Organic Low Fat	2 tbsp	50	2	2	0	6	1	130
Organic Mid-Eastern	2 tbsp	65	2	4	0	6	1	120
TAKE-OUT								
hummus	¼ cup (2.2 oz)	109	3	5	0	12	3	149

HYACINTH BEANS

FOOD	PORTION	CALS	PROT	FAT	CHOL	CARB	FIBER	SOD
dried cooked	1 cup	228	16	1	0	40	–	13

ICE CREAM AND FROZEN DESSERTS (*see also* ICES AND ICE POPS, SHERBET, YOGURT FROZEN)

FOOD	PORTION	CALS	PROT	FAT	CHOL	CARB	FIBER	SOD
chocolate	½ cup (4 fl oz)	143	3	7	22	19	–	50
dixie cup chocolate	1 (3.5 fl oz)	125	2	6	20	16	–	44
dixie cup strawberry	1 (3.5 fl oz)	112	2	5	17	16	–	35

FOOD	PORTION	CALS	PROT	FAT	CHOL	CARB	FIBER	SOD
dixie cup vanilla	1 (3.5 fl oz)	116	2	6	25	14	–	46
freeze dried ice cream chocolate strawberry & vanilla	1 pkg (0.75 oz)	158	2	5	1	24	1	97
strawberry	½ cup (4 fl oz)	127	2	6	19	18	–	40
vanilla	½ cup (4 fl oz)	132	2	7	29	16	–	53
vanilla soft serve	½ cup	111	4	2	10	19	–	62
Breyers								
Butter Pecan	½ cup	150	2	10	20	14	0	110
Carb Smart Chocolate	½ cup	90	2	6	15	13	4	75
Carb Smart Fudge Bar	1 (3.5 oz)	100	3	7	20	9	1	50
Carb Smart Vanilla	½ cup	90	2	6	15	13	4	45
Carb Smart Vanilla Bar Chocolate Coated	1 (3 oz)	170	2	15	15	9	2	45
Cherry Vanilla	½ cup	130	2	6	15	18	0	55
Chocolate Crackle	½ cup	160	2	10	15	15	0	30
Chocolate Extra Creamy	½ cup	140	2	7	30	17	1	50
Coffee	½ cup	130	2	7	20	15	0	45
Cookies & Cream	½ cup	150	2	7	15	19	0	90
Double Churn ½ Fat Chocolate Mocha Silk	½ cup	130	3	5	20	19	1	50
Double Churn ½ Fat Creamy Vanilla	½ cup	100	2	3	10	17	0	65
Double Churn ½ Fat Mint Chocolate Chip	½ cup	130	2	5	10	19	1	50
Double Churn ½ Fat Rocky Road	½ cup	130	3	5	10	22	1	45
Double Churn Fat Free Chocolate Fudge Brownie	½ cup	110	3	0	0	25	4	75
Double Churn Fat Free Creamy Vanilla	½ cup	90	3	0	0	21	3	50
Double Churn Fat Free French Chocolate	½ cup	90	3	0	0	22	4	55
Double Churn No Sugar Added Vanilla	½ cup	80	2	4	10	14	4	45
Dulce De Leche	½ cup	150	2	6	15	21	0	105
French Vanilla	½ cup	140	3	7	45	14	0	35
Heath English Toffee	½ cup	160	2	6	10	25	0	130

FOOD	PORTION	CALS	PROT	FAT	CHOL	CARB	FIBER	SOD
Overload Very Chocolate Cherry	½ cup	120	2	3	5	21	1	50
Overload Waffle Cone	½ cup	130	2	3	5	22	0	95
Peach	½ cup	120	2	5	15	17	0	30
Sandwich Mrs. Fields Brownie	1 (6 oz)	450	5	19	20	64	2	140
Sandwich Mrs. Fields Cookie	1 (3 oz)	190	2	8	10	29	0	125
Sandwich Oreo	1 (3 oz)	170	2	6	10	26	1	190
Snicker	½ cup	170	3	8	20	20	0	80
Strawberry	½ cup	120	2	5	15	15	0	35
Strawberry Cheesecake Sara Lee	½ cup	150	2	6	10	20	0	75
Vanilla Fudge Brownie	½ cup	150	2	7	15	20	1	50
Vanilla Lactose Free	½ cup	130	2	7	20	14	0	20
Celestial Seasonings								
Tea Dreams Cinnamon Apple Spice	½ cup	140	0	6	0	24	1	55
Tea Dreams Vanilla Ginger Spice Chai	½ cup	140	0	6	0	24	1	70
Tea Dreams Bars Chocolate Caramel Chai	1 (2.7 oz)	240	tr	15	0	28	2	65
Ciao Bella								
Gelato Chocolate	1 pkg (3.5 oz)	210	4	13	39	22	1	53
Gelato Hazelnut	1 pkg (3.5 oz)	210	3	13	39	21	1	61
Gelato Vanilla	1 pkg (3.5 oz)	184	3	11	39	19	0	61
Clemmy's								
Butter Pecan Sugar Free	½ cup	200	1	17	70	13	4	40
Chocolate Sugar Free	½ cup	200	2	16	80	19	3	30
Ice Cream Os Snack Size Sugar Free	1	100	1	7	10	12	2	25
Ice Cream Os Sugar Free	1	180	1	13	20	22	3	45
Toasted Almond Sugar Free	½ cup	220	2	16	75	20	4	70
Vanilla Bean Sugar Free	½ cup	200	1	15	80	18	4	30
Dippin' Dots								
Banana Split	½ cup	170	3	10	32	16	0	22
Chocolate	½ cup	165	3	10	29	15	0	16

FOOD	PORTION	CALS	PROT	FAT	CHOL	CARB	FIBER	SOD
Fudge Fat Free No Sugar Added	½ cup	92	4	0	2	18	0	95
Horchata	½ cup	170	3	10	32	16	0	22
Java Delight	½ cup	170	3	10	32	16	0	22
Root Beer Float	½ cup	111	1	3	13	20	0	34
Vanilla	½ cup	170	3	10	32	16	0	22
Fat Boy								
Casco Nut Sundae On A Stick	1 (3 oz)	310	7	24	15	21	2	40
Casco Nut Sundae On A Stick Cherry Cordial	1 (3 oz)	300	3	22	15	26	1	45
Sandwich Chocolate	1 (3 oz)	210	4	9	20	31	1	150
Sandwich Egg Nog	1 (3 oz)	220	4	10	35	31	tr	160
Sandwich Jr. Vanilla	1 (1.6 oz)	120	2	5	15	17	0	25
Sandwich Vanilla	1 (3 oz)	220	4	10	20	30	1	160
Glace De Vino								
Chocolate Amarreto Cream Sherry	½ cup	180	2	7	20	21	0	50
Raspberry Merlot Cheesecake	½ cup	180	2	7	20	22	0	50
Good Humor								
Bar Chocolate Eclair	1 (3 oz)	160	2	8	5	21	1	35
Bar Cookies & Cream	1 (3 oz)	190	2	11	10	21	1	75
Bar King Heath	1 (4 oz)	310	3	20	20	31	1	85
Bar Vanilla Chocolate Coated	1 (4 oz)	260	3	17	20	24	1	50
Cone King Giant	1 (8 oz)	390	7	21	30	44	2	135
Cone King Vanilla	1 (4.6 oz)	250	4	13	15	30	1	100
Cone Sundae	1 (4.3 oz)	260	4	15	15	29	1	80
Sandwich Oreo	1 (4.5 oz)	240	4	10	10	36	2	310
Sandwich Vanilla	1 (3 oz)	130	2	2	5	26	2	80
Sandwich Giant Vanilla	1 (6 oz)	220	4	4	0	43	1	150
Swirlwind	1 (6 oz)	160	4	3	10	31	0	110
Haagen-Dazs								
Bailey's Irish Cream	½ cup (3.6 oz)	260	5	17	100	21	0	50
Bar Chocolate & Dark Chocolate	1 (3 oz)	290	4	20	65	24	2	30
Bar Vanilla & Almonds	1 (3 oz)	310	5	22	65	22	tr	65

FOOD	PORTION	CALS	PROT	FAT	CHOL	CARB	FIBER	SOD
Bar Vanilla & Milk Chocolate	1 (3 oz)	290	4	21	75	22	0	55
Butter Pecan	½ cup (3.7 oz)	310	5	23	110	21	tr	110
Caramel Cone	½ cup (4 oz)	320	4	19	100	32	0	190
Cherry Vanilla	½ cup (3.5 oz)	240	4	15	100	23	0	60
Chocolate Chip Cookie Dough	½ cup (3.6 oz)	310	4	20	95	29	0	125
Chocolate Peanut Butter	½ cup (3.8 oz)	360	8	24	100	27	2	100
Cookies & Cream	½ cup (3.6 oz)	270	5	17	105	23	0	95
Dulce De Leche	½ cup (3.7 oz)	290	5	17	100	28	0	95
Five Coffee	½ cup (3.6 oz)	220	5	12	70	23	0	70
Five Milk Chocolate	½ cup (3.6 oz)	220	6	12	75	22	tr	75
Five Mint	½ cup (3.6 oz)	220	5	12	70	24	0	50
Five Passion Fruit	½ cup (3.6 oz)	220	4	11	70	25	0	45
Five Vanilla	½ cup (3.7 oz)	270	5	18	120	21	0	70
Green Tea	½ cup (3.6 oz)	250	5	17	105	20	0	50
Mango	½ cup (3.7 oz)	250	4	14	85	28	tr	50
Reserve Amazon Valley Chocolate	½ cup (3.7 oz)	290	5	19	105	25	0	45
Reserve Caramelized Hazelnut Gianduja	½ cup (3.5 oz)	290	4	18	90	27	0	65
Reserve Fleur De Sel Caramel	½ cup (3.7 oz)	280	4	17	85	28	0	85
Reserve Hawaiian Lehua Honey & Sweet Cream	½ cup (3.8 oz)	270	4	17	100	26	0	60
Rocky Road	½ cup (3.6 oz)	300	5	18	90	29	1	75

FOOD	PORTION	CALS	PROT	FAT	CHOL	CARB	FIBER	SOD
Strawberry	½ cup (3.7 oz)	250	4	16	95	23	tr	65
Vanilla Honey Bee	½ cup (3.6 oz)	270	5	17	110	23	1	50
Healthy Choice								
Bar Fudge Low Fat No Sugar Added	1 (2.6 oz)	100	4	2	5	16	5	80
Hershey's								
Banana Split	½ cup (2.5 oz)	160	2	9	35	18	0	55
Chocolate	½ cup (2.5 oz)	140	3	8	30	15	tr	55
Cookies And Cream	½ cup (2.5 oz)	160	2	9	35	16	0	70
Fudge Royale	½ cup (2.5 oz)	180	2	9	35	19	0	80
Mint Moose Tracks	½ cup (2.5 oz)	200	3	14	35	21	tr	75
Raspberry	½ cup (2.5 oz)	170	2	9	35	21	0	55
Tally-Ho Low Fat Butter Pecan	½ cup (2.5 oz)	90	3	2	10	14	0	95
Vanilla	½ cup (2.5 oz)	150	3	9	35	14	0	60
Julie's								
Organic Gluten Free Sandwich Vanilla	1 (2.6 oz)	220	3	11	40	30	1	95
Klondike								
Bar Caramel Pretzel	1 (4 oz)	260	3	14	10	30	1	170
Bar Original Vanilla	1 (4.5 oz)	250	3	17	20	22	0	55
Bar Reese's	1 (4 oz)	260	4	16	10	26	1	95
Bar Whitehouse Cherry	1 (4.5 oz)	250	2	17	20	24	0	55
Cone Crunchy Vanilla	1 (4.3 oz)	280	5	16	15	30	1	85
Slim A Bear 100 Calorie Sandwich Vanilla	1 (3 oz)	100	2	2	0	21	2	65
Slim A Bear Bar Vanilla	1 (4 oz)	170	6	9	5	21	4	65
Land O Lakes								
Vanilla	½ cup (2.4 oz)	150	2	8	30	17	0	40

FOOD	PORTION	CALS	PROT	FAT	CHOL	CARB	FIBER	SOD
Vanilla Light	½ cup (2.3 oz)	100	3	3	15	17	0	50
Molli Coolz								
Cup Banana Cream Pie	1	120	2	9	35	9	1	35
Cup Chocolate Fusion	1	140	2	10	25	10	1	55
Cup Chocolate Peanut Butter	1	160	2	12	45	12	0	55
Ionz Cotton Candy	1 cup	100	2	7	35	8	0	30
Ionz S'mores	1 cup	110	2	9	30	7	1	50
Rocks Cherry Blue Raz & Lemon	1 cup	80	tr	2	0	15	0	23
Rocks Lemon Lime	1 cup	80	tr	2	0	15	0	23
Shakers Chocolate	1 (10.2 oz)	250	3	11	35	35	5	72
Natural Choice								
Organic Double Chocolate	½ cup	230	3	14	35	25	0	65
Organic Strawberry	½ cup	210	2	13	35	22	0	65
Organic Vanilla	½ cup	220	2	14	35	22	0	70
Popsicle								
Creamsicle	1 (2.5 oz)	100	1	2	5	20	0	35
Purely Decadent								
Dairy Free Bar Chocolate Coated Vanilla	1 (2.7 oz)	200	2	9	0	26	3	10
Dairy Free Bar Chocolate Coated Vanilla Almond	1 (2.7 oz)	210	2	10	0	28	4	10
Organic Coconut Milk Chocolate	½ cup	150	1	9	0	20	6	5
Organic Coconut Milk Vanilla Bean	½ cup	150	1	8	0	19	6	5
Organic Dairy Free Belgian Chocolate	½ cup	180	1	7	0	30	4	15
Organic Dairy Free Chocolate Obsession	½ cup	210	2	9	0	36	5	15
Organic Dairy Free Gluten Free Cookie Dough	½ cup	230	1	8	0	36	5	75
Organic Dairy Free Mocha Almond Fudge	½ cup	200	3	9	0	32	6	45
Organic Dairy Free Snickerdoodle	½ cup	190	1	6	0	34	5	65
Organic Dairy Free Vanilla	½ cup	170	1	8	0	29	6	20

FOOD	PORTION	CALS	PROT	FAT	CHOL	CARB	FIBER	SOD
Rice Dream								
Bar Vanilla Chocolate Coating	1 (3 oz)	230	1	15	0	24	tr	70
Bar Vanilla Nutty	1 (3.3 oz)	320	5	24	0	27	2	65
Carob Almond	½ cup	180	0	10	0	26	2	70
Frozen Pie Chocolate	1 (3.4 oz)	330	3	19	0	40	2	50
Mint Carob Chip	½ cup	170	1	8	0	25	0	85
Strawberry	½ cup	160	0	8	0	25	2	70
Sheer Bliss								
Bar Pomegranate	1 (3.1 oz)	260	3	16	30	24	tr	55
Blissbites	2 (1.1 oz)	100	1	7	10	9	0	15
Blisswich	1 (3.3 oz)	270	3	10	20	39	tr	55
Freedom	½ cup (4 oz)	290	3	16	65	32	0	60
Mediterranean Coffee	½ cup (4 oz)	260	3	18	65	25	0	65
Pomegranate	½ cup (4 oz)	290	3	16	55	32	0	60
Vanilla	½ cup (4 oz)	300	6	19	65	29	0	65
Skinny Cow								
Bar Dippers Vanilla & Caramel	1	80	2	3	3	11	2	30
Bar Truffle Caramel	1	100	3	2	5	19	3	50
Bar Truffle French Vanilla	1	100	3	2	20	18	3	45
Cone Chocolate w/ Fudge	1	150	4	3	5	29	3	95
Cone Vanilla w/ Caramel	1	150	4	3	5	29	3	80
Fudge Bar	1	100	4	1	3	22	4	45
Sandwich Chocolate Peanut Butter	1	150	4	2	5	30	3	100
Sandwich Cookies 'N Cream	1	150	4	2	3	31	3	105
Sandwich Vanilla	1	140	4	2	1	30	3	95
Sandwich Vanilla No Sugar Added	1	140	4	2	15	30	5	115
SoDelicious								
Dairy Free Sandwich Minis Pomegranate	1 (1.4 oz)	90	2	2	0	18	1	75
Dairy Free Sandwich Mint	1 (2.2 oz)	150	3	3	0	28	2	125
Dairy Free Sandwich Vanilla	1 (2 oz)	150	3	3	0	28	2	105
Dairy Free Sugar Free Chocolate Coated Vanilla Bar	1 (2.2 oz)	150	2	14	0	15	6	50

FOOD	PORTION	CALS	PROT	FAT	CHOL	CARB	FIBER	SOD
Dairy Free Sugar Free Fudge Bar	1 (2 oz)	80	2	5	0	12	6	50
Organic Dairy Free Sandwich Neapolitan	1 (2.2 oz)	150	3	3	0	28	2	110
Soy Dream								
Butter Pecan	½ cup	140	1	9	0	17	tr	130
Sandwich Lil' Dreamers Chocolate	1 (1.4 oz)	100	1	5	0	15	tr	60
Vanilla	½ cup	140	1	7	0	18	tr	140
Starbucks								
Caramel Macchiato	½ cup (3.6 oz)	240	3	13	60	27	0	105
Coffee	½ cup (3.5 oz)	210	3	13	65	21	0	55
Java Chip Frappuccino	½ cup (3.5 oz)	250	3	15	60	25	0	50
Mocha Frappuccino	½ cup (3.5 oz)	220	3	13	55	23	tr	65
Mocha Bar	1	280	4	19	50	26	1	60
Stonyfield Farm								
Gotta Have Java	1 serv (4 oz)	250	3	16	60	22	0	45
Strawberry Licious	1 serv (4 oz)	220	3	13	50	23	0	35
Vanilla Chai	1 serv (4 oz)	240	3	16	60	21	0	45
Straus								
Organic Coffee	4 oz	240	4	15	70	19	0	55
Organic Vanilla Bean	4 oz	240	4	15	70	19	0	55
The Greek Gods								
Pagoto Ice Krema Baklava	½ cup (4 oz)	240	5	12	40	29	1	60
Pagoto Ice Krema Chocolate Fig	½ cup (4 oz)	240	4	11	40	32	0	60
Pagoto Ice Krema Honey Pomegranate	½ cup (4 oz)	230	4	11	40	31	0	60
Turkey Hill								
Banana Split	½ cup	150	2	7	25	19	1	40
Choco Mint Chip	½ cup	160	2	9	25	17	1	45
Chocolate All Natural	½ cup	150	3	8	30	18	0	45
Chocolate Marshmallow	½ cup	160	2	6	20	24	1	100
Coconut Cream Pie	½ cup	170	2	9	30	20	0	95
Cookies 'N Cream	½ cup	150	2	8	25	19	0	60
Duetto Cherry	½ cup	120	1	3	10	21	0	35

FOOD	PORTION	CALS	PROT	FAT	CHOL	CARB	FIBER	SOD
Duetto Lemon	½ cup	120	1	4	10	21	0	35
Duetto Root Beer	½ cup	120	0	3	10	21	0	35
French Vanilla	½ cup	140	2	7	50	16	0	45
Light Banana Split	½ cup	110	2	3	5	19	1	50
Light Dulce De Chocolate	½ cup	120	2	3	5	22	1	110
Light Moose Tracks	½ cup	140	3	6	5	20	1	65
Light Vanilla Bean	½ cup	100	2	2	5	17	1	55
No Sugar Added Cherry Fudge Ripple	½ cup	80	3	0	0	22	4	70
No Sugar Added Vanilla Bean	½ cup	70	3	0	0	19	5	75
Original Vanilla	½ cup	140	2	7	30	16	0	45
Peanut Butter Ripple	½ cup	170	3	11	25	16	1	90
Rocky Road	½ cup	170	3	8	20	23	1	125
Sandwich Chocolate Chunk	1 (3.2 oz)	320	3	15	30	44	1	290
Sandwich Vanilla Bean	1 (2.5 oz)	190	3	7	20	29	1	95
Sandwich Light Vanilla Bean	1 (2.5 oz)	160	3	3	10	32	3	95
Sundae Cone Vanilla Fudge	1 (3.3 oz)	320	6	18	20	35	2	120
Tin Roof Sundae	½ cup	150	2	8	25	19	0	65
TAKE-OUT								
cone vanilla light soft serve	1 (4.6 oz)	164	4	6	28	24	–	92
gelato chocolate hazelnut	½ cup (5.3 oz)	370	9	29	92	26	2	49
gelato vanilla	½ cup (3 oz)	211	3	15	151	18	0	78
ice cream pie no crust	1 slice (3.4 oz)	218	3	14	56	21	1	74
mud pie	⅛ pie (8 oz)	698	9	32	53	96	3	560
sundae caramel	1 (5.4 oz)	303	7	9	25	49	–	195
sundae hot fudge	1 (5.4 oz)	284	6	9	21	48	–	182
sundae strawberry	1 (5.4 oz)	269	6	8	21	45	–	92

ICE CREAM CONES AND CUPS

FOOD	PORTION	CALS	PROT	FAT	CHOL	CARB	FIBER	SOD
brown sugar cone	1 (10 g)	40	1	tr	0	8	tr	32
wafer cone	1	17	tr	tr	0	3	tr	6
waffle cone	1 lg	121	2	2	0	23	1	41
Keebler								
Cone Sugar	1	50	1	1	0	10	0	55
Ice Creme Cone	1	15	0	0	0	4	0	20
Waffle Bowl	1	50	tr	1	0	10	0	25
Waffle Cone	1	50	tr	1	0	10	0	25

FOOD	PORTION	CALS	PROT	FAT	CHOL	CARB	FIBER	SOD
ICE CREAM TOPPINGS								
butterscotch	2 tbsp (1.4 oz)	103	1	tr	–	27	–	143
caramel	2 tbsp (1.4 oz)	103	1	tr	–	27	–	143
marshmallow cream	1 jar (7 oz)	615	3	tr	0	157	–	90
marshmallow cream	1 oz	88	1	tr	0	23	–	13
nuts in syrup	2 tbsp	184	2	9	0	24	1	17
pineapple	1 cup (11.5 oz)	861	1	–	0	226	–	214
pineapple	2 tbsp (1.5 oz)	106	tr	tr	0	28	tr	18
strawberry	2 tbsp (1.5 oz)	107	tr	tr	0	28	–	9
strawberry	1 cup (11.5 oz)	863	1	1	0	225	–	73
Hershey's								
Sundae Syrup Caramel	2 tbsp (1.4 oz)	100	–	0	0	25	0	95
Steel's								
Sugar Free Fudge Sauce	2 tbsp (0.9 oz)	110	1	6	10	13	1	5
ICED TEA								
MIX								
Aquafull								
Zesty Lemon Dietary Supplement	1 pkg (9 g)	20	–	0	0	8	4	15
Crystal Light								
Sugar Free All Flavors as prep	8 oz	5	0	0	0	0	0	0
Lipton								
Tea To Go Green Sugar Free Mandarin Mango	½ pkg (0.7 oz)	0	0	0	0	0	0	0
Nestea								
Lemon Liquid Concentrate as prep	8 oz	80	0	0	0	19	–	0
Peach Liquid Concentrate as prep	8 oz	90	0	0	0	21	–	0
Sugar Free w/ Lemon	2 tsp	5	0	0	0	2	–	0

FOOD	PORTION	CALS	PROT	FAT	CHOL	CARB	FIBER	SOD
Sweetened w/ Lemon	1⅓ tbsp	60	0	0	0	15	–	0
Unsweetened w/ Lemon	2 tsp	5	0	0	0	1	–	0
READY-TO-DRINK								
Bina								
Lemon	8 oz	70	0	0	0	17	–	25
Peach	8 oz	114	0	0	0	29	–	0
Bolthouse Farms								
Perfectly Protein Vanilla Chai Tea w/ Soy	8 oz	160	10	3	0	25	0	60
Bombilla & Gourd								
Organic Eco Teas All Flavors	8 oz	40	0	0	0	11	–	0
Cafe Sepia								
Matcha Latte	1 can (8.6 oz)	130	3	3	10	23	1	50
Delta Blues								
Tea Punch Black Tea Sumptuous Spearmint	8 oz	90	0	0	0	21	0	0
Tea Punch Green Tea Peach & Delectable Lemongrass	8 oz	90	0	0	0	22	–	0
Tea Punch Green Tea Peach Apricot Pineapple Quince	8 oz	100	0	0	0	24	–	0
Fuze								
Antioxidant Tea	8 oz	60	0	0	0	15	–	0
Green Tea	8 oz	60	0	0	0	16	–	0
White Tea	8 oz	60	0	0	0	15	–	0
Gold Peak Tea								
Green Tea Sweetened	1 bottle (16.9 oz)	170	0	0	0	45	–	45
Hawaiian								
Iced Tea	1 can (11.5 oz)	120	0	0	0	35	0	50
Ito En								
Dark Green Tea Oi Ocha	8 oz	0	0	0	0	0	0	20
Golden Oolong	8 oz	0	0	0	0	0	0	20
Green Tea Jasmine	8 oz	0	0	0	0	0	0	20
Green Tea Oi Ocha	8 oz	0	0	0	0	0	0	20
Sencho Shot Japanese Green Tea	1 can (6.4 oz)	0	0	0	0	0	0	20

FOOD	PORTION	CALS	PROT	FAT	CHOL	CARB	FIBER	SOD
Kombucha								
Wonder Drink Asian Pear Ginger	1 bottle (8.5 oz)	65	0	0	0	16	–	0
Wonder Drink Rooibus Red Peach	1 bottle (8.5 oz)	60	0	0	0	15	–	10
Nantucket Nectars								
Half & Half	8 oz	90	0	0	0	22	0	25
Original Lemon	8 oz	80	0	0	0	22	0	25
Nestea								
Green Tea Diet Peach	8 oz	0	0	0	0	0	0	30
Green Tea Peach	1 bottle (20 oz)	220	0	0	0	57	–	75
Lemon	1 bottle (20 oz)	210	0	0	0	56	–	75
Lemon Diet	8 oz	0	0	0	0	0	–	30
Sweetened	8 oz	60	0	0	0	17	–	25
Sweetened Diet Green Tea	8 oz	0	0	0	0	0	0	0
Sweetened Green Tea	8 oz	80	0	0	0	20	–	0
Old Orchard								
Green Tea w/ Lemon & Honey	8 oz	45	0	0	0	12	0	9
Green Tea w/ Pomegranate	8 oz	45	0	0	0	12	0	9
Osteo								
Fruit Tea All Flavors	1 can (12 oz)	120	0	0	0	32	0	5
Pixie								
Black Tea Mate Lemon Ginger	8 oz	35	0	0	0	8	0	15
Yerba Mate Authentic	8 oz	30	0	0	0	7	0	5
POMx								
Green Tea Pomegranate Lychee	8 oz	70	0	0	0	18	–	5
Light Green Tea Pomegranate Hibiscus	8 oz	35	0	0	0	16	–	0
Santa Cruz								
Organic Lemon	8 oz	60	0	0	0	15	0	0
Organic Peppermint	8 oz	60	0	0	0	15	0	0
Organic TeaZer Passionfruit	1 bottle (12 oz)	90	0	0	0	22	0	0
Organic TeaZer Pear	1 bottle (12 oz)	90	0	0	0	21	0	0

FOOD	PORTION	CALS	PROT	FAT	CHOL	CARB	FIBER	SOD
Snapple								
Black Tea Lemon	8 oz	80	0	0	0	21	–	65
Diet Lemon Tea	8 oz	10	0	0	0	0	–	5
Diet Lemonade Iced Tea	8 oz	10	0	0	0	2	–	5
Diet Peach	8 oz	0	0	0	0	0	–	5
Diet Plum-A-Granate	8 oz	5	0	0	0	0	0	5
Green Tea Mango Metabolism	8 oz	60	0	0	0	15	–	5
Peach	8 oz	90	0	0	0	23	–	5
Red Tea Pomegranate Raspberry	8 oz	80	0	0	0	21	–	60
White Tea Apple Plum	8 oz	80	0	0	0	21	–	60
Sokenbicha								
All Flavors	1 bottle	0	0	0	0	0	0	10
SSips								
Diet Green Tea w/ Honey & Ginseng	1 box (7 oz)	0	0	0	0	0	0	10
Green Tea w/ Honey & Ginseng	1 box (7 oz)	60	0	0	0	15	–	10
Lemon	8 oz	100	0	0	0	24	0	10
Sweet Leaf								
Diet Mint & Honey Green Tea	8 oz	0	tr	0	0	tr	0	0
Lemon & Lime Unsweet	8 oz	0	0	0	0	0	0	0
Original Sweet	8 oz	70	0	0	0	18	–	10
Pomegranate Green Tea	8 oz	60	tr	0	0	16	–	0
Swiss Tea								
Diet	8 oz	0	0	0	0	1	0	20
Diet Decafe	8 oz	0	0	0	0	0	0	15
Green Tea w/ Ginseng & Honey	8 oz	80	0	0	0	20	0	10
Sweet Tea Southern Style	8 oz	90	0	0	0	23	0	10
W/ Lemon	8 oz	100	0	0	0	24	0	15
White Tea Sweetened w/ Raspberry	8 oz	90	0	0	0	24	0	15
Teas' Tea								
Green Hoji	8 oz	0	0	0	0	0	0	30
Lemongrass Green	8 oz	0	0	0	0	0	0	20
Pure Black	8 oz	0	0	0	0	0	0	15
Pure Green	8 oz	0	0	0	0	0	0	20

FOOD	PORTION	CALS	PROT	FAT	CHOL	CARB	FIBER	SOD
True Brew								
Cranberry Orange	8 oz	72	0	0	0	18	0	–
Green Tea	8 oz	64	0	0	0	16	0	–
Sweet Tea	8 oz	76	0	0	0	19	0	–
Turkey Hill								
Decaffeinated	8 oz	80	0	0	0	20	–	15
Diet Decaffeinated	8 oz	0	0	0	0	0	0	15
Nature's Accents Blueberry Oolong	8 oz	100	0	0	0	24	–	10
Nature's Accents Chai Spiced Zero Calorie	8 oz	0	0	0	0	1	–	10
Nature's Accents Green Tea	8 oz	70	0	0	0	17	–	20
Southern Brew Extra Sweet	8 oz	90	0	0	0	21	–	10
VidaTea								
All Flavors	1 can	90	0	0	0	24	–	–
VitaZest								
Green Tea Vitamin Enriched	8 oz	0	0	0	0	0	0	0
Weil For Tea								
Gyokuro	1 can (8.6 oz)	0	0	0	0	0	0	30
Turmeric	1 can (8.6 oz)	0	0	0	0	0	0	15
ICES AND ICE POPS								
Breeze Freeze								
100% Fruit Juice	1 (8 oz)	54	0	0	0	13	0	24
Fruit Granita	1 (8 oz)	120	1	0	0	28	tr	15
Breyers								
Pure Fruit Pop Lemon Lime	1 (1.75 oz)	40	0	0	0	10	–	0
Pure Fruit Pop Pomegranate Blends	1 (1.75 oz)	40	0	0	0	10	–	0
Dippin' Dots								
Cherry Berry	½ cup	90	0	0	0	23	0	0
Watermelon	½ cup	90	0	0	0	23	0	0
Haagen-Dazs								
Fat Free Sorbet Mango	½ cup (4 oz)	120	0	0	0	37	0	10
Fat Free Sorbet Raspberry	½ cup (3.7 oz)	120	0	0	0	30	2	0
Fat Free Sorbet Zesty Lemon	½ cup (4 oz)	110	0	0	0	29	tr	25
Lowfat Sorbet Chocolate	½ cup (3.7 oz)	130	2	1	0	28	2	70

FOOD	PORTION	CALS	PROT	FAT	CHOL	CARB	FIBER	SOD
Luigi's								
Italian Ice Cherry	1 (6 oz)	130	0	0	0	32	tr	15
Italian Ice Lemon Strawberry	1 (6 oz)	120	0	0	0	31	tr	10
Italian Ice No Sugar Added Lemon	1 (6 oz)	60	0	0	0	20	0	10
Italian Ice Pina Colada	1 (6 oz)	130	0	0	0	33	0	40
Swirl Blue Ribbon Lemonade	1 (6 oz)	150	0	0	0	39	0	10
Mr. J								
All Flavors	1 bar (2.25 oz)	50	tr	tr	–	12	–	5
Natural Choice								
Organic Vegan Fruit Bars Coconut	1 (2.75 oz)	90	0	4	0	16	1	10
Organic Vegan Fruit Bars Pink Lemonade	1 (2.75 oz)	50	0	0	0	13	0	5
Organic Vegan Grape	1 (2.75 oz)	50	0	0	0	13	0	5
Organic Vegan Sorbet Blueberry	½ cup	110	0	0	0	29	tr	10
Organic Vegan Sorbet Lemon	½ cup	110	0	0	0	30	0	15
Organic Vegan Sorbet Mango	½ cup	110	0	0	0	29	1	10
PickleSickle								
Pop	1 (2 oz)	3	0	0	0	1	0	245
Popsicle								
Creamsicle Pop No Sugar Added	2 (1.65 oz)	45	1	1	<5	10	2	25
Creamsicle Pop Sugar Free	2 (1.65 oz)	40	1	2	0	10	6	5
Diet Soda Pops	1 (1.6 oz)	15	0	0	0	3	–	0
Firecracker	1 (1.6 oz)	35	0	0	0	9	–	0
Fudgsicle Bar	1 (2.5 oz)	100	2	2	0	17	1	75
Fudgsicle Pops No Sugar Added	1 (1.65 oz)	40	2	1	0	10	2	45
Lifesavers Pop	1 (3.5 oz)	90	0	0	0	22	–	10
Pop Ups Orange Burst	1 (2.75 oz)	90	1	1	5	18	0	20
Rainbow Pops	1 (1.65 oz)	40	0	0	0	10	–	5
Snow Cone	1 (7 oz)	30	0	0	0	7	–	5

FOOD	PORTION	CALS	PROT	FAT	CHOL	CARB	FIBER	SOD
Power Of Fruit								
Fruit Bar Banana Berry	1 (1.75 oz)	27	tr	tr	0	7	1	2
Fruit Bar Original	1 (1.75 oz)	28	tr	tr	0	7	1	1
Fruit Bar Tropical	1 (1.75 oz)	30	tr	tr	0	8	1	1
SoDelicious								
Dairy Free Creamy Orange Bar	1 (2.2 oz)	80	1	2	0	18	2	30
Sweet Nothings								
Bar Mango Raspberry	1 (2.6 oz)	100	1	0	0	23	0	10
Turkey Hill								
Venice Mango	½ cup	100	0	0	0	23	0	30
Venice Pomegranate Blueberry w/ Acai	½ cup	100	0	0	0	25	0	5

INDIAN FOOD (see ASIAN FOOD)

JACKFRUIT

FOOD	PORTION	CALS	PROT	FAT	CHOL	CARB	FIBER	SOD
canned in syrup	½ cup (3.1 oz)	82	tr	tr	0	21	1	10
fresh sliced	1 cup (5.8 oz)	157	3	1	0	38	3	3

JALAPENO (see PEPPERS)

JAM/JELLY/PRESERVES

FOOD	PORTION	CALS	PROT	FAT	CHOL	CARB	FIBER	SOD
apple butter	1 tbsp (0.6 oz)	31	tr	tr	0	8	tr	3
jam all flavors	1 pkg (0.5 oz)	39	tr	tr	0	10	tr	4
jam all flavors	1 tbsp (0.7 oz)	56	tr	tr	0	14	tr	6
jam apricot	1 tbsp (0.7 oz)	48	tr	tr	0	13	tr	8
jam diet all flavors	1 tbsp (0.5 oz)	18	tr	tr	0	8	tr	0
jelly all flavors	1 tbsp (0.7 oz)	51	tr	0	0	13	tr	6
jelly reduced sugar all flavors	1 tbsp (0.7 oz)	34	tr	tr	0	9	tr	0
jelly diet all flavors	1 tbsp (0.7 oz)	25	tr	tr	0	10	1	0
orange marmalade	1 tbsp (0.7 oz)	49	tr	0	0	13	tr	11

FOOD	PORTION	CALS	PROT	FAT	CHOL	CARB	FIBER	SOD
preserves all flavors	1 tbsp (0.7 oz)	56	tr	tr	0	14	tr	6
Beth's Farm Kitchen								
Apple Butter	2 tbsp (1 oz)	15	0	0	0	4	1	0
Jam Gooseberry	2 tbsp (1 oz)	45	0	0	0	11	1	0
Jam Sour Cherry	2 tbsp (1 oz)	15	0	0	0	4	1	0
Jam Strawberry Rhubarb	2 tbsp (1 oz)	40	0	0	0	11	0	0
Marmalade Bitter Orange	2 tbsp (1 oz)	40	0	0	0	10	0	0
Cascadian Farm								
Organic Fruit Spread Blackberry	1 tbsp	45	0	0	0	11	–	0
Organic Fruit Spread Raspberry	1 tbsp	45	0	0	0	11	–	0
Organic Sweet Orange Marmalade	1 tbsp	45	0	0	0	11	–	0
Chukar Cherries								
Preserves No Sugar Added	1 tbsp	24	0	0	0	18	tr	97
Preserves Red Sour Cherry Cherry Amaretto	1 tbsp	40	0	0	0	10	tr	0
Preserves Vanilla Peach	1 tbsp	28	0	0	0	19	tr	109
Columbia Empire Farms								
Marionberry Seedless Preserves	1 tbsp	60	0	0	0	14	–	5
Comfort Care								
Country Apple Butter	1 tbsp (1 oz)	40	0	0	0	11	1	0
Delicia								
Fruit Spread Black Cherry	1 tbsp (0.7 oz)	40	0	0	0	10	–	0
Gedney								
State Fair Preserves Strawberry Rhubarb	1 tbsp	50	0	0	0	12	0	0
Hero								
Swiss Preserves Black Cherry	1 tbsp (0.7 oz)	50	tr	0	0	13	2	2
Jake & Amos								
Jam Fig	1 tbsp (0.5 oz)	35	0	0	0	9	0	0
Jam Hot Pepper	1 tbsp	43	0	0	0	9	–	3
Jam Rhubarb	1 tbsp (0.7 oz)	40	0	0	0	12	0	0

FOOD	PORTION	CALS	PROT	FAT	CHOL	CARB	FIBER	SOD
Polaner								
All Fruit w/ Fiber Grape	1 tbsp (0.6 oz)	30	0	0	0	9	3	0
Revolution Foods								
Organic Jelly Grape	1 tbsp (0.7 oz)	60	0	0	0	14	0	5
Organic Preserves Strawberry	1 tbsp (0.7 oz)	60	0	0	0	14	0	0
Robert Rothchild Farm								
Preserves Cherry Acai	1 tbsp	35	0	0	0	9	0	0
Sarabeth's								
Spreadable Fruit Blood Orange Marmalade	1 tbsp (0.7 oz)	35	0	0	0	8	1	0
Spreadable Fruit Chunky Apple	1 tbsp (0.7 oz)	30	0	0	0	7	–	0
Spreadable Fruit Orange Apricot Marmalade	1 tbsp (0.7 oz)	30	0	0	0	8	–	0
Spreadable Fruit Pineapple Mango	1 tbsp (0.7 oz)	35	0	0	0	9	0	0
Spreadable Fruit Strawberry Peach	1 tbsp (0.7 oz)	30	0	0	0	8	–	0
Spreadable Fruit Strawberry Rhubarb	1 tbsp (0.7 oz)	40	0	0	0	10	tr	<5
Trappist								
Jelly Pomegranate	1 tbsp (0.7 oz)	50	0	0	0	14	–	5
Tree Of Life								
Organic Fruit Spread Grape	1 tbsp (0.6 oz)	30	8	0	0	8	0	0
Organic Fruit Spread Peach	1 tbsp (0.6 oz)	30	0	0	0	8	0	0
Welch's								
Grape Jelly	1 tbsp	50	0	0	0	13	–	15

JAPANESE FOOD (*see* ASIAN FOOD, SUSHI)

JELLY (*see* JAM/JELLY/PRESERVES)

JELLYFISH

FOOD	PORTION	CALS	PROT	FAT	CHOL	CARB	FIBER	SOD
pickled	½ cup (1 oz)	10	2	tr	1	0	0	2810

FOOD	PORTION	CALS	PROT	FAT	CHOL	CARB	FIBER	SOD
JERKY								
beef	1 oz	122	10	8	14	3	1	664
pork	1 oz	122	10	8	14	3	1	664
venison	1 oz	119	10	7	39	4	0	888
Applegate Farms								
Natural Joy Stick	1 (1 oz)	100	9	7	25	0	tr	700
Dakota Gourmet								
Fruit Jerky Strawberry Kiwi	1	70	tr	0	0	16	1	15
Frank's RedHot								
Chile'N Lime Steak Strips	1 oz	80	10	4	30	2	0	370
Original Beef	1 oz	80	11	1	20	5	0	750
Gary West								
Beef Strips Hickory Smoked	1 oz	70	12	1	30	5	0	780
Buffalo Strips	½ pkg (1 oz)	60	11	0	0	3	0	460
Elk Strips	½ pkg (1 oz)	70	13	1	10	4	0	640
Ostrim								
Stick Beef & Ostrich	1 (1.5 oz)	80	14	2	25	3	–	430
Outpost								
Beef	1 oz	70	13	1	30	4	0	790
Beef Steak	1 pkg (0.9 oz)	60	8	3	20	2	0	550
Beef Stick	1 (0.4 oz)	60	2	5	10	2	0	190
Primal								
Meatless Vegan Hickory Smoke	1 pkg (1 oz)	99	10	3	0	8	1	344
Meatless Vegan Mesquite Lime	1 pkg (1 oz)	74	10	2	0	7	0	347
Meatless Vegan Texas BBQ	1 pkg (1 oz)	81	10	1	0	11	1	383
Meatless Vegan Thai Peanut	1 pkg (1 oz)	74	10	2	0	8	1	353
Slim Jim								
Beef	7 pieces	130	11	8	35	3	0	770
Beef Jerky Hickory Smoked	1 oz	80	12	2	30	4	0	470
Classic Handipack	1 box	210	8	19	50	3	tr	610
Giant Caddy Pepperoni	1 pkg	150	6	13	35	3	0	450
Twin Pack Cheese & Pepperoni	1 pkg	150	9	12	40	2	1	620
Tanka								
Natural Buffalo Cranberry Bar	1 (1 oz)	70	7	2	17	7	1	360
Natural Buffalo Cranberry Bite	1 (0.5 oz)	35	4	1	9	3	0	180

FOOD	PORTION	CALS	PROT	FAT	CHOL	CARB	FIBER	SOD
Tony's Smokehouse								
Salmon	1 pkg (0.5 oz)	40	7	1	12	2	1	247
JICAMA								
fresh	1 sm (12.8 oz)	139	3	tr	0	32	18	15
raw sliced	1 cup	46	1	tr	0	11	6	5
JUJUBE								
dried	1 oz	82	1	tr	0	21	–	3
JUTE								
cooked	1 cup	32	3	tr	0	6	2	10
KALE								
chopped cooked w/o salt	1 cup	36	2	1	0	7	3	30
fresh cooked w/ fat	1 cup	69	2	4	0	7	2	339
scotch chopped cooked w/o salt	1 cup	36	2	1	0	7	2	58
Allens								
Seasoned	½ cup	35	3	1	0	5	1	830
Glory								
Fresh Greens	1 serv (2.8 oz)	40	3	1	0	8	2	35
Seasoned canned	½ cup	35	2	1	0	5	1	490
KANGAROO								
kangaroo	3 oz	120	24	2	56	–	–	–
KEFIR								
kefir	8 oz	98	8	2	10	12	0	257
Evolve								
Plain	8 oz	120	11	3	10	15	5	190
Strawberry	8 oz	180	10	2	10	31	5	180
Helios								
Organic Blueberry	8 oz	160	11	2	10	25	3	125
Organic Nonfat Plain w/ Omega 3s	8 oz	80	9	0	18	10	0	90
Organic Plain	8 oz	120	8	4	15	12	2	85
Organic Raspberry	8 oz	160	8	4	15	26	2	85
Lifeway								
BioKefir Shot Digestion Vanilla	1 bottle (3.5 oz)	60	5	0	0	10	2	50

FOOD	PORTION	CALS	PROT	FAT	CHOL	CARB	FIBER	SOD
BioKefir Shot Heart Health Blackberry	1 bottle (3.5 oz)	60	5	0	0	10	–	50
Greek Style	8 oz	210	8	14	55	12	–	120
Lowfat Blueberry	8 oz	140	11	2	10	20	–	125
Lowfat Cappuccino	8 oz	140	11	2	10	20	–	125
Lowfat Pomegranate	8 oz	140	11	2	10	20	–	125
Nonfat Peach	8 oz	180	11	0	5	33	3	125
Nonfat Plain	8 oz	90	11	0	5	12	–	120
Nonfat Raspberry	8 oz	150	11	0	0	27	–	125
Organic Lowfat Plain	8 oz	110	11	2	10	12	–	125
Organic Lowfat Wildberry	8 oz	160	11	2	10	25	3	125
Original	8 oz	150	8	8	30	12	0	125
Plain Lowfat	8 oz	110	11	2	10	12	–	125
Plain Whole Milk	8 oz	160	10	8	30	12	–	125
Probugs Goo-Berry Pie	1 bottle (5 oz)	130	9	5	19	15	2	78
Slim6 Mixed Berry	8 oz	110	14	2	10	8	2	125
Slim6 Plain	8 oz	110	14	2	10	8	2	125
Nancy's								
Organic Lowfat Blackberry	1 cup	180	7	3	15	34	2	80
Organic Lowfat Plain	1 cup	110	8	3	15	14	1	105
Organic Lowfat Raspberry	1 cup	180	7	3	15	35	3	80
Yakult								
Drink	1 bottle (2.7 oz)	50	1	0	–	12	0	20

KETCHUP

FOOD	PORTION	CALS	PROT	FAT	CHOL	CARB	FIBER	SOD
banana	1 tsp	10	0	0	0	2	0	75
ketchup	1 tbsp	15	tr	tr	0	4	0	167
ketchup	1 pkg (0.2 oz)	6	tr	tr	0	2	tr	71
low sodium	1 tbsp	15	tr	tr	0	4	0	3
Fischer & Wieser								
Chipotle Chili	1 tbsp (0.7 oz)	15	0	0	0	3	–	120
Heinz								
Ketchup	1 tbsp	15	0	0	0	4	0	190
Organic	1 tbsp	20	0	0	0	5	0	190
Muir Glen								
Organic	1 tbsp	20	0	0	0	4	0	230

FOOD	PORTION	CALS	PROT	FAT	CHOL	CARB	FIBER	SOD
Nature's Hollow								
Sugar Free	1 tbsp (0.7 oz)	0	0	0	0	2	0	130
OrganicVille								
No Added Sugar	1 tbsp (0.6 oz)	20	0	0	0	4	0	125
Texas Sassy								
Tequila Ketchup	1 tbsp (0.5 oz)	20	0	0	0	5	–	5
Tree Of Life								
Organic	1 tbsp (0.6 oz)	20	0	0	0	4	0	210
Walden Farms								
Calorie Free	1 tbsp (0.5 oz)	0	0	0	0	0	0	170
Wholemato								
Organic Agave	1 tbsp	15	0	0	0	3	0	230
KIDNEY								
beef simmered	3 oz	134	23	4	609	0	0	80
lamb braised	3 oz	116	20	3	480	1	0	128
pork braised	3 oz	128	22	4	408	0	0	68
veal braised	3 oz	139	22	5	672	0	0	94
Rumba								
Beef	4 oz	120	19	4	320	2	0	200
KIDNEY BEANS								
canned	½ cup	108	7	1	0	19	6	379
dried cooked w/o salt	½ cup	112	8	tr	0	20	6	1
B&M								
Red Kidney Baked Beans	½ cup (4.6 oz)	200	8	3	<5	36	6	460
Progresso								
Cannellini	½ cup (4.6 oz)	110	8	0	0	20	6	340
Van Camp's								
New Orleans	½ cup	90	6	0	0	19	6	450
KIWI								
fresh	1 lg (3.2 oz)	56	1	tr	0	13	3	3
fresh	1 med (2.6 oz)	46	1	tr	0	11	2	2

FOOD	PORTION	CALS	PROT	FAT	CHOL	CARB	FIBER	SOD
Chiquita								
Fresh	1 (2.7 oz)	46	1	0	0	11	2	2
FruitziO								
Freeze Dried	1 pkg (0.88 oz)	40	0	0	0	8	1	0
KIWI JUICE								
Auna								
Kiwifruit Juice	1 bottle (12 oz)	120	0	0	0	33	4	25
KNISH								
Gabila's								
Potato	1 (4.5 oz)	170	6	6	0	29	5	440
TAKE-OUT								
cheese	1 (2.1 oz)	205	6	12	56	19	1	268
meat	1 (1.8 oz)	174	7	11	53	13	1	202
potato	1 (2.1 oz)	212	5	12	59	21	1	210
potato	1 lg (7 oz)	332	8	12	72	49	1	470
KOHLRABI								
raw sliced	1 cup	36	2	tr	0	8	4	27
sliced cooked w/o salt	1 cup	48	3	tr	0	11	2	35
TAKE-OUT								
creamed	1 cup	150	5	9	6	14	1	555
KRILL								
fresh	1 oz	22	3	1	–	tr	0	119
KUMQUATS								
canned in syrup	1	13	tr	tr	0	3	1	1
fresh	1	13	tr	tr	0	3	1	2
LAMB								
cubed lean & fat braised	4 oz	253	38	10	122	0	0	79
cubed lean broiled	4 oz	211	32	8	102	0	0	86
ground broiled	4 oz	321	28	22	110	0	0	92
leg roasted	4 oz	213	19	15	74	0	0	182
loin chop lean & fat broiled	1 chop (4 oz)	222	17	16	72	0	0	278
rib chop lean & fat broiled	1 chop (1.6 oz)	165	10	14	46	0	0	109
rib roast baked	4 oz	386	25	31	109	0	0	84

FOOD	PORTION	CALS	PROT	FAT	CHOL	CARB	FIBER	SOD
shank lean & fat braised	4 oz	360	42	20	157	0	0	107
shoulder chop lean & fat cooked	1 chop (5.5 oz)	274	22	20	91	0	0	388
shoulder w/ bone braised	4 oz	231	19	17	77	0	0	192
LAMB DISHES								
TAKE-OUT								
keema w/ coconut milk	1 serv (8 oz)	380	13	28	88	18	6	392
moroccan pilaf w/ bulgur	1 serv	327	–	13	54	–	–	303
moussaka	4 in sq (16 oz)	659	35	43	96	32	8	737
shepherd's pie	1 (21.3 oz)	742	42	31	103	76	9	2092
stew w/ potatoes & vegetables	1 cup	260	22	6	58	29	4	728
LAMBSQUARTERS								
chopped cooked w/ salt	1 cup	58	6	1	0	9	4	477
LECITHIN								
lecithin	1 tbsp	104	0	14	0	0	0	–
Bob's Red Mill								
Lecithin Granules	1 tbsp	60	0	4	0	1	0	0
Tree Of Life								
Granules	1 tbsp (0.3 oz)	55	0	4	0	1	0	2
LEEKS								
chopped cooked w/o salt	¼ cup	8	tr	tr	0	2	tr	3
cooked	1 (4.4 oz)	38	1	tr	0	9	1	12
freeze dried	1 tbsp	1	tr	0	0	tr	0	0
LEMON								
fresh	1 med (4 oz)	22	1	tr	0	12	5	3
peel	1 tsp	1	tr	0	0	tr	tr	0
peel	1 tbsp	3	tr	tr	0	1	1	0
wedge	1 (7 g)	2	tr	tr	0	1	tr	0
True Lemon								
Crystallized Lemon	1 pkg (1 g)	0	0	0	0	tr	–	0
LEMON CURD								
lemon curd made w/ egg	2 tsp	29	tr	1	–	4	0	–
Robert Rothchild Farm								
Lemon Curd & Tart Filling	1 tbsp	50	0	2	10	8	0	5

FOOD	PORTION	CALS	PROT	FAT	CHOL	CARB	FIBER	SOD
LEMONGRASS								
fresh	1 tbsp	5	tr	tr	0	1	–	0
LEMON JUICE								
bottled	1 oz	6	1	tr	0	2	tr	6
bottled	1 tbsp	3	tr	tr	0	1	tr	3
fresh	1 oz	8	tr	0	0	3	tr	0
from 1 lemon	1.6 oz	12	tr	0	0	4	tr	0
from wedge	6 g	1	tr	0	0	1	0	0
Canarino								
Italian Hot Lemon Beverage as prep	1 cup	0	0	0	0	0	0	0
Essn								
Sparkling Meyer Lemon Juice	1 can (8.4 oz)	170	1	0	0	41	–	20
Natalie's Orchid Island Juice								
100% Juice	1 tsp	1	0	0	0	0	0	0
Santa Cruz								
Organic 100% Juice	1 tsp	0	0	0	0	0	0	0
LEMONADE								
MIX								
Hansen's								
Fruit Stix Strawberry Lemonade	½ pkg (2 g)	5	0	0	0	1	–	20
READY-TO-DRINK								
Apple & Eve								
Organic	8 oz	130	0	0	0	32	–	5
EarthWise								
Harvest Lemonade	8 oz	100	0	0	0	26	0	5
Mike's								
Hard Lemonade	1 bottle (12 oz)	220	–	0	0	32	–	–
Minute Maid								
Lemonade	1 can (12 oz)	150	0	0	0	42	–	50
Nantucket Nectars								
Lemonade	8 oz	110	0	0	0	28	0	20
Natalie's Orchid Island Juice								
Lemonade	8 oz	130	0	0	0	33	0	0

FOOD	PORTION	CALS	PROT	FAT	CHOL	CARB	FIBER	SOD
Odwalla								
PomaGrand	8 oz	110	0	0	0	28	0	10
Pure Squeezed	8 oz	120	0	0	0	30	0	10
Raaw								
Carrot Lemonade	8 oz	110	1	0	0	27	1	60
Santa Cruz								
Organic Sparkling	8 oz	110	0	0	0	27	0	0
Simply								
Lemonade	8 oz	120	0	0	0	30	–	15
SSips								
Lemonade	8 oz	110	0	0	0	27	0	5
Sweet Leaf								
Half & Half Lemonade Tea	8 oz	85	0	0	0	20	–	10
Original	8 oz	90	tr	0	0	24	–	0
Tropicana								
Light	1 cup	10	0	0	0	2	0	5
Orchard Style	8 oz	120	0	0	0	31	0	20
Twister Strawberry	8 oz	140	tr	0	0	35	0	20
Twister Light	8 oz	50	0	0	0	12	0	10
Turkey Hill								
Lemonade	8 oz	120	0	0	0	29	–	10
Uncle Matt's								
Organic	8 oz	120	tr	0	0	30	0	10
LENTILS								
dried cooked	1 cup	230	18	1	0	40	16	4
Near East								
Lentil Pilaf as prep	1 cup	200	11	3	9	36	8	672
TastyBite								
Jodhpur Lentils	½ pkg (5 oz)	106	6	4	0	12	7	664
Madras Lentils	½ pkg (5 oz)	120	6	5	3	14	5	450
TruRoots								
Organic Sprouted Green not prep	¼ cup (1.4 oz)	140	10	1	0	25	7	10
TAKE-OUT								
lentil loaf	1 slice (1.6 oz)	83	4	4	0	10	3	40
middle eastern lentil salad	1 serv (4.5 oz)	158	–	3	0	–	–	382

FOOD	PORTION	CALS	PROT	FAT	CHOL	CARB	FIBER	SOD
yemiser selatta ethiopian lentil salad	1 serv (3 oz)	115	4	7	0	11	2	536
LETTUCE (*see also* SALAD)								
arugula	6 leaves (0.4 oz)	3	tr	tr	0	tr	tr	3
arugula shredded	1 cup	5	1	tr	0	1	tr	5
boston	1 head (5.7 oz)	21	2	tr	0	4	2	8
boston chopped	6 leaves	7	1	tr	0	1	1	3
cornsalad field salad	1 cup (1.9 oz)	7	1	tr	0	1	1	2
iceberg	6 med leaves	7	tr	tr	0	1	1	5
iceberg	1 lg head (26.5 oz)	106	7	1	0	22	9	76
iceberg shredded	1 cup	10	1	tr	0	2	1	7
looseleaf outer leaves	6 (5 oz)	22	2	tr	0	4	2	40
looseleaf shredded	1 cup	5	tr	tr	0	1	1	10
red leaf	6 leaves (3.6 oz)	16	1	tr	0	2	1	26
red leaf shredded	1 cup	4	tr	tr	0	1	tr	7
romaine	3 leaves (3 oz)	14	1	tr	0	3	2	7
romaine heart	6 leaves (1.3 oz)	6	tr	tr	0	1	1	3
romaine shredded	1 cup	8	1	tr	0	2	1	4
Dole								
Classic Romaine	1½ cups (3 oz)	15	1	0	0	4	1	10
Earthbound Farms								
Organic Baby Romaine Salad	2 cups	15	1	0	0	2	1	50
Fresh Express								
5 Lettuce Mix	3 cups	15	1	0	0	1	1	20
Lettuce Trio	2½ cups	15	1	0	0	3	1	10
Organic Baby Arugula	3 cups	20	2	1	0	3	1	25
Organic Hearts Of Romaine	1½ cups	15	1	0	0	2	1	5
Premium Romaine	2 cups	15	1	0	0	3	2	10
Shreds Iceberg	1½ cups	15	1	0	0	3	1	10
Sweet Butter	2½ cups	10	1	0	0	2	1	0

FOOD	PORTION	CALS	PROT	FAT	CHOL	CARB	FIBER	SOD
Mann's								
Green Leaf Singles	6 leaves (3 oz)	15	2	0	0	3	2	30
Ocean Mist								
Butter Leaf Shredded	1 cup (2 oz)	7	1	0	0	1	1	3
Green Or Green Leaf Shredded	1 cup (1.3 oz)	5	0	0	0	1	0	10
Iceberg	⅙ head (3 oz)	15	1	0	0	3	1	10
Ready Pac								
Baby Arugula	4 cups (3 oz)	20	2	0	0	3	1	25
Shredded Iceberg	1 cup (3 oz)	10	1	0	0	3	1	10
Simply Lettuce	2½ cups (3 oz)	15	1	0	0	3	1	10
LILY ROOT								
dried	1 oz	89	2	1	–	21	tr	25
fresh	1 oz	32	1	tr	–	8	tr	3
LIMA BEANS								
CANNED								
lima beans	½ cup	95	6	tr	0	18	6	405
Allens								
Baby Butter Beans	½ cup	120	7	1	0	22	6	460
Medium Green	½ cup	140	9	1	0	26	7	270
East Texas Fair								
Green	½ cup	120	7	0	0	23	8	370
Hanover								
Butter Beans In Sauce	½ cup	100	7	0	0	18	5	390
DRIED								
cooked	½ cup	150	6	tr	0	20	5	14
FROZEN								
C&W								
Baby	½ cup	110	6	0	0	20	5	240
Green Giant								
Baby & Butter Sauce as prep	⅔ cup	100	5	2	<5	18	5	420
LIME								
fresh	1 (2.4 oz)	20	tr	tr	0	7	1	1
wedge	1 (8 g)	2	tr	tr	0	1	tr	0

FOOD	PORTION	CALS	PROT	FAT	CHOL	CARB	FIBER	SOD
True Lime								
Crystallized Lime	1 pkg	0	0	0	0	0	0	0
LIME JUICE								
bottled	1 oz	6	tr	tr	0	2	tr	5
fresh	1 oz	8	tr	tr	0	3	tr	1
from 1 lime	1.1 oz	11	tr	tr	0	4	tr	1
Angostura								
Lime Mixer	1 tsp	5	0	0	0	2	0	0
Natalie's Orchid Island Juice								
100% Juice	1 tsp	0	0	0	0	0	0	0
Sabor Latino								
Limeade	8 oz	160	0	0	0	39	–	5
Santa Cruz								
Organic 100% Juice	1 tsp	0	0	0	0	0	0	0
Simply								
Limeade	8 oz	120	0	0	0	31	–	15
Sweet Leaf								
Limeade Cherry	8 oz	90	tr	0	0	24	–	0
Turkey Hill								
Limonade	8 oz	120	0	0	0	29	–	10
LING								
blue raw	3.5 oz	83	17	1	–	0	0	–
fresh baked	3 oz	95	21	1	–	0	0	147
fresh fillet baked	5.3 oz	168	37	1	–	0	0	261
LINGCOD								
baked	3 oz	93	19	1	57	0	0	64
fillet baked	5.3 oz	164	34	2	101	0	0	114
LIQUOR (*see* ALCOHOL DRINKS, BEER AND ALE, CHAMPAGNE, MALT, WINE)								
LITCHI JUICE								
Ceres								
100% Juice	8 oz	120	0	0	0	30	1	10
LIVER (*see also* PATE)								
beef braised	1 slice (2.4 oz)	130	20	4	269	3	0	54
beef pan-fried	1 slice (2.8 oz)	142	21	4	309	4	0	62
chicken fried	3 oz	146	22	5	479	1	0	78

FOOD	PORTION	CALS	PROT	FAT	CHOL	CARB	FIBER	SOD
chicken simmered	3 oz	142	21	6	479	1	0	65
duck raw	1 (1.5 oz)	60	8	2	227	2	0	62
goose raw	1 (3.3 oz)	125	15	4	484	6	0	132
lamb braised	3 oz	187	26	7	426	2	0	48
lamb fried	3 oz	202	22	11	419	3	0	105
moose braised	3 oz	132	21	4	331	3	–	60
pork braised	3 oz	140	22	4	302	3	0	42
turkey simmered	1 liver (2.9 oz)	227	17	17	322	1	0	46
veal braised	1 slice (2.8 oz)	154	23	5	409	3	0	62
veal pan fried	1 slice (2.4 oz)	129	18	4	325	3	0	57
Organic Prairie								
Beef	2 oz	80	11	2	155	2	0	40
Perdue								
Chicken Fresh	4 oz	130	19	6	395	0	0	80
Rumba								
Beef	4 oz	160	22	5	365	7	0	80
TAKE-OUT								
calves liver w/ onions	1 serv (5 oz)	177	24	4	335	10	1	390
LLAMA								
llama	3 oz	120	22	3	60	–	–	–
LOBSTER								
northern cooked	1 cup	142	30	1	104	2	–	551
northern cooked	3 oz	83	17	1	61	1	–	323
northern raw	1 lobster (5.3 oz)	136	28	1	143	1	–	–
northern raw	3 oz	77	77	1	81	tr	–	–
spiny steamed	3 oz	122	22	2	76	3	–	193
spiny steamed	1 (5.7 oz)	233	43	3	146	5	–	370
TAKE-OUT								
newburg	1 cup	485	46	27	455	13	–	127
LOGANBERRIES								
fresh	½ cup (2.5 oz)	40	1	tr	0	9	4	1
frzn thawed	½ cup (2.6 oz)	40	1	tr	0	10	4	1

FOOD	PORTION	CALS	PROT	FAT	CHOL	CARB	FIBER	SOD
LONGANS								
fresh	1	2	tr	0	0	tr	–	0
LOQUATS								
fresh	1 sm (0.5 oz)	6	tr	tr	0	2	tr	0
fresh	1 lg (0.7 oz)	9	tr	tr	0	2	tr	0
fresh cubed	½ cup (2.6 oz)	35	tr	tr	0	9	1	1
LOTUS								
root raw sliced	10 slices	45	2	tr	0	14	–	33
root sliced cooked	10 slices	59	1	tr	0	14	–	40
seeds dried	1 oz	94	4	1	0	18	–	1
LOX (*see* SALMON)								
LUPINES								
dried cooked	1 cup	197	26	5	0	16	–	7
LYCHEES								
canned in syrup	1 (0.7 oz)	19	tr	tr	0	5	tr	0
canned in syrup	½ cup (4.4 oz)	114	1	tr	0	29	1	1
dried	1 (2.5 g)	7	tr	tr	0	2	tr	0
fresh	1 (0.3 oz)	6	tr	tr	0	2	tr	0
fresh cut up	½ cup (3.3 oz)	63	1	tr	0	16	1	1
Polar								
Lychee	1	110	tr	0	0	27	1	45
MACA ROOT								
Navitas Naturals								
Powder Gelatanized	1 tsp (5 g)	20	1	0	0	3	1	0
Raw Powder	1 tsp (5 g)	20	1	0	0	4	1	0
MACADAMIA NUTS								
dry roasted w/ salt	11 nuts (1 oz)	200	2	22	0	4	1	80
oil roasted	1 oz	204	2	22	0	4	–	3
Chukar Cherries								
Extra Dark Chocolate Covered	3 tbsp (1.4 oz)	216	2	20	0	14	3	4

FOOD	PORTION	CALS	PROT	FAT	CHOL	CARB	FIBER	SOD
Emily's								
Milk Chocolate Covered	4 (1.5 oz)	260	3	19	<5	21	2	20
Fisher								
Macadamia Nuts	¼ cup (1 oz)	200	2	21	0	4	3	110
Hawaiian Host								
White Choco	3 pieces (1.4 oz)	230	1	15	0	22	0	40
Mauna Loa								
Dry Roasted Salted	¼ cup (1 oz)	230	2	24	0	4	2	105
Dry Roasted Unsalted	¼ cup (1 oz)	230	2	24	0	4	2	0
Honey Roasted	¼ cup (1 oz)	200	2	19	0	9	2	85
Kona Coffee	¼ cup (1 oz)	180	1	15	<5	12	1	75
Maui Onion & Garlic	1 pkg (1.2 oz)	230	2	23	0	5	3	190
MACE								
ground	1 tsp	8	tr	1	0	1	tr	1
MACKEREL								
CANNED								
jack	1 cup	296	44	12	150	0	0	720
jack	1 can (12.7 oz)	563	84	23	285	0	0	1368
Polar								
Jack	⅓ cup	90	13	4	55	0	0	280
FRESH								
atlantic cooked	3 oz	223	20	15	64	0	0	71
atlantic raw	3 oz	174	16	12	60	0	0	76
jack baked	3 oz	171	22	9	51	0	0	94
jack fillet baked	6.2 oz	354	45	18	106	0	0	194
king baked	3 oz	114	22	2	58	0	0	172
king fillet baked	5.4 oz	207	40	4	105	0	0	312
pacific baked	3 oz	171	22	9	51	0	0	94
pacific fillet baked	6.2 oz	354	45	18	106	0	0	194
spanish cooked	3 oz	134	20	5	62	0	0	56
spanish fillet cooked	1 (5.1 oz)	230	34	9	107	0	0	96
spanish raw	3 oz	118	16	5	65	0	0	50
SMOKED								
atlantic	3.5 oz	296	19	24	93	0	0	384

FOOD	PORTION	CALS	PROT	FAT	CHOL	CARB	FIBER	SOD
MAHI MAHI								
fresh baked	4 oz	192	18	13	49	1	0	464
MALANGA								
dasheen mashed	1 cup	226	3	tr	0	53	8	743
dasheen pieces boiled	1 cup	212	3	tr	0	50	8	694
pieces fried	1 cup	304	1	11	0	52	8	442
root raw	1 (10.7 oz)	299	5	1	0	72	5	64
MALT								
malt liquor	1 bottle (12 oz)	148	1	0	0	13	tr	14
nonalcoholic	1 bottle (12 oz)	133	1	tr	0	29	0	47
MALTED MILK								
chocolate as prep w/ milk	1 cup	179	8	5	16	27	1	136
chocolate flavor powder	3 heaping tsp (0.7 oz)	79	1	1	0	18	1	53
natural flavor as prep w/ milk	1 cup	186	9	6	21	24	tr	181
natural flavor powder	3 heaping tsp (0.7 oz)	87	2	2	7	16	tr	104
MAMMY APPLE								
fresh	1	431	4	4	0	106	–	127
MANGO								
dried	½ cup (1.8 oz)	74	1	tr	0	41	3	3
dried	1 slice (5 g)	16	tr	tr	0	4	tr	0
fresh	1 (7.3 oz)	135	1	1	0	35	4	4
fresh sliced	½ cup (3 oz)	54	tr	tr	0	14	2	2
pickled	1 slice (1 oz)	38	tr	tr	0	10	tr	1
C&W								
Chunks	¾ cup	90	tr	0	0	24	3	0
Crispy Green								
Crispy Mangoes Freeze-Dried	1 pkg (0.35 oz)	40	1	0	0	8	1	0
Crunchies								
Freeze Dried	¼ cup (6 g)	20	0	0	0	5	1	0

FOOD	PORTION	CALS	PROT	FAT	CHOL	CARB	FIBER	SOD
Del Monte								
SunFresh In Extra Light Syrup	½ cup (4.4 oz)	70	0	0	0	19	tr	15
Kopali								
Organic Dried	1 pkg (1.8 oz)	140	0	0	0	38	4	0
Peeled Snacks								
Fruit Picks Go-Mango-Man-Go	1 pkg (1.4 oz)	120	2	0	0	28	2	0
Phillippine Brand								
Dried	6 pieces (1.5 oz)	160	tr	0	0	19	1	26
Dried Green	1 pkg (0.7 oz)	75	0	0	0	19	1	5
Polar								
Sliced	3 pieces (5 oz)	100	0	0	0	24	2	20
Sunsweet								
Philippine dried	6 pieces (1.4 oz)	130	1	0	0	32	1	85
MANGO JUICE								
nectar canned	1 cup (8.8 oz)	128	tr	tr	0	33	1	13
Ceres								
100% Juice	8 oz	120	0	0	0	30	1	10
GoodBelly								
Mango Probiotic Drink	8 oz	100	tr	0	0	25	1	15
Old Orchard								
Nectar Cocktail	8 oz	120	0	0	0	30	–	15
Snapple								
Juice Drinks Mango Madness	8 oz	100	0	0	0	26	–	10
MANGOSTEEN								
canned in syrup	½ cup (3.4 oz)	72	tr	1	0	18	2	7
MARGARINE								
margarine butter blend	1 tbsp (0.5 oz)	101	tr	11	2	tr	0	89
squeeze	1 pkg (0.2 oz)	36	tr	4	0	0	0	39

FOOD	PORTION	CALS	PROT	FAT	CHOL	CARB	FIBER	SOD
squeeze liquid	1 tbsp (0.5 oz)	102	tr	11	0	0	0	111
stick	1 stick (4 oz)	810	tr	91	0	1	0	1066
stick	1 tbsp (0.5 oz)	100	tr	11	0	tr	0	132
tub diet	1 tbsp (0.5 oz)	26	0	3	0	tr	0	110
tub fat free	1 tbsp (0.5 oz)	27	tr	tr	0	1	0	85
tub light	1 tbsp (0.5 oz)	59	tr	7	0	tr	0	90
tub salted	1 tbsp (0.5 oz)	101	tr	11	0	tr	0	93
whipped salted	1 tbsp (0.3 oz)	67	tr	8	0	tr	0	62
Benecol								
Spread Light	1 tbsp	50	0	5	0	0	0	110
Spread Regular	1 tbsp	70	0	8	0	0	0	110
Brummel & Brown								
Creamy Fruit Spread Strawberry	1 tbsp	50	0	4	0	3	–	45
Spread w/ Natural Yogurt	1 tbsp (0.5 oz)	45	0	5	0	0	0	90
Country Crock								
Light	1 tbsp (0.5 oz)	50	0	5	0	0	0	85
Regular	1 tbsp (0.5 oz)	90	0	7	0	0	0	110
Spread w/ Calcium + Vitamin D	1 tbsp (0.5 oz)	50	0	5	0	0	0	95
Earth Balance								
Butter Blend Salted	1 tbsp	100	0	11	15	0	0	100
Buttery Spread Original	1 tbsp	100	0	11	0	0	0	120
Buttery Spread Soy Garden	1 tbsp	100	0	11	0	0	0	120
Buttery Sticks Vegan	1 tbsp	100	0	11	0	0	0	120
Land O Lakes								
Soft	1 tbsp (0.5 oz)	100	0	11	0	0	0	125
Stick	1 tbsp (0.5 oz)	100	0	11	0	0	0	105

FOOD	PORTION	CALS	PROT	FAT	CHOL	CARB	FIBER	SOD
Move Over Butter								
Spread	1 tbsp	50	0	6	0	0	0	75
Promise								
Buttery Spread	1 tbsp (0.5 oz)	80	0	8	0	0	0	85
Buttery Spread Activ	1 tbsp	70	0	8	<5	0	0	85
Fat Free	1 tbsp	5	0	0	0	0	0	90
Light	1 tbsp	45	0	5	0	0	0	85
Light Activ	1 tbsp	45	0	5	<5	0	0	85
Smart Balance								
Butter Blend Stick	1 tbsp (0.5 g)	100	0	11	15	0	0	100
Buttery Spread 37% Light	1 tbsp (0.5 oz)	45	0	5	0	0	0	85
Buttery Spread 67%	1 tbsp (0.5 oz)	80	0	9	0	0	0	90
Buttery Spread Low Sodium	1 tbsp (0.4 oz)	65	0	7	0	0	0	30
Buttery Spread Omega Plus	1 tbsp (0.5 oz)	80	0	9	0	0	0	90
Buttery Spread Omega-3 w/ Extra Virgin Olive Oil	1 tbsp (0.4 oz)	60	0	7	0	0	0	70
Buttery Spread w/ Flax Oil	1 tbsp (0.5 oz)	80	0	9	0	0	0	85
Spray Buttery Burst w/ Organic Soy	5 sprays (1 g)	0	0	0	0	0	0	24

MARINADE (see SAUCE)

MARJORAM

FOOD	PORTION	CALS	PROT	FAT	CHOL	CARB	FIBER	SOD
dried	1 tsp	2	tr	tr	0	tr	tr	0

MARLIN

FOOD	PORTION	CALS	PROT	FAT	CHOL	CARB	FIBER	SOD
raw	3 oz	110	20	3	–	0	0	–

MARSHMALLOW

FOOD	PORTION	CALS	PROT	FAT	CHOL	CARB	FIBER	SOD
chocolate coated	1 (0.4 oz)	41	tr	1	0	8	tr	7
coconut coated	1 (0.4 oz)	33	tr	1	0	7	tr	11
marshmallow regular	1 (0.3 oz)	23	tr	tr	0	6	0	6
miniatures	10 (0.3 oz)	22	tr	tr	0	6	0	6
miniatures	1 cup (1.8 oz)	159	1	tr	0	41	tr	40

FOOD	PORTION	CALS	PROT	FAT	CHOL	CARB	FIBER	SOD
MATZO								
brie	1 piece (0.5 oz)	54	1	3	21	5	tr	47
egg	1 (1 oz)	109	3	1	23	22	1	6
matzo ball	1 med (1.2 oz)	48	2	2	36	6	tr	12
plain	1 (1 oz)	111	3	tr	0	23	1	1
whole wheat	1 (1 oz)	98	4	tr	0	22	3	1
Holiday Candies								
Dark Chocolate Coated	1 oz	130	2	5	0	20	1	0
Manischewitz								
Egg & Onion	1 (1 oz)	100	3	1	10	23	2	200
Matzo Ball Mix	2 tbsp	50	1	0	0	11	1	700
Yehuda								
Organic	1 (1 oz)	110	4	1	0	23	3	5
MAYONNAISE								
diet	1 tbsp	36	tr	3	4	3	0	78
imitation	1 tbsp	35	tr	3	4	2	0	75
mayonnaise	1 tbsp	99	tr	11	5	1	0	78
Baconnaise								
Lite	1 tbsp (0.5 oz)	30	0	3	5	2	0	105
Regular	1 tbsp (0.5 oz)	80	0	9	10	1	0	85
Cains								
All Natural	1 tbsp	100	0	11	5	0	0	75
Light	1 tbsp	50	0	5	5	2	0	130
Dietz & Watson								
Mixed Pepper Mayo	1 tbsp (0.5 oz)	100	0	11	5	1	0	85
Hellman's								
Light	1 tbsp (0.5 oz)	35	0	4	<5	tr	–	125
Real	1 tbsp	90	0	10	5	0	0	90
Real Canola No Cholesterol	1 tbsp	90	0	10	5	0	0	90
Reduced Fat	1 tbsp	20	0	2	0	2	–	125
W/ Extra Virgin Olive Oil	1 tbsp	50	0	5	5	tr	–	120
Hollywood								
Canola	1 tbsp	100	0	11	5	0	0	100
Safflower	1 tbsp	100	0	11	5	0	0	100

FOOD	PORTION	CALS	PROT	FAT	CHOL	CARB	FIBER	SOD
Kraft								
Mayo	1 tbsp	90	0	10	<5	0	0	70
Mayo w/ Olive Oil	1 tbsp	45	0	4	<5	2	0	95
Miracle Whip								
Free	1 tbsp	15	0	0	0	3	–	125
Light	1 tbsp	25	0	2	0	3	0	140
Original	1 pkg (0.4 oz)	35	0	3	<5	2	–	85
NatureNaise								
Organic Spread	1 tbsp (0.5 oz)	40	1	3	0	2	–	105
Smart Balance								
Omega Plus Light	1 tbsp (0.5 oz)	50	0	5	5	2	–	115
Vegenaise								
Grapeseed Oil	1 tbsp (0.5 oz)	90	0	9	0	0	0	85
Organic	1 tbsp (0.5 oz)	90	0	9	0	0	0	85
Original	1 tbsp (0.5 oz)	90	0	9	0	0	0	85

MEAT SUBSTITUTES (*see also* BACON SUBSTITUTES, CANADIAN BACON SUBSTITUTES, CHICKEN SUBSTITUTES, HAMBURGER SUBSTITUTES, MEATBALL SUBSTITUTES, SAUSAGE SUBSTITUTES, TURKEY SUBSTITUTES)

FOOD	PORTION	CALS	PROT	FAT	CHOL	CARB	FIBER	SOD
Amy's								
Veggie Loaf w/ Mashed Potatoes & Vegetables	1 pkg (10 oz)	290	9	8	0	47	7	690
Gardein								
BBQ Pulled Shreds	1 serv (4.5 oz)	160	19	2	0	16	1	480
Beefless Tips	1 serv (3.5 oz)	120	18	3	0	7	3	440
Seasoned Bites	1 serv (4.4 oz)	130	20	3	0	8	2	410
Gardenburger								
BBQ Riblets w/ Sauce	1 serv (5 oz)	240	17	5	0	33	5	580
Helen's Kitchen								
GardenSteak Tofu Steak	1 (3 oz)	150	12	2	0	14	3	190

FOOD	PORTION	CALS	PROT	FAT	CHOL	CARB	FIBER	SOD
Loma Linda								
Dinner Cuts	2 slices (3.2 oz)	90	18	1	0	4	2	500
Swiss Stake	1 piece (3.2 oz)	130	9	6	0	9	3	430
Morningstar Farms								
Meal Starters Steak Strips	12 pieces (3 oz)	140	23	3	0	5	1	720
Veat								
Gourmet Bites	1 serv (2.5 oz)	90	8	3	0	8	1	420
Vegetarian Fillet	1 (1.8 oz)	170	15	5	0	19	1	90
Vjana								
Cowgirl Veggie Steaks	1 (3.7 oz)	260	29	14	0	6	4	890
Veggie Doner Kebab	½ cup (3 oz)	210	18	14	0	3	2	810
Veggie Gyros	24 pieces (3 oz)	220	26	11	0	5	2	1050
Worthington								
Bolono	3 slices (2 oz)	80	11	3	0	3	2	660
Choplets	2 slices (3.2 oz)	90	18	1	0	4	2	500
Corned Beef Vegetarian	3 slices (2 oz)	140	10	9	0	5	0	460
Dinner Roast	1 slice (3 oz)	180	14	11	0	6	3	580
Multigrain Cutlets	2 slices (3.2 oz)	100	17	1	0	5	3	290
Prime Stakes	1 piece (3.2 oz)	120	9	6	0	7	1	440
Vegetable Skallops	½ cup (3 oz)	90	17	1	0	4	3	390
Wham	2 slices (2 oz)	110	10	7	0	3	0	400
Yves								
Meatless Beef Skewers	1 (2.8 oz)	100	14	1	0	10	3	400
Meatless Bologna	4 slices	60	14	3	0	2	0	460
Meatless Ground Round Original	⅓ cup	60	10	1	0	5	2	270
Meatless Pepperoni	6 slices	90	14	1	0	4	0	390

FOOD	PORTION	CALS	PROT	FAT	CHOL	CARB	FIBER	SOD
MEATBALL SUBSTITUTES								
meatless	2 (1.3 oz)	71	8	3	0	3	2	198
Franklin Farms								
Portabella Veggiballs Gluten Free	3 (3 oz)	140	16	1	0	18	4	470
Gardenburger								
Mama Mia Meatballs	6 (3 oz)	110	12	5	0	7	4	400
Loma Linda								
Tender Rounds	6 (2.8 oz)	120	13	5	0	6	1	340
Veggie Patch								
Meatless	4 (3 oz)	120	16	5	0	7	4	480
Vjana								
Veggie Cevapcici	4 (2.8 oz)	240	23	14	0	5	3	680
MEATBALLS								
beef cocktail	1 (0.2 oz)	18	2	1	6	0	0	28
beef lg	1 (1.5 oz)	111	11	7	37	0	0	167
beef med	1 (1 oz)	74	7	5	25	0	0	111
chicken cocktail	1 (0.2 oz)	12	1	tr	6	1	0	32
chicken lg	1 (1.5 oz)	71	8	3	36	3	tr	192
chicken med	1 (1 oz)	47	6	2	24	2	tr	128
turkey med	1 (1 oz)	47	6	2	24	2	tr	128
venison	1 (1.5 oz)	69	8	3	37	3	tr	168
Butterball								
Seasoned Italian frzn	6 (3 oz)	170	21	6	50	6	1	560
Coleman								
Chicken Buffalo Style	4	160	12	12	60	1	0	390
Chicken Chipotle Cheddar	4 (2.6 oz)	180	12	14	55	1	0	450
Chicken Italian w/ Parmesan	7 (2.6 oz)	150	14	10	60	1	1	550
Chicken Pesto Parmesan	4 (2.6 oz)	170	13	12	60	1	0	350
Chicken Spinach Fontina Cheese & Roasted Garlic	4 (2.6 oz)	130	13	9	55	0	0	470
Chicken Sun-Dried Tomato Basil & Provolone	4 (2.6 oz)	150	13	9	65	2	0	500
DelGrosso								
Italian Style	3 (3 oz)	180	13	12	65	5	0	960
Hans All Natural								
Chicken Buffalo Style	4	160	21	12	60	1	0	390

FOOD	PORTION	CALS	PROT	FAT	CHOL	CARB	FIBER	SOD
Chicken Sweet Basil Parmesan	4	170	13	12	60	1	0	350
Honeysuckle White								
Turkey Italian Style frzn	3 (3 oz)	190	17	10	65	6	1	600
Mama Lucia								
Homestyle	4	207	14	20	50	8	1	610
Italian Style	4	280	11	23	50	8	0	640
Sausage Beef	8	220	14	17	50	3	1	690
Organic Classics								
Italian Beef	3 (3 oz)	180	17	11	50	5	1	430
Perdue								
Turkey Italian Style	4 (3 oz)	180	15	10	45	5	–	520
Shady Brook								
Turkey Meatballs Appetizer Size + Sweet & Sour Sauce	6 + 2 tbsp sauce	235	17	10	65	17	tr	770
Tyson								
Italian Style Chicken	6 (3 oz)	180	13	11	45	6	2	610
TAKE-OUT								
albondigas w/ sauce	3 + sauce (5.3 oz)	372	21	27	102	11	1	1194
porcupine + tomato sauce	3 + sauce	160	11	7	34	14	1	591
swedish w/ cream sauce	3 + sauce (4.7 oz)	215	17	12	86	9	tr	678
sweet & sour	3 + sauce (4.5 oz)	188	15	11	67	8	1	609

MELON

FOOD	PORTION	CALS	PROT	FAT	CHOL	CARB	FIBER	SOD
sprite	1 (10.6 oz)	110	1	0	0	29	1	190

MEXICAN FOOD (*see* SALSA, SPANISH FOOD, TORTILLA)

MILK

FOOD	PORTION	CALS	PROT	FAT	CHOL	CARB	FIBER	SOD
CANNED								
condensed sweetened	1 cup (10.7 oz)	982	24	27	104	166	0	389
condensed sweetened	1 tbsp (0.7 oz)	61	2	2	6	10	0	24
evaporated nonfat	1 cup (9 oz)	200	19	1	10	29	0	294
evaporated nonfat	1 tbsp (0.5 oz)	12	1	tr	1	2	1	18

FOOD	PORTION	CALS	PROT	FAT	CHOL	CARB	FIBER	SOD
Borden								
Sweetened Condensed Low Fat	2 tbsp	120	3	2	5	23	0	40
Carnation								
Evaporated	2 tbsp (1 oz)	40	2	2	10	3	–	30
Evaporated Fat Free	2 tbsp (1 oz)	25	2	0	0	4	–	30
Evaporated Lowfat 2%	2 tbsp (1 oz)	25	2	1	5	3	–	35
DRIED								
buttermilk	1 tbsp (0.2 oz)	25	2	tr	4	3	0	34
buttermilk	¼ cup (1 oz)	111	10	2	20	14	0	149
nonfat instant	1 tbsp (0.6 oz)	61	6	tr	3	9	0	93
nonfat instant	1 pkg (3.2 oz)	326	32	1	16	47	0	500
whole milk	¼ cup (1.1 oz)	159	8	9	31	12	0	119
Alba								
Instant Non-Fat as prep	1 cup	80	8	0	0	11	0	120
Bob's Red Mill								
Buttermilk Sweet Cream as prep	8 oz	60	5	1	10	7	0	85
Non Fat as prep	8 oz	80	7	0	0	11	0	110
Carnation								
Instant Nonfat as prep	1 cup	80	8	0	<5	12	0	125
Organic Valley								
Buttermilk	3 tbsp	110	10	1	0	16	0	45
Nonfat	3 tbsp	90	9	0	0	13	0	130
Sanalac								
Powder	¼ cup (0.8 oz)	80	8	0	5	13	0	105
REFRIGERATED								
1%	1 cup (8.6 oz)	102	8	3	12	12	0	107
2%	1 cup (8.6 oz)	122	8	5	20	11	0	100
buffalo	7 oz	224	8	16	–	10	–	80
buttermilk lowfat	1 cup (8.6 oz)	98	8	2	10	12	0	257
camel	7 oz	160	10	8	–	10	–	60

FOOD	PORTION	CALS	PROT	FAT	CHOL	CARB	FIBER	SOD
donkey	7 oz	86	4	2	–	12	–	–
fat free	1 cup (8.6 oz)	83	8	tr	5	12	0	103
goat	1 cup (8.6 oz)	168	9	10	27	11	0	122
human	1 cup (8.6 oz)	172	3	11	34	17	0	42
indian buffalo	1 cup (8.6 oz)	237	9	17	46	13	0	127
mare	7 oz	98	4	4	–	12	–	–
sheep	1 cup (8.6 oz)	265	15	17	66	13	0	108
whole	1 cup (8.6 oz)	146	8	8	24	11	0	98
Active Lifestyle								
Fat Free w/ Plant Sterols	8 oz	90	8	0	<0	13	0	125
Dairy Ease								
Fat Free Lactose Free	1 cup (8 oz)	90	8	0	5	12	0	125
Reduced Fat 2% Lactose Free	1 cup (8 oz)	130	9	5	15	12	0	130
Whole Lactose Free	1 cup (8 oz)	160	8	9	20	11	0	125
Farmland								
Buttermilk	8 oz	160	12	4	20	19	0	190
Fat Free	8 oz	80	8	0	5	12	0	130
Special Request 1% Plus Omega-3	8 oz	130	11	3	10	17	0	170
Special Request Skim Plus	8 oz	110	11	0	5	17	0	170
Special Request Skim Plus 100% Lactose Free	8 oz	110	11	0	5	17	0	170
Whole	8 oz	160	12	4	20	19	0	190
Friendship								
Buttermilk Lowfat	1 cup	120	9	4	15	12	0	125
Horizon								
Fat Free	8 oz	90	9	0	<5	12	0	130
Lowfat 1%	8 oz	100	8	3	10	12	0	125
Reduced Fat 2%	8 oz	120	8	5	20	12	0	125
Whole	8 oz	150	8	8	35	12	0	125
Land O Lakes								
1%	1 cup (8 oz)	100	8	3	15	13	0	125
2%	1 cup (8 oz)	120	8	5	20	12	0	125

FOOD	PORTION	CALS	PROT	FAT	CHOL	CARB	FIBER	SOD
Skim	1 cup (8 oz)	90	8	0	<5	13	0	125
Whole	1 cup (8 oz)	150	8	8	35	12	0	125
Organic Valley								
Buttermilk Lowfat 1%	1 cup	100	8	3	15	12	0	250
Fat Free	1 cup	90	8	0	5	13	0	125
Lactose Free Fat Free	1 cup	90	8	0	0	14	0	130
Whole Nonhomogenized	1 cup	150	8	8	35	12	0	125
Over The Moon								
Fat Free	8 oz	100	10	0	5	15	0	150
Low Fat	8 oz	120	10	3	15	14	0	150
Smart Balance								
1% Lowfat w/ HeartRight	1 cup (8 oz)	120	10	3	5	14	–	150
1% Lowfat w/ Omega-3s & Vitamin E	1 cup (8 oz)	140	11	3	5	15	–	170
Fat Free w/ Omega-3s & Vitamin E	1 cup (8 oz)	120	10	0	5	15	–	160
Straus								
Organic Reduced Fat 2% Cream Top	8 oz	130	10	5	25	13	0	130
SunMilk								
Heart Healthy 1% Sunflower Oil	8 oz	120	11	2	<5	15	0	160
Heart Healthy 2% Sunflower Oil	8 oz	120	10	3	<5	15	0	150
Turkey Hill								
Cool Moos Whole Milk	8 oz	160	8	3	10	27	0	140
Valio								
100% Lactose Free 0% Fat	8 oz	80	11	0	<5	7	0	125
100% Lactose Free 2% Fat	8 oz	120	11	5	20	7	0	125
Welsh Farms								
Fat Free	8 oz	80	8	0	5	12	0	130
SHELF-STABLE								
Parmalat								
2% Reduced Fat	8 oz	130	8	5	20	12	0	130
Fat Free	8 oz	80	8	0	5	12	0	130
Lactose Free 2% Reduced Fat	8 oz	130	8	5	20	12	0	130

FOOD	PORTION	CALS	PROT	FAT	CHOL	CARB	FIBER	SOD
MILK DRINKS								
chocolate milk	1 cup (8.8 oz)	208	8	8	30	26	2	150
chocolate milk lowfat	1 cup (8.8 oz)	158	8	3	8	26	1	152
Bravo!								
Blenders Creamy Double Chocolate	1 bottle (11 oz)	180	17	4	20	19	2	350
Blenders Creamy French Vanilla	1 bottle (11 oz)	160	17	4	20	20	2	260
Cocio								
Chocolate Milk	8 oz	140	6	4	15	20	0	80
Dove								
Bravo! Dark Chocolate	1 bottle	310	8	16	60	37	2	140
Bravo! Milk Chocolate	1 bottle	310	8	16	60	36	1	105
Farmland								
Really Really Good! Chocolate Milk	8 oz	160	8	3	10	25	0	150
Horizon Organic								
Lowfat Chocolate Milk	8 oz	170	8	3	15	27	tr	140
Strawberry	8 oz	200	8	5	20	31	0	130
Land O Lakes								
2% Swiss Chocolate	1 cup (8.4 oz)	190	8	5	20	26	tr	220
Chocolate Skim	1 cup (8 oz)	160	8	0	<5	31	tr	220
Strawberry	1 cup (8 oz)	190	7	8	30	22	0	220
Lifeway								
BioKefir Shot Heart Heart Black Cherry	1 bottle (3.5 oz)	60	5	0	0	10	–	50
Nesquik								
Chocolate Powder No Sugar Added as prep w/ lowfat milk	1 cup (8 oz)	160	1	5	21	18	1	168
Chocolate Powder as prep w/ lowfat milk	1 cup (8 oz)	180	tr	5	21	27	tr	120
Ready-To-Drink Banana	1 cup (8 oz)	200	7	5	20	30	0	120
Ready-To-Drink Chocolate	1 cup (8 oz)	200	8	5	15	32	tr	150
Ready-To-Drink Strawberry	1 cup (8 oz)	200	8	5	15	33	0	120
Ready-To-Drink Vanilla	1 cup (8 oz)	200	8	5	15	30	0	120

FOOD	PORTION	CALS	PROT	FAT	CHOL	CARB	FIBER	SOD
Strawberry Powder as prep w/ lowfat milk	1 cup (8 oz)	190	0	4	21	27	0	96
Strawberry Powder not prep	2 tbsp (0.6 oz)	60	0	0	0	15	0	0
Over The Moon								
Chocolate Milk Fat Free	8 oz	150	11	0	5	27	tr	250
Parmalat								
Chocolate Milk 2% Reduced Fat	1 cup	190	8	5	20	28	1	130
Sipahh								
Straw Banana	1 straw	15	0	0	0	3	–	0
Straw Cookies and Cream	1 straw	15	0	0	0	3	–	0
Turkey Hill								
Cool Moos 2% Reduced Fat	8 oz	120	8	5	20	12	0	125
Cool Moos Chocolate	8 oz	180	8	3	10	32	0	210
MILK SUBSTITUTES								
soy milk	1 cup	79	7	5	0	4	–	30
Brazsoy								
Condensed Soy Milk	1 serv (0.7 oz)	54	1	1	0	10	0	11
Soy Cream	1 tbsp (0.5 oz)	27	0	3	0	0	0	15
Living Harvest								
Hempmilk Original	1 cup	130	4	3	0	20	1	120
Hempmilk Vanilla	1 cup	130	4	3	0	20	1	120
Lundberg								
Organic Drink Rice Original	8 oz	120	1	3	0	22	tr	85
Manitoba Harvest								
Hemp Bliss Chocolate	8 oz	160	5	7	0	17	1	120
Hemp Bliss Original	1 cup	110	5	7	0	7	1	95
Hemp Bliss Vanilla	8 oz	150	5	7	0	14	1	120
Odwalla								
Soy Smart Chai	8 oz	150	6	4	–	22	–	30
Soy Smart Vanilla	8 oz	120	6	4	–	15	–	55
Soymilk Plain	8 oz	110	7	4	0	12	3	65
Soymilk Vanilla Being	8 oz	100	4	3	0	13	3	65
Organic Valley								
Soy Original	1 cup	100	7	3	0	11	3	95
Soy Unsweetened	1 cup	80	7	4	0	3	1	110

FOOD	PORTION	CALS	PROT	FAT	CHOL	CARB	FIBER	SOD
Pearl								
Organic Soymilk Coffee	8 oz	150	6	4	0	24	0	190
Organic Soymilk Green Tea	8 oz	110	7	4	0	13	1	95
Organic Soymilk Original	8 oz	110	7	4	0	12	1	110
Rice Dream								
Carob	8 oz	150	1	3	0	30	tr	80
Heartwise Vanilla	8 oz	140	1	2	0	30	3	80
Horchata	8 oz	130	7	4	0	16	2	150
Original	8 oz	120	1	3	0	24	0	100
Original Enriched	8 oz	120	1	3	0	23	0	100
Vanilla Enriched	8 oz	130	1	3	0	26	0	105
Silk								
Chocolate	1 cup (8 oz)	140	5	4	0	23	2	100
Plain	8 oz	100	7	4	0	8	1	120
Soy Heart Health	1 cup	80	6	2	0	10	1	95
Soy Plain Light	1 cup	70	6	2	0	8	1	120
Soy Plus DHA Omega-3	1 cup	110	7	5	0	8	1	120
Soy Pumpkin Spice	1 cup	170	6	4	0	28	0	150
Soy Unsweetened	1 cup	80	7	4	0	4	1	85
Vanilla	1 cup (8 oz)	100	6	4	0	10	1	95
Soy Dream								
Classic Vanilla	8 oz	140	7	4	0	18	2	135
Original Enriched	8 oz	100	7	4	0	8	2	135
WildWood								
Organic Probiotic Soymilk Blueberry	8 oz	190	7	3	0	33	4	60
Organic Probiotic Soymilk Pomegranate	8 oz	180	7	3	0	31	4	55
Organic Soymilk Plain	8 oz	100	7	4	0	8	1	80
Organic Soymilk Unsweetened	8 oz	72	7	4	0	3	1	70
ZenSoy								
Soy Milk Cappuccino	8 oz	150	7	4	0	22	1	160
Soy Milk Chocolate	8 oz	170	7	4	0	27	2	160
Soy Milk Plain	8 oz	90	7	4	0	9	1	80
Soy Milk Vanilla	8 oz	110	7	4	0	14	1	80
Soy On The Go Vanilla w/ Omega 3	1 pkg (8.25 oz)	110	7	4	0	14	1	80

FOOD	PORTION	CALS	PROT	FAT	CHOL	CARB	FIBER	SOD
MILKFISH (AWA)								
baked	4 oz	215	30	10	76	0	0	104
MILKSHAKE								
chocolate	1 serv (10.6 oz)	357	9	8	33	63	1	333
malted milkshake	1 serv (10 oz)	402	9	14	51	62	1	201
vanilla	1 (11 oz)	351	12	9	38	56	0	297
Buffy's Cool Cow								
Chocolate	1 pkg (8 oz)	150	9	3	5	23	tr	135
Vanilla	1 pkg (8 oz)	150	9	3	5	24	0	135
Lean Body								
Hi-Protein Chocolate Ice Cream	1 (17 oz)	260	40	9	25	9	5	600
Molli Coolz								
Shakers Vanilla as prep w/ skim milk	1 (10.2 oz)	240	3	10	35	30	5	96
Nesquik								
Ready-To-Drink Chocolate	1 cup (8 oz)	170	8	5	15	26	tr	180
Silhouette Solution								
Colossal Chocolate not prep	1 pkg (1.05 oz)	110	15	3	35	8	2	230
Vanilla Creme not prep	1 pkg (1.02 oz)	100	15	2	40	8	2	230
MILLET								
cooked	1 cup (6.1 oz)	207	6	2	0	41	2	3
Arrowhead Mills								
Organic Hulled not prep	¼ cup	150	4	2	0	33	1	0
MINERAL WATER (*see* WATER)								
MISO								
dried	1 oz	86	7	3	–	10	1	2130
miso	½ cup	284	16	8	0	39	7	5036
MOLASSES								
blackstrap	1 tbsp (0.7 oz)	47	0	0	0	12	–	11

FOOD	PORTION	CALS	PROT	FAT	CHOL	CARB	FIBER	SOD
molasses	1 tbsp (0.7 oz)	58	0	tr	0	15	0	7
molasses	¼ cup (3 oz)	244	0	tr	0	63	0	31
Tree Of Life								
Blackstrap Unsulphured	1 tbsp	45	0	0	0	11	–	15
MONKFISH								
baked	3 oz	82	16	2	27	0	0	20
MOOSE								
roasted	4 oz	142	31	1	83	0	0	73
MOTH BEANS								
dried cooked	1 cup	207	14	1	0	37	–	17
MOUSSE								
TAKE-OUT								
chocolate	½ cup	454	8	32	283	32	1	77
fish timbale	1 cup	329	22	25	210	3	0	394
MUFFIN								
MIX								
Betty Crocker								
Banana Nut as prep	1	120	2	3	0	22	0	240
Blueberry as prep	1	120	2	3	0	23	–	230
Cornbread Muffin as prep	1	160	2	6	48	24	tr	210
Fiber One Banana Nut as prep	1	170	2	7	36	27	5	230
Fiber One Blueberry as prep	1	160	2	6	36	30	5	240
Lemon Poppyseed as prep	1	200	2	8	36	29	–	210
Duncan Hines								
Blueberry Streusel as prep	1	210	3	8	35	32	3	230
Cinnamon Swirl 100% Whole Grain as prep	1	220	3	8	35	34	3	230
Triple Chocolate Chunk 100% Whole Grain as prep	1	240	4	11	35	35	3	290
Glory								
Golden Sweet Corn as prep	1	170	2	5	36	27	1	360

FOOD	PORTION	CALS	PROT	FAT	CHOL	CARB	FIBER	SOD
Martha White								
Whole Grain Apple Cinnamon not prep	¼ cup (1.2 oz)	140	2	4	5	24	1	150
Whole Grain Blueberry not prep	¼ cup (1.2 oz)	140	2	4	5	24	1	150
Yellow Corn not prep	¼ cup (1.2 oz)	140	2	3	0	26	1	230
Miracle Muffins								
Banana w/ Splenda as prep	1	86	9	3	0	12	7	130
VitaMuffin								
Deep Chocolate as prep	1 (2 oz)	100	4	2	0	26	9	140
Golden Corn as prep	1 (2 oz)	100	3	0	0	24	5	125
READY-TO-EAT								
Do Goodie								
Gluten Free Banana Nut	1	180	2	9	45	24	1	220
Foods By George								
Gluten Free Blueberry	1 (2.8 oz)	220	3	8	25	33	1	450
Hostess								
100 Calorie Pack Mini Banana Streusel	1 pkg (1.2 oz)	100	2	4	10	19	4	120
100 Calorie Pack Mini Blueberry Streusel	1 pkg (1.2 oz)	100	2	3	10	20	4	120
Udi's								
Gluten Free Double Chocolate	1 (4 oz)	350	4	15	80	52	3	250
Uncle Wally's								
Apple Cinnamon Rich & Moist	1 (4 oz)	380	4	18	70	51	1	320
Blueberry Rich & Moist	1 (4 oz)	370	4	18	60	49	1	330
Cheesecake Rich & Moist	1 (4 oz)	390	5	19	70	50	0	360
Chocolate Passion Fat Free	½ (2 oz)	120	3	0	0	28	0	260
Corn Rich & Moist	1 (4 oz)	400	5	18	70	55	1	330
Cranberry Apple Smart Portion	1 (1.1 oz)	80	2	1	0	17	2	130
Cranberry Orange Supreme Fat Free	½ (2 oz)	140	2	0	0	32	1	210
Fiber One Banana Chocolate Chip	1 (2.3 oz)	180	3	5	30	36	7	190
Fiber One Wild Blueberry & Oats	1 (2.3 oz)	170	3	4	30	33	7	200

FOOD	PORTION	CALS	PROT	FAT	CHOL	CARB	FIBER	SOD
Honey Raisin Bran Fat Free	½ (2 oz)	140	2	0	0	32	1	210
My Sweet Multi Bran Sugar Free	1 (2 oz)	120	3	3	10	28	1	280
Pineapple Coconut Rich & Moist	1 (4 oz)	390	4	19	70	51	1	340
Sweet Chocolate Dreams Sugar Free	1 (2 oz)	130	3	3	15	29	1	290
Wild Blueberry Bliss Fat Free	½ (2 oz)	110	2	0	0	25	1	210
VitaMuffin								
Banana Nut	1 (2 oz)	100	5	2	0	19	5	120
Banana Nut Sugar Free	1 (2 oz)	90	5	3	0	21	5	125
VitaTop								
Apple Crumb	1 (2 oz)	100	3	1	0	25	8	105
BlueBran	1 (2 oz)	100	4	1	0	20	5	140
CranBran	1 (2 oz)	100	4	1	0	22	5	140
Deep Chocolate	1 (2 oz)	100	4	2	0	26	9	140
Golden Corn	1 (2 oz)	100	3	1	0	27	10	120
Raisin Bran	1 (2 oz)	100	4	1	0	22	5	140
TAKE-OUT								
blueberry	1 (5 oz)	546	7	27	56	69	2	485
corn	1 lg (5 oz)	424	8	12	36	71	5	890
oat bran	1 lg (5 oz)	375	10	10	0	67	6	546
pumpkin w/ raisins & nuts	1 med (4 oz)	351	5	8	81	67	2	297
MULBERRIES								
fresh	20 (1 oz)	13	tr	tr	0	3	1	3
fresh	½ cup (2.5 oz)	30	1	tr	0	7	1	7
Kopali								
Organic Dark Chocolate Covered	½ pkg (1 oz)	140	2	6	0	20	2	8
Organic Dried	1 pkg (1.7 oz)	240	5	1	0	38	6	36
Navitas Naturals								
Dried	1 oz	91	3	0	0	21	3	25
MULLET								
striped cooked	3 oz	127	21	4	54	0	0	61
striped raw	3 oz	99	16	3	42	0	0	55

FOOD	PORTION	CALS	PROT	FAT	CHOL	CARB	FIBER	SOD
MUNG BEANS								
dried cooked	1 cup	213	14	1	0	39	–	4
TruRoots								
Organic Sprouted not prep	¼ cup (1.4 oz)	140	10	1	0	30	7	10
MUNGO BEANS								
dried cooked	1 cup	190	14	1	1	33	–	13
MUSHROOMS								
CANNED								
caps	8 (1.6 oz)	12	1	tr	0	2	1	200
caps pickled	6 (0.8 oz)	5	1	tr	0	1	tr	53
chanterelle	3.5 oz	12	1	1	0	tr	6	165
pickled	1 cup	33	4	tr	0	5	1	351
pieces	½ cup	20	1	tr	0	2	1	332
straw	1 cup	58	7	1	0	8	5	699
Green Giant								
Pieces & Stems	½ cup	25	2	0	0	4	1	440
Jake & Amos								
Pickled Dill Mushrooms	1 serv (1 oz)	5	0	0	0	1	tr	244
Polar								
Straw	½ cup	20	3	0	0	4	2	460
Whole Button	½ cup	30	3	0	0	4	2	320
Whole Shiitake	½ cup	30	1	1	0	4	tr	620
DRIED								
chanterelle	1 oz	25	5	tr	0	tr	17	9
shiitake	1 (3.6 g)	11	tr	tr	0	3	tr	0
tree ear	½ cup (0.4 oz)	36	1	tr	0	10	–	8
wood ear mok yee	½ cup (0.4 oz)	25	2	tr	–	8	4	6
Ocean Spring								
Fresh Crispy Mixed Mushrooms	1 serv (0.9 oz)	113	–	4	–	18	1	46
FRESH								
brown italian or crimini sliced	1 cup	19	2	tr	0	3	tr	4
brown italian or crimini whole	1 (0.7 oz)	5	1	tr	0	1	tr	1
chanterelle	3.5 oz	11	2	tr	0	tr	6	3

FOOD	PORTION	CALS	PROT	FAT	CHOL	CARB	FIBER	SOD
enoki raw	1 lg (5 g)	2	tr	tr	0	tr	tr	0
enoki sliced	1 cup	29	2	tr	0	5	2	2
enoki whole	1 cup	28	2	tr	0	5	2	2
maitake diced	1 cup	26	1	tr	0	5	2	1
maitake whole	1 (6.6 g)	2	tr	tr	0	tr	tr	0
morel	3.5 oz	9	2	tr	0	0	7	2
oyster	1 sm (0.5 oz)	5	1	tr	0	1	tr	3
oyster sliced	1 cup	30	3	tr	0	6	2	15
portabella raw	1 cap (3 oz)	22	2	tr	0	4	1	5
portabella sliced grilled	1 cup (4.2 oz)	42	5	1	0	6	3	12
shiitake cooked	4 (2.5 oz)	40	1	tr	0	10	2	3
shiitake pieces cooked	1 cup	81	2	tr	0	21	3	6
white	1 (0.6 oz)	4	1	tr	0	1	tr	1
white sliced cooked	1 cup	28	4	tr	0	4	2	13
white sliced raw	½ cup	8	1	tr	0	1	tr	2
Giorgio								
Mushrooms	3 oz	20	2	0	0	3	1	10
Golden Gourmet								
Beech Brown	4 oz	20	3	1	0	7	–	1
Beech White	4 oz	13	3	1	0	6	–	1
King Trumpet	4 oz	20	3	0	0	7	–	2
Maitake	4 oz	20	3	1	0	8	–	1
Hokto								
Organic Bunashimeji Beech Mushrooms	1 pkg (3.5 oz)	30	3	1	0	3	3	0
Organic Maitake Hen Of The Wood	1 pkg (3.5 oz)	30	2	1	0	4	3	0
FROZEN								
Farm Rich								
Breaded	5 (3 oz)	120	3	2	0	23	1	430
TAKE-OUT								
battered fried	1 lg (0.6 oz)	39	1	3	1	3	tr	29
creamed	1 cup	171	6	11	7	15	3	853
stuffed	1 (0.8 oz)	67	3	4	3	6	1	142
MUSKRAT								
roasted	3 oz	199	26	10	–	0	0	81
MUSSELS								
blue raw	1 cup	129	18	3	42	6	–	429

FOOD	PORTION	CALS	PROT	FAT	CHOL	CARB	FIBER	SOD
blue raw	3 oz	73	10	2	24	3	–	243
fresh blue cooked	3 oz	147	20	4	48	6	–	313
Polar								
Mussels	2 oz	60	10	3	15	tr	0	90
MUSTARD								
dry mustard	1 tsp	15	1	1	0	1	–	tr
hot chinese	1 tsp	3	tr	tr	0	tr	tr	56
organic yellow	1 tsp	5	0	0	0	0	0	70
seed	1 tsp	15	1	1	0	1	1	0
yellow prepared	1 tbsp	3	tr	tr	0	tr	tr	57
Bone Suckin'								
Fat Free Gluten Free	1 tbsp	25	0	0	0	5	0	95
Dave's Gourmet								
Insanity	1 tsp (5 g)	5	0	0	0	1	–	55
Dietz & Watson								
Champagne Dill	1 tsp (5 g)	5	0	0	0	0	0	120
Yellow	1 tsp (5 g)	0	0	0	0	0	0	80
D'Oni								
Bold As Love Honey Habanero	1 tsp	5	0	0	0	2	–	45
French's								
Classic Yellow	1 tsp	0	0	0	0	0	0	55
Honey	1 tsp	10	0	0	0	1	–	30
Honey Dijon	1 tsp	10	0	0	0	1	–	40
Horseradish	1 tsp	5	0	0	0	0	0	80
Spicy Brown	1 tsp	5	0	0	0	0	0	80
Gulden's								
Spicy Brown	1 tsp	5	0	0	0	0	0	50
Hellman's								
Deli	1 tsp	5	0	0	0	tr	0	55
Dijonnaise	1 tsp	5	0	0	0	1	0	70
Honey Mustard	1 tsp	10	0	0	0	2	0	25
Jack & Amos								
Sweet Dipping	1 tbsp (0.5 oz)	30	1	1	10	5	0	10
Robert Rothchild Farm								
Champagne Garlic	1 tsp	6	0	0	0	1	0	120
School House Kitchen								
Sweet Smooth Hot	1 tsp	15	0	1	0	1	0	10

FOOD	PORTION	CALS	PROT	FAT	CHOL	CARB	FIBER	SOD
Texas Sassy								
Mustard Sauce	2 tbsp (1 oz)	15	0	0	0	3	–	260
Vivi's								
Classic	1 tbsp (0.5 oz)	15	0	0	0	4	0	190
Sizzlin' Chipotle	1 tbsp (0.5 oz)	15	0	0	0	4	0	200
Zatarain's								
Creole	1 tsp (7 g)	10	0	1	0	tr	0	150
MUSTARD GREENS								
canned	1 cup	23	3	tr	0	3	3	428
fresh as prep w/ fat	1 cup	50	3	3	0	3	3	459
fresh chopped boiled w/o salt	1 cup	21	3	tr	0	3	3	22
fresh raw chopped	1 cup	15	2	tr	0	3	2	14
frozen chopped boiled w/o salt	1 cup	28	3	tr	0	5	4	38
Allen's								
Seasoned	½ cup	45	4	1	0	6	1	830
Glory								
Seasoned	½ cup	35	2	0	0	3	1	490
Sylvia's								
Specially Seasoned	½ cup	30	2	0	0	5	2	220
NATTO								
House								
Natto	2 oz	120	10	6	0	5	0	25
NAVY BEANS								
canned	1 cup	296	20	1	0	54	–	1173
dried cooked	1 cup	259	16	1	0	48	–	2
NECTARINE								
fresh	1 lg (5.5 oz)	69	2	1	0	16	3	0
fresh	1 sm (4.5 oz)	57	1	tr	0	14	2	0
fresh sliced	1 cup (5 oz)	63	2	tr	0	15	2	0
Chiquita								
Fresh	1 (5 oz)	63	2	0	0	15	2	0
NECTARINE JUICE								
Sun Shower								
100% Juice	8 oz	93	1	0	0	21	2	15

FOOD	PORTION	CALS	PROT	FAT	CHOL	CARB	FIBER	SOD
NEUFCHATEL								
neufchatel	1 oz	72	3	6	21	1	0	95
neufchatel	1 pkg (3 oz)	215	8	19	63	3	0	284
Organic Valley								
Soft	2 tbsp	70	2	6	20	2	0	140
NONI JUICE								
Lakewood								
Noni Pure Juice	2 oz	8	0	0	0	2	0	5
Snapple								
Juice Drink Low Calorie Metabolism Noni Berry	8 oz	15	0	0	0	2	–	5
Tree Of Life								
100% Juice Concentrate	2 tbsp	15	0	0	0	4	0	10
NOODLES								
cellophane	1 cup	492	tr	tr	0	121	–	14
chow mein	1 cup (1.6 oz)	237	4	14	0	25	2	189
egg	1 cup (38 g)	145	5	2	36	27	–	8
egg cooked	1 cup (5.6 oz)	213	8	2	53	40	2	11
japanese soba cooked	1 cup (4 oz)	113	6	tr	0	24	–	68
japanese somen cooked	1 cup (6.2 oz)	231	7	tr	0	48	–	283
korean acorn noodles not prep	2 oz	195	7	tr	–	41	tr	–
rice cooked	1 cup (6.2 oz)	192	2	tr	0	44	2	33
spinach/egg cooked	1 cup (5.6 oz)	211	8	3	53	39	4	19
Gluten Free Cafe								
Asian Noodles	1 pkg (9.2 oz)	340	8	10	0	53	5	720
House								
Shirataki Tofu Noodles	2 oz	20	1	1	0	3	2	15
Shirataki Yam Noodles	2 oz	5	0	0	0	1	0	0
Krasdale								
Egg Wide not prep	1 cup (2 oz)	210	8	2	0	41	2	0

FOOD	PORTION	CALS	PROT	FAT	CHOL	CARB	FIBER	SOD
La Choy								
Chow Mein Noodles	½ cup (1 oz)	130	3	5	0	19	tr	230
Rice	½ cup	130	2	4	0	21	tr	350
Light 'N Fluffy								
Egg Extra Wide not prep	⅙ pkg (2 oz)	210	8	3	70	40	2	15
No Yolks								
Dumplings	2 oz	210	8	1	0	41	3	30
NoOodle								
All Natural	1 serv (1.6 oz)	0	0	0	0	1	0	0
Ronzoni								
Healthy Harvest Whole Grain Extra Wide not prep	2 oz	180	8	1	0	41	6	15
Streit's								
Egg Wide not prep	1¾ cups (2 oz)	210	8	3	60	39	2	20
Thai Kitchen								
Stir-Fry Rice Linguini not prep	2 oz	210	4	1	0	46	0	20
NUTMEG								
ground	1 tsp	12	tr	1	0	1	1	0
nutmeg butter	1 tbsp	120	0	14	0	0	0	0
NUTRITION SUPPLEMENTS (*see also* CEREAL BARS, ENERGY BARS, ENERGY DRINKS)								
Cirku								
Beverage Mix Summer Citrus	1 pkg (0.23 oz)	15	0	0	0	3	–	–
Clif								
Shot Bloks Black Cherry	3 (1 oz)	100	0	0	0	24	0	70
Shot Bloks Cola	3 (1 oz)	100	0	0	0	24	0	70
Shot Bloks Margarita	3 (1 oz)	90	0	0	0	24	0	210
Shot Bloks Orange	3 (1 oz)	100	0	0	0	24	0	70
Ensure								
Shake Creamy Milk Chocolate	1 bottle (8 oz)	250	9	6	5	40	1	190
Shake Strawberries & Cream	1 bottle (8 oz)	250	9	6	5	40	0	200
Glowelle								
Beauty Drink All Flavors	1 bottle	100	0	0	0	24	–	25

FOOD	PORTION	CALS	PROT	FAT	CHOL	CARB	FIBER	SOD
Glucerna								
Shake Creamy Chocolate Delight	1 bottle (8 oz)	200	10	7	<5	27	5	210
Shake Homemade Vanilla	1 bottle (8 oz)	200	10	7	<5	26	5	210
Jelly Belly								
Sport Beans Lemon Lime	1 pkg (1 oz)	100	0	0	0	25	–	80
Joint Juice								
Tropical Fruit	1 can (8 oz)	25	0	0	0	6	–	80
Luna								
Electrolyte Splash	1 pkg	80	0	0	0	20	–	200
Moons Energy Chews Watermelon	6 (1 oz)	100	0	0	0	24	0	70
Recovery Smoothie	1 pkg	120	0	0	0	21	1	150
Oxylent								
Oxygenating Multivitamin Drink	1 pkg	10	0	0	0	2	–	35
S/7								
Prenatal Vitamin Drink Berry	1 pkg (0.5 oz)	45	0	1	–	9	–	55
Slim-Fast								
Optima Ready-To-Drink Creamy Milk Chocolate	1 can (11 oz)	190	10	6	5	25	5	200
To Go								
Extreme Berries	½ pkg (3.15 g)	12	tr	tr	–	3	tr	1
NUTS MIXED *(see also individual names)*								
dry roasted w/ peanuts salted	¼ cup	203	6	18	0	9	3	229
dry roasted w/ peanuts w/o salt	¼ cup	203	6	18	0	9	3	4
mixed nuts chocolate covered	¼ cup (1.5 oz)	240	4	17	5	20	2	25
oil roasted w/o peanuts salted	¼ cup	221	6	20	0	8	2	110
oil roasted w/o peanuts w/o salt	¼ cup	221	6	20	0	8	2	4
Back To Nature								
Tuscan Herb Roast	1 oz	170	5	15	0	7	2	100

FOOD	PORTION	CALS	PROT	FAT	CHOL	CARB	FIBER	SOD
Dave's Gourmet								
Burning Nuts	1 oz	200	9	17	–	7	3	135
Emily's								
Roasted Mixed Nuts	¼ cup (1.3 oz)	230	6	20	0	8	2	80
Mauna Loa								
Mixed Nuts	¼ cup (1 oz)	180	5	16	0	6	2	85
NuttZo								
Multi-Nut Butter Organic	2 tbsp (1.1 oz)	180	7	16	–	7	3	70
Planters								
Mixed	30 nuts (1 oz)	170	6	15	0	6	2	110
True North								
Clusters Pecan Almond Peanut	8 (1 oz)	170	5	13	0	13	2	75
OCTOPUS								
dried boiled	3 oz	144	26	2	84	4	0	695
fresh steamed	3 oz	139	25	2	81	4	0	111
smoked	1 oz	40	7	1	23	1	0	111
TAKE-OUT								
ensalada de pulpo	1 cup	299	17	21	52	10	2	232
OHELOBERRIES								
fresh	1 cup	39	1	tr	0	10	–	2
OIL								
almond	1 tbsp	120	0	14	0	0	0	–
almond	1 cup	1927	0	218	0	0	0	–
apricot kernel	1 cup	1927	0	218	0	0	0	–
apricot kernel	1 tbsp	120	0	14	0	0	0	–
avocado	1 tbsp	124	0	14	0	0	0	–
avocado	1 cup	1927	0	218	0	0	0	–
babassu palm	1 tbsp	120	0	14	0	0	0	–
butter oil	1 tbsp	112	tr	13	33	0	0	–
butter oil	1 cup	1795	1	204	524	0	0	–
canola	1 cup	1927	0	218	0	0	0	–
canola	1 tbsp	124	0	14	0	0	0	–
coconut	1 tbsp	117	0	14	0	0	0	0
corn	1 cup	1927	0	218	0	0	0	–

FOOD	PORTION	CALS	PROT	FAT	CHOL	CARB	FIBER	SOD
corn	1 tbsp	120	0	14	0	0	0	–
cottonseed	1 cup	1927	0	218	0	0	0	–
cottonseed	1 tbsp	120	0	14	0	0	0	–
cupu assu	1 tbsp	120	0	14	0	0	0	–
garlic oil	1 tbsp	150	0	17	0	0	0	0
grapeseed	1 tbsp	120	0	14	0	0	0	0
hazelnut	1 tbsp	120	0	14	0	0	0	–
hazelnut	1 cup	1927	0	218	0	0	0	–
mustard	1 cup	1927	0	218	0	0	0	–
mustard	1 tbsp	124	0	14	0	0	0	–
oat	1 tbsp	120	0	14	0	0	0	–
olive	1 tbsp	119	0	14	0	0	0	0
olive	1 cup	1909	0	216	0	0	0	tr
palm	1 tbsp	120	0	14	0	0	0	–
palm	1 cup	1927	0	218	0	0	0	–
palm kernel	1 cup	1879	0	218	0	0	0	–
palm kernel	1 tbsp	117	0	14	0	0	0	–
peanut	1 tbsp	119	0	14	0	0	0	tr
peanut	1 cup	1909	0	216	0	0	0	tr
peppermint	1 tsp	42	–	4	0	0	0	–
poppyseed	1 tbsp	120	0	14	0	0	0	–
pumpkin seed	1 oz	217	0	29	–	0	0	–
rice bran	1 tbsp	120	0	14	0	0	0	–
safflower	1 cup	1927	0	218	0	0	0	–
safflower	1 tbsp	120	0	14	0	0	0	–
sesame	1 tbsp	120	0	14	0	0	0	–
sheanut	1 tbsp	120	0	14	0	0	0	–
soybean	1 cup	1927	0	218	0	0	0	tr
soybean	1 tbsp	120	0	14	0	0	0	0
sunflower	1 cup	1927	0	218	0	0	0	–
sunflower	1 tbsp	120	0	14	0	0	0	–
teaseed	1 tbsp	120	0	14	0	0	0	–
tomatoseed	1 tbsp	120	0	14	0	0	0	–
vegetable	1 cup	1927	0	218	0	0	0	–
vegetable	1 tbsp	120	0	14	0	0	0	–
walnut	1 tbsp	120	0	14	0	0	0	–
walnut	1 cup	1927	0	218	0	0	0	–
wheat germ	1 tbsp	120	0	14	0	0	0	–

FOOD	PORTION	CALS	PROT	FAT	CHOL	CARB	FIBER	SOD
Azukar Organics								
Virgin Coconut	1 tbsp (0.5 oz)	125	0	14	0	0	0	0
Bell Plantation								
Extra Virgin Roasted Peanut	1 tbsp	120	0	14	0	0	0	0
Bragg								
Olive Extra Virgin	1 tbsp	120	0	14	0	2	0	0
Carapelli								
Grapeseed	1 tbsp	120	0	14	0	0	0	0
Olive Extra Virgin	1 tbsp	120	0	14	0	0	0	0
Colavita								
Olive Extra Virgin	1 tbsp (0.5 oz)	120	0	14	0	0	0	0
Crisco								
Cooking Spray Original	⅓ sec spray	0	0	0	0	0	0	0
Frying Oil Blend	1 tbsp	130	0	14	0	0	0	0
Light Olive	1 tbsp	120	0	14	0	0	0	0
Peanut	1 tbsp	120	0	14	0	0	0	0
Pure Vegetable	1 tbsp	120	0	14	0	0	0	0
Gaea								
Olive Carbon Neutral	1 tbsp (0.5 oz)	130	0	14	0	0	0	0
Gourme Mist								
Extra Virgin Olive Cold Pressed	1 sec spray	4	0	tr	0	0	0	0
Hollywood								
Canola Enriched	1 tbsp	120	0	14	0	0	0	0
Peanut Enriched Gold	1 tbsp	120	0	14	0	0	0	0
Safflower Expeller Pressed	1 tbsp	120	0	14	0	0	0	0
House Of Tsang								
Mongolian Fire	1 tsp	45	0	5	0	0	0	0
Wok Oil	1 tbsp	130	0	14	0	0	0	0
Kinloch Plantation								
100% Virgin Pecan	1 tbsp	130	0	14	0	0	0	0
Living Harvest								
Organic Hemp Oil	2 tbsp	250	0	28	0	0	0	0
LouAna								
Canola	1 tbsp (0.5 oz)	120	0	14	0	0	0	0

FOOD	PORTION	CALS	PROT	FAT	CHOL	CARB	FIBER	SOD
Lucini								
Extra Virgin Premium Select	1 tbsp (0.5 oz)	120	0	14	0	0	0	0
Manitoba Harvest								
Hemp Seed Oil	1 tbsp	126	0	14	0	0	0	0
Martinis								
Kalamata Olive Extra Virgin Cold Pressed	1 tbsp (0.5 oz)	120	0	15	0	0	0	0
Mazola								
Corn	1 tbsp	120	0	14	0	0	0	0
Monini								
Grapeseed	1 tbsp (0.5 oz)	120	0	14	0	0	0	0
Navitas Naturals								
Organic Virgin Coconut	1 tbsp (0.5 oz)	120	0	14	0	0	0	0
Nutiva								
Organic Coconut Extra Virgin	1 tbsp	120	0	14	0	0	0	0
Organic Hemp Cold Pressed	1 tbsp	120	0	14	0	0	0	0
Olivo								
Spray Olive Oil 100% Extra Virgin	⅓ sec spray	0	0	0	0	0	0	0
Pam								
Organic Canola	⅓ sec spray	0	0	0	0	0	0	0
Pompeian								
Olive	1 tbsp	130	–	14	0	–	–	–
Robert Rothchild Farm								
Basil Infused	1 tbsp	120	0	14	0	0	0	0
Smart Balance								
Omega Oil	1 tbsp (0.5 oz)	120	0	14	0	0	0	90
Tree Of Life								
Almond Expeller Pressed	1 tbsp (0.5 oz)	120	0	14	0	0	0	0
Avocado Expeller Pressed	1 tbsp (0.5 oz)	120	0	14	0	0	0	0
Macadamia Nut Expeller Pressed	1 tbsp (0.5 oz)	120	0	14	0	0	0	0

FOOD	PORTION	CALS	PROT	FAT	CHOL	CARB	FIBER	SOD
Organic Coconut Expeller Pressed	1 tbsp	120	0	14	0	0	0	0
Walnut Expeller Pressed	1 tbsp (0.5 oz)	120	0	14	0	0	0	0
Wesson								
Canola	1 tbsp	120	0	14	0	0	0	0
OKRA								
CANNED								
pickled	6 pods (2.3 oz)	18	1	tr	0	4	2	150
Allens								
Cut	½ cup	30	1	0	0	6	3	400
McIlhenny								
Spicy Pickled	1 oz	10	0	0	0	2	1	270
Trappey's								
Creole Gumbo	½ cup	35	2	0	0	6	3	290
FRESH								
cooked w/ salt	8 pods	19	2	tr	0	4	2	205
luffa chinese okra cooked	1 cup	39	3	tr	0	8	4	422
sliced cooked w/ salt	½ cup	18	2	tr	0	4	2	193
TAKE-OUT								
batter dipped fried	10 pieces (2.6 oz)	142	2	10	2	12	2	100
OLIVES								
black	2 med (0.3 oz)	8	tr	1	0	tr	tr	70
greek	1 (0.5 oz)	16	tr	1	0	1	tr	132
green	2 extra lg (0.5 oz)	19	tr	2	0	1	tr	205
green	2 lg (0.3 oz)	11	tr	1	0	tr	tr	121
green	1 sm (0.2 oz)	8	tr	1	0	tr	tr	90
green	2 med (0.2 oz)	10	tr	1	0	tr	tr	106
green chopped	¼ cup (1.2 oz)	48	tr	5	0	1	1	517
green olive tapenade	1 tbsp	25	0	3	0	1	0	210
green stuffed	¼ cup (1.3 oz)	47	tr	5	0	1	1	493
green stuffed	2 lg (0.3 oz)	12	tr	1	0	tr	tr	123
green stuffed	2 sm (0.2 oz)	9	tr	1	0	tr	tr	91

FOOD	PORTION	CALS	PROT	FAT	CHOL	CARB	FIBER	SOD
green stuffed	2 med (0.3 oz)	10	tr	1	0	tr	tr	107
ripe	2 lg (0.3 oz)	10	tr	1	0	1	tr	81
ripe	2 sm (0.2 oz)	7	tr	1	0	tr	tr	60
ripe	2 extra lg (0.4 oz)	12	tr	1	0	1	tr	97
ripe sliced	¼ cup (1.2 oz)	35	tr	3	0	2	1	297
spanish stuffed	5 (0.5 oz)	15	0	1	0	1	0	320
Dave's Gourmet								
Olives In Pain	⅛ jar (0.5 oz)	15	0	2	–	0	0	270
Martinis								
Kalamata Pitted	4 (0.5 oz)	40	tr	4	0	tr	tr	148
Peloponnese								
Amfissa	3	45	0	5	0	1	0	200
Ionian Green	3	25	0	3	0	1	0	250
Kalamata Pitted	5	45	0	5	0	1	0	210
Kalamata Spread	1 tsp	15	0	2	0	0	0	160
Progresso								
Tapenade	1 tbsp (0.5 oz)	20	0	2	0	1	0	180
Stonewall Kitchen								
Mixed Olive Spread	1 tbsp	35	0	2	–	5	–	150
Zatarain's								
Cocktail	7 (0.5 oz)	25	0	3	0	0	0	350
Stuffed	6 (0.5 oz)	25	0	3	0	0	0	280
ONION								
CANNED								
cocktail	½ cup	41	2	tr	0	9	2	257
Dietz & Watson								
Sweet Vidalia In Sauce	1 tbsp (0.5 oz)	12	0	0	0	3	0	0
French's								
Original French Fried	2 tbsp	45	0	4	0	3	0	60
McSweet								
Pickled Onions	4 (1 oz)	10	0	0	0	2	0	1060
The Gracious Gourmet								
Balsamic Four Onion Spread	1 tbsp (0.5 oz)	20	0	0	0	6	0	45

FOOD	PORTION	CALS	PROT	FAT	CHOL	CARB	FIBER	SOD
DRIED								
flakes	1 tbsp	17	tr	tr	0	4	1	1
powder	1 tsp	7	tr	tr	0	2	tr	1
shallots	1 tbsp	3	tr	0	0	1	–	1
Bob's Red Mill								
Minced	1 tbsp	40	1	1	0	8	1	4
Seneca								
Crisp Onions	1 tbsp (7 g)	40	0	3	0	4	0	35
FRESH								
cooked w/o salt	1 med (3.3 oz)	41	1	tr	0	10	1	3
cooked w/o salt	1 lg (4.5 oz)	56	2	tr	0	13	2	4
cooked w/o salt	1 sm (2 oz)	26	1	tr	0	6	1	2
cooked w/o salt chopped	1 tbsp	7	tr	tr	0	2	tr	0
raw chopped	1 tbsp	4	tr	tr	0	1	tr	0
raw chopped	½ cup	32	1	tr	0	7	1	3
raw slice	1 (0.5 oz)	6	tr	tr	0	1	tr	1
raw sliced	½ cup	23	1	tr	0	5	1	2
scallions raw	1 med (0.5 oz)	5	tr	tr	0	1	tr	2
scallions raw chopped	¼ cup	8	tr	tr	0	2	1	4
shallots raw chopped	¼ cup	29	1	tr	0	7	–	5
sweet whole raw	1 (11.6 oz)	106	3	tr	0	25	3	26
whole raw	1 med (4 oz)	44	1	tr	0	10	2	4
whole raw	1 sm (2.5 oz)	28	1	tr	0	7	1	3
whole raw	1 lg (5.3 oz)	60	2	tr	0	14	3	6
Bland Farms								
Vidalia Sweet	1 (5 oz)	60	1	0	0	14	3	10
Blue Ribbon								
Yellow	1 med (5.2 oz)	60	2	0	0	14	3	5
Earthbound Farms								
Organic Green Onions	¼ cup	10	0	0	0	2	1	5
Organic Red	1 med (5.2 oz)	60	2	0	0	14	3	5
Ocean Mist								
Green Onions Chopped	¼ cup	10	0	0	0	2	1	5
OsoSweet								
Onion	1 med (5 oz)	60	2	0	0	14	3	5

FOOD	PORTION	CALS	PROT	FAT	CHOL	CARB	FIBER	SOD
FROZEN								
C&W								
Petite Whole	⅔ cup (3 oz)	30	0	0	0	6	tr	10
Farm Rich								
Petals Breaded + Sauce	10 (3 oz)	200	2	12	5	22	1	700
TAKE-OUT								
creamed	1 cup	187	5	9	7	22	2	306
fried	½ cup	57	tr	5	0	3	1	5
rings breaded & fried	8 to 9 (3 oz)	276	4	16	14	31	–	430
OPOSSUM								
roasted	3 oz	188	26	9	–	0	0	–
ORANGE								
CANNED								
Del Monte								
Mandarin In Lite Orange Gel	1 pkg (4.5 oz)	60	0	0	0	14	0	40
SunFresh Mandarin In Light Syrup	½ cup (4.5 oz)	70	tr	0	0	17	0	10
FRESH								
california valencia sections	½ cup (3.2 oz)	44	1	tr	0	11	2	0
california valencia	1 (4.2 oz)	59	1	tr	0	14	3	0
florida	1 (5.3 oz)	69	1	tr	0	17	4	0
florida sections	½ cup (3.2 oz)	43	1	tr	0	11	2	0
navel	1 (4.9 oz)	69	1	tr	0	18	3	1
navel sections	1 cup (5.8 oz)	81	2	tr	0	21	4	2
peel	1 tbsp (0.2 oz)	3	tr	tr	0	1	1	0
Darling								
Mandarine	1 med (3.8 oz)	50	1	0	0	13	3	0
Sunkist								
Cara Cara	1 med (5.4 oz)	80	1	0	0	19	3	0
ORANGE JUICE								
chilled bottled	1 cup (8.7 oz)	112	2	1	0	26	1	2

FOOD	PORTION	CALS	PROT	FAT	CHOL	CARB	FIBER	SOD
fresh	1 cup (8.7 oz)	112	2	1	0	26	1	2
mandarin orange	7 oz	94	2	tr	–	20	–	–
Florida's Natural								
Calcium & Vitamin D	8 oz	110	2	0	0	26	0	0
Izze								
Sparkling Esque Mandarin Orange	1 bottle (12 oz)	50	0	0	0	12	–	10
Land O Lakes								
Juice	1 cup (8 oz)	110	1	0	0	25	0	45
Juice w/ Calcium	1 cup (8 oz)	120	1	0	0	29	0	0
Mott's								
100% Juice Sunkist Orange Sensation	1 bottle (14 oz)	210	0	0	0	50	0	15
Mr. J								
100% Juice Calcium Fortified	1 pkg (4 oz)	60	0	0	0	19	–	–
NutraBalance								
Fortified	1 pkg (4 oz)	60	1	0	0	17	4	25
Ocean Spray								
Juice	8 oz	100	0	0	0	31	–	35
Odwalla								
100% Juice	8 oz	110	1	0	0	25	0	15
Organic Valley								
W/ Calcium	1 cup	110	2	0	0	26	0	0
Simply								
Orange Calcium Fortified	8 oz	110	2	0	0	26	–	0
Orange Original	8 oz	110	2	0	0	26	–	0
Snapple								
Orangeade	8 oz	100	0	0	0	26	–	5
SSips								
Orangeade	8 oz	120	0	0	0	31	–	10
Tree Ripe								
100% Juice + Calcium & Vitamins	8 oz	120	1	0	0	29	0	0
Organic 100% Juice	6 oz	90	0	0	0	22	0	10
Tropicana								
Antioxidant Advantage	8 oz	110	2	0	0	26	0	0
Calcium + Vitamin D	8 oz	110	2	0	0	26	0	0
Fiber	8 oz	120	2	0	0	29	3	0

FOOD	PORTION	CALS	PROT	FAT	CHOL	CARB	FIBER	SOD
Healthy Heart	8 oz	120	2	0	0	26	0	0
Healthy Kids	8 oz	110	2	0	0	26	0	0
Light'n Healthy w/ Calcium	8 oz	50	tr	0	0	13	0	10
No Pulp	8 oz	110	2	0	0	26	0	0
Orangeade	8 oz	111	0	0	0	33	0	0
Organic	8 oz	120	1	0	0	28	0	25
Trop50' Orange Juice Beverage	8 oz	50	tr	0	0	13	0	10
Uncle Matt's								
Organic 100% Juice Pulp Free	8 oz	110	2	0	0	26	0	10
Organic 100% Juice w/ Pulp	8 oz	110	2	0	0	26	0	10
Welsh Farms								
Juice	8 oz	110	0	0	0	27	–	–
TAKE-OUT								
orange julius	1 cup (9.2 oz)	212	14	tr	0	39	tr	196

OREGANO

FOOD	PORTION	CALS	PROT	FAT	CHOL	CARB	FIBER	SOD
crumbled	1 tsp	3	tr	tr	0	1	tr	0
ground	1 tsp	6	tr	tr	0	1	1	0

ORGAN MEATS (*see* BRAINS, GIBLETS, GIZZARDS, HEART, KIDNEY, LIVER, SWEETBREAD)

OSTRICH

FOOD	PORTION	CALS	PROT	FAT	CHOL	CARB	FIBER	SOD
cooked	4 oz	195	29	8	92	0	0	450
cooked diced	1 cup (4.7 oz)	215	35	9	111	0	0	543
Natural Frontier Foods								
Filets	1 (4 oz)	130	28	3	50	0	0	75
Ground Lean	4 oz	130	28	3	50	0	0	75

OYSTERS

FOOD	PORTION	CALS	PROT	FAT	CHOL	CARB	FIBER	SOD
canned eastern	1 cup	112	11	4	89	6	0	181
eastern baked	6 med	47	4	1	22	4	0	96
eastern raw	6 med	50	4	1	21	5	0	150
eastern sauteed	6 med	76	5	5	36	3	0	342
smoked	6	33	3	1	26	2	0	259
Polar								
Whole	¼ cup	70	7	3	3	4	0	150
Whole Smoked	⅓ cup	95	8	5	10	4	0	160

FOOD	PORTION	CALS	PROT	FAT	CHOL	CARB	FIBER	SOD
TAKE-OUT								
breaded & fried	6	368	13	18	108	40	–	677
fritter	1 (1.4 oz)	121	4	6	36	12	tr	276
oysters rockefeller	1 cup	302	18	17	90	22	4	1113
stew	1 cup	208	11	13	78	11	0	892
PANCAKE/WAFFLE SYRUP								
light	¼ cup	98	0	0	0	27	0	120
pancake syrup	1 pkg (2 oz)	156	0	tr	0	41	0	36
pancake syrup	¼ cup	209	0	tr	0	55	0	48
Aunt Jemima								
Butter Lite	¼ cup (2.1 oz)	100	0	0	0	26	1	210
Naturally Fresh								
Maple Mountain Sugar Free	2 tbsp	0	0	0	0	0	0	70
Wholesome Sweeteners								
Organic	¼ cup	240	0	0	0	60	0	90
PANCAKES								
FROZEN								
Aunt Jemima								
Buttermilk	3 (3 oz)	210	6	4	20	40	2	600
Buttermilk Low Fat	3 (3 oz)	210	6	4	20	40	2	560
Whole Grain	3 (3 oz)	230	7	6	20	38	3	480
Dr. Praeger's								
Broccoli	1 (2 oz)	80	2	4	0	9	2	170
Potato	1 (2.2 oz)	100	2	4	15	13	3	190
Golden								
Potato Latkes	1 (1.3 oz)	70	2	3	<5	10	1	190
Zucchini	1 (1.3 oz)	70	2	3	0	8	1	170
Jimmy Dean								
Breakfast Bowls Pancake & Sausage Links	1 pkg	710	13	31	45	93	3	890
Griddle Cake Sandwich Sausage Egg & Cheese	1 (4 oz)	370	8	23	40	32	1	640
Griddle Sticks	1 (2.5 oz)	160	7	6	25	21	0	410
Pillsbury								
Blueberry	3 (4 oz)	230	5	4	10	46	2	430
Buttermilk	3 (4 oz)	240	6	4	10	47	2	470
Original	3 (4 oz)	250	6	4	10	49	2	450

FOOD	PORTION	CALS	PROT	FAT	CHOL	CARB	FIBER	SOD
Ratner's								
Potato Latkes	1 (1.5 oz)	80	2	2	25	15	tr	380
MIX								
Arrowhead Mills								
Gluten Free Pancake & Waffle as prep	2 (5 in)	240	11	6	57	42	0	312
Batter Blaster								
Organic Original Pancake & Waffle Batter not prep	¼ cup (2 oz)	112	3	1	10	23	2	95
Bisquick								
Shake 'N Pour Buttermilk as prep	3	220	6	3	0	42	1	800
TAKE-OUT								
bu chu jun korean w/ vegetables	1 (4 oz)	83	2	4	21	11	1	230
buckwheat	1 (7 in)	142	5	5	45	19	2	366
norwegian lefse	1 (9 in) (2.7 oz)	163	3	5	8	27	2	134
pindaettok korean mung bean	1 (3.9 oz)	204	6	11	3	20	6	33
plain	1 (7 in)	183	4	3	7	35	1	407
potato	1 (1.3 oz)	70	2	4	26	8	1	151
w/ butter & syrup	2 (8.1 oz)	520	8	14	58	91	–	1104
whole wheat	1 (7 in)	183	6	8	47	23	3	489

PANCREAS (*see* SWEETBREAD)

PANINI (*see* SANDWICHES)

PAPAYA

FOOD	PORTION	CALS	PROT	FAT	CHOL	CARB	FIBER	SOD
canned in syrup	½ cup (2.3 oz)	50	tr	tr	0	13	1	2
dried	1 strip (0.8 oz)	59	1	tr	0	15	3	5
fresh	1 lg (13.3 oz)	148	2	1	0	37	7	11
fresh	1 sm (5.3 oz)	59	1	tr	0	15	3	5
fresh cubed	1 cup (4.9 oz)	55	1	tr	0	14	3	4
green cooked	½ cup (2.3 oz)	18	tr	tr	0	5	1	2

FOOD	PORTION	CALS	PROT	FAT	CHOL	CARB	FIBER	SOD
PAPAYA JUICE								
nectar	1 cup (8.8 oz)	142	tr	tr	0	36	2	12
Ceres								
100% Juice	8 oz	120	0	0	0	31	0	15
Lakewood								
Red	8 oz	80	1	0	0	20	2	6
Yellow	8 oz	105	2	0	0	26	2	5
Old Orchard								
Nectar Cocktail	8 oz	120	0	0	0	30	–	15
PAPRIKA								
dried	1 tsp	1	tr	tr	0	tr	tr	2
Bob's Red Mill								
Hungarian	½ tsp	11	0	0	0	2	1	0
PARSLEY								
dried	1 tbsp	4	tr	tr	0	1	1	7
freeze dried	1 tbsp	1	tr	tr	0	tr	tr	2
fresh chopped	¼ cup	5	tr	tr	0	1	1	8
fresh chopped	1 tbsp	1	tr	tr	0	tr	tr	2
fresh sprigs	5 (1.8 oz)	18	1	tr	0	3	2	28
PARSNIPS								
fresh sliced cooked w/o salt	½ cup (2.7 oz)	55	1	tr	0	13	3	8
whole cooked	1 (5.6 oz)	114	2	tr	0	27	6	16
TAKE-OUT								
creamed	1 cup (8 oz)	237	6	11	7	31	5	652
PASSION FRUIT								
fresh	1 (0.6 oz)	17	tr	tr	0	4	2	5
fresh cut up	½ cup (4.1 oz)	114	3	1	0	28	12	33
PASSION FRUIT JUICE								
nectar	1 cup (8.8 oz)	168	tr	tr	0	44	tr	10
yellow lilikoi	1 cup (8.7 oz)	138	1	tr	0	35	1	15
Ceres								
100% Juice	8 oz	130	0	0	0	32	0	15

FOOD	PORTION	CALS	PROT	FAT	CHOL	CARB	FIBER	SOD
EarthWise								
Passionfruit Aloe	8 oz	110	0	0	0	28	0	30
Santa Cruz								
Organic 100% Juice Nectar	8 oz	150	1	0	0	40	0	15

PASTA (*see also* NOODLES, PASTA DINNERS, PASTA SALAD)

FOOD	PORTION	CALS	PROT	FAT	CHOL	CARB	FIBER	SOD
DRY								
corn cooked	1 cup (4.9 oz)	176	4	1	0	39	7	0
elbows not prep	1 cup	389	13	2	0	78	–	8
elbows cooked	1 cup (4.9 oz)	197	7	1	0	40	2	1
shells small cooked	1 cup (4 oz)	162	5	1	0	33	2	1
spaghetti cooked	1 cup (4.9 oz)	197	7	1	0	40	2	1
spinach spaghetti cooked	1 cup (4.9 oz)	182	6	1	0	37	–	20
spirals cooked	1 cup (4.7 oz)	189	6	tr	0	38	2	1
vegetable cooked	1 cup (4.7 oz)	172	6	tr	0	36	6	8
whole wheat all shapes cooked	1 cup	174	7	tr	0	37	4	4
Amish Natural								
Fettuccine Fiber Rich not prep	2 oz	200	6	1	0	42	11	50
Fettuccine not prep	2 oz	201	8	1	0	41	2	5
Fettuccine Whole Wheat not prep	2 oz	210	8	2	0	41	7	5
Barilla								
Plus Rotini not prep	2 oz	210	10	2	0	38	4	25
Rotini Whole Grain not prep	2 oz	200	7	2	0	41	6	0
Spaghetti Whole Grain not prep	1/7 box (2 oz)	200	7	2	0	41	6	0
Tortellini Three Cheese not prep	2/3 cup (2 oz)	230	8	8	35	32	3	500
DeBoles								
Angel Hair Rice Pasta not prep	1/4 pkg (2 oz)	210	4	1	0	46	tr	15

FOOD	PORTION	CALS	PROT	FAT	CHOL	CARB	FIBER	SOD
Elbow Corn Pasta Wheat Free not prep	1/6 pkg (2 oz)	200	4	2	0	43	5	15
Fettuccine not prep	1/4 pkg (2 oz)	210	7	1	0	41	1	0
Organic Angel Hair Whole Wheat not prep	1/4 pkg (2 oz)	210	7	2	0	42	5	10
Organic Eggless Ribbon not prep	1 cup (2 oz)	210	7	1	0	43	1	5
Organic Fettucini Spinach not prep	1/4 pkg (2 oz)	210	7	1	0	43	3	20
Organic Lasagna not prep	1/4 pkg (2.5 oz)	260	9	1	0	54	1	5
Organic Rigatoni Whole Wheat not prep	1 cup (2 oz)	210	7	2	0	42	5	10
Rigatoni not prep	1/4 pkg (2 oz)	210	7	1	0	41	1	0
Dreamfields								
Lasagna not prep	2 pieces (2 oz)	190	7	1	0	42	5	15
Rotini not prep	2/3 cup (2 oz)	190	7	1	0	42	5	15
Gillian's								
Penne Brown Rice Pasta Wheat Gluten Egg Free not prep	2 oz	200	4	2	0	43	2	0
Jovial								
Organic Einkorn All Shapes	2 oz	200	9	2	0	35	4	0
Organic Einkorn White All Shapes	2 oz	200	8	2	0	40	2	0
Organic Gluten Free Brown Rice All Shapes	2 oz	210	5	2	0	43	2	0
Lundberg								
Organic Spaghetti Brown Rice not prep	2 oz	210	4	2	0	44	3	5
Maddy's								
Gluten Free not prep	4 oz	310	5	2	0	66	2	120
Mueller's								
Elbow Macaroni not prep	1/2 cup	210	7	1	0	41	2	0
Ronzoni								
Bow Ties not prep	1 cup (2 oz)	210	7	1	0	42	2	0
Elbows not prep	1/2 cup (2 oz)	210	7	1	0	42	2	0
Garden Delight Radiatore not prep	2 oz	190	7	1	0	40	4	15

FOOD	PORTION	CALS	PROT	FAT	CHOL	CARB	FIBER	SOD
Garden Delight Spaghetti not prep	2 oz	190	7	1	0	40	4	15
Smart Taste Rotini not prep	2 oz	180	6	1	0	43	7	5
Wacky Mac								
Veggie All Shapes not prep	2 oz	200	8	1	0	41	1	15
FRESH								
cooked	2 oz	75	3	1	33	14	–	3
spinach cooked	2 oz	74	3	1	19	14	–	3
Buitoni								
Ravioli Four Cheese 100% Whole Wheat	1¼ cups	320	16	10	65	42	5	690
Monterey Gourmet								
Whole Wheat Ravioli Vegetable & Cheese	1 cup (3.5 oz)	240	12	6	25	35	4	340
Whole Wheat Tortellini Italian Cheese	1 cup (3.5 oz)	290	13	6	35	48	5	290

PASTA DINNERS (*see also* PASTA SALAD)

FOOD	PORTION	CALS	PROT	FAT	CHOL	CARB	FIBER	SOD
CANNED								
Chef Boyardee								
Beef Ravioli	1 cup	240	8	8	15	35	3	900
Beefaroni	1 cup (8.7 oz)	260	10	10	25	33	3	990
Mini Ravioli	1 cup (8.8 oz)	250	8	9	15	35	3	950
Mini-Bites Spaghetti & Meatballs	1 cup (8.8 oz)	240	10	10	15	28	3	750
Spaghetti & Meat Balls	1 cup (9 oz)	270	11	10	20	32	2	900
Hormel								
Kid's Kitchen Microwave Meals Cheezy Mac 'N Beef	1 pkg (7.5 oz)	250	14	6	20	34	1	840
Kid's Kitchen Microwave Meals Cheezy Mac 'N Cheese	1 pkg (7.5 oz)	270	11	14	40	24	1	750
Kid's Kitchen Microwave Meals Mini Beef Ravioli	1 pkg (7.5 oz)	240	8	6	20	38	1	950
Kid's Kitchen Microwave Meals Spaghetti Rings & Franks	1 pkg (7.5 oz)	240	9	8	25	32	1	840

FOOD	PORTION	CALS	PROT	FAT	CHOL	CARB	FIBER	SOD
Lasagna w/ Meat Sauce	1 pkg (7.5 oz)	210	9	5	10	31	3	840
Spaghetti w/ Meat Sauce	1 pkg (7.5 oz)	210	10	5	15	31	3	750
SpaghettiOs								
A to Z's w/ Meatballs	1 cup	260	11	9	20	33	3	990
A to Z's w/ Sliced Franks	1 cup	230	9	6	20	32	2	990
Mini Beef Ravioli In Meat Sauce	1 cup	260	11	5	10	43	5	1060
Pasta	1 cup	180	6	1	5	37	3	630
Plus Calcium	1 cup	170	6	1	5	35	3	620
FROZEN								
4Real								
Mac+Cheese	1 pkg (8 oz)	230	8	5	5	33	2	410
Meat Sauce w/ Beef Ravioli	1 pkg (8 oz)	190	8	4	30	32	2	410
Spaghetti Rings	1 pkg (8 oz)	180	6	1	0	37	2	310
Amy's								
Bowls Baked Ziti	1 pkg	390	9	12	0	62	6	590
Bowls Stuffed Pasta Shells	1 pkg	310	19	13	30	30	5	740
Lasagna Cheese	1 pkg (10.2 oz)	380	20	14	45	44	4	680
Lasagna Tofu Vegetable	1 pkg (9.4 oz)	310	13	11	0	41	6	680
Macaroni & Cheese	1 pkg (8.9 oz)	410	16	16	40	47	3	590
Macaroni & Cheese Light In Sodium	1 pkg (8.9 oz)	400	16	16	40	47	3	290
Macaroni & Soy Cheese	1 pkg (8.9 oz)	370	16	15	0	42	4	500
Rice Mac & Cheese	1 pkg (9 oz)	400	16	16	50	47	1	590
Banquet								
Lasagna Family Entree	1 cup	510	25	16	15	63	3	730
Macaroni & Cheese	1 cup	200	7	6	10	30	3	750
Noodles & Beef	1 cup	160	8	4	30	20	2	900
Birds Eye								
Steamfresh Meals For Two Shrimp Alfredo	½ pkg (11.9 oz)	420	21	12	100	55	4	900
Steamfresh Meals For Two Shrimp Pasta Primavera	½ pkg (11.9 oz)	450	15	24	130	39	3	770

FOOD	PORTION	CALS	PROT	FAT	CHOL	CARB	FIBER	SOD
Blue Horizon Organic								
Penne Alfredo w/ Shrimp	½ pkg (9.9 oz)	430	17	22	115	39	2	380
Penne Alla Vodka w/ Shrimp	½ pkg (9.9 oz)	270	17	6	75	38	3	280
Pesto Farfalle w/ Shrimp	½ pkg (9.9 oz)	280	17	6	70	38	3	430
Scampi Rotini w/ Shrimp	½ pkg (9.9 oz)	410	18	19	85	44	4	640
Caesar's								
Gluten Free Lasagna Cheese In Marinara Sauce	1 pkg (11.5 oz)	520	14	14	50	84	4	570
Gluten Free Lasagna Vegetable In Marinara Sauce	1 pkg (11.5 oz)	510	13	13	45	84	5	510
Gluten Free Manicotti w/ Cheese In Marinara Sauce	1 pkg (11 oz)	380	16	18	105	42	3	640
Gluten Free Stuffed Shells w/ Cheese In Marinara Sauce	1 pkg (11 oz)	370	16	18	65	37	3	660
Cedarlane								
Zone Chicken & Vegetables Pasta & Ginger	1 pkg (10 oz)	340	24	12	140	35	3	650
Zone Lasagna Vegetable	1 pkg (10.9 oz)	310	24	12	15	33	5	910
Celentano								
Cheese Ravioli	4 (4.3 oz)	220	11	5	30	34	2	280
Contessa								
Ravioli Portobello	6 (6.7 oz)	360	14	17	65	39	2	640
Glory								
Macaroni & Cheese	1 pkg	480	21	23	90	47	1	1300
Gluten Free Cafe								
Fettuccini Alfredo	1 pkg (9.2 oz)	400	4	16	45	55	2	390
Pasta Primavera	1 pkg (9.2 oz)	270	4	9	25	42	4	260

FOOD	PORTION	CALS	PROT	FAT	CHOL	CARB	FIBER	SOD
Glutino								
Gluten Free Duo Mushroom Penne	1 pkg (10.5 oz)	380	8	6	5	73	5	720
Gluten Free Macaroni & Cheese	1 pkg (8.8 oz)	430	19	20	45	44	2	1430
Gluten Free Penne Alfredo	1 pkg (9.1 oz)	340	15	8	50	48	3	830
Green Giant								
Skillet Meal Chicken & Cheesy Pasta as prep	1¼ cups	270	15	6	33	42	4	740
Healthy Choice								
Creamy Garlic Shrimp w/ Bow Tie Pasta	1 pkg (11.5 oz)	280	13	5	25	44	5	600
Portabella Marsala Pasta	1 pkg (9 oz)	270	12	7	15	38	5	550
Tomato Basil Penne	1 pkg (10 oz)	280	13	6	15	39	7	600
Helen's Kitchen								
Farfalle & Basil Pasta w/ Tofu Steaks	1 pkg (9 oz)	320	20	11	30	70	5	370
Joy Of Cooking								
Al Dente Cavatappi Bolognese	1 cup (7.7 oz)	280	14	12	55	29	2	700
Best Loved Macaroni & Cheese	1 cup (5.4 oz)	280	10	18	25	36	1	520
Cheese Ravioli Pomodoro	1 cup (7.7 oz)	250	13	7	30	34	3	710
Creamy Fettuccine Carbonara	1 cup (7.5 oz)	330	15	16	100	31	3	620
Kashi								
Chicken Pasta Pomodoro	1 pkg (10 oz)	280	19	6	25	38	6	470
Marie Callender's								
Fettucine Chicken & Broccoli	1 meal	630	30	37	90	43	6	900
Meat Lasagna	1 cup	240	14	9	45	24	2	950
Meals To Live								
Turkey Meatballs w/ Marinara Sauce & Whole Wheat Spaghetti	1 pkg (11 oz)	300	21	5	40	44	9	480

FOOD	PORTION	CALS	PROT	FAT	CHOL	CARB	FIBER	SOD
Milton's								
Lasagna Vegetable w/ Multi-Grain Pasta	1 cup (8 oz)	340	17	16	60	30	5	950
Mon Cuisine								
Vegetarian Spaghetti & Meatballs	1 pkg (10 oz)	360	29	4	0	54	9	440
Moosewood								
Organic Vegetarian Broccoli & Pasta Parmesan	1 pkg (10 oz)	380	14	13	30	52	4	380
Organic Vegetarian Farfalle & Spinach Pesto Sauce	1 pkg (10 oz)	370	14	11	20	56	4	370
Organic Vegetarian Spicy Penne Puttanesca	1 pkg (10 oz)	300	8	10	0	45	2	300
New York Ravioli								
Jolie Kid Shapes Ravioli Cheese	1 cup	330	15	9	35	47	4	270
Jolie Kid Shapes Ravioli Cheese & Broccoli	1 cup	340	15	8	105	53	2	210
Ravioli Four Cheese	1 cup	360	17	6	80	58	2	250
Ravioli Tomato Basil & Mozzarella	1 cup	340	12	5	55	64	2	210
Organic Bistro								
Pasta Puttanesca	1 pkg (12.15 oz)	330	12	6	0	57	9	370
Organic Classics								
Cajun Chicken Tetrazzine w/ Penne Pasta	1 pkg (10 oz)	370	25	10	55	43	3	490
Chicken Cacciatore w/ Penne Pasta	1 pkg (10 oz)	270	20	4	40	37	3	390
Macaroni & Meat Sauce	1 pkg (10 oz)	340	16	9	20	49	3	580
Plum Organics								
Bowtie Pasta	1 pkg (6.9 oz)	230	7	6	15	37	3	15
Cheese Filled Spinach Tortellini	1 pkg (6.9 oz)	190	8	2	10	37	3	270
Putney Pasta								
Ravioli Butternut Squash & Vermont Maple Syrup	1 cup	200	8	4	30	35	1	270

FOOD	PORTION	CALS	PROT	FAT	CHOL	CARB	FIBER	SOD
Ravioli Portobello & Grilled Onion	7 (5.2 oz)	240	11	5	40	39	3	260
Ravioli Whole Wheat Spinach & Cheese	9 (5 oz)	300	13	9	55	42	2	340
Skillet Meal Chicken Piccata	1 serv (9 oz)	300	14	11	30	35	2	350
Skillet Meal Shrimp Pesto	1 serv (9 oz)	540	18	38	100	32	3	410
Tortellini Spinach Mozzarella & Walnuts	1 cup	360	20	8	60	51	2	410
Tortellini Tri-Color Three Cheese	1 cup	340	16	8	55	51	1	500
Stouffer's								
Cheesy Spaghetti Bake	1 pkg (12 oz)	460	21	24	120	39	4	950
Chicken Parmigiana	1 pkg (13.13 oz)	460	18	18	35	56	4	1060
Escalloped Chicken & Noodles	1 pkg (8 oz)	330	14	18	35	28	2	910
Homestyle Chicken & Noodles	1 pkg (12 oz)	340	25	12	65	33	3	950
Italian Sausage Stuffed Rigatoni	1 pkg (9.13 oz)	380	18	14	60	46	2	880
Lasagna Bake w/ Meat Sauce	1 pkg (11.5 oz)	380	18	13	40	47	5	1080
Lasagna Vegetable	1 pkg (10.5 oz)	390	17	18	25	40	4	730
Macaroni & Beef	1 pkg (11.5 oz)	330	19	11	40	38	4	920
Macaroni & Cheese	1 cup (6 oz)	350	15	17	25	34	2	920
Manicotti Cheese	1 pkg (9 oz)	360	18	14	70	41	2	920
Shrimp Scampi	1 pkg (14 oz)	410	21	11	80	57	6	990
Tuna Noodle Casserole	1 pkg (10 oz)	350	18	15	40	35	2	930
Turkey Tettrazini	1 pkg (10 oz)	380	19	20	60	32	1	970
Tabatchnick								
Macaroni & Cheese	1 serv (7.5 oz)	250	9	8	20	34	tr	770

FOOD	PORTION	CALS	PROT	FAT	CHOL	CARB	FIBER	SOD
Taste Above								
Meatless Thai Peanut Coconut Sauce w/ Veggie Chicken & Vermicelli	1 pkg (10 oz)	320	26	19	0	22	8	300
Meatless Tuscan Marinara Sauce w/ Veggie Chicken & Penne Pasta	1 pkg (10 oz)	320	26	19	0	22	8	300
Weight Watchers								
Smart Ones Lasagna w/ Meat Sauce	1 pkg (10.5 oz)	300	17	6	25	43	5	780
Yves								
Meatless Lasagna	1 pkg (10.5 oz)	300	17	3	0	51	4	650
MIX								
Back To Nature								
Crazy Bugs Macaroni & Cheese as prep	1 cup	370	12	10	24	60	2	864
Harvest Wheat Elbows & Cheddar as prep	½ pkg	380	12	12	30	60	2	768
Organic Shells & Cheese as prep	½ pkg	380	12	12	30	60	2	750
Carapelli								
Penne Alfredo as prep	1 cup	240	9	1	5	47	4	960
Spirals Creamy Tomato as prep	1 cup	240	9	1	0	49	4	900
DeBoles								
Organic Macaroni & Cheese Whole Wheat as prep	1 cup	410	11	14	42	60	9	384
Pasta & Cheese as prep	1 cup	420	10	15	51	60	6	384
Rice Shells & Cheddar as prep	½ cup	260	3	8	24	57	1	216
Hamburger Helper								
Cheesy Jambalaya as prep	1 cup	330	4	13	60	30	1	840
Knorr								
Pasta & Sauce Jalapeno Jack as prep	1 cup	230	8	3	3	45	2	504
Pasta Sides w/ Whole Grains Alfredo as prep	⅔ cup	300	10	11	15	42	4	864

FOOD	PORTION	CALS	PROT	FAT	CHOL	CARB	FIBER	SOD
Kraft								
Macaroni & Cheese White Cheddar as prep	⅓ pkg	380	10	15	10	48	0	744
La Bella Vita								
Chicken & Lemon Borsellini as prep	1 cup	270	14	6	70	39	2	430
Near East								
Basil & Herb as prep	1 cup	240	8	5	0	42	3	430
Spicy Tomato as prep	1 cup	230	7	5	0	38	3	600
Pasta Roni								
Angel Hair w/ Herbs as prep	1 cup	310	9	13	5	41	2	820
Chicken as prep	1 cup	300	9	12	5	39	2	1060
Chicken Quesadilla as prep	1 cup	310	10	13	5	40	2	860
Fettuccine Alfredo as prep	1 cup	450	11	25	5	47	2	1140
Nature's Way Mushrooms In Cream Sauce as prep	1 cup	280	9	10	5	39	2	710
Sour Cream & Chives as prep	1 cup	310	8	15	5	38	2	880
Stroganoff as prep	1 cup	350	12	14	10	47	2	970
Road's End Organics								
Mac & Cheese Dairy Free Gluten Free as prep	1 cup	310	8	1	0	63	5	310
Shells & Cheese as prep	1 cup	330	14	1	0	66	7	408
Simply Shari's								
Mac & Cheese Gluten Free as prep	¼ pkg (4 oz)	280	18	6	15	17	2	330
Thai Kitchen								
Stir-Fry Rice Noodles Thai Peanut as prep	½ pkg	310	9	6	0	54	1	330
REFRIGERATED								
Country Crock								
Elbow Macaroni & Cheese	1 cup (8 oz)	370	14	17	40	40	1	940
Four Cheese Pasta	1 cup (8 oz)	380	15	17	40	41	2	1060
NoOodle								
Mamma Mia! Marinara	1 pkg (10 oz)	70	2	3	0	13	4	480
Say Cheese Pleeeze!	1 pkg (10 oz)	100	4	10	25	6	4	190
Terri-Yaki Chicken	1 pkg (10 oz)	80	11	2	25	10	4	650
Ultra-Lite Primavera	1 pkg (10 oz)	30	2	0	0	8	4	360

FOOD	PORTION	CALS	PROT	FAT	CHOL	CARB	FIBER	SOD
Rozzano								
Organic Ravioli Grilled Vegetable	1 cup (3.5 oz)	200	10	6	35	26	2	420
SHELF-STABLE								
Allergaroo								
Gluten Free Spaghetti	1 pkg (8 oz)	220	3	3	0	49	3	510
Gluten Free Spyglass Noodles	1 pkg (8 oz)	230	4	3	0	49	3	510
Betty Crocker								
Bowl Appetit! Cheddar Broccoli Pasta	1 bowl (2.8 oz)	330	11	11	10	49	2	1000
Bowl Appetit! Garlic Parmesan Pasta	1 bowl (2.8 oz)	320	11	9	10	50	1	1010
Healthy Choice								
Fresh Mixers Ziti & Meat Sauce	1 pkg (6.9 oz)	340	15	6	20	56	8	600
Hormel								
Compleats Microwave Meals Chicken & Noodles	1 pkg (9.9 oz)	240	15	8	60	27	2	990
TastyBite								
Peanut Sauce w/ Noodles	1 pkg (10 oz)	530	17	19	0	104	12	595
TAKE-OUT								
bami goreng indonesian noodle dish	1 cup	170	5	3	0	25	4	500
lasagna meatless	1 piece (9 oz)	356	19	11	38	46	3	896
lasagna w/ meat	1 piece (8 oz)	362	22	14	56	37	3	838
lasagna w/ vegetables	1 serv (9 oz)	315	17	10	33	41	4	776
macaroni & cheese w/ ham	1 cup	542	21	33	61	41	3	1375
manicotti cheese filled w/ marinara sauce	1 (5 oz)	229	13	10	83	22	1	615
manicotti cheese filled w/ meat sauce	1 (5 oz)	239	14	11	86	20	3	612
pasta w/ pesto sauce	1 cup	370	10	25	10	27	2	178
ravioli cheese & spinach filled w/ cream sauce	1 cup	362	15	17	160	38	2	962
ravioli cheese w/ tomato sauce	1 cup	335	14	14	158	38	2	1570

FOOD	PORTION	CALS	PROT	FAT	CHOL	CARB	FIBER	SOD
ravioli meat filled w/ marinara sauce	1 cup	372	22	16	168	36	3	1488
rigatoni w/ sausage sauce	¾ cup	260	10	12	59	28	3	106
spaghetti w/ red clam sauce	1 cup	285	13	8	17	41	3	280
spaghetti w/ sauce & meatballs	2 cups	670	34	26	114	80	12	1820
spaghetti w/ white clam sauce	1 cup	456	25	20	50	43	3	461
tortellini cheese w/ tomato sauce	1 cup	332	14	14	158	38	2	1560
tortellini meat filled w/ marinara sauce	1 cup	281	14	10	90	33	2	1294
tortellini spinach filled w/ marinara sauce	1 cup	238	10	8	72	32	2	1190
PASTA SALAD								
MIX								
Suddenly Salad								
Caesar as prep	1 cup (1.8 oz)	310	6	14	0	38	1	640
Classic as prep	¾ cup	250	6	8	0	39	1	840
Creamy Italian as prep	¾ cup	350	7	20	15	36	2	410
Creamy Parmesan as prep	¾ cup	370	5	22	18	33	1	300
TAKE-OUT								
pasta salad w/ crab vegetables mayonnaise	1 cup	317	10	16	32	33	2	866
pasta salad w/ shrimp vegetables & mayonnaise	1 cup (6.2 oz)	335	10	17	65	35	2	982
tortellini salad cheese filled w/ vinaigrette dressing	1 cup	333	12	18	144	30	1	1070
PATE								
chicken liver canned	1 tbsp	26	2	2	51	1	0	50
duck pate	1 oz	96	4	8	–	1	–	–
fish pate	1 oz	76	3	7	–	1	–	286
liver w/ truffle	1 serv (2 oz)	183	6	16	59	4	–	452
mushroom anchovy pate	1 can (2.25 oz)	130	2	11	5	7	1	400
pate de foie gras smoked canned	1 tbsp	60	1	6	20	1	0	91
pork pate	1 oz	107	3	10	51	1	0	189

FOOD	PORTION	CALS	PROT	FAT	CHOL	CARB	FIBER	SOD
pork pate en croute	1 oz	91	3	7	32	3	tr	214
rabbit pate	1 oz	66	5	5	21	1	–	97
shrimp	1 can (2.25 oz)	140	6	10	25	7	0	450
Patchwork								
All Flavors	2 oz	270	5	27	90	5	0	410
PEACH								
CANNED								
halves in light syrup	1 half (3.4 oz)	53	tr	tr	0	14	1	5
halves juice pack	1 half (3.4 oz)	43	1	tr	0	11	1	4
in heavy syrup	½ cup (2.6 oz)	85	1	tr	0	22	2	7
peach sauce	½ cup	120	tr	0	0	32	1	0
pickled	½ cup (4.2 oz)	143	1	tr	0	35	1	1
pickled whole	1 (3.1 oz)	104	1	tr	0	26	1	1
slices juice pack	½ cup (4.4 oz)	55	1	tr	0	14	2	5
slices light syrup	½ cup (4.4 oz)	68	1	tr	0	18	2	6
slices water pack	½ cup (4.3 oz)	29	1	tr	0	7	2	4
spiced in heavy syrup	½ cup (4.2 oz)	91	1	tr	0	24	2	5
Del Monte								
Carb Clever Sliced	½ cup (4.2 oz)	30	1	0	0	7	1	10
Chunks Raspberry Flavor	½ cup (4.4 oz)	80	tr	0	0	20	tr	10
Clingstone Sliced In Light Syrup	½ cup (4.4 oz)	70	0	0	0	17	1	10
Fruit Bowls	½ cup (4.4 oz)	70	0	0	0	17	2	20
Fruit Cup Diced In Water No Sugar Added	1 pkg (3.75 oz)	25	0	0	0	6	–	10
Fruit Naturals Chunks No Sugar Added	½ cup (4.2 oz)	40	1	0	0	12	2	0

FOOD	PORTION	CALS	PROT	FAT	CHOL	CARB	FIBER	SOD
Orchard Select Cinnamon Spiced	½ cup (4.4 oz)	80	tr	0	0	20	tr	10
Orchard Select Sliced Cling No Sugar Added	½ cup (4.2 oz)	40	1	0	0	11	2	10
Peaches In Peach Gel	1 pkg (4.5 oz)	90	0	0	0	22	0	40
Dole								
Yellow Cling Diced Peaches In Light Syrup	1 pkg (4 oz)	80	0	0	0	20	tr	0
Polar								
White	½ cup	70	1	0	0	17	1	10
S&W								
Slices Natural Style	½ cup (4.4 oz)	80	1	0	0	19	1	20
DRIED								
halves	½ cup (2.8 oz)	191	3	1	0	49	7	6
halves	1 (0.5 oz)	31	tr	tr	0	8	1	1
halves cooked w/o sugar	½ cup (4.5 oz)	99	2	tr	0	25	4	3
FruitziO								
Freeze Dried	1 pkg (0.35 oz)	40	0	0	0	9	1	0
Mrs. May's								
Fruit Chips	1 pkg	35	0	0	0	8	1	0
Stoneridge Orchards								
Whole	⅓ cup (1.4 oz)	140	0	0	0	31	1	75
FRESH								
peach	1 med (5.3 oz)	58	1	tr	0	14	2	0
peach	1 lg (6.1 oz)	68	2	tr	0	17	3	0
sliced	½ cup (2.7 oz)	30	1	tr	0	8	1	0
FROZEN								
C&W								
Ultimate Sliced	¾ cup	50	1	0	0	13	2	0
PEACH JUICE								
nectar	1 cup (8.7 oz)	134	1	tr	0	35	2	17

FOOD	PORTION	CALS	PROT	FAT	CHOL	CARB	FIBER	SOD
Ceres								
100% Juice	8 oz	120	0	0	0	30	0	5
Froose								
Playful Peach	1 box (4.2 oz)	80	1	0	0	19	3	15
Izze								
Sparkling Peach	1 bottle (12 oz)	130	0	0	0	32	–	20
OKF								
Sparkling Fresh Peach	1 bottle (8.3 oz)	50	0	0	0	12	3	36
Santa Cruz								
Organic Nectar	8 oz	120	0	0	0	31	0	10
PEANUT BUTTER								
chunky	2 tbsp (1.1 oz)	188	8	16	0	7	3	156
no sugar added	2 tbsp (1.1 oz)	208	8	18	0	5	3	143
reduced sodium	2 tbsp (1.1 oz)	202	8	16	0	7	2	65
smooth	2 tbsp (1.1 oz)	188	8	16	0	7	2	147
Arrowhead Mills								
Organic Creamy	2 tbsp	190	8	17	0	6	2	0
Organic Honey Sweetened Creamy	2 tbsp	190	7	16	0	7	2	100
Organic Natural Crunchy	2 tbsp	190	8	17	0	6	2	0
Better'n Peanut Butter								
Creamy	2 tbsp (1.1 oz)	100	4	2	–	13	2	190
Low Sodium	2 tbsp (1.1 oz)	100	4	2	–	13	2	95
Chet's								
Chocolate	2 tbsp	180	7	14	0	10	2	135
Roasted Nut	2 tbsp	180	7	14	0	9	2	130
Earth Balance								
Creamy or Chunky	1 tbsp	190	7	17	0	7	3	110
Jake & Amos								
Schmier	1 tbsp (0.6 oz)	60	2	3	0	8	0	35

FOOD	PORTION	CALS	PROT	FAT	CHOL	CARB	FIBER	SOD
Jif								
Simply	2 tbsp (1.1 oz)	190	8	16	0	6	2	65
Justin's								
Organic Cinnamon	2 tbsp (1.1 oz)	180	7	15	0	8	3	65
Organic Classic	2 tbsp (1.1 oz)	150	7	17	0	7	2	0
Naturally More								
Natural	2 tbsp	169	10	11	0	8	4	130
Organic	2 tbsp	170	10	11	0	8	4	65
PB2								
Powdered Chocolate	2 tbsp	52	4	13	tr	6	1	60
Powdered Chocolate Chip	2 tbsp	53	6	2	0	3	tr	78
Reese's								
Creamy	2 tbsp (1.1 oz)	190	8	16	–	7	3	140
Peanut Butter Chips	1 tbsp (0.5 oz)	80	2	5	–	8	tr	35
Revolution Foods								
Organic Creamy & Crunchy	1 tbsp (1.1 oz)	200	10	16	0	5	2	120
Santa Cruz								
Organic Creamy	2 tbsp (1.1 oz)	210	8	16	0	6	2	50
Skippy								
Creamy	2 tbsp (1.3 oz)	190	7	16	0	7	2	150
Extra Chunky Super Chunk	2 tbsp (1.1. oz)	190	7	16	0	7	2	120
Reduced Fat Creamy	2 tbsp (1.3 oz)	180	7	12	0	15	2	170
Roasted Honey Nut Creamy	2 tbsp (1.1 oz)	190	7	16	0	7	2	125
Smart Balance								
Omega Creamy & Chunky	2 tbsp (1.1 oz)	200	7	17	0	6	2	110
Wonder								
Peanut Spread	2 tbsp	100	4	3	0	13	0	190
Peanut Spread Low Sodium	2 tbsp	100	4	3	0	13	0	95

FOOD	PORTION	CALS	PROT	FAT	CHOL	CARB	FIBER	SOD
PEANUT BUTTER SUBSTITUTES								
NoNuts								
Golden Peabutter	1 tbsp	93	2	7	0	6	1	1
PEANUTS								
chocolate coated	1	21	1	1	0	2	tr	2
chocolate coated	¼ cup	193	5	12	3	18	2	15
cooked w/ salt	½ cup	286	12	20	0	19	8	676
dry roasted w/ salt	28 (1 oz)	164	7	14	0	6	1	230
dry roasted w/ salt	1 oz	166	7	14	0	6	2	230
dry roasted w/o salt	28 (1 oz)	164	7	14	0	6	2	2
dry roasted w/o salt	¼ cup	214	9	18	0	8	3	2
honey roasted	¼ cup	191	8	16	0	8	3	95
sugar coated	¼ cup	203	6	13	0	18	2	61
yogurt coated	¼ cup	230	6	16	0	18	2	24
Fisher								
Butter Toffee	¼ cup (1 oz)	140	3	6	0	18	1	110
Honey Roasted	¼ cup (1 oz)	170	5	13	0	9	2	125
Lance								
Salted	1 pkg (1.1 oz)	200	9	15	0	6	4	150
Nuts Are Good								
Buffalo	1 oz	120	3	6	0	16	2	180
Pina Colada	1 oz	130	3	7	0	16	1	0
Raspberry	1 oz	130	3	7	0	16	1	0
Vanilla Rum	1 oz	130	3	7	0	17	1	0
Planters								
Five Alarm Chili Dry Roasted	39 (1 oz)	160	8	14	0	5	1	160
Honey Roasted	39 (1 oz)	160	6	12	0	8	2	115
Sunfood								
Organic Wild Jungle	1 oz	174	7	14	0	5	2	5
SunRidge Farms								
Chocolate Toffee	6 (1.4 oz)	200	3	11	5	24	1	45
Yogurt Clusters	4 (1.4 oz)	220	6	15	0	17	1	15
True North								
Clusters	6 (1 oz)	170	6	13	0	9	2	75
PEAR								
CANNED								
halves in heavy syrup	1 (1.7 oz)	36	tr	tr	0	9	1	2

FOOD	PORTION	CALS	PROT	FAT	CHOL	CARB	FIBER	SOD
halves in heavy syrup	½ cup (3.5 oz)	74	tr	tr	0	19	3	5
halves in light syrup	1 (2.7 oz)	43	tr	tr	0	12	1	4
halves juice pack	1 (2.7 oz)	38	tr	tr	0	10	1	3
halves juice pack	½ cup (4.4 oz)	62	tr	tr	0	16	2	5
halves light syrup	½ cup (4.4 oz)	72	tr	tr	0	19	2	6
halves water pack	1 (2.7 oz)	22	tr	tr	0	6	1	2
Del Monte								
Halves In 100% Juice	½ cup (4.4 oz)	60	0	0	0	15	1	10
Halves In Heavy Syrup	½ cup (4.6 oz)	100	0	0	0	24	1	10
Halves In Light Syrup	½ cup (4.4 oz)	80	0	0	0	15	1	10
Orchard Select Sliced Bartlett	½ cup (4.4 oz)	70	0	0	0	17	1	10
Liberty Gold								
Bartlett In Heavy Syrup	½ cup (4.5 oz)	90	0	0	0	23	2	10
S&W								
Halves Light Syrup	½ cup (4.4 oz)	80	0	0	0	19	2	10
DRIED								
halves	½ cup (3.2 oz)	236	2	1	0	63	7	50
halves	1 (0.6 oz)	47	tr	tr	0	13	1	1
halves	5 (3 oz)	229	2	1	0	61	7	5
halves cooked w/o sugar	½ cup (4.5 oz)	162	1	tr	0	43	8	4
Bare Fruit								
Organic	1 pkg (0.6 oz)	46	1	0	0	12	2	0
Brothers-All-Natural								
Crisps Asian Pear	1 pkg (0.35 oz)	40	0	0	0	9	1	0
Crispy Green								
Crispy Asian Pears	1 pkg (0.35 oz)	40	0	0	0	8	1	0

FOOD	PORTION	CALS	PROT	FAT	CHOL	CARB	FIBER	SOD
Crunchies								
Freeze Dried	¼ cup (6 g)	20	0	0	0	5	1	0
FRESH								
asian	1 lg (9.6 oz)	116	1	1	0	30	10	0
asian	1 med (4.3 oz)	51	1	tr	0	13	4	0
pear	1 lg (8.1 oz)	133	1	tr	0	36	7	2
pear	1 sm (5.2 oz)	86	1	tr	0	23	5	1
pear	1 med (6.2 oz)	103	1	tr	0	28	6	2
sliced w/ skin	1 cup (4.9 oz)	81	1	tr	0	22	4	1
Chiquita								
Pear	1 (6.2 oz)	103	1	0	0	28	6	2
PEAR JUICE								
nectar canned	1 cup (8.8 oz)	150	tr	tr	0	39	2	10
Ceres								
100% Juice	8 oz	120	0	0	0	31	2	10
Froose								
Perfect Pear	1 box (4.2 oz)	80	0	0	0	18	3	15
Santa Cruz								
Organic Nectar	8 oz	120	0	0	0	30	0	30
Smart Juice								
Organic 100% Juice	8 oz	110	0	0	0	31	2	10
PEAS								
CANNED								
green	½ cup (4.4 oz)	66	4	tr	0	12	4	310
green low sodium	½ cup (4.4 oz)	66	4	tr	0	12	4	11
Del Monte								
Sweet No Salt Added	½ cup	60	3	0	0	11	4	10
Green Giant								
50% Less Sodium Young Tender Sweet	½ cup	60	4	0	0	11	3	200
Young Tender Sweet	½ cup	60	4	0	0	12	3	400

FOOD	PORTION	CALS	PROT	FAT	CHOL	CARB	FIBER	SOD
Le Sueur								
Very Young Small	½ cup (4.2 oz)	60	4	0	0	12	3	380
S&W								
Petit Pois	½ cup (4.4 oz)	60	3	0	0	10	4	360
DRIED								
split cooked w/o salt	1 cup (6.9 oz)	231	16	1	0	41	16	4
Arrowhead Mills								
Organic Green Split not prep	¼ cup	160	12	1	0	24	4	10
Crunchies								
Freeze Dried Organic	¼ cup (0.5 oz)	50	3	1	0	9	3	3
HamPeas								
Green Split Peas as prep	½ cup	120	8	1	0	21	4	63
Jack Rabbit								
Green Split	¼ cup (1.6 oz)	110	11	0	0	27	11	25
Snapea Crisps								
Baked Original	22 (1 oz)	70	5	8	0	14	2	125
SunRidge Farms								
Wasabi Roasted	¼ cup (1 oz)	120	7	1	0	20	2	75
Tree Of Life								
Wasabi Peas	¼ cup (1.1 oz)	120	5	4	0	17	2	130
FRESH								
green cooked w/o salt	½ cup (2.8 oz)	67	4	tr	0	13	4	2
green raw	½ cup (2.5 oz)	59	4	tr	0	10	4	4
snap peas cooked w/o salt	1 cup (5.6 oz)	67	5	tr	0	11	5	6
snap peas raw	10 (1.2 oz)	14	1	tr	0	3	1	1
snap peas raw	1 cup (2.2 oz)	26	2	tr	0	5	2	3
Mann's								
Snow Peas	1 serv (3 oz)	35	2	0	0	6	2	0

FOOD	PORTION	CALS	PROT	FAT	CHOL	CARB	FIBER	SOD
FROZEN								
creamed	1 cup (4.3 oz)	132	6	6	4	15	4	239
green cooked w/o salt	½ cup (2.8 oz)	62	4	tr	0	11	4	58
Birds Eye								
Steamfresh Garlic Baby Peas & Mushrooms	¾ cup	80	4	2	0	12	3	340
Steamfresh Singles Sweet Peas	1 pkg (3.2 oz)	70	5	0	0	13	4	0
C&W								
Alfredo	½ cup	110	6	5	15	11	4	380
Early Harvest Petite No Salt Added	⅔ cup	70	4	0	0	12	4	0
Sugar Snap	⅔ cup	40	2	0	0	7	2	0
Green Giant								
Early June No Sauce	⅔ cup	50	5	1	0	11	4	95
SHELF-STABLE								
TastyBite								
Agra Peas & Greens	½ pkg (5 oz)	138	4	10	3	9	4	417
PECANS								
candied	1 oz	190	tr	17	0	10	5	75
dry roasted	1 oz	187	2	18	0	6	–	0
dry roasted salted	1 oz	187	2	18	0	6	–	260
halves dry roasted w/ salt	20 (1 oz)	200	3	21	0	4	3	110
halves dried	1 cup	721	8	73	0	20	7	1
oil roasted	1 oz	195	2	20	0	5	–	0
oil roasted salted	1 oz	195	2	20	0	5	–	252
Emily's								
Roasted & Salted	¼ cup (1 oz)	210	3	22	0	4	3	118
Fisher								
Roasted & Salted	¼ cup (1 oz)	200	3	21	0	4	3	110
PECTIN								
liquid	1 oz	3	0	0	0	1	1	0
powder	1 pkg (1.75 oz)	162	0	tr	0	45	4	100
Sure Jell								
Fruit Pectin	1 pkg (1.75 oz)	0	0	0	0	0	0	0

FOOD	PORTION	CALS	PROT	FAT	CHOL	CARB	FIBER	SOD
PEPEAO								
dried	¼ cup	18	tr	tr	0	5	–	4
raw sliced	1 cup	25	tr	tr	0	7	–	9
PEPPER								
black	1 tsp	5	tr	tr	0	1	1	1
cayenne	1 tsp	6	tr	tr	0	1	1	1
white	1 tsp	7	tr	tr	0	2	1	0
McCormick								
Lemon Pepper w/ Garlic & Onion California Style	¼ tsp (0.6 g)	0	0	0	0	0	0	30
PEPPERMINT								
fresh chopped	2 tbsp	2	tr	tr	0	tr	tr	1
PEPPERS								
CANNED								
chili green	1 cup (5.5 oz)	29	1	tr	0	6	2	552
chili green hot chopped	½ cup	17	1	tr	0	4	–	–
chili pepper paste	1 tbsp	6	tr	1	–	1	1	1445
chili red hot	1 (2.6 oz)	18	1	tr	0	4	–	–
chili red hot chopped	½ cup	17	1	tr	0	4	–	–
green halves	½ cup	13	1	tr	0	3	–	958
jalapeno chopped	½ cup	17	1	tr	0	3	–	995
red halves	½ cup	13	1	tr	0	3	–	958
Dietz & Watson								
Sweet Roasted	1 oz	5	0	0	0	1	0	55
Gedney								
Hot & Sweet Jalapeno Peppers	¼ cup	30	0	0	0	5	0	260
Hot Banana Pepper Rings	¼ cup	10	0	0	0	1	0	400
Gertie's Finest								
Piquillo	1 oz	10	1	0	0	2	tr	134
Jake & Amos								
Mild Sweet Stuffed	2 tbsp	15	0	0	0	7	0	265
Pace								
Green Chiles Diced	2 tbsp	10	0	0	0	2	tr	100
DRIED								
ancho	1 (0.6 oz)	48	2	1	0	9	4	7
ancho	1 tsp	3	tr	tr	0	1	tr	0
casabel	1 tsp	3	tr	tr	0	1	tr	–

FOOD	PORTION	CALS	PROT	FAT	CHOL	CARB	FIBER	SOD
chipotle smoked	1 tsp	3	tr	tr	0	1	tr	–
green	1 tbsp	1	tr	tr	0	tr	–	1
guajillo	1 tsp	3	tr	tr	0	1	tr	–
mulato	1 tsp	3	tr	tr	0	1	tr	–
pasilla	1 (7 g)	24	1	1	0	4	2	6
pasilla	1 tsp	3	tr	tr	0	1	tr	1
red	1 tbsp	1	tr	tr	0	tr	–	1
FRESH								
banana	1 (4 in) (1.2 oz)	9	1	tr	0	2	1	4
banana	1 cup (4.4 oz)	33	2	1	0	7	4	16
chili green hot	1	18	1	tr	0	4	–	3
chili green hot chopped	½ cup	30	2	tr	0	7	–	5
chili red chopped	½ cup	30	2	tr	0	7	–	5
chili red hot	1 (1.6 oz)	18	1	tr	0	4	–	3
green	1 (2.6 oz)	20	1	tr	0	5	1	1
green chopped	½ cup	13	tr	tr	0	3	1	1
green chopped cooked	½ cup	19	1	tr	0	5	–	1
green cooked	1 (2.6 oz)	20	1	tr	0	5	–	1
habanero	1 tsp	9	1	tr	0	2	1	2
hungarian	1 (0.9 oz)	8	tr	tr	0	2	0	tr
jalapeno	1 (0.5 oz)	4	tr	tr	0	1	tr	tr
jalapeno sliced	1 cup (3.2 oz)	27	1	1	0	5	3	1
red	1 (2.6 oz)	20	1	tr	0	5	1	1
red chopped	½ cup	13	tr	tr	0	3	1	1
red chopped cooked	½ cup	19	1	tr	0	5	–	1
red cooked	1 (2.6 oz)	20	1	tr	0	5	–	1
serrano	1 (6 g)	2	tr	tr	0	tr	tr	1
serrano chopped	1 cup (3.7 oz)	34	2	tr	0	7	4	11
yellow	1 (6.5 oz)	50	2	tr	0	12	–	3
yellow	10 strips	14	1	tr	0	3	–	1
FROZEN								
green chopped	1 oz	6	tr	tr	0	1	–	1
red chopped	1 oz	6	tr	tr	0	1	–	1
C&W								
Strips	¾ cup	25	1	0	0	4	1	10
PERCH								
FRESH								
cooked	3 oz	99	21	1	98	0	0	67

FOOD	PORTION	CALS	PROT	FAT	CHOL	CARB	FIBER	SOD
cooked	1 fillet (1.6 oz)	54	11	1	53	0	0	36
ocean perch atlantic cooked	1 fillet (1.8 oz)	60	12	1	27	0	0	48
ocean perch atlantic cooked	3 oz	103	20	2	46	0	0	82
ocean perch atlantic raw	3 oz	80	16	1	36	0	0	64
raw	3 oz	77	16	1	76	0	0	52
red raw	3.5 oz	114	18	4	–	0	0	80
FROZEN								
Bell								
Cajun Nuggets	12 (4.5 oz)	170	21	3	75	16	1	300
Fillets Breaded	1 piece (4.5 oz)	170	21	3	75	16	tr	510
Fillets Unbreaded	1 piece (3.5 oz)	80	18	1	75	0	0	20
PERSIMMONS								
dried japanese	1 (1.2 oz)	93	tr	tr	0	25	5	1
fresh	1 (6 oz)	118	1	tr	0	31	6	2
PHEASANT								
breast boneless cooked	½ (4.4 oz)	312	41	15	113	0	0	260
cooked diced	1 cup	332	44	16	120	0	0	277
drumstick & thigh cooked	1 (2.6 oz)	184	24	9	67	0	0	154
PHYLLO								
sheet	1 (0.7 oz)	57	1	1	0	10	tr	92
Ekizian								
Sheets	2 (4 oz)	433	12	9	62	76	3	287
Fillo Factory								
Kataifi Shredded Fillo	1 (2 oz)	180	5	2	0	35	4	140
Organic	2 sheets (1.5 oz)	130	4	1	0	27	1	160
Organic Whole Wheat	2 sheets (1.8 oz)	140	4	1	0	30	2	200
Shells Large	1 (0.7 oz)	80	2	2	0	13	0	55
PICANTE (*see* SALSA)								
PICKLES								
bread & butter	6 slices	39	tr	tr	0	9	1	323
dill	1 lg (4.7 oz)	24	1	tr	0	6	2	1731

FOOD	PORTION	CALS	PROT	FAT	CHOL	CARB	FIBER	SOD
dill low sodium	1 med (2.3 oz)	12	tr	tr	0	3	1	12
dill sliced	6 slices	7	tr	tr	0	2	1	497
sweet gherkin	1 (1.2 oz)	41	tr	tr	0	11	tr	329
tsukemono japanese pickles sliced	¼ cup	10	tr	tr	0	2	1	180
Claussen								
Bread 'N Butter Chips	1 oz	20	0	0	0	4	–	180
Kosher Dills Halves	1 (1 oz)	5	0	0	0	1	0	330
Sweet Gerkins	1 (0.9 oz)	30	0	0	0	7	–	210
Dietz & Watson								
New Half Sours	2 pieces (1 oz)	0	0	0	0	0	0	360
Gedney								
Baby Dills	3 (1 oz)	5	0	0	0	1	0	290
Organic Baby Dills	2 (1 oz)	5	0	0	0	1	0	260
Jake & Amos								
Bread & Butter Chips	2 tbsp	20	0	0	0	5	0	288
Texas Sassy								
Pickle Chips	1 tbsp (0.5 oz)	30	0	0	0	7	–	115
Tree Of Life								
Organic Sweet Bread & Butter Chips	4 (1 oz)	30	0	0	0	8	0	180

PIE (*see also* PIE CRUST, PIE FILLING)

FROZEN

FOOD	PORTION	CALS	PROT	FAT	CHOL	CARB	FIBER	SOD
Mrs. Smith's								
Bake & Serve No Sugar Added Apple	1 slice (4.6 oz)	310	3	16	0	40	4	430
Blueberry Crumb	1 slice (4.2 oz)	320	3	14	0	48	2	280
Cherry	1 slice (4.6 oz)	330	3	16	0	44	1	280
Cinnabon Apple Crumb	1 slice (4.6 oz)	350	3	16	0	49	2	340
Classic Cream Key Lime	1 slice (4.2 oz)	410	5	19	15	56	1	200
Coconut Custard	1 slice (4.4 oz)	300	6	17	65	31	1	260
Deep Dish Berry Burst	1 slice (4.2 oz)	340	3	15	0	51	3	240

FOOD	PORTION	CALS	PROT	FAT	CHOL	CARB	FIBER	SOD
Dutch Apple Crumb	1 slice (4.6 oz)	370	3	17	0	52	2	250
Pumpkin Custard	1 slice (4.6 oz)	300	5	15	40	38	2	280
Soda Shoppe Boston Cream	1 slice (2.7 oz)	220	2	9	30	32	0	160
Soda Shoppe Chocolate Cream	1 slice (4.6 oz)	350	4	17	15	47	1	270
Soda Shoppe Lemon Meringue	1 slice (4.2 oz)	300	3	10	40	51	0	190
READY-TO-EAT								
Foods By George								
Gluten Free Pecan Tarts	1 (4 oz)	470	6	26	95	51	3	160
Lance								
Pecan	1 (3 oz)	350	4	17	25	46	3	200
Lifestream								
Pie Oh-My Apple	1 (3.5 oz)	280	3	11	0	43	2	240
Pie Oh-My Pineapple	1 (3.5 oz)	280	3	11	0	45	2	400
TAKE-OUT								
apple one crust	1 slice (5.3 oz)	363	3	14	0	59	2	298
apple tart	1 (4.2 oz)	370	4	19	0	48	1	382
apple two crust	1 slice (5.3 oz)	356	3	17	0	51	2	399
apricot tart	1 (4.2 oz)	356	4	17	0	48	2	362
apricot two crust	1 slice (5.3 oz)	417	5	19	0	59	3	332
banana cream	1 slice (5.1 oz)	387	6	20	73	47	1	346
blackberry one crust	1 slice (4.4 oz)	341	4	17	0	44	4	346
blackberry two crust	1 slice (5.3 oz)	394	4	19	0	54	5	318
blueberry one crust	1 slice (4.8 oz)	292	3	12	0	45	3	211
blueberry tart	1 (4.2 oz)	346	3	17	0	47	2	341
blueberry two crust	1 slice (5.3 oz)	348	3	15	0	52	2	488
cherry one crust	1 slice (4.8 oz)	312	3	12	0	50	2	258

FOOD	PORTION	CALS	PROT	FAT	CHOL	CARB	FIBER	SOD
cherry two crust	1 slice (5.3 oz)	390	3	17	0	60	1	369
chess	1 slice (3 oz)	365	5	18	128	48	1	205
chocolate cream	1 slice (5 oz)	380	7	18	73	50	2	320
coconut creme	1 slice (5 oz)	429	3	24	0	54	2	367
custard	1 slice (4.8 oz)	286	7	16	45	28	2	326
grasshopper	1 slice (3.5 oz)	341	4	19	96	33	1	260
key lime	1 slice (5 oz)	420	4	14	25	71	tr	210
lemon meringue	1 slice (4.8 oz)	367	2	12	62	65	2	200
lemon meringue tart	1 (4.1 oz)	298	4	14	68	41	1	276
mince two crust	1 slice (5.3 oz)	434	4	16	0	72	4	381
peach two crust	1 slice (5.3 oz)	334	3	15	0	49	1	405
pear two crust	1 slice (5.3 oz)	400	4	18	0	57	3	354
pecan	1 slice (4 oz)	456	5	21	36	65	4	483
pineapple two crust	1 slice (5.3 oz)	394	4	18	0	55	2	328
plum two crust	1 slice (5.3 oz)	441	4	21	0	61	2	46
prune one crust	1 slice (5.3 oz)	450	6	14	0	77	2	357
pumpkin	1 slice (5.4 oz)	323	6	15	31	42	4	434
raisin tart	1 (4.2 oz)	348	4	16	0	49	2	265
raisin two crust	1 slice (5.3 oz)	376	4	16	0	55	2	334
raspberry one crust	1 slice (4.8 oz)	330	3	13	5	52	6	212
raspberry two crust	1 slice (5.3 oz)	422	4	20	0	58	5	340

FOOD	PORTION	CALS	PROT	FAT	CHOL	CARB	FIBER	SOD
rhubarb two crust	1 slice (5.3 oz)	444	5	23	0	55	2	412
shoo-fly	1 slice (4 oz)	404	4	13	36	69	1	239
strawberry rhubarb two crust	1 slice (5.3 oz)	422	5	21	20	53	2	382
strawberry two crust	1 slice (6 oz)	386	4	16	0	58	3	284
sweet potato	1 piece (5.4 oz)	276	6	14	57	32	2	205
PIE CRUST								
baked	1/6 crust (1 oz)	147	1	9	0	14	tr	185
chocolate wafer	1/8 crust (1.2 oz)	177	2	11	0	19	1	235
chocolate wafer tart shell	1 (0.8 oz)	111	1	7	0	12	tr	148
deep dish frzn	1/8 crust (1.8 oz)	266	3	16	0	27	1	200
graham cracker	1/6 crust (1.2 oz)	172	1	9	0	23	1	199
graham cracker tart shell	1 (0.8 oz)	109	1	5	0	14	tr	126
puff pastry shell	1 (1.4 oz)	223	3	15	0	18	1	101
tart shell	1 (1 oz)	149	1	10	0	14	tr	188
Honey Maid								
Graham Cracker Crumbs as prep	1/8 pie	160	1	9	0	18	0	192
Keebler								
Graham Reduced Fat	1/8 pie (0.7 oz)	100	1	4	0	15	tr	100
Ready Crust Chocolate	1/8 pie (0.7 oz)	100	1	5	0	14	tr	110
Ready Crust Graham	1/10 pie (0.9 oz)	130	1	6	0	18	tr	140
Ready Crust Shortbread	1/8 pie (0.7 oz)	110	1	5	0	14	0	110
Mrs. Smith's								
Deep Dish Shell frzn	1 slice (1 oz)	130	2	7	0	14	0	110
Nilla Wafers								
Pie Crust	1/6 (1 oz)	140	1	8	5	18	0	85
Pepperidge Farm								
Puff Pastry Sheets frzn	1/6 sheet	170	3	11	0	14	tr	200
Puff Pastry Shell frzn	1	190	4	13	0	16	tr	230

FOOD	PORTION	CALS	PROT	FAT	CHOL	CARB	FIBER	SOD
Pillsbury								
Crusts Just Unroll	⅛ (1 oz)	110	tr	7	<5	12	0	140
Deep Dish frzn	⅛ (0.7 oz)	90	1	5	<5	11	0	85
Pet Ritz Deep Dish frzn	⅛ (0.6 oz)	90	1	5	<5	11	0	85
PIE FILLING								
apple	1 cup	155	tr	tr	0	41	2	6
blueberry	1 cup	474	1	1	0	116	7	31
cherry	1 cup	317	2	2	0	76	2	143
lemon	1 cup	923	13	18	348	185	1	226
pumpkin pie mix canned	1 cup (9.5 oz)	281	3	tr	0	71	22	562
Chukar Cherries								
Triple Cherry	½ cup	190	tr	1	0	47	2	0
Comstock								
Country Cherry Original	⅓ cup (3.1 oz)	90	0	0	0	23	1	25
Farmer's Market								
Organic Pumpkin Pie Mix	½ cup	100	0	0	0	25	2	0
PIEROGI								
potato	1 (1.3 oz)	70	3	2	22	11	1	95
Mrs. T's								
Mini Potato & Cheddar	7 (3 oz)	130	4	2	5	25	1	360
Potato & Cheddar	4 (4 oz)	170	6	3	5	32	1	510
Potato & Onion	3 (4 oz)	160	5	2	5	32	1	390
Potato Broccoli & Cheddar	3 (4 oz)	190	6	5	5	31	2	530
Sauerkraut	3 (4 oz)	140	4	2	5	28	3	670
Sour Cream & Chive	3 (4 oz)	190	5	5	10	32	1	480
PIGEON PEAS								
dried cooked	1 cup	204	11	1	0	39	–	9
dried cooked w/ salt	½ cup (2.9 oz)	102	6	tr	0	20	6	202
PIGNOLIA (*see* PINE NUTS)								
PIG'S FEET								
cooked	1	201	19	14	93	0	0	204
pickled	1	177	12	14	70	tr	0	803
Hormel								
Pigs Feet	2 oz	80	7	6	45	0	0	590

FOOD	PORTION	CALS	PROT	FAT	CHOL	CARB	FIBER	SOD
PIKE								
northern cooked	3 oz	96	21	1	43	0	0	42
northern cooked	½ fillet (5.4 oz)	176	38	1	78	0	0	76
northern raw	3 oz	75	16	1	33	0	0	33
roe raw	1 oz	37	7	tr	103	tr	–	–
walleye baked	3 oz	101	21	1	94	0	0	56
walleye fillet baked	4.4 oz	147	30	2	137	0	0	81
PILLNUTS								
canarytree dried	1 oz	204	3	23	0	1	–	1
PIMIENTOS								
canned	1 tbsp	3	tr	tr	0	1	–	2
canned	1 slice	0	tr	0	0	tr	–	0
PINE NUTS								
pine nuts dried	¼ cup (1.2 oz)	277	5	23	0	4	1	1
pinyon dried	1 oz	178	3	17	0	5	3	20
pinyon dried	20 (2 g)	13	tr	1	0	tr	tr	1
Fisher								
Pine Nuts	¼ cup (1 oz)	190	4	19	0	4	1	0
PINEAPPLE								
CANNED								
in heavy syrup crushed sliced or chunks	1 cup (8.9 oz)	198	1	tr	0	51	2	3
in heavy syrup sliced	1 (1.7 oz)	38	tr	tr	0	10	tr	0
in juice crushed sliced or chunks	1 cup (8.7 oz)	149	1	tr	0	39	2	2
in light syrup crushed sliced or chunks	1 cup (8.8 oz)	131	1	tr	0	34	2	3
in light syrup sliced	1 (1.7 oz)	25	tr	tr	0	6	tr	0
in water crushed sliced or chunks	1 cup (8.6 oz)	79	1	tr	0	20	2	2
juice pack sliced	1 (1.6 oz)	28	tr	tr	0	7	tr	0
water pack sliced	1 (1.6 oz)	15	tr	tr	0	4	tr	0
Del Monte								
Chunks In Heavy Syrup	½ cup (4.3 oz)	90	0	0	0	24	1	10

FOOD	PORTION	CALS	PROT	FAT	CHOL	CARB	FIBER	SOD
Chunks In Its Own Juice	½ cup (4.3 oz)	70	0	0	0	17	1	10
Crushed In Heavy Syrup	½ cup (4.3 oz)	90	0	0	0	24	1	10
Crushed In Its Own Juice	½ cup (4.3 oz)	70	0	0	0	17	1	10
Fruit Naturals Chunks	½ cup (4.4 oz)	70	tr	0	0	18	tr	5
Slices In Heavy Syrup	2 (4 oz)	60	0	0	0	16	1	10
Gefen								
Chunks In Juice	½ cup (4.9 oz)	80	0	0	0	19	1	0
Liberty Gold								
Chunks In Natural Juice	½ cup (4.7 oz)	80	tr	0	0	21	2	10
Slices Natural Juice	½ cup	80	tr	0	0	21	1	10
DRIED								
dried	1 piece (1 oz)	71	1	tr	0	19	2	1
Brothers-All-Natural								
Crisps	1 pkg (0.53 oz)	60	0	0	0	14	1	0
Crispy Green								
Crispy Pineapple	1 pkg (0.35)	35	0	0	0	9	1	0
Crunchies								
Freeze Dried	1 pkg (9 g)	35	0	0	0	8	tr	0
Kopali								
Organic	1 pkg (1.7 oz)	170	0	0	0	43	2	24
Mrs. May's								
Fruit Chips	1 pkg	35	0	0	0	8	1	0
Sunsweet								
Philippine	⅓ cup (1.4 oz)	130	0	0	0	33	2	95
FRESH								
chunks	1 cup (5.8 oz)	82	1	tr	0	22	2	2
slice	1 slice (3 oz)	42	tr	tr	0	11	1	1
whole	1 (2 lbs)	452	5	1	0	119	13	9

FOOD	PORTION	CALS	PROT	FAT	CHOL	CARB	FIBER	SOD
Chiquita								
Bites	1 piece (2.8 oz)	40	1	0	0	9	tr	15
Cut Up	1 cup (5.8 oz)	82	1	0	0	22	2	2
FROZEN								
chunks sweetened	1 cup (8.6 oz)	211	1	tr	0	54	3	5
PINEAPPLE JUICE								
canned unsweetened w/ vitamin C	1 cup (8.8 oz)	132	1	tr	0	32	1	5
frzn unsweetened as prep w/ water	1 cup (8.8 oz)	130	1	tr	0	32	1	2
Ceres								
100% Juice	8 oz	120	0	0	0	29	2	5
Fizzy Lizzy								
Pineapple	1 bottle (12 oz)	100	0	0	0	25	–	0
Sundia								
Purely	½ cup	60	1	0	0	15	1	0
Walnut Acres								
Organic	8 oz	130	0	0	0	32	–	5
PINK BEANS								
dried cooked	1 cup	252	15	1	0	47	–	3
PINTO BEANS								
dried cooked	1 cup	245	15	1	0	45	15	2
Arrowhead Mills								
Organic Dried not prep	¼ cup	150	9	0	0	27	10	0
HamBeens								
Dried as prep	½ cup	120	7	1	0	22	6	63
Tree Of Life								
Organic	½ cup (4.6 oz)	120	8	0	0	23	<9	120
TAKE-OUT								
stewed w/ viandas	1 cup	222	11	8	8	27	6	668
PISTACHIOS								
dry roasted w/ salt	49 nuts (1 oz)	161	6	13	0	8	3	115

FOOD	PORTION	CALS	PROT	FAT	CHOL	CARB	FIBER	SOD
dry roasted w/o salt	49 nuts (1 oz)	162	6	13	0	8	3	3
in shells	½ cup	165	6	13	0	8	3	89
Fisher								
Shelled	¼ cup (1 oz)	160	6	13	0	8	3	110
Love'n Bake								
Pistachio Paste	2 tbsp	160	4	11	0	14	2	0
True North								
Sea Salted In Shells	½ cup	170	6	14	0	7	4	270
Wonderful								
Roasted & Salted In Shells	½ cup	170	6	14	0	8	3	160
PITANGA								
fresh	1	2	tr	tr	0	1	–	0
fresh	1 cup	57	1	1	0	13	–	5
PIZZA (*see also* PIZZA CRUST)								
4Real								
Cheese	1 (4.2 oz)	220	11	4	5	38	5	350
Cheesy Pizza Quesadilla	1 (2.5 oz)	160	11	5	5	15	1	350
Turkey Pepperoni	1 (4.2 oz)	220	11	4	5	38	5	350
A.C. LaRocco								
Thin Crust Whole Grain Cheese & Garlic	⅓ pie (4.8 oz)	250	12	8	15	40	9	340
Thin Crust Whole Grain Greek Sesame	⅓ pie (4.4 oz)	250	12	8	17	40	9	350
Thin Crust Whole Grain Tomato & Feta	⅓ pie (4.8 oz)	250	12	8	15	40	9	340
Ultra Thin Sprouted Grain Bruschetta	½ pie (3.5 oz)	170	11	8	16	17	1	290
Ultra Thin Sprouted Grain Old World Veggie	½ pie (3.6 oz)	170	11	7	15	19	2	260
Amy's								
Cheese & Pesto Whole Wheat Crust	⅓ pie (4.6 oz)	360	13	18	15	37	4	680
Margherita	1 pie (6.2 oz)	360	16	17	10	47	3	720
Non Dairy Cheese Rice Crust	1 pie (6 oz)	460	10	28	0	46	4	680
Pocket Sandwich Spinach Feta	1 (4.5 oz)	260	11	9	20	34	3	590

FOOD	PORTION	CALS	PROT	FAT	CHOL	CARB	FIBER	SOD
Roasted Vegetable No Cheese	⅓ pie (4 oz)	270	6	9	0	42	2	490
Single Serve Spinach Light In Sodium	1 (7.2 oz)	440	19	18	20	54	3	390
Soy Cheese	⅓ pie (4.3 oz)	290	12	11	0	37	2	590
Toaster Pops Cheese Pizza	5–6 pieces (1.9 oz)	160	5	6	5	21	1	220
Bellatoria								
Fire Grilled Flatbread Buffalo Chicken	⅓ pie (5.8 oz)	340	20	17	45	34	5	1050
Fire Grilled Flatbread Chicken Ranch w/ Uncured Bacon	¼ pie (4.5 oz)	270	19	13	45	25	3	750
Ultra Thin Crust Margherita	⅓ pie (4.9 oz)	280	14	16	30	23	1	500
Ultra Thin Crust Ultimate Pepperoni	¼ pie (4.3 oz)	300	16	18	45	21	1	790
Cedarlane								
Zone Cheese	1 (6.5 oz)	380	27	14	30	39	6	700
Dayeinu								
Passover Pizza	1 slice (4 oz)	325	15	8	18	49	5	480
DiGiorno								
Crispy Flatbread Tuscan Chicken	⅓ pie (4.6 oz)	280	14	14	35	25	2	680
For One Thin Crust Grilled Chicken & Vegetable	1 (8.4 oz)	520	28	17	45	64	4	850
For One Traditional Crust Supreme	1 (9.9 oz)	790	31	36	50	85	6	1460
Four Cheese	⅙ pie (4.7 oz)	310	15	11	25	40	2	850
Garlic Bread Pepperoni	⅙ pie (5 oz)	380	17	17	25	40	3	690
Rising Crust Four Cheese	⅓ pie (4 oz)	270	13	9	20	34	2	710
Rising Crust Italian Sausage	⅙ pie (5 oz)	350	15	14	30	40	2	960
Rising Crust Spinach Mushroom Garlic	⅙ pie (5 oz)	290	15	9	15	42	2	790
Rising Crust Three Meat	⅙ pie (5 oz)	350	16	15	30	41	2	1010
Stuffed Crust Pepperoni	⅕ pie (5.3 oz)	380	19	16	40	40	3	1040

FOOD	PORTION	CALS	PROT	FAT	CHOL	CARB	FIBER	SOD
Thin Crispy Crust Pepperoni	⅕ pie (4.4 oz)	320	16	15	35	31	2	790
Thin Crispy Crust Spinach Mushroom Garlic	⅕ pie (4.6 oz)	250	12	9	20	32	3	540
Ultimate Topping Four Meat	⅕ pie (5 oz)	380	19	19	50	34	2	1140
Ultimate Topping Supreme	⅕ pie (5.3 oz)	360	16	18	45	35	2	1010
Farm Rich								
Slices Pepperoni	2 (3.5 oz)	280	14	14	30	22	1	720
Foods By George								
Gluten Free Cheese	1 pie (6.5 oz)	400	20	15	30	44	2	860
Glutino								
Gluten Free Duo Cheese	1 (6.1 oz)	420	10	12	25	68	2	560
Gluten Free Spinach & Feta	1 (6.1 oz)	430	10	16	25	62	4	1000
Health Is Wealth								
Vegetarian Mini Pizza Bagels	4 (3.1 oz)	150	8	0	0	28	3	490
Hot Pockets								
Croissant Five Cheese	1 (4.5 oz)	350	14	17	20	35	2	750
Croissant Pepperoni	1 (4.5 oz)	380	11	22	25	32	2	810
Sausage	1 (4.5 oz)	330	10	16	20	36	2	630
Jeno's								
Crisp 'N Tasty Cheese	1 pie (6.8 oz)	440	16	21	15	47	2	1060
Crisp 'N Tasty Pepperoni	1 (6.7 oz)	490	16	26	20	50	2	1170
Crisp 'N Tasty Supreme	1 (7.2 oz)	490	17	25	20	49	2	1150
Kraft								
Rising Crust Three Meat	⅓ pie (4.4 oz)	320	15	14	30	25	2	880
Lean Pockets								
Pepperoni	1 (4.5 oz)	260	15	7	20	35	3	900
Sausage & Pepperoni	1 (4.5 oz)	280	12	7	25	39	2	630
Lunchables								
Pepperoni Sausage	1 pkg	440	16	12	30	68	3	590
Pizza Deep Dish Cheese	1 pkg	370	10	11	15	60	5	500
Red Baron								
Classic Crust 4 Cheese	1 pie (8.6 oz)	740	33	39	65	62	3	1480

FOOD	PORTION	CALS	PROT	FAT	CHOL	CARB	FIBER	SOD
Simply Shari's								
Gluten Free Cheese	½ pie (5 oz)	290	15	11	65	35	2	780
Gluten Free Pepperoni	½ pie (5 oz)	320	17	13	75	35	2	1000
Gluten Free Pesto Margherita	½ pie (5 oz)	340	14	15	60	36	3	840
Gluten Free Spinach Feta	¼ pkg (5 oz)	280	13	10	65	35	2	890
Gluten Free Vegetable Margherita	¼ pie (5 oz)	220	5	5	40	38	3	700
Stouffer's								
Corner Bistro Flatbread Chicken Bacon & Spinach	1 pkg (9.13 oz)	640	31	29	65	65	3	990
Corner Bistro Flatbread Margherita	1 pkg (9.13 oz)	540	22	22	40	65	4	800
Corner Bistro Flatbread Shrimp & Roasted Garlic	1 pkg (9.33 oz)	600	33	19	115	75	5	610
French Bread Grilled Vegetable	1 pkg (11.63 oz)	340	13	12	15	44	4	570
French Bread Sausage	1 pkg (4.2 oz)	420	15	21	25	43	4	730
French Bread Sausage & Pepperoni	1 pkg (4.2 oz)	460	17	24	30	42	4	880
French Bread White Pizza	1 pkg (10.13 oz)	470	22	23	40	44	4	900
Totino's								
Crisp Crust Canadian Bacon	½ pie (5.1 oz)	320	13	15	10	34	1	910
Crisp Crust Combination	½ pie (5.3 oz)	380	14	21	15	34	1	940
Crisp Crust Pepperoni Trio	½ pie (5 oz)	370	13	21	15	33	1	980
Crisp Crust Three Meat	½ pie (5.2 oz)	350	13	18	15	34	1	870
Pizza Rolls Combination	6 (3 oz)	220	8	11	10	24	1	470
Pizza Rolls Supreme	6 (3 oz)	210	7	9	10	25	2	390
Pizza Rolls Mega Ultimate Combination	3 (3.3 oz)	200	8	8	10	25	1	480
TAKE-OUT								
cheese	16 in pie	3384	151	144	294	372	23	6584
cheese	⅛ of 16 in pie	423	19	18	37	46	3	823
cheese deep dish individual	1 (5.5 oz)	460	15	24	20	47	2	750

FOOD	PORTION	CALS	PROT	FAT	CHOL	CARB	FIBER	SOD
cheese & vegetables	⅛ of 16 in pie	428	17	16	19	55	3	967
ground beef	16 in pie	3753	151	172	299	392	20	8642
ham & pineapple	⅛ of 16 in pie	439	19	16	29	55	3	1110
no cheese	⅛ of 16 in pie	262	6	7	0	43	2	356
pepperoni	⅛ of 16 in pie	469	19	22	37	49	3	1080
white pizza	⅛ of 16 in pie	484	20	17	38	61	2	903
PIZZA CRUST								
crust	1 slice (1.7 oz)	130	4	2	0	25	1	230
whole wheat	⅛ crust (2 oz)	120	4	2	0	24	4	250
Boboli								
100% Whole Wheat	⅕ crust (2 oz)	150	6	3	0	27	5	280
Original	⅛ crust (1.8 oz)	140	5	3	0	24	1	270
Original Mini	½ crust (2.5 oz)	190	6	3	0	35	1	380
Thin Crust	⅕ crust (2 oz)	170	6	4	0	28	1	330
French Meadow Bakery								
Gluten Free	¼ pie (1.9 oz)	160	2	4	0	29	1	310
Martha White								
Mix not prep	¼ pkg	160	5	1	0	32	1	250
Pillsbury								
Classic	⅙ crust (2.3 oz)	160	5	2	0	31	tr	470
Udi's								
Gluten Free	½ crust (4.2 oz)	300	7	9	0	47	2	580
PLANTAINS								
cooked mashed	1 cup	232	2	tr	0	62	5	10
sliced cooked	1 cup	179	1	tr	0	48	4	8

FOOD	PORTION	CALS	PROT	FAT	CHOL	CARB	FIBER	SOD
Grab Em Snacks								
Chips Black Pepper	1 oz	150	tr	8	0	19	2	180
TAKE-OUT								
mofongo	1 serv	320	9	3	7	71	5	1019
ripe fried	1 serv (2.8 oz)	214	1	7	–	38	4	–
sweet baked w/ ice cream	1 serv	285	2	8	0	57	3	65
PLUM JUICE								
Nantucket Nectars								
Red Plum	8 oz	120	0	0	0	30	0	25
Sunsweet								
PlumSmart Light	8 oz	60	0	0	0	15	3	20
PlumSmart w/ Extra Fiber	8 oz	160	0	0	0	36	3	55
PLUMS								
canned in heavy syrup	1 cup	163	1	tr	0	42	3	35
canned purple juice pack	1 cup	146	1	tr	0	38	2	3
canned purple water pack	1 cup	102	1	tr	0	27	2	2
dried japanese	1	9	tr	tr	0	2	tr	96
fresh	1	30	tr	tr	0	8	1	0
pickled	1	34	tr	tr	0	9	tr	0
Chiquita								
Fresh	1 (2.3 oz)	30	0	0	0	8	1	0
Oregon								
Whole In Heavy Syrup	½ cup (4.6 oz)	100	1	0	0	25	2	25
Sunsweet								
Plumsweets Dried	14 pieces (1 oz)	120	1	6	0	19	2	5
POI								
poi	1 cup	240	1	0	0	65	1	29
POKEBERRY SHOOTS								
cooked	½ cup	16	2	tr	0	3	–	–
fresh	½ cup	18	2	tr	0	3	–	–
POLENTA								
Bob's Red Mill								
Corn Grits Polenta not prep	¼ cup	130	3	1	0	27	2	0

FOOD	PORTION	CALS	PROT	FAT	CHOL	CARB	FIBER	SOD
POLLACK								
altantic fillet baked	5.3 oz	178	38	2	137	0	0	166
atlantic baked	3 oz	100	21	1	77	0	0	94
POMEGRANATE								
fresh	1 (5.4 oz)	105	1	tr	0	26	1	5
Navitas Naturals								
Pomegranate Powder	1 tbsp (0.5 oz)	50	0	0	0	13	0	35
POMEGRANATE JUICE								
Apple & Eve								
Organic	8 oz	130	0	0	0	33	–	25
Arthur's								
Pom Plus	1 bottle (11 oz)	220	1	0	0	54	1	25
Frutzzo								
Organic 100% Juice	1 bottle (12 oz)	130	0	0	0	32	0	25
Langers								
100% Juice	8 oz	150	0	0	0	37	–	15
Odwalla								
PomaGrand 100% Juice	8 oz	160	0	0	0	40	0	30
Old Orchard								
100% Pure	8 oz	140	0	0	0	34	–	15
POM								
100% Juice	8 oz	160	0	0	0	40	0	10
Pomegranate Blueberry	8 oz	160	0	0	0	39	0	20
Pomegranate Mango	8 oz	140	0	0	0	36	0	10
Smart Juice								
Organic 100% Juice	8 oz	149	1	0	0	37	1	25
Tart Is Smart								
Concentrate	0.5 oz	37	0	0	0	9	0	2
POMPANO								
smoked	2 oz	109	12	6	33	0	0	215
steamed or poached	4 oz	156	18	9	47	0	0	55
TAKE-OUT								
battered & fried	4 oz	304	20	21	67	8	tr	132
breaded & fried	4 oz	242	16	15	63	10	1	438

FOOD	PORTION	CALS	PROT	FAT	CHOL	CARB	FIBER	SOD
POPCORN								
air popped	1 cup (0.3 oz)	31	1	tr	0	6	2	0
caramel coated	1 cup (1.2 oz)	152	1	5	–	28	2	72
caramel coated w/ peanuts	⅔ cup (1 oz)	114	2	2	0	23	1	84
cheese	1 cup (0.4 oz)	58	1	4	1	6	1	98
oil popped	1 cup (0.4 oz)	55	1	3	0	6	1	97
Deep River Snacks								
Sharp White Cheddar	1 oz	150	3	10	5	13	2	200
Divvies								
Caramel Corn Vegan	½ cup	80	tr	3	0	14	tr	35
I.M. Healthy								
Roasted Sweet Corn Original Lightly Salted	1 oz	120	3	5	0	20	2	46
Jay's								
Caramel	¾ cup	110	tr	0	0	26	1	80
Ok-Ke-Doke Cheese	1 oz	160	2	11	10	13	2	270
Lance								
White Cheddar	1 pkg (0.7 oz)	100	1	11	0	8	2	250
Mrs. Fields								
Clusters Butter Toffee Crunch	⅔ cup	170	2	5	<5	31	3	180
Orville Redenbacher's								
Microwave Smart Pop 94% Fat Free	1 cup	15	4	0	0	3	1	240
Popcorn Indiana								
Kettle Corn Original	2 cups (1 oz)	130	1	5	0	21	2	130
Kettle Corn Smoked Cheddar	2 cups (1 oz)	120	2	4	0	22	2	95
Movie Theater	2 cups (1 oz)	150	2	10	20	14	3	190
Sea Salt	3 cups (1 oz)	130	3	6	0	18	3	190
PopCorners								
Butter	1 oz	120	2	4	0	21	tr	280
Jalapeno	1 oz	130	2	5	0	19	tr	115
Kettle	1 oz	120	2	4	0	21	tr	105
SeaSalt	1 oz	130	2	3	0	22	0	170
White Cheddar	1 oz	130	2	5	0	19	tr	115

FOOD	PORTION	CALS	PROT	FAT	CHOL	CARB	FIBER	SOD
Poppycock								
Cashew Lovers	½ cup (1.1 oz)	148	2	6	5	21	tr	90
Original	½ cup (1.1 oz)	160	2	8	10	20	1	90
Pecan Delight	½ cup (1.1 oz)	150	1	8	10	20	0	90
Smart Balance								
Movie Style as prep	1 cup	35	–	2	0	3	1	24
Smart 'N Healthy as prep	1 cup	20	4	0	0	6	1	0
Snyder's Of Hanover								
Butter	0.6 oz	100	1	8	0	6	1	150
The Whole Earth								
Organic Kettle Corn Salty & Sweet	2 cups (1 oz)	120	2	5	0	20	2	130
Tree Of Life								
Organic Lightly Salted	4 cups	100	3	2	0	21	5	350
Utz								
Butter	2 cups	170	2	12	0	13	2	250
Cheese	2 cups	160	2	11	5	14	3	300
Puff'n Corn Original Hulless	2 cups	150	1	17	0	11	0	150
POPOVER								
home recipe as prep w/ 2% milk	1 (1.4 oz)	87	4	3	46	11	–	82
home recipe as prep w/ whole milk	1 (1.4 oz)	90	4	3	47	11	–	82
mix as prep	1 (1.2 oz)	67	3	2	–	10	–	143
POPPY SEEDS								
poppy seeds	1 tbsp	47	2	4	0	2	1	2
Bob's Red Mill								
Poppy Seeds	3 tbsp	170	6	14	0	6	3	0
Love'n Bake								
Poppy Seed Filling	2 tbsp	120	2	5	0	18	tr	15
PORGY								
fresh	3 oz	77	18	tr	–	0	0	52

FOOD	PORTION	CALS	PROT	FAT	CHOL	CARB	FIBER	SOD
PORK (*see also* HAM, JERKY, PORK DISHES)								
FRESH								
boneless loin lean & fat roasted	3.5 oz	195	26	9	80	0	0	46
center loin chop bone in broiled	1 (3 oz)	178	22	9	71	0	0	46
center rib chop lean & fat bone in broiled	1 (3 oz)	189	21	11	57	0	0	46
country style ribs bone in lean & fat braised	3.5 oz	288	28	19	110	0	0	61
dehydrated oriental style	1 cup (0.8 oz)	135	3	14	15	tr	0	151
fresh ham rump half lean & fat roasted	4 oz	278	32	16	106	0	0	69
fresh ham shank half lean & fat roasted	4 oz	319	28	22	102	0	0	65
fresh ham whole lean & fat roasted	4 oz	302	30	19	104	0	0	66
ground cooked	4 oz	328	28	23	104	0	0	81
ham hock cooked	1	167	14	12	56	0	0	128
shoulder chop bone in braised	1 (3 oz)	229	23	15	84	0	0	49
sirloin roast lean & fat bone in roasted	4 oz	231	27	13	89	0	0	57
spareribs bone in roasted	3 oz	304	18	26	89	0	0	77
tail simmered	3 oz	336	15	30	110	0	0	21
tenderloin roast boneless lean & fat roasted	4 oz	145	26	4	73	0	0	49
top loin chop boneless lean & fat broiled	1 (3.5 oz)	195	27	9	73	0	0	44
Boar's Head								
Smoked Shoulder Butt Roast	3 oz	170	13	13	55	tr	–	760
Dietz & Watson								
Chops Boneless Smoked	3 oz	110	15	3	40	3	0	750
Shoulder Butt	3 oz	150	15	9	50	1	0	740
Spare Ribs Canadian Center Cut	1 serv (5 oz)	300	16	20	76	15	0	500
Hatfield								
Chop Center Cut Boneless	1 (4 oz)	130	19	4	45	2	0	620

FOOD	PORTION	CALS	PROT	FAT	CHOL	CARB	FIBER	SOD
Organic Prairie								
Chop Bone In	1 (3.3 oz)	220	26	13	80	0	0	55
Smithfield								
Boneless Smoked Pork Chop	3 oz	110	15	4	45	4	0	820
Smoked Pork Chop	3 oz	100	14	3	30	2	0	1070
Tyson								
Baby Back Ribs Buffalo	4 oz	300	16	24	80	4	0	1080
Ground Reduced Fat	4 oz	260	18	20	65	0	0	320
Half Loin Boneless	4 oz	190	20	12	45	0	0	270
Loin Chops Bone-In Center Cut	4 oz	190	20	13	45	0	0	330
Spareribs	4 oz	290	16	24	80	0	0	330
Stew Meat	4 oz	130	21	5	65	0	0	300
FROZEN								
Organic Prairie								
Ribs Boneless Country Style	1 (4 oz)	160	23	7	75	0	0	55
Tenderloin	4 oz	150	23	6	75	0	0	55
TAKE-OUT								
char siu chinese style	1 piece (0.4 oz)	28	2	2	7	2	0	72
chicharrones pork cracklings fried	1 cup	492	34	38	100	1	0	2102
chop breaded & fried	1 lg (5 oz)	441	30	26	126	19	1	835
chop breaded & fried	1 med (3.4 oz)	304	20	18	87	13	1	577
chop stewed	1 lg (4.6 oz)	315	36	18	106	0	0	63

PORK DISHES

FOOD	PORTION	CALS	PROT	FAT	CHOL	CARB	FIBER	SOD
A La Carte Gourmet								
Pork Loin w/ Cream Spinach Feta Stuffing	1 serv (5 oz)	200	20	9	85	8	tr	600
Hormel								
Always Tender Loin Filet Honey Mustard	1 serv (4 oz)	140	20	5	45	4	0	510
Always Tender Tenderloin Apple Burbon	1 serv (4 oz)	140	19	4	50	5	0	500
Pork Roast Au Jus	1 serv (2 oz)	90	8	3	25	10	0	510
Tyson								
Roast Pork w/ Vegetables	1 serv (4 oz)	190	21	4	60	18	2	190

FOOD	PORTION	CALS	PROT	FAT	CHOL	CARB	FIBER	SOD
Ventera								
Pork Carnitas	1 serv (5 oz)	190	23	8	70	6	1	390
TAKE-OUT								
kalua pork	1 cup (7 oz)	497	43	34	157	1	0	3498
pork satay w/ peanut sauce	5 sticks (3.5 oz)	214	12	13	74	14	3	318
pulled pork w/ barbecue sauce	1 serv (5 oz)	240	14	14	55	15	1	680
spareribs barbecue w/ sauce	2 med (2.8 oz)	248	17	18	70	3	tr	267
tourtiere	1 piece (4.9 oz)	451	15	34	–	21	–	–

PORK RINDS *(see* SNACKS)

POT PIE

FOOD	PORTION	CALS	PROT	FAT	CHOL	CARB	FIBER	SOD
Amy's								
Broccoli	1 (7.5 oz)	430	11	22	45	46	4	630
Shepherd's	1 (8 oz)	160	5	4	0	27	5	590
Shepherd's Pie Light In Sodium	1 (8 oz)	160	5	4	0	27	5	290
Vegetable	1 (7.5 oz)	360	10	13	0	50	4	640
Banquet								
Beef	1	450	14	27	30	36	2	730
Chicken	1	370	10	21	35	34	2	850
Chicken w/ Broccoli	1	350	10	20	30	32	2	800
Turkey	1	390	10	21	35	36	2	840
Bell & Evans								
Chicken	1 cup (7.9 oz)	520	16	29	80	48	2	630
Hot Pockets								
Pot Pie Express Chicken	1 (4.5 oz)	330	8	18	15	34	2	760
Marie Callender's								
Beef	½ pie	540	16	32	25	46	3	700
Cheeesy Chicken	½ pie	600	17	37	30	46	3	850
Chicken	1	670	19	41	35	55	3	1000
Creamy Mushroom & Chicken	½ pie	560	15	35	30	45	3	700
Turkey	1	670	19	41	25	56	4	1000
Mon Cuisine								
Vegan	1 pkg (9 oz)	650	21	39	0	60	8	850

FOOD	PORTION	CALS	PROT	FAT	CHOL	CARB	FIBER	SOD
Pepperidge Farm								
Chili Beans & Cornbread	1 cup	360	11	17	20	40	3	890
Reduced Fat Roasted White Meat Chicken	1 cup	470	14	21	25	56	0	900
Roasted White Meat Chicken	1 cup	510	13	32	30	43	3	870
Stouffer's								
Chicken White Meat	1 pkg (10 oz)	660	19	37	50	62	2	1060
TAKE-OUT								
beef	1 (14.6 oz)	938	34	57	67	72	5	1660
chicken	1 (14.6 oz)	897	37	52	113	69	6	1080
ham	1 serv (11 oz)	752	28	45	38	58	4	1937
oyster	1 serv (11.5 oz)	817	19	53	89	67	3	1056
puerto rican pastelon de carne	1 piece (5 oz)	666	22	48	93	35	2	1476
st. stephen's day pie	1 serv (16.7 oz)	549	35	29	198	38	6	474
tuna	1 (27 oz)	1715	71	102	92	126	10	1953
vegetarian w/ meat substitute	1 (8 oz)	511	17	32	20	39	5	543

POTATO (*see also* CHIPS, KNISH, PANCAKES)

FOOD	PORTION	CALS	PROT	FAT	CHOL	CARB	FIBER	SOD
CANNED								
potatoes	½ cup	54	1	tr	0	12	–	–
Butterfield								
Whole White	3.5 pieces (5.8 oz)	90	2	0	0	20	2	330
Del Monte								
Savory Sides Au Gratin	½ cup	80	2	3	0	13	1	470
S&W								
New Whole	2 (5.5 oz)	60	1	0	0	13	2	360
Sunshine								
Whole White	3 pieces (5.9 oz)	90	2	0	0	20	2	330
FRESH								
baked skin only	1 skin (2 oz)	115	2	tr	0	27	2	12
baked w/ skin	1 (6.5 oz)	220	5	tr	0	51	–	16

FOOD	PORTION	CALS	PROT	FAT	CHOL	CARB	FIBER	SOD
baked w/o skin	½ cup	57	1	tr	0	13	1	3
baked w/o skin	1 (5 oz)	145	3	tr	0	34	2	8
boiled	½ cup	68	1	tr	0	16	1	3
microwaved	1 (7 oz)	212	5	tr	0	49	–	16
microwaved w/o skin	½ cup	78	2	tr	0	18	–	5
raw w/o skin	1 (3.9 oz)	88	2	tr	0	20	–	7
Masser's								
Roasted Russet Triple Washed	1 (5.3 oz)	110	3	0	0	26	2	0
Melissa's								
Dutch Yellow Baby diced	¾ cup (3.9 oz)	80	2	0	0	20	2	35
FROZEN								
french fries	10 strips	111	2	4	0	17	2	15
french fries thick cut	10 strips	109	2	4	0	17	–	23
hash browns	½ cup	170	2	9	–	22	–	27
potato puffs	½ cup	138	2	7	0	19	–	462
potato puffs	1	16	tr	1	0	2	–	52
Birds Eye								
Steamfresh Roasted Red Potatoes w/ Garlic Butter Sauce	1¼ cups (5.1 oz)	190	3	7	20	30	3	390
Cascadian Farm								
Organic Country Style	¾ cup	50	1	0	0	12	1	10
Organic Hash Browns	1 cup	60	2	0	0	14	1	10
Funster								
BBQ Lite	14 pieces (3 oz)	140	2	3	0	25	<2	500
Cheddar	14 pieces (3 oz)	135	2	3	0	25	<2	385
Original	14 pieces (3 oz)	135	2	3	0	25	2	230
Green Giant								
Roasted Potatoes w/ Garlic & Herb Sauce as prep	½ cup	90	2	2	0	15	1	420
Health Is Wealth								
Twice Baked Cheddar Cheese	1 (5 oz)	200	4	10	10	25	2	340
Vegetarian Potato Skins	2 (2.7 oz)	110	5	7	15	8	1	440

FOOD	PORTION	CALS	PROT	FAT	CHOL	CARB	FIBER	SOD
Joy Of Cooking								
Elegant Scalloped	1 cup (8 oz)	300	9	17	50	21	2	710
Red Skin Mashed	1 cup (4.2 oz)	160	3	9	25	17	2	720
McCain								
5 Minute Fries	1 serv (3 oz)	120	1	5	0	16	1	290
Farmer's Kitchen Oven Baked Crinkles	12 pieces (2 oz)	50	1	1	0	11	1	130
Purely Potatoes Whole Baby Skin On	1 serv (3 oz)	100	2	0	0	16	tr	25
MIX								
au gratin as prep	½ cup	160	6	9	29	14	–	528
instant mashed flakes as prep w/ whole milk & butter	½ cup	118	2	6	15	16	–	349
instant mashed flakes not prep	½ cup	78	2	tr	0	18	–	24
instant mashed granules as prep w/ whole milk & butter	½ cup	114	2	5	15	15	–	270
instant mashed granules not prep	½ cup	372	8	1	0	86	–	67
scalloped	½ cup	105	4	5	14	13	–	409
Betty Crocker								
Au Gratin as prep	⅔ cup	150	2	5	0	24	1	624
Cheddar & Bacon as prep	⅔ cup	120	2	3	0	21	1	696
Cheesy Scalloped as prep	½ cup	120	2	3	0	21	1	600
Julienne as prep	⅔ cup	140	2	5	0	20	1	624
Mashed Four Cheese as prep	½ cup	170	2	7	6	21	1	480
Mashed Sour Cream & Chives as prep	½ cup	170	2	7	6	21	1	456
Scalloped as prep	½ cup	130	2	4	0	20	1	624
Seasoned Skillets Hash Browns as prep	½ cup	120	2	4	0	19	2	456
Idahoan								
Mashed Buttery Homestyle as prep	½ cup	110	2	3	0	20	1	450
Mashed Buttery Yukon as prep	½ cup	110	2	3	0	21	2	400

FOOD	PORTION	CALS	PROT	FAT	CHOL	CARB	FIBER	SOD
Mashed Original as prep	½ cup	170	2	7	0	24	2	456
Mashed Roasted Garlic & Parmesan as prep	½ cup	110	3	2	0	21	2	560
REFRIGERATED								
Bob Evans								
Mashed Potatoes Original	½ cup (4.4 oz)	150	3	7	15	20	2	410
Country Crock								
Garlic Mashed	⅔ cup (5 oz)	160	2	7	10	22	2	430
Homestyle Mashed	⅔ cup (5 oz)	160	2	9	15	18	1	510
Loaded Mashed	⅔ cup (5 oz)	200	4	11	25	22	2	410
Diner's Choice								
Mashed	⅔ cup	110	2	5	10	15	3	500
Reser's								
Potato Express Red Skinned Mashed	½ cup	140	3	5	15	22	2	310
Simply Potatoes								
Traditional Mashed	½ cup (4.4 oz)	120	2	6	20	15	2	420
SHELF-STABLE								
TastyBite								
Bombay Potatoes	½ pkg (5 oz)	105	5	4	0	13	3	412
TAKE-OUT								
au gratin w/ cheese	½ cup	178	7	10	18	17	–	548
baked topped w/ cheese sauce	1	475	15	29	19	47	–	381
baked topped w/ cheese sauce & bacon	1	451	18	26	30	44	–	973
baked topped w/ cheese sauce & broccoli	1 (12 oz)	403	14	21	20	47	–	485
baked topped w/ cheese sauce & chili	1	481	23	22	31	56	–	701
baked topped w/ sour cream & chives	1	394	7	22	23	50	–	182
cheese fries w/ ranch dressing	1 serv	3010	–	–	–	–	–	–
french fries	1 reg	235	3	12	0	29	–	124
hash browns	½ cup (2.5 oz)	151	2	9	9	16	–	290
indian yogurt potatoes	1 serv	315	7	9	18	52	0	216

FOOD	PORTION	CALS	PROT	FAT	CHOL	CARB	FIBER	SOD
mashed	½ cup	111	2	4	2	18	–	309
o'brien	1 cup	157	5	3	7	30	–	421
potato pancakes	1 (1.3 oz)	101	2	7	35	11	–	188
potato salad	½ cup	179	3	10	85	14	2	661
red new boiled	5 sm (5 oz)	120	3	0	0	27	2	5
scalloped	½ cup	127	4	5	7	18	–	435
twice baked w/ cheese	1 half (10 oz)	392	8	18	54	48	4	810
POTATO STARCH								
potato starch	1 oz	96	tr	tr	0	24	–	1
Bob's Red Mill								
Potato Starch	1 tbsp	40	0	0	0	10	0	0
POUT								
ocean baked	3 oz	86	18	1	57	0	0	66
ocean fillet baked	4.8 oz	139	29	2	91	0	0	107
PRETZELS								
chocolate covered	1 (0.4 oz)	47	1	1	1	8	tr	110
soft	1 lg (5 oz)	483	12	4	4	99	2	2008
twists salted	10 (2.1 oz)	229	6	2	0	48	2	1029
twists w/o salt	10 (2.1 oz)	229	5	2	0	48	2	173
whole wheat	2 sm (1 oz)	103	3	1	0	23	2	58
yogurt covered	1 cup (3 oz)	391	7	13	1	61	1	588
yogurt covered	1 (4 g)	19	tr	1	0	3	tr	29
Better Balance								
Cinnamon Toast Gluten Free	1 oz	120	10	5	0	9	3	150
Golden Butter Twists Gluten Free	1 oz	110	10	5	0	12	2	220
Jalapeno Mustard Gluten Free	1 oz	120	10	5	0	9	3	150
Braids								
Honey Wheat	7 (1 oz)	110	3	2	0	23	1	280
Mini Knots	17 (1 oz)	110	3	1	0	23	tr	340
Glenny's								
Organic Original Salted	8 (1 oz)	110	3	0	0	23	1	480
Organic Sourdough	6 (1 oz)	110	3	0	0	23	1	480
Glutino								
Gluten Free All Shapes	44 (1.4 oz)	190	1	8	0	28	0	540

FOOD	PORTION	CALS	PROT	FAT	CHOL	CARB	FIBER	SOD
New York Style								
Pretzel Flatz Original Salt	12	110	3	1	0	23	1	250
Rold Gold								
Braided Twists	1 oz	110	2	1	0	22	1	410
Braided Twists Honey Wheat	1 oz	110	2	1	0	23	1	230
Dipped Twists Fudge Coated	1 oz	140	2	6	0	18	2	140
Mini Sticks Honey Mustard & Onion	1 oz	140	2	6	0	19	1	120
Pretzel Waves Cheddar	1 oz	130	2	5	0	20	1	290
Pretzel Waves Dark Chocolate Drizzle	1 oz	130	2	4	0	20	2	300
Pretzel Waves Vanilla Yogurt Drizzle	1 oz	130	2	5	0	21	tr	250
Sourdough Hard	1	100	2	1	0	21	1	500
Sticks Classic	1 oz	100	2	0	0	23	1	580
Tiny Twists	1 oz	100	3	0	0	23	1	420
Salba Smart								
Omega-3 Enriched	1 oz	110	2	2	0	21	1	330
Snyder's Of Hanover								
100 Calorie Pack Snaps	1 pkg (0.9 oz)	100	3	1	0	22	tr	340
Dips Milk Chocolate	1 oz	140	2	6	<5	19	tr	100
Dips Special Dark Chocolate	1 oz	140	2	5	<5	22	2	130
Gluten Free Sticks	30 (1 oz)	110	0	2	0	25	tr	260
Mini Unsalted	1 oz	110	3	0	0	25	tr	75
MultiGrain Sticks Lightly Salted	1 oz	120	3	2	0	23	3	160
MultiGrain Twists	1 oz	120	3	2	0	22	2	170
Nibblers Sourdough	1 oz	120	3	0	0	25	tr	200
Old Tyme	1 oz	120	3	1	0	24	1	120
Organic Honey Wheat	1 oz	130	3	2	0	24	1	210
Organic Oat Bran	1 oz	120	3	0	0	25	2	320
Pieces Garlic Bread	1 oz	140	3	7	0	18	1	160
Pieces Honey Mustard & Onions	1 oz	140	2	7	0	18	tr	240
Pieces Hot Buffalo Wing	1 oz	140	2	7	0	17	tr	380
Pretzel Sandwich Peanut Butter	1 oz	140	4	7	0	16	tr	140

FOOD	PORTION	CALS	PROT	FAT	CHOL	CARB	FIBER	SOD
Rods	1 oz	120	3	1	0	24	1	290
Snaps	1 oz	120	3	1	0	25	1	270
Sourdough Unsalted	1 oz	100	3	0	0	22	1	90
Sticks 12 Multi Grain	1 oz	130	3	2	0	22	3	180
Superpretzel								
Mozzarella	2 (1.8 oz)	130	6	4	5	20	1	420
Pretzelfils Pizza	2 (1.8 oz)	130	5	2	5	22	1	180
Soft	1 (2.25 oz)	160	5	1	0	34	1	130
Soft Bites	5 (1.9 oz)	150	3	1	0	32	1	912
Softstix	2 (1.8 oz)	130	4	3	1	22	1	260
Tom Sturgis								
Little Cheesers	17 (1 oz)	120	3	2	0	22	2	380
Little Ones	17 (1 oz)	110	2	2	0	22	tr	550
Utz								
Braided Twists Baked Honey Wheat	1 oz	110	3	2	0	23	1	280
Chocolate Covered	6 (1.1 oz)	140	2	5	0	22	tr	220
Hard	1	90	2	0	0	18	tr	470
Special	1 oz	110	3	1	0	21	1	470
Special Multigrain	1 oz	110	3	1	0	21	2	340
Sticks Organic Whole Grain	1 oz	120	3	2	0	22	3	200
PRUNE JUICE								
jarred	1 cup	182	2	tr	0	45	3	10
Lakewood								
Organic	8 oz	165	1	0	0	40	3	5
Old Orchard								
Healthy Balance	8 oz	70	0	0	0	12	5	35
Sunsweet								
100% Juice	8 oz	180	2	0	0	43	3	30
Tree Of Life								
Organic 100% Juice	8 oz	180	1	0	0	43	2	480
PRUNES								
cooked w/o sugar	½ cup	133	1	tr	0	35	4	1
dried	1	20	tr	tr	0	5	1	0
Del Monte								
Dried Pitted	5 (1.5 oz)	100	1	0	0	24	3	5
Earthbound Farms								
Organic Dried Plums	5	110	1	0	0	25	3	0

FOOD	PORTION	CALS	PROT	FAT	CHOL	CARB	FIBER	SOD
Love'n Bake								
Prune Lekvar	2 tbsp	90	0	0	0	21	1	120
Sunsweet								
Ones	4 (1.4 oz)	100	1	0	0	24	3	5
Pitted	5 (1.4 oz)	100	1	0	0	24	3	5
Pitted 60 Calorie Pack	1 pkg (0.9 oz)	60	1	0	0	16	2	0
PUDDING								
READY-TO-EAT								
Jell-O								
100 Calorie Pack Fat Free Chocolate Vanilla Swirl	1 pkg (4 oz)	100	2	0	0	23	tr	190
100 Calorie Pack Fat Free Tapioca	1 pkg (4 oz)	100	1	0	0	23	0	210
Sugar Free Dulce De Leche	1 pkg (3.7 oz)	60	1	1	0	13	0	178
Vanilla	1 serv (4 oz)	110	1	2	0	23	0	190
Kozy Shack								
Banana	1 pkg (4 oz)	130	3	5	15	19	0	120
Chocolate No Sugar Added	1 pkg (4 oz)	60	3	1	10	10	4	130
Old Fashioned Tapioca	1 pkg (4 oz)	130	3	3	10	23	0	130
Original Rice	1 pkg (4 oz)	130	4	3	15	21	0	120
Real Chocolate	1 pkg (4 oz)	140	4	4	10	24	1	135
Rice No Sugar Added	1 pkg (4 oz)	70	4	1	10	11	3	120
Soy Chocolate	1 pkg (4.4 oz)	120	4	2	0	23	2	80
Soy Vanilla	1 pkg (4.4 oz)	110	4	2	0	21	1	80
Tapioca No Sugar Added	1 pkg (4 oz)	70	4	1	5	11	4	135
Vanilla	1 pkg (4 oz)	130	3	3	15	21	0	135
Vanilla No Sugar Added	1 pkg (4 oz)	90	3	3	10	10	4	115
SoYummi								
GoLite Bavarian Cream	1 pkg (3.5 oz)	86	3	3	0	12	–	–
Mousse All Flavors	1 pkg (4.4 oz)	137	4	4	0	21	2	–
Swiss Miss								
Chocolate	1 pkg	150	3	4	0	27	0	190
Low Fat Chocolate	1 pkg	130	3	2	0	26	0	180
Pie Lover's Banana Cream	1 pkg	130	2	4	<5	23	0	170

FOOD	PORTION	CALS	PROT	FAT	CHOL	CARB	FIBER	SOD
Pie Lover's Lemon Meringue	1 pkg	140	0	3	0	28	0	600
Swirl Chocolate Vanilla	1 pkg	140	2	4	0	27	0	160
ZenSoy								
Banana	1 pkg (4 oz)	100	2	1	0	21	1	75
Chocolate	1 pkg (4 oz)	130	3	1	0	29	2	75
Vanilla	1 pkg (4 oz)	110	2	1	0	23	1	75
TAKE-OUT								
blancmange	1 serv (4.7 oz)	154	4	5	–	25	tr	–
bread w/ raisins	1 cup	306	11	9	124	47	2	472
coconut	1 cup	291	8	9	15	45	2	451
corn	1 cup	328	11	13	185	43	4	703
guinataan coconut milk pudding	1 cup (9 oz)	331	2	11	0	59	3	20
indian pudding	½ cup	156	5	4	40	25	1	220
noodle pudding kugel	1 cup	297	9	10	144	44	2	94
plum pudding	1 slice (1.5 oz)	125	2	5	22	20	1	83
pumpkin	½ cup (4.6 oz)	139	3	4	4	24	tr	204
queen of puddings	1 serv (4.4 oz)	266	6	10	–	41	tr	–
rice pudding	1 cup	302	8	4	14	60	1	133
sweet potato	½ cup	107	2	3	1	19	3	310
tapioca	1 cup	236	10	7	156	35	0	312
yorkshire	1 serv (3 oz)	177	6	8	57	22	tr	168
PUFFERFISH								
raw	3 oz	72	17	0	–	0	0	120
PUMMELO								
fresh	1	228	5	tr	0	59	–	7
sections	1 cup	71	1	tr	0	18	–	2
PUMPKIN								
butter	1 tbsp	32	0	0	0	8	–	0
canned w/o salt	1 cup (8.6 oz)	83	3	1	0	20	7	12
cooked mashed w/o salt	1 cup (8.6 oz)	49	2	tr	0	12	3	2
flowers cooked w/o salt	1 cup (4.7 oz)	20	1	tr	0	4	1	8
leaves cooked w/o salt	1 cup (2.5 oz)	15	2	tr	0	2	2	6

FOOD	PORTION	CALS	PROT	FAT	CHOL	CARB	FIBER	SOD
Jake & Amos								
Pumpkin Butter	1 tbsp (0.5 oz)	5	0	0	0	1	0	0
Tree Of Life								
Organic Puree	½ cup (4.3 oz)	50	1	0	0	10	4	5
TAKE-OUT								
indian sago	1 serv (2.3 oz)	75	2	5	0	6	3	222
pumpkin fritters	1 (1.2 oz)	84	1	3	3	14	tr	94
PUMPKIN SEEDS								
kernels dried	¼ cup (1.1 oz)	180	10	16	0	3	2	2
kernels roasted w/o salt	¼ cup (1 oz)	169	9	14	0	4	2	5
whole roasted w/o salt	¼ cup (0.5 oz)	71	3	3	0	9	3	3
Mrs. May's								
Pumpkin Crunch	1 oz	164	9	11	0	8	1	41
Tree Of Life								
Seeds Roasted & Salted	¼ cup (2 oz)	300	13	24	0	8	4	330
PURSLANE								
cooked	1 cup	21	2	tr	0	4	–	51
fresh	1 cup	7	1	tr	0	1	–	20
QUAIL								
cooked bone removed	1 (2.7 oz)	177	19	11	65	0	0	163
QUICHE								
Mrs. Smith's								
Pour-A-Quiche Bacon & Onion	1 serv (4.3 oz)	230	14	16	195	6	0	700
TAKE-OUT								
cheese	⅛ (9 in) pie	566	17	44	240	27	1	459
lorraine	⅛ (9 in) pie	568	17	44	242	27	1	695
mushroom	1 slice (3 oz)	256	9	18	–	17	1	–
spinach	⅛ (9 in) pie	342	11	26	157	17	1	326
QUINCE								
fresh	1	53	tr	tr	0	14	–	4

FOOD	PORTION	CALS	PROT	FAT	CHOL	CARB	FIBER	SOD
QUINCE JUICE								
Smart Juice								
Organic 100% Juice	8 oz	110	1	0	0	31	0	7
QUINOA								
cooked	1 cup (6.5 oz)	222	8	4	0	39	5	13
quinoa not prep	¼ cup (1.5 oz)	156	6	3	0	27	3	2
Alti Plano Gold								
Natural	1 pkg	170	6	3	0	30	5	120
Ancient Harvest Quinoa								
Flakes not prep	¼ cup	159	5	2	0	28	3	8
Organic Inca Red not prep	¼ cup	163	6	3	0	29	4	5
Organic Traditional not prep	¼ cup	172	6	3	0	31	3	1
Simply Shari's								
Quinoa + Marinara Gluten Free as prep	¼ pkg (4 oz)	175	10	2	5	35	5	225
TruRoots								
Organic not prep	¼ cup (1.6 oz)	172	5	3	0	31	3	1
RABBIT								
domestic w/o bone roasted	3 oz	167	25	7	70	0	0	40
wild w/o bone stewed	3 oz	147	28	3	104	0	0	38
RACCOON								
roasted	3 oz	217	25	12	–	0	0	–
RADICCHIO								
raw shredded	½ cup	5	tr	tr	0	1	–	4
RADISHES								
chinese dried	½ cup	157	5	tr	0	37	–	161
chinese raw	1 (12 oz)	62	2	tr	0	14	–	71
chinese raw sliced	½ cup	8	tr	tr	0	2	–	9
chinese sliced cooked	½ cup	13	tr	tr	0	3	–	10
daikon dried	½ cup	157	5	tr	0	37	–	161
daikon raw	1 (12 oz)	62	2	tr	0	14	–	71
daikon raw sliced	½ cup	8	tr	tr	0	2	–	9
daikon sliced cooked	½ cup	13	tr	tr	0	3	–	10

FOOD	PORTION	CALS	PROT	FAT	CHOL	CARB	FIBER	SOD
red raw	10	7	tr	tr	0	2	–	11
red sliced	½ cup	10	tr	tr	0	2	–	14
white icicle raw	1 (0.5 oz)	2	tr	tr	0	tr	–	3
white icicle raw sliced	½ cup	7	1	tr	0	1	–	8
Cadis								
Fresh	6 (2.6 oz)	12	1	tr	0	2	–	18
TAKE-OUT								
korean kimchee	½ cup	31	2	1	–	6	–	–
moo namul saengche korean salad	1 serv (3.7 oz)	34	1	tr	0	8	2	547

RAISINS

FOOD	PORTION	CALS	PROT	FAT	CHOL	CARB	FIBER	SOD
cinnamon coated	¼ cup	108	1	tr	0	29	1	4
cooked	¼ cup	162	1	tr	0	42	1	5
golden seedless	¼ cup	109	1	tr	0	29	1	4
jumbo golden	¼ cup	130	1	0	0	31	2	10
milk chocolate coated	¼ cup	176	2	7	1	31	2	16
milk chocolate coated	28 (1 oz)	109	1	4	1	19	1	10
seedless	55 (1 oz)	86	1	tr	0	23	1	3
sultanas	1 oz	88	1	0	–	23	2	–
Amazin' Raisin								
All Flavors	1 pkg (1 oz)	84	1	0	0	22	2	4
Bob's Red Mill								
Unsulfured	⅓ cup	130	1	0	0	31	3	5
Earthbound Farms								
Organic Jumbo Flame Seedless	¼ cup	120	1	0	0	32	2	0
Emily's								
Milk Chocolate Covered	29 (1.4 oz)	180	2	8	<5	26	2	15
Fool								
Cinnamon Raisin Spread	1 tbsp	20	0	0	0	5	1	0
Godiva								
Milk Chocolate Covered	1 pkg (1.2 oz)	150	2	7	<5	21	1	20
Revolution Foods								
Organic	1 pkg (1.2 oz)	100	1	0	0	28	1	0
Sun-Maid								
Chocolate Covered	30 (1.4 oz)	170	2	6	5	26	1	20

FOOD	PORTION	CALS	PROT	FAT	CHOL	CARB	FIBER	SOD
Golden	¼ cup (1.4 oz)	130	1	0	0	31	2	10
Jumbo	¼ cup (1.4 oz)	130	1	0	0	31	2	10
Seedless	¼ cup (1.4 oz)	130	1	0	0	31	2	10
Snack Box	1 (1 oz)	90	1	0	0	22	2	5
RAMBUTAN								
canned in syrup	1 (0.3 oz)	7	tr	tr	–	2	tr	1
canned in syrup	1 cup (4.3 oz)	123	1	tr	0	31	1	16
puerto rican fresh	5 (1.6 oz)	34	tr	tr	–	8	tr	9
Polar								
In Syrup	½ cup	68	0	0	0	17	tr	10
RASPBERRIES								
black fresh	1 cup	70	2	1	0	16	9	1
canned in heavy syrup	½ cup	116	1	tr	0	30	4	4
canned water pack	1 cup	43	1	1	0	10	5	2
fresh	1 cup	64	1	1	0	15	8	1
fresh	1 pt	162	4	2	0	37	20	3
frzn sweetened	1 cup	129	1	tr	0	33	6	1
frzn unsweetened	1 cup	65	2	1	0	15	8	1
C&W								
Ultimate Red	¾ cup	70	2	0	0	15	7	0
Cascadian Farm								
Organic frzn	1¼ cup	60	1	0	0	17	6	0
Oregon								
In Heavy Syrup	½ cup	120	tr	0	0	30	5	10
Stoneridge Orchards								
Dried Whole	⅓ cup (1.4 oz)	130	1	1	0	32	3	0
RASPBERRY JUICE								
Old Orchard								
Organic 100% Juice	8 oz	120	0	0	0	29	–	25
RED BEANS								
Allens								
Red Beans	½ cup	100	6	1	0	19	9	310

FOOD	PORTION	CALS	PROT	FAT	CHOL	CARB	FIBER	SOD
RELISH								
hamburger	½ cup	158	1	1	0	42	–	1338
hamburger	1 tbsp	19	tr	tr	0	5	–	164
hot dog	1 tbsp	14	tr	tr	0	4	–	164
hot dog	½ cup	111	2	1	0	28	–	1332
piccalilli	1.4 oz	13	tr	tr	–	2	1	–
sweet	1 tbsp	19	tr	tr	0	5	–	122
sweet	½ cup	159	tr	1	0	43	–	990
tomato	¼ cup (2.8 oz)	119	1	tr	0	28	1	1894
Cascadian Farm								
Organic Sweet Relish	1 tbsp (0.5 oz)	15	1	0	0	4	0	65
Claussen								
Sweet Pickle	1 tbsp (0.5 oz)	15	0	0	0	3	0	85
Gedney								
Hot Dog	1 tbsp	18	0	0	0	4	0	100
Organic Sweet	1 tbsp	15	0	0	0	4	0	120
Jake & Amos								
Chow Chow Sweet & Sour	1 serv (4 oz)	140	4	0	0	31	5	110
Corn	2 tbsp	40	1	0	0	8	0	55
Green Tomato	1 serv (1 oz)	25	0	0	0	7	–	90
Patak's								
Brinjal Eggplant Sweet Spicy	1 tbsp	70	0	4	0	8	1	250
Garlic	1 tbsp	45	0	3	0	4	0	300
Lime Mild	1 tbsp	30	0	3	0	0	0	530
Mango Mild	1 tbsp	40	0	4	0	1	0	660
Peloponnese								
Sun Dried Tomato	1 tbsp	25	0	2	0	2	0	200
Texas Sassy								
Pickle Relish	1 tbsp (0.5 oz)	30	0	0	0	7	–	115
Tree Of Life								
Organic Sweet Pickle	1 tbsp (0.5)	15	0	0	0	4	0	120
RENNIN								
tablet	1 (0.9 g)	1	0	0	–	tr	–	234

FOOD	PORTION	CALS	PROT	FAT	CHOL	CARB	FIBER	SOD
RHUBARB								
fresh	½ cup	13	1	tr	0	3	–	2
frozen	½ cup	60	tr	tr	0	3	–	1
frzn as prep w/ sugar	½ cup	139	tr	tr	0	37	–	2
RICE (*see also* RICE CAKES, WILD RICE)								
arborio	½ cup	100	2	0	0	22	–	5
brown long grain cooked	1 cup (6.8 oz)	216	5	2	0	45	4	10
brown medium grain cooked	1 cup (6.8 oz)	218	5	2	0	46	4	2
glutinous cooked	1 cup (6.1 oz)	169	4	tr	0	37	2	9
starch	1 oz	98	tr	0	0	24	–	17
white long grain cooked	1 cup (5.5 oz)	205	4	tr	0	45	1	2
white long grain instant cooked	1 cup (5.8 oz)	162	3	tr	0	35	1	5
white medium grain cooked	1 cup (6.5 oz)	242	4	tr	0	53	1	0
white short grain cooked	1 cup (6.5 oz)	242	4	tr	0	53	–	0
Amy's								
Bowls Brown Rice Black-Eyed Peas & Veggies	1 pkg (8.9 oz)	290	11	11	0	38	8	580
Bowls Brown Rice & Vegetables	1 pkg (9.9 oz)	260	9	9	0	36	5	270
Arrowhead Mills								
Organic Brown Basmati not prep	¼ cup	140	3	2	0	31	2	0
Organic Long Grain Brown not prep	¼ cup	160	3	1	0	32	1	0
Betty Crocker								
Bowl Appetit! Teriyaki Rice	1 bowl (2.5 oz)	260	7	3	0	54	2	1160
Birds Eye								
Steamfresh Whole Grain Brown Rice as prep	1 cup (4.8 oz)	150	4	1	0	31	2	5

FOOD	PORTION	CALS	PROT	FAT	CHOL	CARB	FIBER	SOD
Carolina								
White Medium Grain as prep	1 cup	160	3	0	0	35	1	0
Country Crock								
Cheddar Broccoli Rice	1 cup (7 oz)	270	8	11	20	35	1	790
Gourmet House								
Indian Basmati as prep	¾ cup	160	3	0	0	35	0	0
Italian Arborio as prep	¾ cup	160	3	0	0	37	tr	0
Organic Brown as prep	¾ pkg	150	3	1	0	32	1	0
Organic White as prep	¾ cup	150	3	0	0	35	0	0
Goya								
Yellow Rice not prep	¼ cup (1.6 oz)	160	4	0	0	35	tr	250
Green Giant								
Rice Pilaf	1 pkg (9.9 oz)	200	5	3	5	40	3	1080
White & Wild & Green Beans	1 pkg (9.9 oz)	260	6	5	0	48	3	1260
Knorr								
Asian Side Dish Chicken Fried Rice as prep	1 cup	240	7	1	0	48	1	864
Rice Sides Rice Medley as prep	1 cup	250	6	5	<5	45	1	780
Rice Sides Sesame Chicken w/ Whole Grains as prep	⅔ cup	300	7	9	0	51	3	864
Lundberg								
Eco-Farmed Black Japonica not prep	¼ cup	170	5	2	0	38	3	0
Eco-Farmed California Brown Basmati not prep	¼ cup	160	4	2	0	34	2	0
Eco-Farmed White California Arborio not prep	¼ cup	160	6	0	0	43	1	3
Organic Brown Golden Rose not prep	¼ cup	160	3	1	0	34	1	0
Organic Rice Sensations Ginger Miso not prep	½ cup	116	3	1	0	24	1	150
Organic Risotto Porcini Mushroom not prep	½ cup	143	4	1	0	35	1	535

FOOD	PORTION	CALS	PROT	FAT	CHOL	CARB	FIBER	SOD
Organic White Sushi Rice not prep	¼ cup	150	4	0	0	36	1	0
Organic Wild Blend not prep	¼ cup	150	4	2	0	35	3	0
RiceXpress Chicken Herb	½ pkg (4.4 oz)	250	4	5	0	47	6	670
RiceXpress Santa Fe Grill	½ pkg (4.4 oz)	260	5	5	0	50	3	472
Risotto Butternut Squash not prep	½ cup	143	4	1	0	31	1	496
Mahatma								
Jasmine as prep	¾ cup	160	3	0	0	36	0	0
White as prep	¾ cup	150	3	0	0	35	0	0
Whole Grain Brown as prep	¾ cup	150	3	1	0	32	1	0
Marrakesh Express								
Pilaf Tomato & Basil as prep	1 cup	190	6	0	0	41	0	570
Risotto Parmesan as prep	1 cup	200	5	1	0	42	1	870
Minute								
Brown as prep	⅔ cup	150	3	2	0	34	2	10
Ready To Serve Brown & Wild Rice	1 pkg (4.4 oz)	230	5	5	0	42	5	135
Ready To Serve Pilaf	1 pkg (4.4 oz)	220	5	4	0	41	2	1350
Ready To Serve Spanish Rice	1 pkg (4.4 oz)	230	6	5	0	41	2	420
Ready To Serve Whole Grain Brown	1 pkg (4.4 oz)	230	5	4	0	40	2	175
Steamers Broccoli & Cheese	1 cup (6.4 oz)	200	6	4	5	37	1	720
Steamers Fried Rice	1 cup (6.5 oz)	280	5	6	5	50	2	770
White as prep	1 cup	200	5	0	0	45	0	5
Near East								
Long Grain & Wild Original as prep	1 cup	220	5	4	9	43	2	840
Pilaf Curry as prep	1 cup	220	4	4	9	44	2	696
Pilaf Original as prep	1 cup	220	4	4	9	43	1	816
Pilaf Sesame Ginger as prep	1 cup	270	5	4	6	55	1	528

FOOD	PORTION	CALS	PROT	FAT	CHOL	CARB	FIBER	SOD
Pilaf Spanish Rice as prep	1 cup	310	5	7	21	54	2	1104
Whole Grains Brown Rice as prep	1 cup	210	5	4	9	41	3	696
Patak's								
Basmati	1 pkg	430	9	5	0	87	2	440
Coconut	1 pkg	500	10	12	0	87	4	880
Yellow	1 pkg	440	10	5	0	89	2	1140
Rice A Roni								
Beef as prep	1 cup	310	7	9	0	51	2	1110
Chicken as prep	1 cup	310	7	9	0	51	2	1160
Express Asian Fried	1 cup	280	6	6	0	51	2	710
Fried Rice as prep	1 cup	320	7	11	0	49	2	1490
Garden Vegetable as prep	1 cup	270	6	10	0	41	2	910
Long Grain & Wild as prep	1 cup	250	5	7	0	43	1	760
Lower Sodium Chicken as prep	1 cup	270	7	5	0	51	2	730
Parmesan Chicken as prep	1 cup	370	8	15	5	51	3	1360
Red Beans & Rice as prep	1 cup	290	8	7	0	51	5	1170
Savory Whole Grain Blends Spanish as prep	1 cup	250	5	8	0	42	3	760
Spanish as prep	1 cup	260	6	7	0	44	2	1340
River Rice								
Brown as prep	¾ cup	150	3	0	0	32	1	0
Stahlbush Island Farms								
Organic Brown Rice & Black Beans frzn	1 cup (6.2 oz)	200	8	2	0	39	7	10
Success								
Boil-In-Bag Jasmine as prep	¾ cup	150	3	0	0	36	0	0
Boil-In-Bag White as prep	1 cup	190	4	0	0	43	0	0
Ready To Serve Brown	1 cup	170	3	5	0	28	2	5
TastyBite								
Pilaf Multigrain	½ pkg (5 oz)	200	9	5	0	33	4	440
Pilaf Tandoori	½ pkg (5 oz)	183	3	3	0	37	1	458
Thai Kitchen								
Jasmine not prep	2 tbsp (1.5 oz)	160	3	0	0	36	tr	0

FOOD	PORTION	CALS	PROT	FAT	CHOL	CARB	FIBER	SOD
Uncle Ben's								
Boil-In-Bag Whole Grain Brown Rice	1 cup	170	4	2	0	36	2	0
Long Grain & Wild Herb Roasted Chicken as prep	1 cup	190	5	1	0	39	3	640
Long Grain & Wild Sun-Dried Tomato Florentine as prep	1 cup	180	6	1	0	39	3	580
Ready Rice Spanish	1 cup (5 oz)	200	4	3	0	40	2	620
Ready Rice Whole Grain Medley	1 cup (5 oz)	210	5	4	0	41	4	730
Ready Rice Whole Grain Medley Roasted Garlic	1 cup (4.9 oz)	200	5	3	0	38	3	560
Whole Grain White as prep	1 cup	170	4	1	0	38	4	5
Water Maid								
Medium Grain as prep	¾ cup	160	3	0	0	36	1	0
Zatarain's								
Black Eyed Peas & Rice as prep	1 cup	220	9	1	0	46	4	1330
Caribbean Rice Mix as prep	1 cup	160	3	2	0	34	tr	820
Cheddar Broccoli as prep	1 cup	220	5	2	<5	45	tr	820
Yellow as prep	1 cup	190	4	0	0	43	tr	930
TAKE-OUT								
coconut rice	1 serv	500	6	42	–	30	2	27
congee	½ cup (4.1 oz)	44	1	–	–	10	–	–
dirty rice w/ chicken giblets	1 cup (6.9 oz)	291	11	10	107	38	1	457
nasi goreng indonesian rice & vegetables	1 cup (4.9 oz)	130	4	0	0	28	1	530
pea palau rice & peas fried in ghee	1 serv	144	4	5	21	21	2	145
pilaf	½ cup	84	4	3	22	11	3	362
rice & black beans	1 cup (5.1 oz)	220	7	6	–	36	5	613
risotto	1 serv (6.6 oz)	426	6	18	–	65	3	–
spanish	¾ cup	363	11	27	35	19	–	1339

FOOD	PORTION	CALS	PROT	FAT	CHOL	CARB	FIBER	SOD
RICE CAKES								
Hain								
Mini Munchies Apple Cinnamon	9 (0.5 oz)	60	1	1	0	14	tr	<5
Lundberg								
Eco-Farmed Apple Cinnamon	1 (0.7 oz)	80	2	1	0	18	tr	0
Eco-Farmed Brown Rice Salt Free	1 (0.7 oz)	70	1	0	0	14	tr	0
Eco-Farmed Toasted Sesame	1 (0.7 oz)	70	2	0	0	15	1	65
Organic Caramel Corn	1 (0.7 oz)	80	1	1	0	18	1	40
Organic Green Tea w/ Lemon	1 (0.7 oz)	80	1	0	0	17	1	0
Organic Mochi Sweet	1 (0.7 oz)	70	1	0	0	15	tr	55
Quaker								
Mini Delights Chocolatey Drizzle	1 pkg (0.7 oz)	90	1	4	0	14	1	85
Riceworks								
Sweet Chili	10 (1 oz)	140	2	6	0	19	1	170
Wasabi	10 (1 oz)	140	2	6	0	19	1	140
ROCKFISH								
pacific cooked	1 fillet (5.2 oz)	180	36	3	66	0	0	114
pacific cooked	3 oz	103	20	2	38	0	0	65
pacific raw	3 oz	80	16	1	29	0	0	51
ROE *(see also individual fish names)*								
fresh baked	1 oz	58	8	2	136	1	0	33
ROLL								
FROZEN								
Joy Of Cooking								
Ciabatta Olive Oil Rosemary	1 (1.7 oz)	120	4	2	0	21	1	240
French Baguettes Mini	1 (1.6 oz)	100	3	0	0	20	1	220
Pillsbury								
Dinner Rolls Crusty Sourdough	1 (1.2 oz)	90	4	1	0	17	tr	200
Dinner Rolls Crusty French	1 (1.2 oz)	90	3	1	0	15	tr	190
Dinner Rolls Whole Wheat	1 (1.2 oz)	90	4	1	0	17	3	170

FOOD	PORTION	CALS	PROT	FAT	CHOL	CARB	FIBER	SOD
READY-TO-EAT								
bialy	1 (2.2 oz)	138	14	0	0	32	1	167
brioche sweet roll	1 (3.5 oz)	410	10	23	190	41	3	495
cheese	1 (2.3 oz)	238	5	12	50	29	1	236
cinnamon raisin	1 (2.1 oz)	223	4	10	40	31	1	230
dinner	1 (1 oz)	78	3	1	0	14	1	134
egg	1 (1.2 oz)	107	3	2	16	18	1	191
french	1 (1.3 oz)	105	3	2	0	19	1	231
garlic	1 (1.5 oz)	133	5	3	2	22	1	229
hamburger or hot dog	1 (1.5 oz)	120	4	2	0	21	1	206
hamburger or hot dog multi grain	1 (1.5 oz)	113	4	3	0	19	2	197
hamburger or hot dog reduced calorie	1 (1.5 oz)	84	4	1	0	18	3	190
hamburger or hot dog whole wheat	1 (1.5 oz)	114	4	2	0	22	3	206
hard	1 (2 oz)	167	6	2	0	30	1	310
hoagie or submarine roll whole wheat	1 (4.7 oz)	359	12	6	0	69	10	645
hot cross bun	1	202	5	4	–	38	1	–
mexican bolillo	1 (4.1 oz)	305	10	2	1	60	2	358
oat bran	1 (1.2 oz)	78	3	2	0	13	1	136
oatmeal	1 (1.3 oz)	103	3	2	7	17	1	145
pumpernickel	1 (1.3 oz)	100	4	1	0	19	2	205
rye	1 med (1.3 oz)	103	4	1	0	19	2	321
sourdough	1 (1.6 oz)	130	5	1	0	25	1	292
wheat	1 (1 oz)	76	2	2	0	13	1	95
whole wheat	1 med (1.3 oz)	96	3	2	0	18	3	172
Arnold								
Whole Grains Sandwich 100% Whole Wheat	1 (2.2 oz)	160	8	2	0	26	4	310
Calise								
Kaiser 100% Whole Wheat	1 (2.5 oz)	190	8	3	0	33	3	370
Ecce Panis								
Focaccia	1 (3.2 oz)	260	8	5	0	49	2	480
French Meadow Bakery								
Gluten Free Italian	1 (4.4 oz)	340	3	9	0	63	8	470

FOOD	PORTION	CALS	PROT	FAT	CHOL	CARB	FIBER	SOD
J.J. Cassone								
Sandwich	1 (2.5 oz)	190	7	2	0	38	2	400
Mrs Baird's								
Home Bake	1 (1 oz)	80	2	2	0	13	tr	110
Natural Ovens								
Better Wheat Buns	1 (2.2 oz)	170	7	3	0	30	4	140
Nature's Own								
100% Whole Grain Sugar Free	1 (1.9 oz)	110	6	2	0	23	4	240
Butter Buns	1 (1.7 oz)	120	5	2	5	23	1	115
Pepperidge Farm								
Deli Flats Soft 100% Whole Wheat	1 (1.5 oz)	100	6	2	0	19	5	170
Hamburger 100% Whole Wheat	1 (1.5 oz)	120	6	2	0	18	2	190
Hoagie Soft w/ Sesame Seeds	1	210	7	6	0	35	2	350
Hot & Crusty Sourdough	1	100	4	1	0	21	1	190
Hot Dog	1	140	5	3	0	26	tr	190
Hot Dog Whole Grain White	1	110	6	1	0	21	2	220
Parker House Dinner	1	80	3	2	0	14	tr	95
Premium Wheat	1	220	8	5	0	36	1	310
Sandwich Buns Sesame Seeds	1 (1.6 oz)	130	5	3	0	22	1	220
Rudi's Organic Bakery								
100% Whole Wheat	1 (2.3 oz)	160	7	2	0	29	5	240
Hot Dog Spelt	1 (2 oz)	140	5	2	0	28	2	260
Hot Dog Wheat	1 (2 oz)	150	5	2	0	28	2	260
Hot Dog White	1 (2 oz)	150	5	2	0	28	tr	280
S. Rosen's								
Brat & Sausage Rolls	1 (2.1 oz)	160	6	3	0	28	1	340
Klassic Kaiser	1 (2.6 oz)	230	6	3	0	46	1	420
Stroehmann								
Hot Dog Wheat	1 (1.8 oz)	140	5	3	0	25	2	240
Udi's								
Gluten Free Cinnamon	1 (3 oz)	260	3	7	0	48	2	270
Weight Watchers								
Sandwich Wheat	1 (2 oz)	140	6	2	0	28	5	300

FOOD	PORTION	CALS	PROT	FAT	CHOL	CARB	FIBER	SOD
REFRIGERATED								
crescent	1 (1 oz)	78	3	1	0	14	1	134
Pillsbury								
Crescent Big & Buttery	1 (1.7 oz)	170	3	10	0	20	tr	370
Crescent Butter Flake	1 (1 oz)	110	2	6	0	11	0	220
Crescent Original	1 (1 oz)	110	2	6	0	11	0	220
Crescent Reduced Fat	1 (1 oz)	90	2	5	0	12	0	220
ROSE APPLE								
fresh	3.5 oz	32	1	tr	0	7	–	–
ROSE HIP								
fresh	1 oz	26	1	0	0	5	–	42
ROSELLE								
fresh	1 cup	28	1	tr	0	6	–	3
ROSEMARY								
dried	1 tsp	4	tr	tr	0	1	1	1
fresh	1 tbsp	1	tr	tr	0	tr	tr	0
ROUGHY								
orange baked	3 oz	75	16	1	22	0	0	69
RUBS (*see* HERBS/SPICES)								
RUTABAGA								
cooked mashed	1 cup	94	3	1	0	21	4	602
cubed cooked	1 cup	66	2	tr	0	14	3	427
Glory								
Cut Fresh	1 cup	50	2	0	0	11	4	30
Sunshine								
Diced	½ cup	30	tr	0	0	7	1	220
SABLEFISH								
baked	3 oz	213	15	17	53	0	0	61
fillet baked	5.3 oz	378	26	30	95	0	0	108
smoked	1 oz	72	5	6	18	0	0	206
smoked	3 oz	218	15	17	55	0	0	626
SAFFLOWER								
seeds dried	1 oz	147	5	11	0	10	–	–
SAFFRON								
dried	1 tsp	2	tr	tr	0	tr	tr	1

FOOD	PORTION	CALS	PROT	FAT	CHOL	CARB	FIBER	SOD
SAGE								
ground	1 tsp	2	tr	tr	0	tr	tr	0
SALAD (*see also* SALAD TOPPINGS)								
Dole								
Field Greens	1½ cups (3 oz)	20	1	0	0	4	2	15
Earthbound Farms								
Organic Baby Arugula Salad	2 cups	20	2	0	0	3	1	25
Organic Baby Lettuce Salad	2 cups	15	1	0	0	3	1	60
Organic Baby Spinach Salad	2 cups	10	2	0	0	7	7	100
Organic Fresh Herb Salad	2 cups	15	2	0	0	4	2	70
Organic Mixed Baby Greens	2 cups	15	2	0	0	4	2	70
Fresh Express								
50/50 Mix	3 cups	10	2	0	0	5	4	65
Asian Supreme w/ Dressing as prep	2½ cups	170	3	10	0	17	2	380
Caesar Lite w/ Dressing as prep	2½ cups	100	2	7	10	8	2	360
Caesar w/ Dressing as prep	2½ cups	150	2	13	10	8	2	370
Fancy Field Greens	3 cups	20	1	0	0	3	2	15
Gourmet Cafe Caribbean Chicken as prep	1 pkg (3.5 oz)	120	4	6	10	14	1	190
Gourmet Cafe Chicken Caesar w/ Crostini as prep	1 pkg (3.5 oz)	150	8	11	25	5	1	390
Gourmet Cafe Chopped Turkey Chef as prep	1 pkg (3.5 oz)	120	5	9	15	7	tr	300
Gourmet Cafe Orchard Harvest as prep	1 pkg (3.5 oz)	230	5	18	10	13	2	270
Gourmet Cafe Tuscan Pesto Chicken as prep	1 pkg (3.5 oz)	130	7	8	15	6	1	280
Gourmet Cafe Waldorf Chicken as prep	1 pkg (3.5 oz)	190	7	10	20	19	2	350
More Carrots American	1½ cups	15	1	0	0	3	1	10
Organic Italian	2½ cups	15	1	0	0	3	1	5

FOOD	PORTION	CALS	PROT	FAT	CHOL	CARB	FIBER	SOD
Original Iceberg Garden With Zip	1½ cups	15	1	0	0	3	4	0
Pacifica! Veggie Supreme w/ Dressing as prep	3 cups	220	4	15	10	18	2	340
Spring Mix	3 cups	15	1	0	0	3	2	40
Sweet Baby Greens	3 cups	10	1	0	0	2	1	10
Veggie Lover's	2 cups	20	1	0	0	4	1	15
Lifestyle Foods								
Asian w/ Chicken	1 pkg (8.9 oz)	340	13	16	30	36	3	710
Casear	1 pkg (5 oz)	210	5	11	25	22	2	570
Garden	1 pkg (6.6 oz)	180	4	12	10	14	2	670
Greek	1 pkg (6 oz)	130	3	11	10	6	2	1040
Mann's								
Rainbow	1 serv (3 oz)	25	2	0	0	5	2	25
Ready Pac								
All American	2 cups (3 oz)	15	1	0	0	3	1	15
American Blue Cheese Mix as prep	1¾ cups (3.5 oz)	110	2	8	10	8	1	250
Baby Romaine Blend	4½ cups (3 oz)	20	2	0	0	3	2	90
Baby Spinach Mix as prep	2 cups (3.5 oz)	140	4	3	0	24	2	270
Chef	1 pkg (7.7 oz)	270	15	20	55	10	2	890
Cobb	1 pkg (7.2 oz)	300	13	23	140	7	2	950
Garden	2 cups (3 oz)	15	1	0	0	3	1	10
Grand Asian Mix as prep	1¼ cups (3.5 oz)	130	3	6	0	19	2	260
Spinach Bacon	1 pkg (4.7 oz)	240	12	12	130	19	3	750
Spring Mix	4½ cups	20	2	0	0	4	2	25
Spring Mix Spinach	5 cups (3 oz)	20	2	0	0	4	2	45
Veggie Medley	2 cups (3 oz)	15	1	0	0	4	1	15
TAKE-OUT								
7-layer salad	2 cups	557	11	51	119	15	3	612
caesar	4 cups	734	22	61	173	28	7	1119
chef salad w/o dressing	3 cups	535	52	32	280	9	–	1487

FOOD	PORTION	CALS	PROT	FAT	CHOL	CARB	FIBER	SOD
cobb w/ dressing	4 cups	645	32	49	294	23	11	1512
greek w/ dressing	4 cups	424	28	29	475	14	4	1638
mixed salad greens shredded	1 cup	9	1	tr	0	2	1	16
somen w/ lettuce egg fish pork	2 cups	550	40	17	429	57	4	1229
spinach w/o dressing	4 cups	429	20	19	308	45	6	909
tossed w/ avocado w/o dressing	2 cups	90	2	6	0	9	5	35
tossed w/ chicken w/o dressing	3 cups	194	33	4	86	5	2	108
tossed w/ egg w/o dressing	2 cups	93	7	5	183	6	2	92
tossed w/ shrimp w/o dressing	1½ cups (8.3 oz)	106	15	2	179	7	–	489
tossed w/ shrimp & egg w/o dressing	3 cups	185	30	5	430	5	2	1006
tossed w/o dressing	2 cups	22	1	tr	0	5	2	30
waldorf	1 cup	242	2	21	7	15	3	119
wilted lettuce w/ bacon dressing	1 cup	99	3	8	11	3	1	159

SALAD DRESSING (*see also* SALAD TOPPINGS)

MIX

Good Seasons

FOOD	PORTION	CALS	PROT	FAT	CHOL	CARB	FIBER	SOD
Italian as prep	2 tbsp	130	0	13	0	3	–	336
Italian not prep	⅛ pkg (3 g)	5	0	0	0	1	–	320
J&D's								
Bacon Ranch as prep	2 tbsp	120	0	12	12	3	–	240
READY-TO-EAT								
blue cheese	1 tbsp	77	1	8	–	1	–	–
french	1 tbsp	67	tr	6	–	3	–	214
french reduced calorie	1 tbsp	22	0	1	1	4	–	128
italian	1 tbsp	69	tr	7	–	2	–	116
italian reduced calorie	1 tbsp	16	tr	2	1	1	–	118
japanese ginger salad dressing	2 tbsp	90	–	–	–	–	–	–
russian	1 tbsp	76	tr	8	–	2	–	133
russian reduced calorie	1 tbsp	23	tr	1	1	5	–	141
sesame seed	1 tbsp	68	1	7	0	1	–	153
thousand island	1 tbsp	59	tr	6	–	2	–	109

FOOD	PORTION	CALS	PROT	FAT	CHOL	CARB	FIBER	SOD
thousand island reduced calorie	1 tbsp	24	tr	2	2	3	–	153
Bernstein's								
Chunky Blue Cheese	2 tbsp	120	1	13	5	2	0	180
Creamy Caesar	2 tbsp	120	0	13	15	1	0	200
Italian Restaurant Recipe	2 tbsp	120	1	12	5	1	0	360
Light Fantastic Roasted Garlic Balsamic	2 tbsp	45	0	4	0	3	0	320
Red Wine & Garlic Italian	2 tbsp	110	0	1	0	2	0	250
Bragg								
Ginger & Sesame	2 tbsp	150	0	12	0	2	0	230
Organic Vinaigrette	2 tbsp	150	0	15	0	3	0	120
Cains								
Caesar Creamy	2 tbsp	170	0	19	5	1	0	170
Caesar Fat Free	2 tbsp	30	0	0	0	6	0	600
Caesar Light	2 tbsp	70	2	6	5	5	0	490
Chianti Vinaigrette	2 tbsp	130	0	12	0	5	0	220
Creamy Dill Cucumber Fat Free	2 tbsp	35	0	0	0	8	0	370
French	2 tbsp	120	0	11	0	6	0	170
French Light	2 tbsp	80	0	5	0	10	0	170
Greek	2 tbsp	160	0	17	5	2	0	190
Italian Fat Free	2 tbsp	15	0	0	0	4	0	490
Ranch	2 tbsp	180	0	19	5	1	0	270
Ranch Light	2 tbsp	80	0	6	5	6	0	310
Follow Your Heart								
Lemon Herb	2 tbsp (1 oz)	100	0	11	0	1	0	220
Sesame Miso	2 tbsp (1 oz)	64	1	6	0	3	0	151
Thousand Island	2 tbsp (1 oz)	80	0	8	0	3	tr	230
Gotta Luv It								
Chipotle Lime	2 tbsp	110	0	11	0	3	0	100
Raspberry Balsamic Vinaigrette	2 tbsp	150	0	14	0	6	0	0
Sweet & Tangy Italian	2 tbsp	140	0	15	0	2	0	0
Jake & Amos								
Bacon	2 tbsp (1 oz)	90	1	5	25	10	1	35
Kraft								
Honey Dijon	2 tbsp	100	0	9	0	6	0	250
Italian Creamy	2 tbsp	100	0	11	0	2	0	250
Light Done Right Caesar	2 tbsp	60	1	5	10	3	0	320

FOOD	PORTION	CALS	PROT	FAT	CHOL	CARB	FIBER	SOD
Light Done Right Red Wine Vinaigrette	2 tbsp	45	0	4	0	3	0	310
Ranch Garlic	2 tbsp	120	0	12	0	3	0	360
Special Collection Classic Italian Vinaigrette	2 tbsp	60	0	4	0	5	0	430
Special Collection Parmesan Romano	2 tbsp	140	1	14	10	2	0	360
Special Collection Tangy Tomato Bacon	2 tbsp	100	0	6	0	10	0	350
Thousand Island w/ Bacon	2 tbsp	100	0	8	0	7	0	220
LiteHouse								
Bleu Cheese Bacon	2 tbsp	150	1	16	15	1	0	240
Organic Vinaigrette Raspberry Lime	2 tbsp	40	0	2	0	5	0	55
Ranch Homestyle	2 tbsp	120	0	12	10	2	0	240
Ranch Lite	2 tbsp	70	0	6	5	2	0	220
Sesame Ginger	2 tbsp	35	0	0	0	8	0	230
Spinach Salad	2 tbsp	50	1	0	0	11	0	260
Vinaigrette Huckleberry	2 tbsp	20	0	0	0	4	0	90
Vinaigrette Lite Honey Dijon	2 tbsp	130	0	13	10	3	0	250
Lucini								
Delicate Cucumber & Shallots	2 tbsp (1 oz)	120	0	12	–	2	–	170
Fig & Walnut Savory Balsamic	2 tbsp (1 oz)	110	0	10	–	4	–	180
Roasted Hazelnut & Extra Virgin Olive Oil	2 tbsp (1 oz)	120	1	11	–	3	–	190
Marie's								
Blue Cheese Lite Chunky	2 tbsp	80	1	6	5	7	4	280
Blue Cheese Vinaigrette	2 tbsp	120	2	11	5	4	0	200
Caesar	2 tbsp	170	1	19	15	1	0	170
Coleslaw	2 tbsp	120	0	13	10	8	0	170
Creamy Ranch	2 tbsp	170	1	19	15	1	0	150
Red Wine Vinaigrette	2 tbsp	60	0	5	0	6	0	210
Sesame Ginger	2 tbsp	70	0	8	0	7	0	250
Naturally Fresh								
Balsamic Vinaigrette	2 tbsp	10	0	0	0	2	0	250
Bleu Cheese	2 tbsp	170	1	18	15	1	0	120
Bleu Cheese Bacon	2 tbsp	170	1	18	15	1	0	150

FOOD	PORTION	CALS	PROT	FAT	CHOL	CARB	FIBER	SOD
Bleu Cheese Lite	2 tbsp	100	1	10	10	1	0	130
Buffalo Ranch	2 tbsp	110	0	10	10	4	0	350
Classic Oriental	2 tbsp	100	0	11	0	9	0	140
Ginger	2 tbsp	70	1	7	0	1	0	370
Greek Feta	2 tbsp	100	0	12	5	1	0	270
Honey French	2 tbsp	100	0	11	0	5	0	310
Honey Mustard	2 tbsp	140	1	13	10	5	0	180
Orange Miso	2 tbsp	100	0	9	5	4	0	135
Ranch Classic	2 tbsp	150	1	16	10	1	0	240
Ranch Lite	2 tbsp	80	1	8	5	2	0	240
Slaw	2 tbsp	90	0	10	10	6	0	150
Newman's Own								
Lighten Up Light Balsamic Vinaigrette	2 tbsp (1 oz)	45	0	4	0	2	0	470
OrganicVille								
Herbs De Provence	2 tbsp (1 oz)	100	0	11	0	tr	0	190
Miso Ginger	2 tbsp (1 oz)	100	0	10	0	1	0	250
Orange Cranberry	2 tbsp (1 oz)	100	0	10	0	3	0	190
Pomegranate	2 tbsp (1 oz)	100	0	10	0	2	0	55
Ranch Non Dairy	2 tbsp (1 oz)	90	tr	9	0	1	0	240
Sesame Goddess	2 tbsp (1 oz)	130	1	13	0	2	0	290
Petrini's								
Italian Original	2 tbsp (1 oz)	106	tr	12	0	tr	tr	210
Italian Ranch	2 tbsp (1 oz)	140	0	14	5	1	–	190
School House Kitchen								
Balsamic Vinaigrette Basico	2 tbsp	160	0	17	0	3	0	260
Soy Vay								
Cha-Cha Chinese Chicken	3 tbsp	190	2	15	0	11	0	250
Texas Sassy								
Vinaigrette	2 tbsp (1 oz)	80	0	8	–	4	–	10
Three Acre Kitchen								
Balsamic Vinaigrette	2 tbsp (1.1 oz)	130	0	14	–	3	–	75
Vino De Milo								
Gorgonzola Pear Riesling	2 tbsp	80	0	7	0	2	0	75
Pomegranate Port	2 tbsp	90	0	7	0	5	0	0
Walden Farms								
Sesame Ginger Calorie Free	2 tbsp (1 oz)	0	0	0	0	0	0	260

FOOD	PORTION	CALS	PROT	FAT	CHOL	CARB	FIBER	SOD
Wild Thymes Farm								
Salad Refreshers Black Currant	1 tbsp	36	tr	3	0	3	tr	4
Salad Refreshers Meyer Lemon	1 tbsp	35	0	3	0	3	tr	4
Salad Refreshers Morello Cherry	1 tbsp	34	tr	3	0	3	tr	6
Salad Refreshers Pomegranate	1 tbsp	33	0	3	0	3	0	4
Vinaigrette Mandarin Orange Basil	1 tbsp	43	0	4	0	2	tr	6
Vinaigrette Raspberry Pear	1 tbsp	43	0	4	0	1	tr	7
Vinaigrette Roasted Apple Shallot	1 tbsp	42	0	4	0	2	tr	6
Vinaigrette Toasted Sesame Wasabi	1 tbsp	42	tr	4	0	1	tr	55
Wishbone								
Bountifuls Berry Delight	2 tbsp	35	0	0	0	8	–	210
Bountifuls Tuscan Romano Basil	2 tbsp	25	0	1	0	4	–	340
Western	2 tbsp (1 oz)	160	0	12	0	11	0	230
Western Fat Free	2 tbsp (1 oz)	50	0	0	0	12	0	280
Western Light Just 2 Good	2 tbsp (1 oz)	70	0	2	0	13	0	270
TAKE-OUT								
vinegar & oil	1 tbsp	72	0	8	0	tr	–	tr
SALAD TOPPINGS								
Fresh Gourmet								
Crispy Onions Garlic Pepper	1½ tbsp	35	–	2	0	4	–	50
Tortilla Strips Lightly Salted	2 tbsp	35	–	2	0	5	0	25
Wonton Strips Wasabi Ranch	2 tbsp	35	1	2	0	4	0	45
McCormick								
Salad Toppins	1.3 tbsp (7 g)	35	2	2	0	3	0	70
Salad Toppins Garden Vegetable	1.3 tbsp (7 g)	35	2	2	0	3	0	50
Naturally Fresh								
Fruit & Nut Mix	½ tbsp	45	1	4	0	2	1	20

FOOD	PORTION	CALS	PROT	FAT	CHOL	CARB	FIBER	SOD
Glazed Almond & Pecan Pieces	½ tbsp	40	1	3	0	3	1	0
SALBA								
Salba Smart								
Ground	2 tbsp	65	3	4	0	5	4	2
Whole Grain	1 tbsp	65	3	4	0	5	4	2
SALMON								
CANNED								
w/ bone	½ cup	106	15	5	39	0	0	410
Chicken Of The Sea								
Pink	¼ cup (2.2 oz)	90	12	5	40	0	0	270
Polar								
Pink	¼ cup	90	12	5	40	0	0	270
Sockeye Red	¼ cup	110	13	7	40	0	0	270
Tonnino								
Wild Sockeye In Olive Oil	2 oz	220	16	17	–	tr	tr	450
Wild Planet								
Salmon Wild Alaskan Pink	2 oz	65	12	2	25	0	0	220
Salmon Wild Alaskan Sockeye	2 oz	85	12	4	24	0	0	196
FRESH								
atlantic farmed baked	4 oz	233	25	14	71	0	0	69
coho wild poached	4 oz	209	31	9	65	0	0	30
pink baked	4 oz	169	29	5	76	0	0	97
roe raw	1 oz	59	7	3	–	tr	–	–
sockeye baked	4 oz	245	31	12	99	0	0	75
FROZEN								
Gorton's								
Fillets Classic Grilled	1 (3 oz)	100	15	3	35	2	–	270
SeaPak								
Burgers	1 (3.2 oz)	110	18	3	60	1	0	380
Herb Butter Fillet	1 (5 oz)	350	23	26	105	3	0	280
SMOKED								
lox	1 oz	33	5	1	7	0	0	567
Kasilof Fish Co.								
Wild Alaska Fillet	1 pkg (2 oz)	90	11	4	62	4	0	336

FOOD	PORTION	CALS	PROT	FAT	CHOL	CARB	FIBER	SOD
TAKE-OUT								
guisado salmon stew	1 serv (7.4 oz)	320	26	16	66	18	3	1130
roulette w/ spinach stuffing	1 serv (4 oz)	160	13	6	45	10	tr	400
salmon cake	1 (4.2 oz)	264	16	16	56	14	1	671
salmon loaf	1 slice (3.7 oz)	206	16	11	120	9	tr	819
SALSA								
black bean & corn	2 tbsp	15	1	0	0	3	tr	45
citrus	2 tbsp (1 oz)	10	0	0	0	2	0	7
peach	2 tbsp	15	0	0	0	4	0	90
tomatoless corn & chile	2 tbsp	45	1	0	0	10	tr	95
Amy's								
Organic Black Bean & Corn	2 tbsp (1 oz)	15	1	0	0	3	tr	170
Organic Medium	2 tbsp (1 oz)	10	0	0	0	2	0	190
Bone Suckin'								
Fat Free Gluten Free	2 tbsp	40	0	0	0	10	0	110
Chi-Chi's								
Fiesta Mild	2 tbsp	10	0	0	0	2	0	150
Chukar Cherries								
Peach Cherry	1 tbsp	13	0	0	0	3	tr	65
Clint's								
Texas Medium	2 tbsp (1 oz)	5	0	0	0	1	–	70
Dave's Gourmet								
Insanity	2 tbsp (1 oz)	15	tr	0	0	2	–	170
Dei Fratelli								
Casera Mild	2 tbsp (1.1 oz)	5	0	0	0	2	0	230
DelGrosso								
Chunky Hot	2 tbsp (1.1 oz)	10	0	0	0	3	tr	250
Chunky Mild	2 tbsp (1.1 oz)	10	0	0	0	3	tr	110
Emerald Valley								
Organic Fiesta	1 tbsp (1 oz)	20	tr	0	0	4	tr	125
Organic Green	2 tbsp (1 oz)	10	0	0	0	2	tr	110
Jake & Amos								
Black Bean	2 tbsp (1 oz)	15	0	0	0	3	0	60
Peach	2 tbsp (1 oz)	20	0	0	0	6	0	40
Jala-Fresca								
Green Stuff Medium	2 tbsp	10	0	0	0	2	0	240

FOOD	PORTION	CALS	PROT	FAT	CHOL	CARB	FIBER	SOD
Muir Glen								
Organic Medium	2 tbsp	10	0	0	0	3	0	130
Number 9								
Black Bean & Corn	2 tbsp (1.1 oz)	20	1	0	0	4	1	90
Hot	2 tbsp (1.1 oz)	15	1	0	0	2	1	85
Mild	2 tbsp (1.1 oz)	15	1	0	0	2	1	90
OrganicVille								
Mild	2 tbsp (1 oz)	15	0	0	0	3	0	135
Pineapple	2 tbsp (1 oz)	15	0	0	0	4	0	130
Pace								
Black Bean & Corn	2 tbsp	25	1	0	0	5	1	150
Organic Picante	2 tbsp	10	0	0	0	2	tr	220
Thick & Chunky	2 tbsp	10	0	0	0	2	tr	230
Ready Pac								
Pico De Gallo	2 tbsp (1 oz)	5	0	0	0	2	0	15
Robert Rothchild Farm								
Tomatillo & Pepper	2 tbsp	20	0	0	0	5	tr	95
Salba Smart								
Organic Omega-3 Enriched	2 tbsp	12	0	0	0	2	1	126
Snyder's Of Hanover								
Sweet	2 tbsp	20	0	0	0	5	0	95
Utz								
Sweet	2 tbsp	10	0	0	0	2	tr	160
Walnut Acres								
Organic Fiesta Cilantro	2 tbsp	10	0	0	0	2	0	135
Organic Sweet Southwestern Peach	2 tbsp	20	0	0	0	5	0	85
SALSIFY								
fresh sliced cooked	½ cup	46	2	tr	0	10	–	11
SALT SUBSTITUTES								
gomasio sesame salt	2 tsp	34	1	3	–	2	1	388
AlsoSalt								
Butter Flavored	¼ tsp	1	0	0	0	0	0	0
Garlic Flavored	¼ tsp	1	0	0	0	0	0	0
Original	¼ tsp	1	0	0	0	0	0	0
French's								
No Salt	¼ cup	0	0	0	0	0	0	0
Nu-Salt								
Salt Substitute	1 pkg (1 g)	0	0	0	0	0	0	0

FOOD	PORTION	CALS	PROT	FAT	CHOL	CARB	FIBER	SOD
SALT/SEASONED SALT								
kosher	¼ tsp	0	0	0	0	0	0	730
salt	1 dash (0.4 g)	0	0	0	0	0	0	155
salt	1 tbsp (0.6 oz)	0	0	0	0	0	0	6976
salt	1 tsp (6 g)	0	0	0	0	0	0	2325
sea salt coarse	1 tsp	0	0	0	0	0	0	1320
sea salt fine	¼ tsp	0	0	0	0	0	0	440
BaconSalt								
Original	¼ tsp (1 g)	0	0	0	<5	0	0	135
Peppered	¼ tsp (1 g)	0	0	0	<5	0	0	130
Bob's Red Mill								
Garlic Salt Blend	¼ tsp	0	0	0	0	0	0	335
Sea Salt	¼ tsp	0	0	0	0	0	0	390
Falksalt								
Flake Salt All Flavors	¼ tsp (1.5 g)	0	0	0	0	0	0	580
Lawry's								
Original Seasoned Salt	¼ tsp	0	0	0	0	0	0	380
Maine Coast								
Sea Salt w/ Sea Veg	¼ tsp	0	0	0	0	0	0	396
McCormick								
Grinder Garlic Sea Salt	¼ tsp	0	0	0	0	0	0	125
Grinder Sea Salt	¼ tsp	0	0	0	0	0	0	400
Morton								
Iodized	¼ tsp	0	0	0	0	0	0	590
NutraSalt								
African Medley	1 serv (1g)	0	0	0	0	0	0	55
Sea Salt	1 serv (1g)	0	0	0	0	0	0	118
Seasoned Salt	1 serv (1g)	0	0	0	0	0	0	85
Ocean's Flavor								
Natural Sea Salt	¼ tsp	0	0	0	0	0	0	211
Spice Hunter								
Celery Salt	¼ tsp	0	0	0	0	0	0	270
Garlic Salt	¼ tsp	0	0	0	0	0	0	290
SANDWICHES								
Alexia								
Panini Tuscan Four Cheese w/ Roasted Tomato & Basil	1 pkg (6 oz)	380	18	15	25	42	6	900
Panini Tuscan Grilled Chicken w/ Mozzarella	1 pkg (6 oz)	400	23	18	35	37	5	650

FOOD	PORTION	CALS	PROT	FAT	CHOL	CARB	FIBER	SOD
Panini Tuscan Grilled Steak w/ Mushrooms & Onions	1 pkg (6 oz)	370	22	12	40	43	5	350
Panini Tuscan Smoked Chicken w/ Fire Roasted Vegetables & Parmesan	1 pkg (6 oz)	410	22	19	35	37	5	700
Amy's								
Pocket Sandwich Tofu Scramble	1 (4 oz)	180	11	6	0	23	tr	520
Pocket Sandwich Vegetable Pie	1 (5 oz)	300	8	9	0	45	3	490
Wrap Indian Somosa	1 (5 oz)	250	8	9	0	35	4	680
Aunt Jemima								
Biscuit Sausage Egg & Cheese	1 (4 oz)	340	12	21	110	27	1	830
Croissant Sausage Egg & Cheese	1 (4 oz)	350	13	23	145	22	1	680
Griddlecake Sausage Egg & Cheese	1 (4.4 oz)	350	13	20	150	30	tr	900
Aunt Trudy's								
Fillo Pocket Cheese & Tomato	1 (5 oz)	320	11	15	20	36	2	490
Fillo Pocket Classic Samosa	1 (5 oz)	280	6	10	0	43	3	350
Fillo Pocket Mediterranean Olive & Veggies	1 (5 oz)	270	6	10	0	41	2	550
Organic Fillo Pocket Roasted Sweet Potato	1 (5 oz)	310	5	12	0	45	4	270
Cedarlane								
Wrap Low Fat Couscous & Vegetable Veggie	1 (6 oz)	220	14	3	0	36	3	580
DiGiorno								
Flatbread Melts Chicken Parmesan	1 (6 oz)	380	19	14	35	45	2	750
Fillo Factory								
Organic Fillo Pocket Asian Vegetable	1 (5 oz)	240	5	10	0	34	3	390
Gardenburger								
Wrap Black Bean Chipotle	1 (4.7 oz)	240	13	8	10	32	6	600
Wrap Pizza 100% Meatless Margherita	1 (4.7 oz)	240	12	8	10	34	5	590

FOOD	PORTION	CALS	PROT	FAT	CHOL	CARB	FIBER	SOD
Guiltless Gourmet								
Wrap Black Bean Chipotle	1 (5.7 oz)	270	9	3	0	51	7	570
Wrap California Veggie	1 (5.7 oz)	300	10	5	0	53	6	260
Wrap Mediterranean Spinach	1 (5.7 oz)	270	10	5	<5	45	4	270
Hot Pockets								
Bacon Egg & Cheese	1 (2.2 oz)	160	6	8	40	17	1	240
Barbecue Beef	1 (4.5 oz)	310	11	10	25	42	1	800
Biscuit Sausage Egg & Cheese	1 (4.5 oz)	270	10	11	80	32	2	750
Calzone Four Meat & Four Cheese	½ (4.2 oz)	300	11	13	25	35	2	750
Calzone Pepperoni & Three Cheese	½ (4.2 oz)	330	11	15	25	39	2	780
Chicken Melt	1 (4.5 oz)	300	12	11	30	36	1	610
Croissant Chicken Parmesan	1 (4.5 oz)	340	9	15	10	41	3	810
Croissant Turkey Bacon Club	1 (4.5 oz)	320	12	15	25	34	1	640
Ham & Cheese	1 (4.5 oz)	290	11	11	30	36	1	660
Meatballs & Mozzarella	1 (4.5 oz)	300	11	12	25	36	2	760
Philly Steak & Cheese	1 (4.5 oz)	270	12	9	25	34	2	870
Steak Fajita	1 (4.5 oz)	280	10	12	25	33	2	750
Turkey & Ham w/ Cheese	1 (4 .5 oz)	280	12	10	30	35	1	660
Jimmy Dean								
Bagel Sausage Egg & Cheese	1 (4.8 oz)	380	13	21	115	34	1	770
Biscuit Sausage Egg & Cheese	1 (4.5 oz)	440	13	31	120	27	1	850
Croissant Sausage Egg & Cheese	1 (4.5 oz)	430	13	29	115	30	1	740
D-Lights Croissants Turkey Sausage Egg White & Cheese	1 (4.8 oz)	300	17	12	35	31	4	910
D-Lights Honey Wheat Muffin Canadian Bacon Egg White & Cheese	1 (4.5 oz)	230	15	6	15	30	2	790
Muffin Sausage Egg & Cheese	1 (4.6 oz)	350	13	21	110	28	1	720

FOOD	PORTION	CALS	PROT	FAT	CHOL	CARB	FIBER	SOD
Lean Pockets								
Bacon Egg & Cheese	1 (2.2 oz)	150	6	5	40	18	1	230
Barbecue Beef	1 (4.5 oz)	290	11	7	25	46	2	700
Chicken Cheddar & Broccoli	1 (4.5 oz)	260	11	7	20	40	2	490
Chicken Fajita	1 (4.5 oz)	240	10	7	20	35	3	660
Chicken Parmesan	1 (4.5 oz)	290	11	7	25	45	3	500
Ham & Cheese	1 (4.5 oz)	270	12	7	25	39	2	560
Meatballs & Mozzarella	1 (4.5 oz)	260	14	7	20	35	4	880
Philly Steak & Cheese	1 (4.5 oz)	270	11	7	25	38	1	600
Sausage Egg & Cheese	1 (2.2 oz)	140	6	5	30	18	1	220
Steak Fajita	1 (4.5 oz)	250	10	7	20	36	4	670
Three Cheese & Chicken Quesadilla	1 (4.5 oz)	260	13	7	20	34	3	690
Turkey & Ham w/ Cheddar	1 (4.5 oz)	280	12	7	25	40	2	640
Turkey Broccoli & Cheese	1 (4.5 oz)	270	10	7	25	39	2	450
Lunchables								
Chicken Dunks	1 pkg	310	12	6	30	52	0	550
Cracker Stackers Bologna & American	1 pkg (4.1 oz)	390	14	22	60	34	1	890
Cracker Stackers Ham & Swiss	1 pkg (4.5 oz)	340	20	18	70	23	1	1130
Sub Ham + American	1 pkg	350	13	11	20	49	2	670
Sub Turkey + Cheddar	1 pkg	360	11	8	20	62	4	600
Oscar Mayer								
Deli Creations Honey Ham & Swiss	1 pkg (6.8 oz)	440	28	14	55	51	4	1490
Deli Creations Steakhouse Cheddar	1 pkg (7.1 oz)	450	29	15	60	50	3	1420
Deli Creations Turkey & Cheddar Dijon	1 pkg (6.7 oz)	430	26	15	50	48	5	1410
PBJammerz								
Peanut Butter & Jelly All Flavors	1 (2 oz)	220	8	13	0	22	3	150
Pillsbury								
Toaster Scrambles Cheese Egg & Bacon	1 (1.6 oz)	180	4	12	25	15	0	330
Toaster Scrambles Cheese Egg & Sausage	1 (1.6 oz)	180	4	12	25	15	0	320

FOOD	PORTION	CALS	PROT	FAT	CHOL	CARB	FIBER	SOD
Stouffer's								
Corner Bistro Panini Philly Style Steak & Cheese	1 pkg (6 oz)	340	20	16	40	33	3	680
Corner Bistro Panini Southwestern Chicken	1 pkg (6 oz)	360	20	16	45	31	3	920
Van's								
Breakfast In A Pocket Sandwich Ham Egg & Cheese	1 (4.5 oz)	370	11	22	80	30	tr	550
Breakfast In A Pocket Sandwich Veggie Egg & Cheese	1 (4.5 oz)	340	10	19	80	31	1	510
Breakfast Panini Huevos Rancheros	1 (4.5 oz)	270	11	11	125	33	5	330
Breakfast Panini Sausage Egg & Cheese	1 (4.5 oz)	290	14	13	105	28	3	730
TAKE-OUT								
bacon & egg	1 (6.2 oz)	388	21	21	421	28	1	938
bacon lettuce & tomato w/ mayo	1 (5.8 oz)	344	12	17	21	35	3	945
beef barbecue w/ bun	1 (6.7 oz)	417	32	12	69	42	2	647
calzone beef & cheese	1 (14 oz)	1476	62	76	187	131	6	1726
calzone cheese	1 (15 oz)	1632	80	93	254	117	5	2519
chicken fillet	1 (6.4 oz)	515	24	29	60	39	–	957
chicken fillet w/ cheese	1 (8 oz)	632	29	39	78	42	–	1238
chicken salad	1 (5 oz)	333	19	16	49	28	2	565
crab cake w/ bun	1	308	21	8	97	36	2	578
crispy chicken fillet w/ lettuce tomato & mayo	1 (7.7 oz)	537	27	26	64	49	3	1424
croque monsieur	1 (12.4 oz)	765	41	46	152	43	2	1018
egg salad	1 (5.6 oz)	485	14	35	329	28	1	706
french dip w/ roll	1 (6.8 oz)	357	26	13	54	34	1	562
fried egg	1 (3.4 oz)	226	10	9	206	26	1	439
grilled cheese	1 (2.9 oz)	290	9	16	22	28	1	764
gyro	1 (13.7 oz)	593	44	12	82	74	4	874
ham & egg	1 (4.4 oz)	272	15	11	222	27	2	802
ham w/ cheese lettuce & mayo	1 (5.4 oz)	369	19	18	57	32	2	1525
hot turkey w/ gravy	1	389	40	10	88	32	2	1349
peanut butter	1 (3.3 oz)	342	12	17	0	38	3	568

FOOD	PORTION	CALS	PROT	FAT	CHOL	CARB	FIBER	SOD
peanut butter & banana	1	617	10	14	0	43	4	451
peanut butter & jelly	1 (3.3 oz)	327	10	14	0	42	3	483
reuben w/ sauerkraut & cheese	1 (6.4 oz)	463	21	29	81	30	4	1377
roast beef w/ gravy	1 (7.8 oz)	386	30	16	69	30	2	1083
sloppy joe pork on bun	1 (6.5 oz)	318	23	9	50	34	2	908
tuna melt	1 (5.3 oz)	350	20	16	34	30	1	832
tuna salad w/ lettuce	1 (5.9 oz)	289	19	7	22	37	2	785
turkey w/ mayo	1 (5 oz)	329	29	11	67	26	1	565
SAPODILLA								
fresh	1	140	1	2	0	34	–	20
fresh cut up	1 cup	199	1	3	0	48	–	29
SAPOTES								
fresh	1	301	5	1	0	76	–	21
SARDINES								
CANNED								
atlantic in oil w/ bone	2	50	6	3	34	0	0	121
atlantic in oil w/ bone	1 can (3.2 oz)	192	23	11	131	0	0	465
pacific in tomato sauce w/ bone	1 (1.3 oz)	68	6	5	23	0	0	157
pacific in tomato sauce w/ bone	1 can (13 oz)	658	61	44	225	0	0	1532
King Oscar								
In Extra Virgin Olive Oil	1 can (3.75 oz)	150	14	11	120	0	0	340
Skinless Boneless In Soya Oil	3 pieces (1.9 oz)	120	13	7	20	0	0	350
Polar								
In Mustard	1 can (4.5 oz)	170	17	7	75	10	0	610
In Tomato Sauce	1 can (4.5 oz)	120	17	4	70	5	0	600
In Water	1 can (3 oz)	100	20	3	50	tr	0	140
Wild Planet								
Sardines Wild In Extra Virgin Olive Oil	2 oz	110	10	8	25	0	0	260

FOOD	PORTION	CALS	PROT	FAT	CHOL	CARB	FIBER	SOD
Sardines Wild In Marinara Sauce	2 oz	60	11	2	25	0	0	220
Sardines Wild In Oil w/ Lemon	2 oz	110	10	8	25	0	0	250
Sardines Wild In Spring Water	2 oz	73	13	2	48	0	0	194
FRESH								
raw	3.5 oz	135	19	5	–	0	0	100
SAUCE (*see also* BARBECUE SAUCE, CURRY, GRAVY, SPAGHETTI SAUCE)								
adobo fresco	2 tbsp	81	1	8	0	7	1	6175
bearnaise	1 oz	177	1	19	21	1	tr	257
cheese mix as prep w/ milk	1 cup	307	16	17	53	23	–	1566
enchilada sauce green	¼ cup	46	1	4	11	3	1	113
enchilada sauce red	¼ cup	79	1	8	22	2	1	86
fish sauce chinese	1 tbsp	9	2	0	–	tr	0	1224
fish sauce vietnamese nuoc mam	1 tbsp	6	1	0	0	1	0	1390
hoisin	1 tbsp	35	1	1	0	7	tr	258
moroccan tagine	½ cup (4 oz)	70	2	3	0	10	1	1140
mushroom mix as prep w/ milk	1 cup	228	11	10	34	24	–	1533
oyster	1 tbsp	8	tr	0	0	2	0	437
plum sauce	0.5 oz	42	0	0	–	10	0	281
satay peanut sauce	1 oz	77	2	6	0	3	1	138
sour cream mix as prep w/ milk	1 cup	509	19	30	91	45	–	1007
stroganoff mix as prep	1 cup	271	12	11	38	34	–	1829
sweet & sour mix as prep	1 cup	294	1	tr	0	73	–	779
teriyaki	1 tbsp	15	1	0	0	3	–	690
teriyaki mix as prep	1 cup	131	4	1	0	28	–	4791
white sauce mix as prep w/ milk	1 cup	241	10	13	34	21	–	796
Ahh!Gourmet								
Perky Savory Coffee Sauce	4 tbsp	71	tr	0	0	17	tr	57
Ritzy Kumquat Plum Sauce	4 tbsp	98	tr	0	0	24	1	507
Spicy Garlicky Sweet Sauce Paste	4 tbsp	101	2	4	0	16	2	503
Spicy Ginger Soy Sauce Paste	4 tbsp	137	2	8	0	15	2	612

FOOD	PORTION	CALS	PROT	FAT	CHOL	CARB	FIBER	SOD
Asian Creations								
Marvelous Mango	¼ cup	20	0	0	0	6	0	20
Pad Thai Pizzazz	2 oz	110	2	6	0	14	tr	310
Peanut Passion	¼ cup	130	4	9	0	12	1	420
Bear-Man								
Sap-Happy Golden Bear	2 tbsp	60	0	0	0	20	0	350
Bone Suckin'								
Hiccuppin' Hot	1 tsp	10	0	0	0	2	0	25
Yaki Stir Fry	1 tbsp	30	0	0	0	7	0	260
Burbon Chicken								
Marinade Original	1 tbsp (0.6 oz)	5	0	0	0	1	–	410
Cains								
Tartar	2 tbsp	160	0	16	15	2	0	160
Chef Hymie Grande								
New Mexico Sweet Basting Sauce	2 tbsp (1.2 oz)	35	0	0	0	8	–	15
China Pride								
Duck Sauce Sweet & Pungent	2 tbsp	80	0	0	0	19	1	260
Dave's Gourmet								
Hot Sauce Roasted Garlic	1 tsp (5 g)	0	0	0	0	0	0	90
Insanity Sauce	1 tsp (5 g)	10	0	1	–	0	0	0
Jammin' Jerk	1 tsp (5 g)	5	0	0	0	1	–	15
Steak Sauce	1 tbsp (0.6 oz)	20	0	0	0	5	–	220
Dei Fratelli								
Sloppy Joe Sauce	¼ cup (2.2 oz)	35	1	0	0	9	1	360
DelGrosso								
Sloppy Joe Sauce	¼ cup (2.2 oz)	60	1	1	0	13	1	260
D'Oni								
Happy Together Orange Chili Garlic	2 tbsp	50	0	0	0	12	–	80
Moondance Marinade	1 tbsp	10	–	0	0	0	–	150
Ethnic Gourmet								
Punjab Saag Spinach	4 oz	60	2	3	5	6	1	500
Simmer Sauce Calcutta Masala	4 oz	90	2	5	5	10	1	500
Simmer Sauce Delhi Korma	4 oz	100	2	7	10	9	2	500

FOOD	PORTION	CALS	PROT	FAT	CHOL	CARB	FIBER	SOD
Fischer & Wieser								
Bourbon Charred Pineapple	1 tbsp (0.7 oz)	35	0	0	0	8	0	0
Chipotle Original Roasted Raspberry	1 tbsp (0.7 oz)	40	0	0	0	10	1	60
Chipotle Roasted Blackberry	1 tbsp (0.7 oz)	35	0	0	0	9	–	70
Grilling Chipotle Plum	1 tbsp (0.7 oz)	40	0	0	0	10	–	15
Grilling Spicy Garlic Steak	1 tbsp (0.7 oz)	20	1	1	0	2	0	270
Habanero Mango Ginger	1 tbsp (0.7 oz)	40	0	0	0	11	–	0
Marinade All Purpose Vegetable & Meat	1 tbsp (0.7 oz)	35	0	3	0	3	0	290
Onion Glaze Sweet & Savory	1 tbsp (0.7 oz)	45	0	0	0	11	–	5
Soppin' Big Bold Red	1 tbsp (0.7 oz)	35	1	0	0	7	–	380
Fortun's								
Asian Style Pepper	¼ cup (2 oz)	40	1	1	0	5	0	500
Lemon Dill Caper w/ White Wine	¼ cup (2 oz)	20	0	1	0	3	0	370
Marsala & Mushroom	¼ cup (2 oz)	40	1	1	0	5	0	340
Spicy Mustard w/ Brandy	¼ cup (2 oz)	35	0	2	5	2	0	450
Stroganoff	¼ cup (2 oz)	45	1	3	5	3	0	580
Frank's								
RedHot Chile & Lime Sauce	1 tsp	0	0	0	0	0	0	200
RedHot Original Cayenne Pepper Sauce	1 tsp	0	0	0	0	0	0	200
RedHot X-tra Hot	1 tsp	0	0	0	0	0	0	210
French's								
Worcestershire	1 tsp	0	0	0	0	1	0	50
Good Clean Food								
Simmer Sauce Balsamic Mushroom	⅜ cup (3 oz)	100	2	6	5	9	tr	250
Simmer Sauce Cacciatore	⅜ cup (3 oz)	70	2	4	–	7	2	350
Simmer Sauce Creole	⅜ cup (3 oz)	45	2	2	5	7	1	330
Simmer Sauce Dill	⅜ cup (3 oz)	60	2	4	5	5	–	250

FOOD	PORTION	CALS	PROT	FAT	CHOL	CARB	FIBER	SOD
Simmer Sauce French Tarragon	⅜ cup (3 oz)	90	2	6	5	8	tr	290
Simmer Sauce Mediterranean	⅜ cup (3 oz)	50	1	3	–	6	1	180
Hot Squeeze								
Original	2 tbsp (1 oz)	110	1	0	0	27	–	310
House Of Tsang								
General Tsao	1 tsp	45	0	1	0	10	0	230
Hoisin	1 tsp	15	0	0	0	4	0	120
Kobe Steak Grill	1 tbsp	50	0	4	0	2	0	560
Korean Teriyaki Stir Fry	1 tbsp	35	0	2	0	5	0	460
Peanut Sauce Bangkok Padang	1 tbsp	45	1	3	0	4	0	250
Spicy Brown Bean	1 tbsp	15	0	0	0	3	0	130
Sweet & Sour	1 tbsp	35	0	0	0	8	0	50
Sweet Ginger Sesame	1 tbsp	40	0	1	0	8	0	401
Thai Peanut	1 tbsp	50	1	3	0	4	0	280
Kikkoman								
Black Bean w/ Garlic	1 tbsp (1.2 oz)	50	3	1	0	6	2	1120
Hoisan	2 tbsp (1.2 oz)	80	1	2	0	17	0	460
Katsu	1 tbsp (0.6 oz)	20	0	1	0	5	–	290
Marinade Quick & Easy Honey & Mustard	1 tbsp (0.6 oz)	30	1	0	0	6	–	420
Oyster	1 tbsp (0.6 oz)	25	0	0	0	5	0	860
Peanut Sauce Thai Style	2 tbsp (1.2 oz)	80	2	4	0	10	tr	650
Plum	2 tbsp (1.2 oz)	80	0	1	0	18	0	280
Stir-Fry	1 tbsp (0.6 oz)	20	tr	0	0	4	–	520
Sweet & Sour	2 tbsp (1.2 oz)	35	0	0	0	9	–	190
Teriyaki Less Sodium	1 tbsp (0.5 oz)	15	tr	0	0	3	–	320
Teriyaki Sauce & Marinade	1 tbsp (0.5 oz)	15	1	0	0	2	–	610

FOOD	PORTION	CALS	PROT	FAT	CHOL	CARB	FIBER	SOD
Teriyaki Takumi Original	1 tbsp (0.6 oz)	30	1	0	0	6	–	450
Knorr								
Alfredo Mix as prep	2 oz	60	2	3	5	5	–	390
Bearnaise Mix as prep	2 oz	35	2	1	5	5	–	190
Demi-Glace Mix as prep	2 oz	30	1	1	0	4	–	500
Green Peppercorn Mix as prep	2 oz	35	1	1	5	5	–	390
Hollandaise Mix as prep	2 oz	35	2	1	5	5	–	170
Mango Habanero	1 oz	20	tr	0	0	6	–	95
Sweet Red Chili	1 oz	80	1	0	0	19	–	300
White Mix as prep	2 oz	20	tr	1	0	3	–	290
La Choy								
Sweet & Sour	2 tbsp (1.2 oz)	60	0	0	0	14	0	110
Teriyaki	1 tbsp (0.6 oz)	40	tr	0	0	10	0	570
Latino Chef								
Chimichurri Sun Dried Tomato	2 tbsp	120	2	10	0	8	2	210
Sofrito	2 tbsp	20	0	1	0	3	–	160
Lawry's								
Marinade Szechuan Sweet & Sour BBQ	1 tbsp (0.5 oz)	35	0	0	0	8	–	460
Marinade Tuscan Sun-Dried Tomato	1 tbsp (0.5 oz)	15	0	0	0	2	–	350
Lea & Perrins								
Worcestershire	1 tsp (0.2 oz)	5	0	0	0	1	–	65
Loney's								
Bar-B-Q Chicken as prep	¼ cup (2.1 oz)	15	tr	0	0	3	0	200
Manwich								
Sloppy Joe Original	¼ cup (2.2 oz)	30	1	0	0	7	1	380
McCormick								
Cocktail For Seafood Original	¼ cup (2.1 oz)	90	1	1	0	19	1	970
Seafood Sauce Asian	2 tbsp (1.2 oz)	50	tr	2	0	7	0	470
Seafood Sauce Cajun Style	1 tbsp (1.1 oz)	15	0	0	0	3	0	370

FOOD	PORTION	CALS	PROT	FAT	CHOL	CARB	FIBER	SOD
Seafood Sauce Scampi	1 tbsp (1 oz)	160	0	17	0	2	0	220
Tartar Fat Free	2 tbsp (1.1 oz)	30	0	0	0	7	1	250
Tartar Original	2 tbsp (1 oz)	140	0	14	20	3	0	190
Mrs. Dash								
10 Minute Marinade Lemon Herb Peppercorn	1 tbsp (0.5 oz)	25	0	2	–	2	–	0
10 Minute Marinade Mesquite Grille	1 tbsp (0.5 oz)	25	0	2	–	2	–	0
10 Minute Marinade Spicy Teriyaki	1 tbsp (0.5 oz)	25	0	1	–	5	–	0
10 Minute Marinade Zesty Garlic Herb	1 tbsp (0.5 oz)	25	0	2	–	3	–	0
Naturally Fresh								
Seafood Cocktail	2 tbsp	25	0	0	0	5	0	210
Tartar Sauce	2 tbsp	130	0	14	10	2	0	85
Old Bay								
Tartar Sauce	2 tbsp (1.1 oz)	130	0	12	15	3	0	210
Old El Paso								
Enchilada Mild	¼ cup	25	0	1	0	4	0	250
OrganicVille								
Island Teriyaki	1 tbsp (0.5 oz)	25	tr	1	0	4	0	240
Pace								
Taco Sauce Green	1 tbsp	5	0	0	0	1	0	100
Taco Sauce Red	2 tbsp	10	0	0	0	2	0	130
Patak's								
Jalfrezi Sweet Peppers & Coconut	½ cup	140	2	8	0	15	1	620
Korma Rich Creamy Coconut	½ cup	240	2	20	15	13	1	750
Rogan Josh Spicy Tomato & Cardamom	½ cup	90	2	4	0	12	2	750
Tikka Masala Tangy Lemon & Cilantro	½ cup	120	1	8	0	12	1	900
Progresso								
Bruschetta	2 tbsp (1 oz)	10	0	1	0	1	0	100

FOOD	PORTION	CALS	PROT	FAT	CHOL	CARB	FIBER	SOD
Road's End Organics								
Alfredo Style Dairy Free Gluten Free	⅓ pkg	35	3	0	0	5	1	240
Cheddar Style Dairy Free	⅓ pkg	35	2	0	0	6	1	260
Robert Rothchild Farm								
Anne Mae's Smoky Sweet Chipotle	2 tbsp	35	tr	0	0	9	0	80
Saucy Susan								
Peach Apricot	2 tbsp (1.3 oz)	80	0	0	0	19	2	260
Simply Boulder								
Coconut Peanut	2 tbsp (1 oz)	90	2	7	0	6	0	140
Lemon Pesto	2 tbsp (1 oz)	50	0	5	0	3	0	200
Zesty Pineapple	2 tbsp (1 oz)	45	0	3	0	7	0	85
Soy Vay								
Hoisin Garlic Asian Glaze & Marinade	1 tbsp	40	1	1	0	7	0	400
Veri Veri Teriyaki	1 tbsp	35	0	1	0	6	0	490
Steel's								
Cocktail w/ Dill & Lemon Sugar Free Gluten Free	¼ cup (2.4 oz)	35	2	0	0	9	2	85
Hoisin No Sugar Added Gluten Free	2 tbsp (1 oz)	30	1	0	0	6	1	330
Tabasco								
Pepper Sauce	1 tsp	0	0	0	0	0	0	40
Texas Sassy								
Marinade Salsa	1 tbsp (0.5 oz)	15	0	0	0	3	–	45
Pickle Sauce	1 tbsp (0.5 oz)	30	0	0	0	7	–	115
Thai Kitchen								
Premium Fish Sauce	1 tbsp (0.5 oz)	10	2	0	0	0	0	1360
The Gracious Gourmet								
Pesto Lemon Artichoke	2 tbsp (1 oz)	50	1	5	0	2	1	180
The Wizard's								
Organic Worcestershire Vegetarian Wheat Free	1 tsp	0	0	0	0	1	0	115

FOOD	PORTION	CALS	PROT	FAT	CHOL	CARB	FIBER	SOD
Three Acre Kitchen								
Marinade Balsamic w/ Juniper & Rosemary	1 tbsp (0.5 oz)	50	0	5	–	2	–	85
Walden Farms								
Calorie Free Scampi Sauce	2 tbsp (1 oz)	0	0	0	0	0	0	130
Wild Thymes Farm								
Marinade Hawaiian Teriyaki	1 tbsp	19	1	1	0	3	tr	280
Marinade Korean Ginger Scallion	1 tbsp	20	tr	1	0	3	tr	300
Marinade New Orleans Creole	1 tbsp	11	tr	0	0	3	tr	61
WildWood								
Aioli	1 tbsp	80	0	9	0	0	0	80
Pesto Basil & Pine Nuts	¼ cup	230	5	23	8	2	1	360
Wingers								
Hotter Than Hot	1 tsp	0	0	0	0	0	0	120
World Harbors								
Buccaneer Blends Pirate's Original	1 tbsp (0.6 oz)	20	0	0	0	4	0	115
Chimichurri	2 tbsp (1.2 oz)	40	0	0	0	9	0	180
Fajita	2 tbsp (1.1 oz)	45	0	0	0	10	0	290
Jerk	2 tbsp (1 oz)	70	0	0	0	18	0	200
Lemon Pepper & Garlic	2 tbsp (1 oz)	35	0	0	0	8	0	140
Thai	2 tbsp (1 oz)	40	0	0	0	8	0	350
TAKE-OUT								
cucumber yogurt sauce	1½ tbsp	20	2	0	2	3	0	20
SAUERKRAUT								
canned	½ cup	22	1	tr	0	5	–	780
Ba-Tampte								
Kosher	2 tbsp (1 oz)	5	0	0	0	1	1	180
Dei Fratelli								
Sauerkraut	2 tbsp (1 oz)	5	0	0	0	1	tr	190
Gedney								
Sauerkraut	½ cup	15	0	0	0	3	0	1020
Tree Of Life								
Organic	½ cup (3.6 oz)	15	0	0	0	3	<3	1000

FOOD	PORTION	CALS	PROT	FAT	CHOL	CARB	FIBER	SOD
SAUSAGE								
beef & pork	1 link (2.3 oz)	196	8	17	51	1	0	560
beef & pork w/ cheddar cheese	1 link (2.7 oz)	228	10	20	49	2	0	653
bierschinken	3.5 oz	174	18	11	–	tr	–	753
bierwurst	3.5 oz	258	16	21	–	0	0	–
blutwurst uncooked	3.5 oz	424	13	39	–	0	0	680
bockwurst	3.5 oz	276	12	25	–	0	0	700
bratwurst chicken cooked	1 (3 oz)	148	16	9	60	0	0	60
bratwurst pork cooked	1 link (2.5 oz)	226	10	19	44	2	0	778
brotwurst pork & beef	1 link (2.5 oz)	226	10	19	44	2	0	778
chipolata	3.5 oz	342	14	32	66	1	0	747
chorizo	1 link (2.1 oz)	273	14	23	53	1	0	741
fleischwurst	3.5 oz	305	12	29	–	0	0	829
free range chicken breakfast	2 links (2.7 oz)	110	14	6	45	1	0	570
gelbwurst uncooked	3.5 oz	363	12	33	–	0	0	640
italian pork cooked	1 (2.4 oz)	230	13	18	38	3	1	809
jagdwurst	3.5 oz	211	16	16	–	0	0	818
knockwurst pork & beef	1 (2.5 oz)	221	8	20	43	2	0	670
mettwurst uncooked	3.5 oz	483	13	45	–	0	0	1090
plockwurst uncooked	3.5 oz	312	19	45	–	0	0	–
polish kielbasa	2 oz	127	7	10	39	2	0	672
pork cooked	2 links (1.7 oz)	163	9	14	40	0	0	360
regensburger uncooked	3.5 oz	354	13	31	–	0	0	–
turkey italian smoked	1 (2 oz)	88	8	5	30	3	1	520
venison patty	1 (1 oz)	84	3	8	15	1	0	292
vienna canned	1 link (0.5 oz)	37	2	3	14	tr	0	155
vienna canned	1 can (4 oz)	260	12	22	98	3	0	1095
weisswurst uncooked	3.5 oz	305	11	27	–	0	0	620
zungenwurst (tongue)	3.5 oz	285	17	24	–	0	0	–
Applegate Farms								
Organic Andouille	1 (3 oz)	120	13	6	60	3	1	620
Organic Spinach & Feta	1 (3 oz)	120	13	7	60	2	0	470

FOOD	PORTION	CALS	PROT	FAT	CHOL	CARB	FIBER	SOD
Armour								
Sizzle & Serve Turkey	3 (1.8 oz)	130	9	9	35	2	0	380
Banquet								
Brown'N Serve Lite Maple	3 (2 oz)	130	9	9	35	4	0	450
Brown'N Serve Lite Original	3 (2.1 oz)	120	9	9	25	2	0	430
Brown'N Serve Turkey	3 (2.1 oz)	110	9	7	40	2	0	390
Butterball								
Bratwurst Turkey	1 (3.2 oz)	140	17	8	60	1	–	460
Breakfast Turkey	3 (3 oz)	130	15	7	55	0	0	530
Polska Kielbasa Turkey	2 oz	100	8	6	30	4	0	610
Sweet Italian Turkey	1 (3.2 oz)	140	16	8	60	1	–	360
Coleman								
Bratwurst	1 (3 oz)	240	11	21	55	tr	0	650
Chicken Spicy Chorizo	1 (3 oz)	150	15	8	65	1	0	490
Dietz & Watson								
Italian	1 (2 oz)	160	8	14	30	1	0	480
Italian Chicken	1 (3.4 oz)	130	15	8	50	0	0	680
Jerk Chicken	1 (3.4 oz)	130	15	8	50	0	0	680
Polska Kielbasa	1 (2 oz)	150	4	13	30	1	0	550
Scrapple Philadelphia	2 oz	120	6	8	40	7	1	320
Hans All Natural								
Breakfast Links Skinless Chicken	2 (1.7 oz)	60	8	4	40	0	0	370
Chicken Spinach & Feta	1 (2.7 oz)	130	13	8	45	1	0	350
Healthy Ones								
Smoked	2 oz	80	7	3	25	6	0	480
High Plains Bison								
Bratwurst Beer & Cheddar	1 (3.2 oz)	280	14	21	55	3	0	820
Cocktail	1 (2 oz)	180	9	15	40	1	0	410
Wild Rice & Asiago	1 (3.2 oz)	260	13	21	60	6	0	610
Honeysuckle White								
Turkey Roll Mild Italian	2.5 oz	100	13	5	40	1	0	460
Jimmy Dean								
Fully Cooked Original Links	3 (2.4 oz)	240	9	22	45	1	0	450
Fully Cooked Original Patties	2 (2.4 oz)	240	9	23	50	1	0	610
Fully Cooked Turkey Links	3 (2.4 oz)	120	13	7	55	1	0	490
Fully Cooked Turkey Patties	2 (2.4 oz)	120	13	7	55	1	0	490
Original Links	3 (2 oz)	170	7	14	35	1	0	350

FOOD	PORTION	CALS	PROT	FAT	CHOL	CARB	FIBER	SOD
Original Patties cooked	2 (2.4 oz)	240	9	23	50	1	0	610
Pork All Natural cooked	2 oz	190	12	15	55	1	0	520
Pork Light cooked	2 oz	140	9	11	35	1	0	350
Johnsonville								
Bratwurst Original	1 (3 oz)	270	15	22	60	2	–	810
Breakfast Patty Original	2 (2 oz)	180	10	15	40	1	–	450
Grilling Chorizo	1 (3 oz)	280	16	22	55	3	–	840
Italian Mild	1 (3 oz)	270	15	22	60	3	–	710
Original Summer	1 (2 oz)	170	9	15	45	1	0	680
Polish	1 (2.7 oz)	240	9	21	60	2	–	640
Pork	2 oz	180	10	15	40	1	–	440
Smoked Turkey	1 (3 oz)	110	10	6	45	4	0	710
Jones								
All Natural Light	3 (2.1 oz)	130	9	9	35	3	–	350
Libby's								
Vienna Sausage BBQ	3	140	5	12	40	4	1	430
Perdue								
Turkey Breakfast	2 oz	80	9	5	30	0	0	350
Turkey Sweet Italian cooked	1 link (2.8 oz)	150	15	8	70	4	–	440
Wampler								
Bratwurst as prep	1 (2.5 oz)	230	12	20	50	0	0	610
Breakfast Links as prep	2 (1.2 oz)	130	7	11	30	0	0	250
Breakfast Patties as prep	1 (1.1 oz)	120	5	11	25	0	0	135
Italian as prep	1 (2.5 oz)	230	12	20	50	0	0	610
READY-TO-EAT								
smoked beef cooked	1 (1.4 oz)	134	–	12	29	–	–	–

SAUSAGE DISHES

FOOD	PORTION	CALS	PROT	FAT	CHOL	CARB	FIBER	SOD
TAKE-OUT								
italian sausage w/ peppers & onions	1 cup	210	17	11	70	14	–	1120
sausage roll	1 (2.3 oz)	311	5	24	–	22	1	–

SAUSAGE SUBSTITUTES

FOOD	PORTION	CALS	PROT	FAT	CHOL	CARB	FIBER	SOD
meatless	1 link (0.9 oz)	64	5	5	0	2	1	222
meatless	1 patty (1.3 oz)	98	7	7	0	4	1	337

FOOD	PORTION	CALS	PROT	FAT	CHOL	CARB	FIBER	SOD
Gardenburger								
Veggie Breakfast	1 patty (1.5 oz)	45	5	3	0	3	2	270
Morningstar Farms								
Breakfast Patties	1 (1.3 oz)	80	8	3	0	4	1	250
Worthington								
Saucettes Breakfast Links	1 (1.3 oz)	90	6	6	0	1	1	200
Yves								
Veggie Brats Classic	1 (3.3 oz)	160	19	5	0	5	1	640
SAVORY								
ground	1 tsp	4	tr	tr	0	1	tr	0
SCALLOP								
raw	3 oz	75	14	1	28	2	–	137
Mrs. Paul's								
Fried	13 (3.7 oz)	260	12	11	25	28	tr	700
TAKE-OUT								
breaded & fried	2 lg	67	6	3	19	3	–	144
SCONE								
TAKE-OUT								
apricot	1	232	5	7	34	39	–	201
blueberry	1 (3 oz)	270	7	9	10	41	2	600
cheese	1 (3.5 oz)	364	10	18	–	44	2	–
orange poppy	1 (3 oz)	260	6	6	30	47	2	400
plain	1 (3.5 oz)	362	8	14	–	54	2	–
raisin	1 (3 oz)	270	6	8	10	43	2	490
SCUP								
fresh baked	3 oz	115	21	3	–	0	0	46
SEA BASS (*see* BASS)								
SEA CUCUMBER								
dried	1 oz	74	14	1	17	1	0	1411
fresh	1 oz	20	5	tr	14	tr	0	143
SEA TROUT (*see* TROUT)								
SEA URCHIN								
canned	1 oz	39	4	1	–	3	0	–
fresh	1 oz	36	4	1	–	3	tr	32
roe paste	1 tbsp	19	2	tr	–	3	0	658

FOOD	PORTION	CALS	PROT	FAT	CHOL	CARB	FIBER	SOD
SEAWEED								
agar dried	1 oz	87	2	tr	0	23	–	29
agar fresh	1 oz	tr	tr	tr	0	2	–	3
furikake	1 tbsp (5 g)	15	1	1	1	2	0	239
hijiki rehydrated	1 tbsp (3 g)	1	0	0	0	0	0	7
hijiki dried	1 tbsp	9	1	0	0	2	1	–
irishmoss fresh	1 oz	14	tr	tr	0	4	–	19
kelp fresh	1 oz	12	tr	tr	0	3	–	66
konbu dried	1 piece (5 g)	11	0	0	0	2	1	150
konbu fresh	1 oz	12	tr	tr	0	3	–	66
laver fresh	1 oz	10	2	tr	0	1	–	14
nori fresh	1 oz	10	2	tr	0	1	–	14
nori sheet dried	1 (8 x 8 in)	5	1	0	0	1	1	18
ogo fresh	1 cup (2.8 oz)	24	1	0	0	5	0	60
seahair dried	1 tbsp	13	1	0	0	3	tr	–
spirulina dried	1 oz	83	16	2	0	7	–	309
spirulina fresh	1 oz	7	2	tr	0	1	–	28
tangle fresh	1 oz	12	tr	tr	0	3	–	66
wakame rehydrated	1 tbsp (3 g)	1	0	0	0	0	0	26
Annie Chun's								
Roasted Snacks Sesame	1 pkg (1.5 g)	5	0	0	0	0	0	45
Roasted Snacks Wasabi	1 pkg (1.5 g)	10	0	tr	–	0	0	20
Maine Coast								
Organic Alaria Whole Leaf	⅓ cup	18	1	tr	–	3	3	297
Organic Dulse Whole Leaf	½ cup	19	2	tr	–	3	2	122
Organic Dulse Granules	1 tsp	6	0	0	0	2	–	22
Organic Kelp Whole Leaf	⅓ cup	17	1	tr	–	3	2	312
Organic Kelp Granules	½ tsp	5	0	0	0	2	–	45
Organic Laver Whole Leaf	⅓ cup	22	2	tr	–	3	2	113
SEEDS								
SaviSeed								
Cocoa Kissed	⅕ pkg (1 oz)	170	5	13	0	10	4	80
Karmalized	⅕ pkg (1 oz)	160	6	11	0	11	3	120
Oh Natural	⅕ pkg (1 oz)	190	8	15	0	5	5	170
SEITAN (*see* WHEAT)								
SEMOLINA								
dry	1 cup (5.9 oz)	601	21	2	0	122	7	2

FOOD	PORTION	CALS	PROT	FAT	CHOL	CARB	FIBER	SOD
SESAME								
seeds	1 tsp	16	1	2	0	tr	–	1
sesame butter	1 tbsp	95	3	8	0	4	1	2
sesame crunch candy	20 pieces (1.2 oz)	181	4	12	0	18	–	–
sesame crunch candy	1 oz	146	3	9	0	14	–	–
tahini from roasted & toasted kernels	1 tbsp	89	3	8	0	3	–	17
tahini from stone ground kernels	1 tbsp	86	3	7	0	4	–	11
tahini from unroasted kernels	1 tbsp	85	3	8	0	3	–	0
Arrowhead Mills								
Organic Seeds	¼ cup	210	9	19	0	3	1	15
Organic Tahini	2 tbsp	190	8	18	0	3	tr	10
Mrs. May's								
Black Sesame Crunch	1 oz	165	4	11	0	14	4	43
Peloponnese								
Tahini	1 tbsp	100	4	9	0	2	1	50
Tree Of Life								
Organic Sesame Tahini	2 tbsp	108	5	15	–	8	5	10
Seeds	¼ cup (1.3 oz)	210	6	18	0	8	3	10
SESBANIA								
flower	1	1	tr	0	0	tr	–	0
flowers	1 cup	5	tr	tr	0	1	–	3
flowers cooked	1 cup	23	1	tr	0	5	–	11
SHAD								
american baked	3 oz	214	18	15	–	0	0	56
cooked	1 oz	55	7	3	121	1	0	149
roe baked w/ butter & lemon	1 oz	36	6	1	–	tr	–	21
SHALLOTS (*see* ONION)								
SHARK								
fin dried	1 oz	32	7	tr	–	–	–	5
raw	3 oz	111	18	4	43	0	0	67
TAKE-OUT								
batter-dipped & fried	3 oz	194	16	12	50	5	–	103

FOOD	PORTION	CALS	PROT	FAT	CHOL	CARB	FIBER	SOD
SHEEPSHEAD FISH								
cooked	3 oz	107	22	1	–	0	0	62
cooked	1 fillet (6.5 oz)	234	48	3	–	0	0	136
raw	3 oz	92	17	2	–	0	0	61
SHELLFISH (*see individual names,* SHELLFISH SUBSTITUTES)								
SHELLFISH SUBSTITUTES								
crab imitation	1 cup (4.4 oz)	144	17	1	60	16	tr	1065
scallop imitation	3 oz	84	11	tr	18	9	–	676
shrimp imitation	3 oz	86	11	1	31	8	0	599
surimi	3 oz	84	13	1	25	6	–	122
TAKE-OUT								
crab salad	1 cup	395	18	26	77	21	1	1739
SHELLIE BEANS								
canned	½ cup	37	2	tr	0	8	–	408
SHERBET								
orange	½ cup (4 fl oz)	132	1	2	5	29	–	44
orange	½ gal	2158	17	31	113	469	–	706
orange	1 bar (2.75 fl oz)	91	1	1	3	20	–	30
Ciao Bella								
Lemon	1 pkg (3.5 oz)	120	0	0	0	31	–	0
Mango	1 pkg (3.5 oz)	100	0	0	0	25	1	0
Raspberry	1 pkg (3.5 oz)	110	1	0	0	28	2	0
Dippin' Dots								
Lemon Lime	½ cup	97	1	1	3	22	0	16
Hershey's								
Lemon	½ cup (3.4 oz)	100	tr	1	<5	23	tr	40
Orange	½ cup (3.4 oz)	100	tr	1	<5	23	0	40
Strawberry	½ cup (3.4 oz)	110	tr	1	<5	25	tr	40

FOOD	PORTION	CALS	PROT	FAT	CHOL	CARB	FIBER	SOD
Hola Fruta								
Bar Pomegranate & Blueberry	1 (2.5 oz)	100	1	1	0	22	0	20
Mango	½ cup	130	1	0	<5	31	0	20
Margarita	½ cup	140	1	1	0	30	0	20
Peach	½ cup	130	8	1	0	30	0	35
Pomegranate	½ cup	140	1	1	0	32	0	20
Land O Lakes								
Orange	½ cup (3.2 oz)	130	2	2	5	28	1	35
Turkey Hill								
Fruit Rainbow	½ cup	120	0	1	5	26	0	15
Orange Grove	½ cup	120	1	1	5	26	0	20
SHRIMP (*see also* ASIAN FOOD, EGG ROLLS)								
CANNED								
canned drained	1 can (6 oz)	113	23	2	285	0	0	878
canned drained	1 cup (4.5 oz)	128	26	2	323	0	0	995
canned drained	10 (1.1 oz)	32	7	tr	81	0	0	249
chinese shrimp paste	1 tbsp	46	1	0	9	10	tr	273
Polar								
Tiny Peeled	¼ cup (2 oz)	44	10	0	113	1	0	650
Wild Planet								
Shrimp Wild Pink	2 oz	50	11	1	125	0	0	330
DRIED								
dried	10 (5 g)	13	3	tr	32	0	0	98
dried	1 oz	72	15	1	181	0	0	559
FRESH								
broiled jumbo	3 (1 oz)	44	7	1	55	tr	0	155
broiled small	3 (0.4 oz)	18	3	1	22	tr	0	62
broiled tiny popcorn	3 (3 g)	4	1	tr	5	tr	0	16
prawn broiled	3 (0.6 oz)	27	4	1	33	tr	0	93
steamed jumbo	3 (1 oz)	41	8	1	59	tr	0	177
steamed large	3 (0.6 oz)	25	5	tr	36	tr	0	106
steamed medium	3 (0.5 oz)	21	4	tr	30	tr	0	88
FROZEN								
Blue Horizon Organic								
Garlic Shrimp	1 serv (3.5 oz)	160	15	2	80	21	1	360

FOOD	PORTION	CALS	PROT	FAT	CHOL	CARB	FIBER	SOD
Panko Shrimp	1 serv (3.5 oz)	160	15	2	80	22	1	360
Popcorn Shrimp	1 serv (3.5 oz)	160	15	2	80	21	1	360
Tempura Shrimp	1 serv (3.5 oz)	160	15	2	85	21	1	290
Contessa								
Orange Shrimp	11 to 13 (6 oz)	250	14	8	95	33	5	1150
Ragin' Cajun	8 to 10 (4 oz)	170	11	10	100	9	3	910
Shrimp Scampi	8 to 10 (4 oz)	290	9	27	85	4	2	810
Gorton's								
Popcorn Crunchy Golden	20 (3.2 oz)	240	8	12	55	24	0	630
Temptations Breaded Butterfly	5 (3.5 oz)	250	11	11	55	27	4	430
Temptations Scampi Sauced	1 serv (4 oz)	120	10	6	65	8	tr	630
Mrs. Paul's								
Butterfly	7 (4 oz)	250	12	11	65	27	1	540
SeaPak								
Butterfly	7 (3 oz)	210	10	10	60	20	tr	480
Coconut + Sauce	4 (3.7 oz)	310	12	14	65	36	1	140
Popcorn	15 (3 oz)	210	10	10	60	20	1	480
Scampi	8 (4 oz)	350	15	29	155	2	0	460
Tempura + Sauce	4 (4.1 oz)	240	9	8	35	35	7	570
Van de Kamp's								
Battered	6 (4 oz)	200	14	6	90	22	1	750
Breaded Popcorn	20 (4 oz)	260	11	11	80	30	2	780
TAKE-OUT								
battered jumbo	3 (3 oz)	268	13	17	95	16	1	778
battered large	3 (1.8 oz)	152	7	9	54	9	1	441
battered medium	3 (1.2 oz)	98	5	5	35	6	tr	285
battered small	3 (0.6 oz)	54	3	3	19	3	tr	156
battered tiny popcorn	3 (6 g)	18	1	1	6	1	tr	52
breaded & fried	1 lg (0.6 oz)	44	3	3	30	2	0	81
cocktail w/ cocktail sauce	4 shrimp (3.2 oz)	78	10	1	114	7	2	727

FOOD	PORTION	CALS	PROT	FAT	CHOL	CARB	FIBER	SOD
creole w/o rice	1 cup (8.6 oz)	335	40	13	293	11	2	1134
gingered	4	80	–	tr	140	–	–	920
jambalaya w/ rice	1 cup (8.5 oz)	294	25	9	262	28	2	1001
scampi	1 cup	310	26	22	246	1	0	330
shish kabob w/ vegetables	1 (7.1 oz)	184	26	5	184	9	2	1040
shrimp cake	1 (4.2 oz)	238	16	13	194	14	1	695
shrimp egg patty torta de cameron seco	2 (1.3 oz)	152	9	11	171	3	tr	289
shrimp in garlic sauce	1 cup (7.4 oz)	649	36	54	267	6	tr	1124
shrimp newburg	1 cup (8.6 oz)	605	30	50	417	11	tr	886
shrimp salad	1 cup (6.4 oz)	258	24	16	291	4	1	1043
shrimp w/ crab stuffing	3 (1.7 oz)	94	10	5	76	3	tr	240
tempura	1 (0.9 oz)	65	4	4	43	3	0	119
toast fried	3 pieces (2.5 oz)	219	8	14	35	16	2	678
SMELT								
rainbow cooked	3 oz	106	19	3	76	0	0	65
rainbow raw	3 oz	83	15	2	60	0	0	51
SMOOTHIES (*see also* FRUIT DRINKS, YOGURT DRINKS)								
Arthur's								
Carrot Energizer	1 bottle (11 oz)	200	2	1	0	47	3	60
Green Energy	1 bottle (11 oz)	230	2	1	0	53	3	15
Bolthouse Farms								
Green Goodness	8 oz	140	2	0	0	33	1	25
Mango Lemonade	8 oz	120	tr	0	0	30	tr	0
Passion Fruit Apple Carrot Juice	8 oz	120	2	0	0	29	2	95
C&W								
Berry Blend	½ cup	90	2	2	10	15	2	65
Peach	½ cup	80	2	2	10	15	1	65

FOOD	PORTION	CALS	PROT	FAT	CHOL	CARB	FIBER	SOD
Del Monte								
Ready-To-Blend Mango Pineapple	1 (6 oz)	115	0	0	0	29	3	15
Ready-To-Blend Strawberry Peach	1 (6 oz)	120	0	0	0	30	4	25
Ready-To-Blend Strawberry Peach Lite	1 (6 oz)	80	0	0	0	20	4	20
Horizon Organic								
Tropical Punch	1 bottle (6.2 oz)	120	4	0	0	25	1	75
Jamba Juice								
All Flavors not prep	½ pkg (4 oz)	60	2	0	0	14	2	15
Kidz Dream								
Orange Cream	1 box	120	4	2	0	21	tr	30
Main St. Cafe								
Protein Smoothie Mixed Berry	1 bottle (11 oz)	270	10	2	15	33	1	300
Protein Smoothie Peach	1 bottle (11 oz)	260	10	2	15	54	1	300
Protein Smoothie Strawberry	1 bottle (11 oz)	280	10	2	15	58	1	300
Nutiva								
Organic HempShake Amazon Acai not prep	4 tbsp	100	9	3	0	15	8	5
Organic HempShake Chocolate not prep	4 tbsp	80	7	2	0	19	12	5
Odwalla								
Bluberry B Monster	8 oz	140	0	0	0	33	0	10
Citrus C Monster	8 oz	150	2	0	0	36	0	15
Mango Tango	8 oz	150	1	1	0	34	0	10
Sambazon								
Acai Amazon Cherry	8 oz	156	5	0	0	16	1	5
Acai Mango Banana	8 oz	190	2	5	0	38	3	90
Acai Mango Uprising	8 oz	190	2	5	0	38	3	90
Acai Protein Warrior Vanilla	8 oz	215	8	6	0	33	3	142
Acai Shaman's Immunity	8 oz	90	1	0	0	24	1	28
Acai Soy Energy	8 oz	210	6	6	0	25	4	142
Acai Strawberry Sensation	8 oz	210	1	4	0	42	2	10

FOOD	PORTION	CALS	PROT	FAT	CHOL	CARB	FIBER	SOD
Acai Supergreens Revolution	8 oz	200	2	4	0	40	3	12
Organic Acai	1 bottle	155	1	3	0	31	2	16
Soy Fusion								
Berry	1 box (8.45 oz)	120	2	1	–	24	–	20
Matcha Green Tea	1 box (8.45 oz)	110	3	2	–	19	–	120
Tropicana								
Fruit Smoothie Mixed Berry	1 bottle (11 oz)	220	1	0	0	54	2	30
Fruit Smoothie Tropical Fruit	1 bottle (11 oz)	220	1	0	0	53	1	15
V8								
Splash Tropical Colada	8 oz	100	3	0	0	21	1	50
SNACKS								
cheese puffs	1 oz	122	2	3	0	21	3	364
oriental mix	1 oz	155	6	12	0	9	–	235
pork skins	1 oz	154	17	9	27	0	0	521
pork skins barbecue	1 oz	152	16	9	33	1	–	756
Barbara's Bakery								
Cheese Puffs Bakes Original	¾ cup	160	2	11	0	13	–	190
Cheese Puffs Original	¾ cup (1 oz)	150	2	10	0	16	–	130
Better Balance								
Kruncheeze White Cheddar Gluten Free	1 oz	130	9	6	0	10	2	200
Carole's								
Soycrunch Cinnamon & Raisins	½ cup	110	6	1	0	19	2	0
Soycrunch Original	½ cup	120	5	2	0	16	2	0
Soycrunch Toffee	½ cup	110	7	2	0	15	2	15
Cheetos								
Crunchy	1 pkg (1.25 oz)	200	2	13	5	19	1	370
Cheez It								
Right Bites Party Mix	1 pkg (0.74 oz)	100	2	4	0	15	tr	200

FOOD	PORTION	CALS	PROT	FAT	CHOL	CARB	FIBER	SOD
Fullbites								
Bold Cheddar	1 pkg (1.3 oz)	150	8	6	<5	21	5	270
Savory BBQ	1 pkg (1.3 oz)	150	8	5	0	22	5	220
Kay's Naturals								
Snack Mix Sweet BBQ Gluten Free	1 oz	120	10	5	0	11	2	230
Lance								
Cheese Puffs	9 (1 oz)	170	2	12	0	13	0	380
Gold-N-Chees	1 oz	150	2	8	0	17	tr	240
Lifestyle Foods								
Awake	1 pkg (5 oz)	170	3	0	2	55	5	65
Essential	1 pkg (5.6 oz)	200	9	10	2	21	3	230
Miami	1 pkg (7.5 oz)	180	5	0	0	36	3	70
Power Up	1 pkg (6.7 oz)	670	18	33	0	77	9	430
Medora Snacks								
Corners Sea Salt	1 oz	130	2	3	0	22	0	170
Pucci Garlic	1 oz	120	4	4	5	17	1	420
Pucci Tomato Basil	1 oz	120	4	4	5	17	1	440
Sotos Cheese Olive Oil & Lemon	1 oz	120	2	4	0	19	2	420
Michael Season's								
Cheese Puffs & Curls	1½ cups	180	3	13	5	13	2	270
Robert's American Gourmet								
Booty Barbeque	1 oz	130	2	5	0	20	1	90
Booty Pirate's	1 oz	130	2	5	0	18	1	150
Booty Veggie	1 oz	130	1	6	0	17	1	150
Smart Puffs	1 oz	130	2	6	0	17	0	150
Tings	1 oz	160	1	8	0	17	0	85
Silhouette Solution								
Puffs BBQ	1 pkg (1.06 oz)	120	15	4	0	8	0	420
Snikiddy								
Puffs Grilled Cheese	1 pkg (0.6 oz)	80	2	3	0	10	1	160

FOOD	PORTION	CALS	PROT	FAT	CHOL	CARB	FIBER	SOD
Puffs Rockin' Ranch	1 pkg (0.6 oz)	83	1	0	0	11	1	160
Snyder's Of Hanover								
CheddAirs	1 oz	130	3	5	0	20	tr	140
MultiGrain Cheese Puffs	1 oz	130	2	6	0	19	2	200
SunRidge Farms								
Mocha Marble Crunch	¼ pkg (1.4 oz)	220	5	16	0	17	3	25
Sweet Emotions								
Chocolate Passion	1 pkg (0.5 oz)	60	1	3	0	10	2	200
Cinnamon Joy	1 pkg (0.5 oz)	60	1	3	0	10	2	200
T.G.I. Friday's								
Mozzarella Sticks	20 (1 oz)	150	2	9	0	14	1	250
Utz								
Cheese Balls	50 (1 oz)	150	2	9	0	16	tr	260
Cheese Curls	18 (1 oz)	150	2	9	0	16	tr	260
Onion Rings	41 (1 oz)	130	1	5	0	20	0	500
Party Mix	1 oz	150	2	7	0	19	1	250
Pork Cracklins	0.5 oz	90	6	7	15	0	0	300
Pork Rinds Original	0.5 oz	80	9	5	15	0	0	210
SNAIL								
cooked	3 oz	233	41	1	110	13	–	350
raw	3 oz	117	20	tr	55	7	–	175
TAKE-OUT								
escargot cooked	5	25	4	0	15	1	0	25
SNAKE								
fresh	3 oz	78	17	tr	–	3	0	57
SNAPPER								
cooked	1 fillet (6 oz)	217	45	3	80	0	0	96
cooked	3 oz	109	22	1	40	0	0	48
raw	3 oz	85	17	1	31	0	0	54
SODA								
club	12 oz	0	0	0	0	0	0	75
cola	12 oz	151	tr	tr	0	39	–	14
cream	12 oz	191	0	0	0	49	–	43
diet cola	12 oz	2	tr	0	0	tr	–	21

FOOD	PORTION	CALS	PROT	FAT	CHOL	CARB	FIBER	SOD
ginger ale	12 oz	124	tr	0	0	32	–	25
grape	12 oz	161	0	0	0	42	–	57
lemon lime	12 oz	149	0	0	0	38	–	41
orange	12 oz	177	0	0	0	46	–	49
pepper type	12 oz	151	0	tr	0	38	–	38
quinine	12 oz	125	0	0	0	32	–	15
root beer	12 oz	152	tr	0	0	39	–	49
shirley temple	1 serv	159	0	0	0	41	0	34
tonic water	12 oz	125	0	0	0	32	–	15
Ale 8 One								
Soft Drink	1 bottle (12 oz)	120	0	0	0	30	–	15
Barq's								
Diet French Vanilla Creme	8 oz	1	0	0	0	tr	0	44
Diet Red Creme	8 oz	4	0	0	0	0	0	43
Diet Root Beer	8 oz	1	0	0	0	tr	0	48
Floatz	8 oz	127	0	0	0	34	0	44
French Vanilla Creme	8 oz	112	0	0	0	30	0	44
Red Creme	8 oz	115	0	0	0	31	0	43
Root Beer	8 oz	111	0	0	0	30	0	48
Cape Cod Dry								
Cranberry	8 oz	120	0	0	0	29	–	0
Diet Cranberry	8 oz	10	0	0	0	2	–	0
Carver's								
Ginger Ale	8 oz	94	0	0	0	24	0	22
Celsius								
Cola	1 bottle (12 oz)	5	–	–	–	–	–	6
Coca-Cola								
C2	8 oz	45	0	0	0	12	–	30
Classic	8 oz	97	0	0	0	27	0	33
W/ Lime	8 oz	98	0	0	0	27	0	25
Coke								
Cherry	8 oz	104	0	0	0	28	0	28
Diet	8 oz	1	0	0	0	tr	0	28
Diet Cherry	8 oz	1	0	0	0	tr	0	28
Diet Plus	8 oz	0	0	0	0	0	0	30
Diet Vanilla	8 oz	1	0	0	0	tr	0	28
Diet w/ Lime	8 oz	2	0	0	0	tr	0	28
Vanilla	8 oz	100	0	0	0	28	0	25

FOOD	PORTION	CALS	PROT	FAT	CHOL	CARB	FIBER	SOD
DRY								
Juniper Berry	1 bottle (12 oz)	55	0	0	0	15	–	0
Vanilla Bean	1 bottle (12 oz)	60	0	0	0	16	–	0
Fanta								
Apple	8 oz	121	0	0	0	33	0	39
Citrus	8 oz	91	0	0	0	25	0	16
Orange	8 oz	111	0	0	0	35	0	35
Fresca								
Soda	8 oz	2	0	0	0	tr	0	24
Fresh Ginger								
Ginger Ale Jasmine Green Tea	1 bottle (12 oz)	160	0	0	0	40	0	5
Ginger Ale Original	1 bottle (12 oz)	160	0	0	0	40	0	0
Ginger Ale Pomegranate w/ Hibiscus	1 bottle (12 oz)	160	0	0	0	41	0	10
Goya								
Ginger Beer	1 bottle (12 oz)	190	0	0	0	43	0	30
GuS								
Dry Cola	1 bottle (12 oz)	95	0	0	0	24	–	10
Dry Crimson Grape	1 bottle (12 oz)	90	0	0	0	22	–	10
Dry Pomegranate	1 bottle (12 oz)	98	0	0	0	24	–	10
Star Ruby Grapefruit	1 bottle (12 oz)	90	0	0	0	22	–	10
Hansen's								
Blackberry	1 bottle	150	tr	0	0	37	–	55
Health Cola								
Soda	1 bottle (12 oz)	140	0	0	0	35	–	0
HotLips								
Apple	1 bottle	136	0	0	0	34	–	50
Boysenberry	1 bottle	152	1	0	0	37	–	1
Pear	1 bottle	142	tr	1	0	34	–	35

FOOD	PORTION	CALS	PROT	FAT	CHOL	CARB	FIBER	SOD
Inca Kola								
Diet	8 oz	1	0	0	0	tr	0	34
Soda	8 oz	96	0	0	0	26	0	31
Jones Soda								
Blue Bubble Gum	1 bottle (12 oz)	190	0	0	0	48	0	25
Cream	1 bottle (12 oz)	190	0	0	0	48	0	25
Crushed Melon	1 bottle (12 oz)	190	0	0	0	48	0	25
FuFu Berry	1 bottle (12 oz)	190	0	0	0	46	0	70
Green Apple	1 bottle (12 oz)	180	0	0	0	46	0	25
Orange Cream	1 bottle (12 oz)	180	0	0	0	46	0	25
Lucozade								
Soda	7 oz	136	0	0	0	36	0	–
Manzana Mia								
Soda	8 oz	99	0	0	0	27	0	47
Mello Yellow								
Diet	8 oz	3	0	0	0	tr	0	25
Soda	8 oz	118	0	0	0	32	0	33
Mr. Pibb								
Diet	8 oz	1	0	0	0	tr	0	26
Northern Neck								
Diet Ginger Ale	8 oz	4	0	0	0	0	0	24
Ginger Ale	8 oz	94	0	0	0	24	0	22
Nutrisoda								
Calm Sparkling Wild Berry & Citron	1 can (8.7 oz)	0	0	0	0	1	–	0
Flex Sparkling Black Cherry & Apple	1 can (8.7 oz)	5	0	0	0	1	–	0
Immune Sparkling Tangerine & Lime	1 can (8.7 oz)	15	2	0	0	1	–	0
Slender Sparkling Guava & Grapefruit	1 can (8.7 oz)	10	0	0	0	1	–	15
Oogave Natural								
All Flavors	8 oz	68	0	0	0	17	0	0

FOOD	PORTION	CALS	PROT	FAT	CHOL	CARB	FIBER	SOD
Orangina								
Sparkling Citrus	8 oz	100	0	0	0	26	–	40
Pepsi								
Cola	8 oz	100	0	0	0	28	–	20
Diet	8 oz	0	0	0	0	0	0	25
Diet Vanilla	8 oz	0	0	0	0	0	0	25
One	8 oz	1	0	0	0	0	–	25
Wild Cherry	8 oz	100	0	0	0	28	–	20
Pibb								
Zero	8 oz	2	0	0	0	tr	0	31
Polar								
Birch Beer	8 oz	110	0	0	0	28	–	0
Bitter Lemon Mixer	8 oz	120	0	0	0	29	–	0
Collins Mixer	8 oz	90	0	0	0	22	–	0
Cream	8 oz	120	0	0	0	30	–	0
Diet Pomegranate Dry	8 oz	10	0	0	0	2	–	0
Orange	8 oz	130	0	0	0	32	–	0
Pomegranate Dry	8 oz	120	0	0	0	30	–	0
Seltzer All Flavors	8 oz	0	0	0	0	0	0	0
Strawberry	8 oz	120	0	0	0	30	–	0
Tonic Water	8 oz	90	0	0	0	23	–	0
Vichy Water	8 oz	0	0	0	0	0	0	300
Red Flash								
Soda	8 oz	105	0	0	0	28	0	21
Reed's								
Ginger Brew Original	1 bottle (12 oz)	145	0	0	0	37	0	5
Santa Cruz								
Organic Cherry	1 can (12 oz)	140	0	0	0	34	0	20
Organic Ginger Ale	1 can (12 oz)	150	0	0	0	37	0	10
Organic Root Beer	1 can (12 oz)	150	0	0	0	36	0	10
Organic Vanilla Creme	1 can (12 oz)	160	0	0	0	38	0	10
Sprite								
Diet Zero	8 oz	0	0	0	0	0	0	25
ReMix Aruba Jam	8 oz	97	0	0	0	26	–	44
Soda	8 oz	96	0	0	0	26	0	47
Steaz								
Organic Green Tea Soda Cola	8 oz	90	0	0	0	23	–	35

FOOD	PORTION	CALS	PROT	FAT	CHOL	CARB	FIBER	SOD
Organic Green Tea Soda Diet Black Cherry	8 oz	20	0	0	0	5	–	20
Organic Green Tea Soda Ginger Ale	8 oz	90	0	0	0	23	–	35
Organic Green Tea Soda Lemon	8 oz	90	0	0	0	23	–	35
Stirrings								
Ginger Ale	8 oz	120	0	0	0	31	0	0
Tab								
Soda	8 oz	1	0	0	0	tr	–	28
Tava								
Sparkling Brazilian Samba	8 oz	0	0	0	0	0	0	35
Sparkling Mediterranean Fiesta	8 oz	0	0	0	0	0	0	40
Thomas Kemper								
Black Cherry	1 bottle (12 oz)	170	0	0	0	40	–	40
Ginger Ale	1 bottle (12 oz)	150	0	0	0	36	–	45
Orange Cream	1 bottle (12 oz)	170	0	0	0	42	–	50
Root Beer	1 bottle (12 oz)	160	0	0	0	41	–	45
Root Beer Low Calorie	1 bottle (12 oz)	20	0	0	0	5	–	70
Vanilla Cream	1 bottle (12 oz)	150	0	0	0	38	–	55
Tropicana								
Twister Orange	1 can (12 oz)	180	0	0	0	52	–	35
Vignette								
Wine Country Soda Chardonnay	1 bottle (12 oz)	130	0	0	0	33	–	20
Wine Country Soda Pinot Noir	1 bottle (12 oz)	130	0	0	0	31	–	15
Virgil's								
Micro Brewed Root Beer	1 bottle (12 oz)	160	0	0	0	42	–	0

FOOD	PORTION	CALS	PROT	FAT	CHOL	CARB	FIBER	SOD
SOLE								
cooked	1 fillet (4.5 oz)	148	31	2	86	0	0	133
cooked	3 oz	99	21	1	58	0	0	89
lemon raw	3.5 oz	85	17	1	–	0	0	80
TAKE-OUT								
breaded & fried	3.2 oz	211	13	11	31	15	–	484
SORGHUM								
sorghum	1 cup (6.7 oz)	651	22	6	0	143	–	12
SOUFFLE								
Garden Lites								
Roasted Vegetable	1 pkg (7 oz)	140	8	2	0	24	3	350
Heavenly Souffle								
Chocolate	1 (2.6 oz)	262	3	16	103	29	0	128
TAKE-OUT								
cheese	1 cup	194	9	15	134	6	tr	307
chicken	1 cup (5.6 oz)	278	20	18	218	9	tr	560
corn	1 cup	257	10	11	152	34	3	666
lime chilled	1 cup	388	11	18	306	48	2	102
seafood	1 cup	245	17	15	231	9	tr	668
spinach	1 cup	124	6	8	97	7	1	170
SOUP								
CANNED								
shrimp cream of as prep	1 cup (8.6 oz)	120	5	6	22	11	tr	908
Allens								
Chicken Broth	1 cup	10	1	0	0	1	0	620
Amy's								
Organic Butternut Squash Light In Sodium	1 cup (8.6 oz)	100	2	3	0	20	2	290
Organic Chunky Tomato Bisque	1 cup (8.4 oz)	120	2	4	10	21	2	680
Organic Chunky Tomato Bisque Light In Sodium	1 cup (8.6 oz)	120	2	4	10	21	2	340
Organic Cream Of Mushroom	¾ cup (6.5 oz)	150	3	9	10	13	2	590

FOOD	PORTION	CALS	PROT	FAT	CHOL	CARB	FIBER	SOD
Organic Lentil Light In Sodium	1 cup (8.6 oz)	180	8	5	0	25	6	290
Organic No Chicken Noodle Soup	1 cup (8.6 oz)	100	5	3	0	13	2	540
Organic Pasta & 3 Bean	1 cup (8.6 oz)	150	5	4	0	22	4	680
Organic Southwestern Vegetable	1 cup (8.7 oz)	140	4	4	0	21	4	680
Organic Split Pea	1 cup (8.6 oz)	100	7	0	0	19	3	670
Split Pea Light In Sodium	1 cup (8.6 oz)	100	7	0	0	19	4	280
Tom Kha Phak Thai Coconut	1 cup (7 oz)	140	4	10	0	9	2	580
Butterball								
Chicken Broth 99% Fat Free	1 cup	10	tr	0	0	2	0	840
Campbell's								
25% Less Sodium Chicken Noodle as prep	1 cup	60	3	2	15	8	1	660
25% Less Sodium Cream Of Mushroom as prep	1 cup	110	2	8	5	8	2	650
98% Fat Free Cream Of Broccoli as prep	1 cup	70	2	2	<5	10	2	700
98% Fat Free Cream Of Celery as prep	1 cup	60	1	3	5	8	1	580
98% Fat Free Cream Of Chicken as prep	1 cup	70	2	3	10	10	1	590
Cheddar Cheese as prep	1 cup	110	2	5	5	12	1	890
Chicken & Stars as prep	1 cup	70	3	2	5	11	1	480
Chicken Alphabet as prep	1 cup	70	3	2	5	12	1	480
Chicken Noodle O's as prep	1 cup	90	3	3	20	15	1	480
Chunky Beef and Country Vegetables	1 cup	150	10	3	15	21	4	890
Chunky Chicken Mushroom Chowder	1 cup	210	7	12	10	19	3	910
Chunky Grilled Chicken w/ Vegetables & Pasta	1 cup	100	8	2	15	15	2	880
Chunky Healthy Request Chicken Noodle	1 cup (8.4 oz)	120	8	3	10	17	2	410

FOOD	PORTION	CALS	PROT	FAT	CHOL	CARB	FIBER	SOD
Chunky Hearty Vegetable w/ Pasta	1 cup	120	4	2	5	23	4	870
Chunky New England Clam Chowder	1 cup	210	7	9	10	25	5	890
Chunky Roadhouse Beef & Bean Chili	1 cup	230	15	8	30	25	8	870
Chunky Sirloin Burger w/ Country Vegetables	1 cup	180	10	7	15	20	4	900
Curly Noodle as prep	1 cup	80	4	2	15	11	1	480
Double Noodle Chicken as prep	1 cup	110	3	2	10	20	1	480
Goldfish Pasta Meatball as prep	1 cup	90	4	3	10	11	1	480
Healthy Request Chicken Rice as prep	1 cup	70	2	2	5	13	1	480
Healthy Request Cream Of Chicken as prep	1 cup (8.4 oz)	80	2	3	5	12	1	410
Healthy Request Italian Style Wedding	1 cup	120	7	3	10	15	2	480
Healthy Request Tomato as prep	1 cup	90	2	2	0	10	1	470
Light Chicken Gumbo as prep	1 cup (8.4 oz)	70	2	1	5	12	1	480
Low Sodium Chicken Broth	1 can	25	4	1	5	1	0	140
Mega Noodle as prep	1 cup	90	3	2	15	15	1	480
Microwavable Bowl Chicken Noodle	1 cup	70	4	2	15	10	tr	870
Microwavable Bowl Vegetable	1 cup	110	4	1	<5	22	3	800
Minestrone as prep	1 cup (8.4 oz)	90	4	1	5	17	3	650
Select Harvest Caramelized French Onion	1 cup (8.4 oz)	80	3	3	5	12	1	480
Select Harvest Chicken Tuscany	1 cup	90	7	2	10	12	4	480
Select Harvest Chicken w/ Egg Noodles	1 cup	100	8	3	25	11	1	480
Select Harvest Chicken w/ Whole Grain Pasta	1 cup (8.4 oz)	100	7	2	20	14	1	410

FOOD	PORTION	CALS	PROT	FAT	CHOL	CARB	FIBER	SOD
Select Harvest Italian Style Wedding	1 cup (8.4 oz)	130	7	5	15	13	1	480
Select Harvest Light Minestrone w/ Whole Grain Pasta	1 cup	80	4	1	0	14	4	480
Select Harvest Light Savory Chicken w/ Vegetables	1 cup	80	5	1	10	15	4	480
Select Harvest Light Southwestern Style Vegetable	1 cup	50	2	0	0	13	3	480
Select Harvest Light Vegetable & Pasta	1 cup	60	3	0	0	13	4	480
Select Harvest Light Vegetable Beef & Barley	1 cup (8.4 oz)	80	5	2	5	14	4	480
Select Harvest Tomato w/ Basil	1 cup	80	1	0	0	18	1	750
Select Italian Sausage w/ Pasta & Pepperoni	1 cup	150	7	6	15	18	2	800
Select Mexican Chicken Tortilla	1 cup	130	8	3	10	19	3	850
Select Potato Broccoli Cheese	1 cup	120	3	4	<5	18	4	890
Select Savory Chicken & Long Grain Rice	1 cup	90	7	1	10	15	1	970
Select Split Pea w/ Roasted Ham	1 cup	160	10	1	5	29	5	830
Select Vegetable Beef	1 cup	110	8	2	15	16	3	910
Soup At Hand 25% Less Sodium Chicken w/ Mini Noodles	1 pkg (10.75 oz)	80	4	2	10	11	2	730
Soup At Hand Vegetable Medley	1 pkg (10.75 oz)	100	3	2	<5	19	4	890
Soup At Hand Velvety Potato	1 pkg (10.75 oz)	160	2	7	<5	21	4	870
Tomato as prep	1 cup (8.4 oz)	90	2	0	0	20	1	480
V8 Garden Broccoli	1 cup (8.4 oz)	90	3	2	5	15	3	480
V8 Golden Butternut Squash	1 cup	140	3	2	5	28	3	750

FOOD	PORTION	CALS	PROT	FAT	CHOL	CARB	FIBER	SOD
V8 Sweet Red Pepper	1 cup	120	3	2	5	22	4	620
V8 Tomato Herb	1 cup	90	3	0	0	19	3	750
College Inn								
Beef Broth 99% Fat Free	1 cup (8.4 oz)	25	4	1	0	0	0	900
Beef Broth Fat Free Lower Sodium	1 cup (8.4 oz)	15	4	0	0	0	0	450
Bold Stock Rotisserie Chicken	1 cup (8.4 oz)	30	3	0	0	4	0	720
Bold Stock Tender Beef	1 cup (8.4 oz)	45	7	0	0	4	0	730
Chicken Broth 99% Fat Free	1 cup (8.5 oz)	15	1	1	0	3	0	930
Chicken Broth Light & Fat Free 50% Less Sodium	1 cup (8.4 oz)	5	1	0	0	0	0	450
Chicken Broth w/ Roasted Garlic	1 cup (8.5 oz)	20	1	0	0	3	0	1000
Chicken Broth w/ Roasted Vegetables & Herbs	1 cup (8.5 oz)	20	1	0	0	3	0	1060
Culinary Broth Thai Coconut Curry	1 cup (8.4 oz)	20	0	1	0	5	0	1010
Culinary Broth Wine & Herbs	1 cup (8.4 oz)	5	0	1	0	1	1	920
Garden Vegetable Broth	1 cup (8.4 oz)	25	1	1	0	6	0	590
Turkey Broth	1 cup (8.4 oz)	20	2	1	0	0	0	950
Comfort Care								
Hearty Beef Barley	1 cup (8 oz)	190	12	7	20	23	4	85
Savory Chicken	1 cup (8 oz)	200	13	7	15	25	5	70
Tomato Cheddar Jack	1 cup (8 oz)	90	8	2	5	13	5	140
Dr. McDougall's								
Chunky Tomato Gluten Free Vegan	1 cup (8.6 oz)	90	2	0	0	20	3	440
Vegetable Gluten Free Vegan	1 cup (3.3 oz)	230	4	13	90	25	0	55
Go Appetit								
Carrot Bisque	8 oz	110	6	5	5	13	3	450
Gazpacho	8 oz	100	1	7	0	9	1	400
Mango Melange	8 oz	150	3	5	0	27	1	–
Health Valley								
Beef Broth Fat Free	1 cup	10	2	0	0	0	0	390

FOOD	PORTION	CALS	PROT	FAT	CHOL	CARB	FIBER	SOD
Chicken Broth Fat Free	1 cup	20	5	0	0	0	0	390
Chicken Broth Fat Free No Salt Added	1 cup	35	5	2	0	0	0	130
Chicken Broth Low Fat	1 cup	35	5	2	25	0	0	390
Clam Chowder Manhattan	1 cup	90	3	3	0	13	1	680
Clam Chowder New England	1 cup	110	5	4	10	15	0	680
Corn & Vegetable Fat Free	1 cup	70	5	0	0	17	7	135
Garden Vegetable Fat Free	1 cup	80	3	0	0	18	4	480
Lentil & Carrot Fat Free	1 cup	100	10	0	0	25	7	220
Organic Black Bean	1 cup	130	7	1	0	25	5	380
Organic Cream Of Mushroom	1 cup	90	1	5	0	11	0	660
Organic Minestrone	1 cup	100	4	2	0	20	5	480
Organic Minestrone No Salt Added	1 cup	70	3	0	0	17	3	45
Organic Mushroom Barley	1 cup	70	2	0	0	17	3	380
Organic Mushroom Barley No Salt Added	1 cup	70	2	0	0	17	3	25
Organic Split Pea No Salt Added	1 cup	110	10	0	0	23	8	45
Organic Tomato	1 cup	80	3	0	0	18	1	380
Organic Tomato No Salt Added	1 cup	80	3	0	0	18	1	35
Tomato Vegetable Fat Free	1 cup	80	6	0	0	17	5	240
Vegetable Broth Fat Free	1 cup	20	0	0	0	5	0	330
Healthy Choice								
Bean & Ham	1 cup	180	11	2	<5	29	10	480
Chicken & Dumplings	1 cup	140	9	3	20	21	3	480
Country Vegetable	1 cup (8.6 oz)	100	4	1	5	20	5	480
Old Fashioned Chicken Noodle	1 cup	100	9	2	15	13	2	480
Tomato Basil	1 cup (8.8 oz)	130	4	1	5	28	3	470
Vegetable Beef	1 cup	130	9	1	15	22	4	480
Zesty Gumbo	1 cup	100	6	2	20	16	4	480
Hormel								
Bean & Ham	1 pkg (7.5 oz)	190	9	4	10	29	7	720

FOOD	PORTION	CALS	PROT	FAT	CHOL	CARB	FIBER	SOD
Beef Vegetable	1 pkg (7.5 oz)	100	6	1	10	16	1	790
Chicken Noodle	1 pkg (7.5 oz)	100	7	3	25	12	0	790
Chicken w/ Rice	1 pkg (7.5 oz)	110	4	3	10	18	1	850
New England Clam Chowder	1 pkg (7.5 oz)	140	5	5	20	18	1	800
Imagine								
Lobster Bisque	1 cup	130	5	5	15	15	–	690
Organic Bistro Cuban Black Bean Bisque	1 cup	170	8	4	0	30	6	480
Organic Broth Beef	1 cup	20	2	1	5	1	0	700
Organic Broth Free Range Chicken	1 cup	10	1	0	0	1	0	570
Organic Broth Vegetable	8 oz	20	2	0	0	2	0	550
Organic Creamy Butternut Squash	1 cup	90	0	2	0	18	2	480
Organic Creamy Chicken	1 cup	70	3	2	0	12	1	680
Organic Creamy Sweet Corn	1 cup	120	4	3	0	20	3	450
Organic Sweet Potato	1 cup	110	2	2	0	23	1	400
Lucini								
Roman Tomato Cream	1 cup (8.6 oz)	170	4	9	25	18	4	770
Umbrian Lentil	1 cup (8.6 oz)	160	7	5	0	23	9	770
Manischewitz								
Beef Broth	1 cup (8.4 oz)	150	1	1	0	1	0	790
Chicken Broth	1 cup (8.4 oz)	15	1	1	0	1	0	790
Chicken Broth Low Sodium	1 cup (8.4 oz)	15	1	1	0	1	0	420
Muir Glen								
Organic Garden Vegetable	1 cup	80	3	1	0	16	3	560
Organic Southwest Black Bean	1 cup	140	7	1	0	27	8	670
Original SoupMan								
Italian Wedding	1 cup	120	4	6	10	18	4	600
New England Clam Chowder	1 cup	290	14	19	90	16	1	930

FOOD	PORTION	CALS	PROT	FAT	CHOL	CARB	FIBER	SOD
Organic Butternut Squash	1 cup	250	3	13	50	33	3	560
Tomato Basil	1 cup	140	4	7	15	18	4	1110
Turkey Chili	1 cup	210	18	7	40	18	5	910
Progresso								
40% Less Sodium Italian Style Wedding	1 cup (8.7 oz)	90	5	2	10	11	1	480
50% Less Sodium Garden Vegetable	1 cup (8.8 oz)	100	3	0	0	22	3	450
50% Less Sodium Zesty Chicken Gumbo	1 cup (8.7 oz)	110	7	2	15	18	2	450
High Fiber Creamy Tomato Basil	1 cup (8.8 oz)	130	3	4	5	26	7	690
Light Beef Pot Roast	1 cup (8.4 oz)	80	6	1	15	12	2	690
Light Chicken Vegetable Rotini	1 cup (8.3 oz)	70	6	2	15	10	2	700
Light Italian Style Vegetable	1 cup (8.6 oz)	60	3	0	0	12	4	700
Light Savory Vegetable Barley	1 cup (8.5 oz)	60	2	0	0	14	4	740
Light Vegetable	1 cup (8.4 oz)	60	3	0	0	14	4	470
Light Vegetable & Noodle	1 cup (8.7 oz)	60	2	1	5	13	4	690
Reduced Sodium Chicken Broth	1 cup (8.4 oz)	20	3	0	0	2	–	560
Reduced Sodium Chicken Gumbo	1 cup (8.7 oz)	110	7	2	15	18	2	450
Reduced Sodium Chicken Noodle	1 cup (8.4 oz)	90	6	2	20	13	1	470
Rich & Hearty Beef Pot Roast	1 cup (8.7 oz)	120	8	2	15	20	2	830
Rich & Hearty Chicken & Homestyle Noodles	1 cup (8.6 oz)	100	7	2	25	14	1	940
Rich & Hearty Chicken Pot Pie	1 cup (8.6 oz)	170	8	6	15	21	2	940
Rich & Hearty Savory Beef Barley Vegetable	1 cup (8.6 oz)	130	8	1	15	22	3	970
Rich & Hearty Sirloin Steak & Vegetables	1 cup	130	8	2	15	21	2	870
Rich & Hearty Slow Cooked Vegetable Beef	1 cup (8.6 oz)	120	6	1	15	20	3	840

FOOD	PORTION	CALS	PROT	FAT	CHOL	CARB	FIBER	SOD
Rich & Hearty Steak & Roasted Russet Potatoes	1 cup (8.6 oz)	140	8	2	15	23	2	990
Traditional Beef & Vegetable	1 cup (8.7 oz)	120	8	2	15	18	2	850
Traditional Beef Barley	1 cup (8.5 oz)	120	7	2	10	20	4	720
Traditional Chickarina	1 cup (8.3 oz)	120	8	5	20	12	2	950
Traditional Chicken & Wild Rice	1 cup (8.4 oz)	100	6	2	15	15	1	870
Traditional Homestyle Chicken	1 cup (8.4 oz)	100	6	2	10	14	1	830
Traditional Italian Style Wedding	1 cup (8.4 oz)	100	6	4	10	12	1	840
Traditional Manhattan Clam Chowder	1 cup (8.4 oz)	100	3	2	10	17	2	970
Traditional New England Clam Chowder	1 cup (8.4 oz)	180	6	9	15	20	1	890
Traditional Potato Broccoli & Cheese	1 cup (8.8 oz)	180	5	10	10	18	2	920
Traditional Split Pea w/ Ham	1 cup (8.5 oz)	140	9	1	5	24	4	690
Traditional Turkey Noodle	1 cup (8.4 oz)	80	5	2	15	12	1	980
Vegetable Classics Creamy Mushroom	1 cup (8.1 oz)	130	2	3	10	9	1	820
Vegetable Classics French Onion	1 cup (8 oz)	50	1	2	<5	8	tr	850
Vegetable Classics Hearty Black Bean	1 cup (8.5 oz)	160	8	1	<5	29	8	690
Vegetable Classics Hearty Tomato	1 cup (8.6 oz)	110	2	1	0	23	3	980
Vegetable Classics Lentil	1 cup (8.5 oz)	160	9	2	0	30	5	810
Vegetable Classics Vegetable	1 cup (8.4 oz)	80	5	0	0	15	3	660
World Recipes Caldo De Pollo	1 cup (8.6 oz)	90	5	2	10	14	1	690

FOOD	PORTION	CALS	PROT	FAT	CHOL	CARB	FIBER	SOD
Snow's								
Clam Chowder	1 cup (8.4 oz)	200	5	15	15	13	1	900
Swanson								
50% Low Sodium Beef Broth	1 cup	15	3	0	0	1	0	440
Beef Broth	1 cup	15	2	0	0	1	0	890
Beef Stock	1 cup	30	4	0	0	3	0	500
Chicken Broth	1 cup	10	1	0	5	1	0	860
Chicken Stock	1 cup	20	4	0	0	1	0	510
Vegetable Broth	1 cup	15	0	0	0	3	tr	940
Tabatchnick								
Graden Fresh Vegetable Broth	⅔ cup (5.5 oz)	10	0	0	0	2	0	550
Wisconsin Cheddar Cheese	⅔ cup (5.5 oz)	150	1	11	0	10	0	970
FROZEN								
Kettle Cuisine								
Angus Beef Steak Chili w/ Beans Gluten Free Dairy Free	1 pkg (10 oz)	250	19	12	55	17	4	760
Chicken w/ Rice Noodles Gluten Free	1 pkg (10 oz)	140	14	3	40	15	2	540
Roasted Vegetable Gluten Free Dairy Free	1 pkg (10 oz)	140	3	6	0	19	5	560
Three Bean Chili Gluten Free	1 pkg (10 oz)	220	11	4	0	36	13	450
Tabatchnick								
Cabbage	1 serv (7.5 oz)	90	2	1	0	21	1	160
Chicken Broth w/ Noodles & Dumplings	1 serv (7.25 oz)	150	5	6	65	19	tr	740
Corn Chowder	1 serv (7.5 oz)	130	4	5	10	21	2	390
Organic Vegetarian Chili	1 serv (7.5 oz)	180	12	4	0	28	8	360
Soup Singles Split Pea	1 bowl (10.9 oz)	210	19	1	0	50	20	540
Split Pea	1 serv (7.5 oz)	140	13	0	0	34	13	380

FOOD	PORTION	CALS	PROT	FAT	CHOL	CARB	FIBER	SOD
Vegetable	1 serv (7.5 oz)	90	3	2	0	17	4	350
Vegetable Low Sodium	1 serv (7.5 oz)	90	4	2	0	17	4	45
Wilderness Wild Rice	1 serv (7.5 oz)	80	3	1	0	16	1	220
Yankee Bean	1 serv (7.5 oz)	180	11	2	0	33	10	340
MIX								
beef broth cube	1 cube	6	1	tr	tr	1	–	864
chicken broth cube	1 cube (4.8 g)	9	1	tr	1	1	–	1152
Edward & Sons								
Bouillon Cubes Not-Beef	½ cube	20	1	2	0	1	0	920
Bouillon Cubes Not-Chicken	½ cube	15	1	2	0	1	0	800
Veggie Low Sodium	½ cup	20	1	2	0	1	0	135
HamBeens								
15 Bean as prep	½ cup	120	8	1	0	20	9	70
15 Bean Beef as prep	½ cup	120	8	1	0	20	9	310
15 Bean Cajun as prep	½ cup	120	8	1	0	20	9	100
15 Bean Chicken as prep	½ cup	120	8	1	0	20	9	250
Spanish American Black Bean as prep	½ cup	120	7	1	0	22	8	280
Kikkoman								
Instant Tofu Miso	1 pkg (6 g)	15	tr	0	0	3	0	700
Instant Wakame Seaweed	1 pkg (10 g)	35	3	1	0	3	0	740
Leahey Gardens								
No Beef Noodle	1½ cups	89	7	1	0	16	6	415
No Chicken Noodle	1½ cups	94	7	1	0	16	6	495
Manischewitz								
Lentil as prep	1 cup	150	7	0	0	29	12	530
Matzo Ball Soup	1 cup	40	1	1	0	9	1	1290
Southwestern Black Bean as prep	1 cup	90	4	1	0	16	4	1340
Split Pea w/ Barley as prep	1 cup	110	7	0	0	21	3	780
Vegetable & Pasta as prep	1 cup	90	4	0	0	17	2	650
Miso-Cup								
Golden Vegetable as prep	1 cup	30	2	1	0	3	tr	780
Japanese Restaurant Style as prep	1 cup	60	4	2	0	7	tr	1170

FOOD	PORTION	CALS	PROT	FAT	CHOL	CARB	FIBER	SOD
Organic Traditional w/ Tofu as prep	1 cup	35	2	1	0	4	tr	480
Reduced Sodium as prep	1 cup	25	2	1	0	3	tr	270
Savory Seaweed as prep	1 cup	30	3	1	0	3	tr	690
Nissin								
Chicken Vegetable as prep	1 pkg	290	6	13	<5	38	2	1430
White Cheddar as prep	1 pkg	290	6	13	0	38	2	1120
Silhouette Solution								
Mediterranean Tomato	1 pkg (1.16 oz)	110	15	3	30	8	1	440
Newbury Chicken Cream	1 pkg (1.3 oz)	110	15	3	30	8	1	520
Streit's								
Matzo Ball as prep	1 cup	50	tr	0	0	12	0	880
Thai Kitchen								
Rice Noodle Bowl Lemongrass & Chili as prep	½ pkg	110	2	2	0	23	1	850
Rice Noodle Bowl Thai Ginger as prep	½ pkg	120	2	2	0	23	1	620
REFRIGERATED								
Moosewood								
Organic Creamy Potato & Corn Chowder	1 cup (8.4 oz)	170	5	6	15	28	3	410
Organic Hungarian Vegetable Noodle	1 cup (8.4 oz)	80	2	2	0	13	2	480
Organic Savannah Sweet Potato Bisque	1 cup (8.4 oz)	200	6	11	20	20	2	580
Organic Texas Two Bean Chili	1 cup (8.4 oz)	200	9	4	0	34	8	840
Organic Tuscan White Bean & Vegetable	1 cup (8.4 oz)	130	6	2	0	24	5	760
Organic Classics								
French Onion w/ Croutons	1 cup	140	3	6	0	17	2	790
Seafood Chowder	1 cup	160	11	6	50	17	1	800
TAKE-OUT								
ban mien fish head	1 serv (10 oz)	277	20	10	59	27	4	851
beef stew soup	1 cup (8.8 oz)	221	23	5	60	20	–	461

FOOD	PORTION	CALS	PROT	FAT	CHOL	CARB	FIBER	SOD
bird's nest	1 cup (8.6 oz)	112	13	3	27	8	0	1549
black bean turtle soup	1 cup (6.5 oz)	240	15	1	0	45	10	442
broccoli cheese	1 cup	165	6	9	14	15	2	875
brunswick stew soup	1 cup (8.5 oz)	232	27	6	71	17	–	438
caldo de res beef soup	1 cup	143	12	5	22	12	2	784
chinese velvet corn	1¼ cups	135	–	0	1	–	–	708
corn & cheese chowder	¾ cup	215	9	12	66	21	3	386
duck soup	1 cup (8.6 oz)	412	16	37	88	2	tr	268
egg drop	1 cup	73	8	4	102	1	0	730
gazpacho	1 cup	46	1	tr	0	5	–	63
greek lemon	¾ cup	63	4	2	83	7	2	386
hot & sour	1 serv (14 oz)	173	14	9	79	9	3	1314
matzo ball soup	1 cup	118	7	5	63	10	1	757
minestrone	1 cup	233	9	13	9	22	4	700
miso w/ tofu	1 cup	84	6	3	0	8	2	989
onion soup gratinee	1 serv	492	25	27	77	38	4	1325
oxtail	1 cup	68	3	2	2	9	1	1166
pasta e fagioli	1 cup (8.8 oz)	194	9	5	3	30	–	790
ratatouille	1 cup (7.5 oz)	266	2	25	0	12	–	329
shark fin	1 bowl (10 oz)	164	15	9	84	9	0	1164
shrimp bisque	1 cup	263	22	14	129	13	tr	263
shrimp gumbo	1 cup (8.6 oz)	163	9	7	73	18	3	661
sopa de albondigas	1 cup	171	10	11	50	9	1	187
thai lemon grass	1 bowl	100	10	4	65	5	–	553
vietnamese pho beef noodle	1 serv (7.8 oz)	480	15	12	46	78	1	43
wonton soup	1 cup	183	14	7	53	14	1	769
yookgaejang korean beef	1 cup (8.4 oz)	94	6	6	50	4	1	209
zupa koprowa polish dill soup	1 bowl	54	11	2	55	6	–	524

FOOD	PORTION	CALS	PROT	FAT	CHOL	CARB	FIBER	SOD
SOUR CREAM								
fat free	½ cup (4.5 oz)	95	4	0	12	20	0	180
fat free	1 tbsp	12	1	0	1	3	0	23
reduced fat	½ cup (4.4 oz)	224	9	17	43	9	0	87
reduced fat	1 tbsp (0.5 oz)	29	1	2	6	1	0	11
sour cream	½ cup (4 oz)	222	2	23	60	3	0	92
sour cream	1 tbsp (0.4 oz)	23	tr	2	6	tr	0	10
Breakstone's								
Sour Cream	2 tbsp (1 oz)	60	tr	5	20	1	0	10
Cabot								
Light	2 tbsp	35	1	3	10	2	0	25
No Fat	2 tbsp	20	1	0	0	3	0	40
Sour Cream	2 tbsp	50	1	5	15	1	0	35
Friendship								
All Natural	2 tbsp (1 oz)	60	1	5	20	1	0	15
Light	1 tbsp (1 oz)	40	1	3	10	3	0	25
Nonfat	2 tbsp (1 oz)	25	2	0	0	4	0	20
Horizon Organic								
Lowfat	2 tbsp	35	1	2	10	3	0	25
Sour Cream	2 tbsp	60	1	5	20	1	0	15
Land O Lakes								
Fat Free	2 tbsp (1.1 oz)	20	1	0	0	3	0	50
Light	2 tbsp (1.1 oz)	40	1	3	5	2	0	20
Sour Cream	2 tbsp (1.1 oz)	60	1	6	20	2	0	40
Nancy's								
Organic	2 tbsp	60	1	6	20	2	0	20
Organic Valley								
Lowfat	2 tbsp	40	1	2	10	1	0	15
SOUR CREAM SUBSTITUTES								
imitation	½ cup (4 oz)	239	3	22	0	8	0	117

FOOD	PORTION	CALS	PROT	FAT	CHOL	CARB	FIBER	SOD
Vegan Gourmet								
Alternative Sour Cream	2 tbsp (1 oz)	50	0	5	0	3	2	25
SOURSOP								
fresh	1	416	6	2	0	105	–	87
fresh cut up	1 cup	150	2	1	0	38	–	31
SOY (*see also* CHEESE SUBSTITUTES, ICE CREAM AND FROZEN DESSERTS, MILK SUBSTITUTES, MISO, SMOOTHIES, SOY SAUCE, SOYBEANS, TEMPEH, TOFU, YOGURT FROZEN)								
natto	½ cup (3.1 oz)	187	16	10	0	13	5	6
Bob's Red Mill								
Protein Powder	1 tbsp	20	5	0	0	0	0	60
I.M. Healthy								
SoyNut Butter Chocolate	2 tbsp	190	6	14	0	12	3	0
SoyNut Butter Honey Creamy	2 tbsp	170	7	11	0	10	3	140
SoyNut Butter Original Chunky	2 tbsp	170	7	11	0	10	3	140
SoyNut Butter Original Creamy	2 tbsp	170	7	11	0	10	3	140
SoyNut Butter Unsweetened Creamy	2 tbsp	190	9	15	0	6	5	140
Simple Food								
Soynut Butter Chocolate	2 tbsp	190	10	12	0	8	2	90
Soynut Butter No Sugar No Salt	2 tbsp	200	10	14	0	8	2	0
Soy Wonder								
Creamy Spread	2 tbsp	170	8	11	0	10	1	170
SoyButter								
Spread	2 tbsp	200	7	15	0	8	2	120
SOY DRINKS (*see* MILK SUBSTITUTES, SMOOTHIES)								
SOY SAUCE								
shoyu	1 tbsp	9	1	tr	0	2	–	1029
soy sauce	1 tbsp	7	tr	tr	0	1	–	1024
tamari	1 tbsp	11	2	tr	0	1	–	1005
Angostura								
Lite Soy	1 tbsp (0.5 oz)	10	1	0	0	2	0	390

FOOD	PORTION	CALS	PROT	FAT	CHOL	CARB	FIBER	SOD
Soy Sauce	1 tbsp (0.5 oz)	10	1	0	0	1	0	670
Dave's Gourmet								
Soyabi Sauce	1 tbsp (0.6 oz)	30	0	2	–	4	–	340
House Of Tsang								
Ginger Soy Sauce	1 tbsp	20	0	0	0	4	0	760
Less Sodium	1 tbsp	5	0	0	0	0	0	300
Kikkoman								
Less Sodium	1 tbsp (0.5 oz)	10	1	0	0	1	–	575
Ponzu	1 tbsp (0.5 oz)	10	tr	0	0	2	–	400
Soy Sauce	1 tbsp (0.5 oz)	10	2	0	0	0	0	920
Sushi Sashimi	1 tbsp (0.5 oz)	15	1	0	0	2	–	870
La Choy								
Lite	1 tbsp (0.5 oz)	15	1	0	0	2	0	550
Lee Kum Kee								
Lite	1 tbsp (0.5 oz)	10	tr	0	0	1	–	600
Mitsukan								
Ponzu Citrus Seasoned	1 tbsp (0.5 oz)	10	0	0	0	1	–	580
San-J								
Tamari Organic Gluten Free	2 pkg (0.5 oz)	10	2	0	0	tr	–	940
Soy Vay								
Wasabiyaki	1 tbsp	35	tr	1	0	6	0	420
Tree Of Life								
Organic Shoyu	1 tbsp (0.5 oz)	15	2	0	0	1	0	960
Organic Tamari Wheat Free	1 tbsp (0.5 oz)	15	2	0	0	1	0	940
SOYBEANS								
dried cooked	1 cup	298	29	15	0	17	–	1
dry roasted	½ cup	387	34	19	0	28	–	2
green cooked	½ cup	127	11	6	0	10	4	13

FOOD	PORTION	CALS	PROT	FAT	CHOL	CARB	FIBER	SOD
roasted	½ cup	405	30	22	0	29	–	140
roasted & toasted	1 cup	490	40	26	0	33	–	4
roasted & toasted salted	1 cup	490	40	26	0	33	–	176
sprouts raw	½ cup	43	5	2	0	3	–	5
sprouts steamed	½ cup	38	4	2	0	3	–	5
sprouts stir fried	1 cup	125	13	7	0	9	–	14
Arrowhead Mills								
Organic Dried not prep	¼ cup	160	14	8	0	11	4	0
C&W								
In the Pod	½ cup	110	9	4	0	12	9	0
Crunchies								
Freeze Dried Edamame	⅜ cup (1 oz)	124	11	6	0	9	3	0
Freeze Dried Edamame Grilled	⅜ cup (0.9 oz)	84	3	1	0	13	1	68
Freeze Dried Edamame Salted	¼ cup (0.9 oz)	90	8	4	0	7	3	130
KooLoos								
Soy Nuts & Flaxseed BBQ	1 pkg (1 oz)	130	7	4	0	16	3	220
Soy Nuts & Flaxseed Original	1 pkg (1 oz)	140	7	5	0	15	3	280
Seapoint Farms								
Edamame Dry Roasted Goji Blend	¼ cup	120	11	3	0	15	7	140
Edamame Dry Roasted Lightly Salted	¼ cup	130	14	4	0	10	8	150
Edamame Dry Roasted Wasabi	¼ cup	130	14	5	0	9	7	130
Edamame In Pods frzn	½ cup	100	8	3	0	9	4	30
Edamame In Pods Lightly Salted	½ cup	100	8	3	0	9	4	260
Edamame Shelled	½ cup	100	8	3	0	9	4	30
Organic Edamame In Pods	½ cup	100	8	3	0	9	4	30
Organic Edamame Shelled	½ cup	100	8	3	0	9	4	30
South Beach								
Soy Nuts Dark Chocolate	1 pkg (0.7 oz)	100	3	6	0	9	2	0

SPAGHETTI (*see* PASTA, PASTA DINNERS, PASTA SALAD, SPAGHETTI SAUCE)

FOOD	PORTION	CALS	PROT	FAT	CHOL	CARB	FIBER	SOD
SPAGHETTI SAUCE								
JARRED								
marinara sauce	1 cup	171	4	8	0	25	–	1572
spaghetti sauce	1 cup	272	12	12	0	40	–	1236
Amy's								
Organic Family Marinara	½ cup (4.4 oz)	80	1	5	0	10	3	590
Organic Marinara Low Sodium	½ cup (4.4 oz)	40	1	1	0	7	1	100
Barilla								
Arrabbiata Tomato & Spicy Pepper	½ cup	90	2	3	0	11	3	560
Garden Vegetable	½ cup	70	2	2	0	11	2	460
Green & Black Olive	½ cup	80	2	3	0	10	4	770
Italian Baking Sauce	¼ cup (4.4 oz)	60	2	1	0	12	2	460
Mushroom & Garlic	½ cup	70	3	2	0	12	2	450
Dave's Gourmet								
Pasta Sauce Spicy Heirloom Marinara	½ cup (4.4 oz)	45	1	2	–	7	2	280
Pasta Sauce Wild Mushroom	½ cup (4.4 oz)	60	2	3	–	7	tr	270
Dei Fratelli								
Arrabbiata	½ cup (4.2 oz)	50	2	2	0	8	2	300
Pizza Sauce	¼ cup (2.2 oz)	30	1	2	0	5	1	230
Del Monte								
W/ Mushrooms	½ cup (4.4 oz)	70	2	1	0	14	2	630
DelGrosso								
Garden Style	½ cup (4.4 oz)	70	2	2	0	12	2	580
Mushroom	½ cup (4.4 oz)	70	3	2	0	11	3	510
New York Style	¼ cup (2.1 oz)	35	1	1	0	6	1	310
Original Meat Flavored	½ cup (4.4 oz)	80	3	2	5	12	3	500

FOOD	PORTION	CALS	PROT	FAT	CHOL	CARB	FIBER	SOD
Pizza Sauce Pepperoni	¼ cup (2.2 oz)	40	2	1	0	6	2	270
Three Cheese	½ cup (4.4 oz)	80	2	2	0	13	3	660
Francesco Rinaldi								
Alfredo	¼ cup (2.1 oz)	80	1	6	35	3	0	400
Chunky Eggplant Parmesan	½ cup (4.4 oz)	90	2	5	0	11	tr	650
Chunky Mushroom & Pepper	½ cup (4.4 oz)	80	2	3	0	13	2	660
Hearty Mushroom Pepper & Onion	½ cup (4.4 oz)	80	2	3	0	12	2	640
Hearty Sweet & Tasty Tomato	½ cup (4.4 oz)	100	2	5	0	16	tr	700
Hearty Three Cheese	½ cup (4.4 oz)	80	3	2	0	15	tr	470
Organic Burgundy Marinara	½ cup (4.3 oz)	100	1	7	0	9	tr	820
Premium Vodka	¼ cup (2.1 oz)	60	2	4	10	4	0	290
Traditional Meat Flavored	½ cup (4.4 oz)	80	2	4	5	12	tr	650
Traditional No Salt Added	½ cup (4.4 oz)	70	2	3	0	12	2	40
Traditional Original	½ cup (4.4 oz)	80	2	3	0	12	tr	650
Hunt's								
100% Natural Sauce	¼ cup (2.2 oz)	20	tr	0	0	4	1	410
Italian Sausage	½ cup	60	3	2	0	10	3	590
Meat	½ cup	60	3	1	0	11	3	610
Traditional	½ cup	50	2	1	0	10	2	580
With Mushrooms	½ cup	45	2	1	0	10	3	290
Knorr								
W/ Meat	4 oz	110	6	5	20	9	–	820
Lucini								
Spicy Tuscan	½ cup (4.4 oz)	80	2	5	0	8	2	480

FOOD	PORTION	CALS	PROT	FAT	CHOL	CARB	FIBER	SOD
Tuscan Marinara w/ Roasted Garlic	½ cup (4.4 oz)	60	2	3	0	8	1	310
Mom's								
Artichoke Heart & Asiago Cheese	½ cup (4.2 oz)	90	3	6	5	7	3	360
Fresh Garlic Basil	½ cup (4.2 oz)	30	2	3	0	7	2	420
Martini	½ cup (4.2 oz)	120	3	4	20	6	1	250
Puttanesca	½ cup (4.2 oz)	90	2	6	5	8	2	550
Muir Glen								
Organic Chunky Tomato	¼ cup	15	tr	0	0	4	tr	230
Organic Garlic Roasted Garlic	½ cup	60	2	1	0	12	2	380
Organic Pizza Sauce	¼ cup	40	1	2	0	6	1	290
Organic Tomato Sauce No Salt Added	¼ cup	25	1	0	0	5	1	10
Pomi								
Strained	½ cup (4.4 oz)	30	1	0	0	5	3	10
Prego								
Heart Smart Traditional Italian	½ cup	100	2	3	0	15	3	430
Italian	½ cup	70	2	2	0	13	3	470
Italian Marinara	½ cup	100	2	5	0	11	4	550
Italian Meat	½ cup	130	2	4	5	19	3	570
Italian Roasted Red Pepper & Garlic	½ cup	90	2	4	0	13	3	530
Italian Three Cheese	½ cup	80	3	2	0	14	3	430
Italian Tomato Basil & Garlic	½ cup	80	2	3	0	12	3	420
Organic Mushroom	½ cup	90	2	3	0	13	4	540
Veggie Smart	½ cup (4.2 oz)	90	2	2	0	16	3	360
Progresso								
Lobster Sauce	½ cup (4.3 oz)	100	3	7	5	6	2	430
Pesto Arrabiata	2 tbsp (1 oz)	140	3	11	5	7	2	140
Pesto Basil & Roasted Garlic	2 tbsp (1 oz)	130	2	13	0	3	0	75

FOOD	PORTION	CALS	PROT	FAT	CHOL	CARB	FIBER	SOD
Red Clam	½ cup (4.4 oz)	60	4	1	10	8	1	350
White Clam	½ cup (4.4 oz)	150	9	10	20	5	0	710
Ragu								
Light Tomato & Basil No Sugar Added	½ cup (4.4 oz)	50	2	1	0	9	3	330
Old World Style Margherita	½ cup (4.4 oz)	70	2	2	0	10	2	410
Old World Style Meat	½ cup (4.4 oz)	70	2	3	0	9	2	460
Old World Style Sweet Tomato Basil	½ cup (4.4 oz)	60	2	2	0	10	3	410
Pizza Quick Fresh Italian	2 oz	35	1	1	0	5	–	270
Robert Rothchild Farm								
Artichoke	½ cup	80	2	5	0	8	0	90
S&W								
Tomato Sauce	¼ cup (2.1 oz)	20	1	0	0	4	1	260
Two Guys								
Jersey Tomato Sauce	½ cup (4.6 oz)	60	2	2	0	10	2	190
Vino De Milo								
Mediterranean Pinot Grigio	½ cup	90	2	4	0	12	2	320
Portobello Shiraz	½ cup	40	1	1	0	9	2	340
Tuscan Merlot	½ cup	80	–	3	0	2	2	470
Walden Farms								
Alfredo Sauce Calorie Free	3 tbsp (1.6 oz)	0	0	0	0	0	0	200
Walnut Acres								
Organic Garlic Garlic	½ cup	125	2	1	0	10	1	280
Organic Marinara & Zinfandel	½ cup	125	2	1	0	9	1	330
Organic Roasted Garlic	½ cup	125	2	1	0	11	1	280
Organic Tomato & Basil	½ cup	125	2	1	0	9	1	330
MIX								
Loney's								
Carbonara as prep	¼ cup (2.1 oz)	33	tr	3	9	3	0	240
Rose as prep	¼ cup (2.1 oz)	29	1	3	0	6	0	240

FOOD	PORTION	CALS	PROT	FAT	CHOL	CARB	FIBER	SOD
TAKE-OUT								
bolognese	5 oz	195	11	15	–	4	tr	–
SPANISH FOOD								
FROZEN								
Amy's								
Bowl Mexican Casserole	1 pkg (9.4 oz)	470	11	16	20	70	7	780
Burrito Black Bean	1 (6 oz)	280	9	8	0	44	4	580
Burrito Cheddar Cheese	1 (6 oz)	300	11	9	10	43	6	580
Burrito Southwestern	1 (5.5 oz)	300	12	10	15	43	6	680
Enchilada Black Bean Vegetable	1 (4.7 oz)	180	5	6	0	26	3	390
Cedarlane								
Organic Burrito Low Fat Rice & Cheese	1 (6 oz)	260	13	1	0	48	7	490
Organic Enchilada Low Fat Black Bean & Tofu	1 (9 oz)	220	10	3	0	42	6	390
Roasted Chile Relleno	1 pkg (10 oz)	400	23	20	55	37	5	770
Zone Burrito Beans & Cheese	1 (6 oz)	350	27	13	15	37	8	380
Contessa								
Fajitas Shrimp	2 (8 oz)	230	11	4	45	37	5	940
Paella w/ Chicken & Seafood	1½ cups	200	17	3	50	28	2	780
Seafood Veracruz not prep	1¾ cups	180	15	2	35	27	6	920
El Monterey								
Burrito Bean & Cheese	1 (5 oz)	280	10	8	5	43	5	560
Burrito Beef & Bean	1 (5 oz)	370	10	17	20	42	4	610
Burrito Half Pound Spicy Red Hot Beef & Bean	1 (8 oz)	600	17	29	35	68	7	1120
Burrito Supreme Breakfast Egg Cheese & Sausage	1 (4.5 oz)	300	10	13	75	34	1	630
Burrito Supreme Shredded Steak & Cheese	1 (5 oz)	290	12	9	20	41	1	590
Burrito XX Large Bean & Cheese	1 (10 oz)	590	21	17	10	88	5	950
Burrito XX Large Beef & Bean	1 (10 oz)	730	22	35	40	83	8	1180

FOOD	PORTION	CALS	PROT	FAT	CHOL	CARB	FIBER	SOD
Cruncheros Cheese & Beef	3 (4.5 oz)	330	10	16	20	35	2	560
Cruncheros Taco Beef & Cheese	4 (5.6 oz)	460	12	29	40	38	2	1040
Enchiladas Cheese w/ Sauce	1 serv (8 oz)	250	11	15	35	22	3	990
Enchiladas Shredded Beef w/ Sauce	1 serv (4 oz)	140	6	6	15	15	2	450
Quesadillas Chicken & Cheese	2 (6 oz)	380	17	15	35	43	2	930
Quesadillas Steak & Cheese	2 (6 oz)	400	21	15	55	42	1	860
Tamales Chicken	1 (4.5 oz)	240	8	12	25	27	2	750
Tamales Shredded Beef	1 (4.5 oz)	310	9	19	30	27	3	660
Taquitos Corn Shredded Beef	3 (4.5 oz)	300	11	13	40	31	1	560
Taquitos Flour Char-Broiled Chicken Breast	3 (5 oz)	380	15	19	35	36	1	670
Taquitos Flour Chicken & Cheese	3 (4.5 oz)	350	10	18	15	36	2	650
Taquitos Southwest Chicken In A Seasoned Batter	2 (2.8 oz)	175	6	8	10	20	1	330
Tornados Apple Cinnamon	1 (3 oz)	180	4	5	0	31	0	140
Tornados Sausage Egg & Cheese	1 (3 oz)	230	6	13	40	23	1	410
Tornados Shredded Beef	1 (3 oz)	210	7	10	15	23	1	400
Tornados Steak Egg & Cheese	1 (3 oz)	170	7	6	10	22	0	310
Tornados XXL Southwest Chicken	1 (4.2 oz)	210	7	10	15	28	1	530
Glutenfreeda								
Burrito Breakfast Beef	1 (3.9 oz)	199	10	8	27	23	2	150
Burrito Vegetarian Bean & Cheese	1 (3.9 oz)	196	6	7	12	29	3	188
Health Is Wealth								
Vegetarian Hot Tamale Munchees	6 (3 oz)	160	6	3	5	26	3	330
Helen's Kitchen								
Cheese Enchiladas w/ Tofu Steaks In Spicy Red Sauce	½ pkg (5 oz)	150	5	9	10	20	5	300

FOOD	PORTION	CALS	PROT	FAT	CHOL	CARB	FIBER	SOD
Jose Ole								
Burrito Chicken	1 (5 oz)	270	9	7	20	41	2	630
Burrito Steak & Jalapeno	1 (5 oz)	300	11	9	15	43	3	710
Chimichanga Shredded Beef	1 (5 oz)	350	13	15	25	39	2	510
Meals To Live								
White Chicken Burrito w/ Green Sauce	1 pkg (9 oz)	330	17	5	15	58	15	480
Patio								
Burrito Bean & Cheese	1	280	8	8	5	44	5	630
Burrito Beef & Bean Mild	1	300	10	10	<5	44	5	740
Enchilada & Beef Tamale	1 meal	460	13	14	0	69	5	1210
Enchilada Beef	1 meal	380	11	12	5	55	5	1270
Enchilada Cheese	1 meal	390	12	13	10	58	10	1500
Enchilada Combo Dinner	1 meal	380	11	12	5	57	5	1250
Stouffer's								
Chicken Enchilada w/ Cheese Sauce & Rice	1 pkg (7.13 oz)	280	12	12	40	30	3	720
Tyson								
Meal Kit Chicken Fajita	1 (3.8 oz)	130	8	4	15	17	2	350
Meal Kit Quesadilla Chicken	1 (4 oz)	250	15	10	35	26	3	430
READY-TO-EAT								
taco shell corn	1 (6.5 inch)	98	2	5	0	13	2	77
taco shell flour	1 (7 inch)	173	3	9	0	19	1	168
TAKE-OUT								
arroz con coco	1 cup	532	7	38	4	46	4	108
burrito w/ beans	1 med (5 oz)	295	10	8	6	45	7	501
burrito w/ beans & rice	1 (3.5 oz)	221	7	5	2	37	4	397
burrito w/ beef	1 sm (3.4 oz)	297	18	13	49	25	1	460
burrito w/ beef & beans	1 med (5 oz)	331	17	13	34	36	6	524
burrito w/ beef beans & cheese	1 med (5 oz)	379	21	19	57	30	5	596
burrito w/ chicken & beans	1 med (5 oz)	295	18	9	37	34	5	498
burrito w/ pork & beans	1 med (5 oz)	320	18	12	34	35	6	494

FOOD	PORTION	CALS	PROT	FAT	CHOL	CARB	FIBER	SOD
chiles rellenos meat & cheese filled	1 (5 oz)	213	10	16	109	9	2	430
chimichanga w/ bean cheese lettuce & tomato	1 (4.1 oz)	271	8	18	17	22	3	301
chimichanga w/ beef & rice	1 (10 oz)	634	19	36	35	58	5	573
chimichanga w/ beef beans lettuce & tomato	1 (4.1 oz)	254	9	15	15	22	3	225
chimichanga w/ beef cheese lettuce & tomato	1 (4.1 oz)	337	13	24	37	19	1	348
chimichanga w/ chicken sour cream lettuce & tomato	1 (4 oz)	277	9	20	30	17	1	153
empanada fruit filled	1 (3.8 oz)	452	4	25	0	55	2	281
empanada meat & vegetable	1 (7.8 oz)	881	18	61	40	66	3	697
empanada sweet potato	1 (7.8 oz)	546	8	23	56	76	4	622
enchilada w/ beans	1 (4.1 oz)	179	6	6	4	27	6	297
enchilada w/ beans & cheese	1 (4.6 oz)	233	9	11	21	25	5	381
enchilada w/ beef	1 (4 oz)	214	11	10	30	21	3	179
enchilada w/ beef & beans	1 (4 oz)	195	8	8	15	25	4	303
frijoles	1 cup	278	18	2	0	49	9	606
frijoles w/ cheese	1 cup	225	11	8	37	29	–	882
nachos w/ beans & cheese	1 serv (9.4 oz)	616	25	33	56	57	13	990
nachos w/ beef beans cheese & sour cream	1 serv (19 oz)	1620	59	97	171	133	19	1846
paella	1 serv (7 oz)	308	23	16	92	17	3	580
pupusa meat filled	1 (3.6 oz)	187	8	6	20	26	3	88
quesadilla w/ cheese	1 (5 oz)	498	20	28	60	40	3	1234
quesadilla w/ meat & cheese	1 (6.5 oz)	605	32	35	98	40	2	1268
taco de jueye w/ crab meat	1 (4.2 oz)	266	16	14	79	18	2	800
taco w/ beans lettuce tomato & salsa	1 (2.8 oz)	117	4	5	2	16	4	214
taco w/ chicken lettuce tomato & salsa	1 (2.5 oz)	114	8	5	22	10	1	134
taco w/ fish lettuce tomato & salsa	1 (2.7 oz)	101	8	4	39	10	1	190

FOOD	PORTION	CALS	PROT	FAT	CHOL	CARB	FIBER	SOD
tostada w/ beef lettuce tomato & salsa	1 (2.7 oz)	143	8	8	21	11	2	152
SPICES (*see individual names,* HERBS/SPICES)								
SPINACH								
CANNED								
drained	1 cup	49	6	1	0	7	5	58
Freshlike								
Cut Leaf	½ cup	45	5	1	0	5	3	200
Popeye								
Leaf Spinach	½ cup	30	3	0	0	4	2	190
Leaf Spinach No Salt Added	½ cup	40	4	1	0	5	2	30
S&W								
Leaf	½ cup (4 oz)	30	2	0	0	4	2	360
FRESH								
baby raw	2 cups	20	1	0	0	5	3	80
cooked	1 cup	41	5	tr	0	7	4	126
malabar cooked	1 cup	10	1	tr	0	1	1	24
mustard cooked	1 cup	29	3	tr	0	5	4	25
new zealand cooked	1 cup	22	2	tr	0	4	–	193
raw	1 cup	7	1	tr	0	1	1	24
Fresh Express								
Baby Spinach	3 cups	20	2	0	0	3	2	65
Organic Baby Spinach	3 cups	35	2	0	0	9	4	135
Ready Pac								
Microwave Spinach as prep	½ cup (3 oz)	20	2	0	0	3	1	60
FROZEN								
chopped cooked	1 cup	30	4	tr	0	5	4	92
Birds Eye								
Chopped	⅓ cup	20	2	0	0	2	2	115
Creamed	½ cup (4.4 oz)	90	3	4	10	9	4	500
C&W								
Baby Chopped	1 cup	30	2	0	0	3	1	120
Creamed	½ cup	100	4	7	20	6	4	410
Cascadian Farm								
Organic Cut	⅓ cup	25	2	0	0	3	1	160
Cedarlane								
Organic Spanakopita Spinach & Feta Pie	½ pkg (5 oz)	260	12	8	20	38	2	650

FOOD	PORTION	CALS	PROT	FAT	CHOL	CARB	FIBER	SOD
Dr. Praeger's								
Spinach Bites	2 (2 oz)	110	3	3	0	17	2	230
Fillo Factory								
Spanakopita Spinach & Cheese Fillo Appetizers	3 (3 oz)	190	6	9	20	20	1	280
Health Is Wealth								
Creamed	½ pkg (4.5 oz)	100	5	4	15	27	2	160
Spinach Munchees	6 (3oz)	180	7	7	0	25	3	320
Seabrook Farms								
Chopped	⅓ cup (2.9 oz)	20	2	0	0	2	2	115
Creamed	½ cup (4.4 oz)	100	4	5	10	10	2	390
Stouffer's								
Creamed	½ pkg (4.5 oz)	200	5	16	25	8	2	490
Tabatchnick								
Creamed	1 serv (3.7 oz)	40	1	1	5	7	1	240
Veggie Patch								
Spinach Bites	3 (2.6 oz)	150	6	8	10	16	3	350
TAKE-OUT								
indian saag	1 serv	28	2	2	0	2	1	44
spanakopita spinach pie	1 serv (3 oz)	148	5	11	60	8	1	289
SPINACH JUICE								
juice	7 oz	14	2	0	0	2	–	146
SPORTS DRINKS (*see* ENERGY DRINKS)								
SPOT								
baked	3 oz	134	20	5	–	0	0	32
SPROUTS								
kidney bean	½ cup	27	4	tr	0	4	–	–
lentil	½ cup	40	3	tr	0	8	–	4
mung bean	½ cup	16	2	tr	0	3	–	3
mung bean canned	½ cup	8	1	tr	0	1	–	–
mung bean cooked	½ cup	13	1	tr	0	3	–	6

FOOD	PORTION	CALS	PROT	FAT	CHOL	CARB	FIBER	SOD
pea	½ cup (2.1 oz)	74	5	tr	0	16	–	12
radish	½ cup	8	1	tr	0	1	–	1
Brassica								
BroccoSprouts	½ cup (1 oz)	16	1	0	0	2	1	3
La Choy								
Bean Sprouts	⅔ cup	15	tr	0	0	3	1	60
TAKE-OUT								
mung bean stir fried	½ cup	31	3	tr	0	7	–	–
SQUAB								
boneless baked	1 (4 oz)	242	26	14	129	0	0	243
SQUASH (*see also* SQUASH SEEDS, ZUCCHINI)								
CANNED								
crookneck sliced	½ cup	14	1	tr	0	3	–	5
Sunshine								
Slice Yellow	½ cup	25	0	0	0	5	2	160
FRESH								
acorn cooked mashed	½ cup	41	1	tr	0	11	3	3
acorn cubed baked	½ cup	57	1	tr	0	15	2	4
butternut baked	½ cup	41	1	tr	0	11	2	4
crookneck sliced cooked	½ cup	18	1	tr	0	4	1	1
hubbard baked	½ cup	51	3	tr	0	11	3	8
hubbard cooked mashed	½ cup	35	2	tr	0	8	3	6
scallop sliced cooked	½ cup	14	1	tr	0	3	1	1
spaghetti cooked	½ cup	23	1	tr	0	5	2	14
Glory								
Yellow Sliced	¾ cup	20	1	0	0	3	1	20
Mann's								
Butternut Cubes	1 serv (3 oz)	40	1	0	0	10	2	0
FROZEN								
butternut cooked mashed	½ cup	47	1	tr	0	12	3	2
crookneck sliced cooked	½ cup	24	1	tr	0	5	–	6
C&W								
Butternut	½ cup	45	1	0	0	10	1	2
McKenzie's								
Southland Butternut	½ cup	70	1	3	0	10	1	270
TAKE-OUT								
fritter	1 (0.8 oz)	81	2	5	15	8	1	79

FOOD	PORTION	CALS	PROT	FAT	CHOL	CARB	FIBER	SOD
squash pie	1 slice (5.4 oz)	291	6	12	66	40	2	259
SQUASH SEEDS								
roasted	1 oz	148	9	12	0	4	5	5
salted & roasted	1 oz	148	9	12	0	4	–	5
seeds dried	1 oz	154	7	13	0	5	2	5
seeds whole roasted	1 oz	127	5	6	0	15	2	5
SQUID								
baked	1 cup	192	26	6	393	5	0	540
canned in its own ink	1 can (4 oz)	122	21	2	308	4	0	360
dried	1 sm (1.5 oz)	147	25	2	371	5	0	255
pickled	1 oz	26	4	tr	63	1	0	431
steamed	1 cup	147	25	2	374	5	0	587
Contessa								
Calamari + Sauce	13 pieces + 2 tbsp sauce	160	5	6	55	21	1	370
Van de Kamp's								
Fried Calamari	15 pieces (4 oz)	270	10	13	105	26	1	650
TAKE-OUT								
arroz con calamares	1 cup	400	14	17	150	47	1	906
calamari breaded & fried	1 cup	296	26	12	378	17	1	584
SQUIRREL								
roasted	3 oz	147	26	4	103	0	0	102
STARFRUIT								
fresh	1	42	1	tr	0	10	–	2
STRAWBERRIES								
canned in heavy syrup	½ cup	117	1	tr	0	30	2	5
fresh halves	1 cup	49	1	tr	0	12	3	2
fresh whole	1 cup	46	1	tr	0	11	3	1
fresh whole	1 pint	114	2	1	0	27	7	4
frzn sweetened sliced	½ cup	122	1	tr	0	33	2	4
frzn sweetened whole	1 cup	199	1	tr	0	54	5	3
frzn whole unsweetened	1 cup	77	1	tr	0	20	5	4
organic fresh whole	8 med	45	1	0	0	12	4	0
C&W								
Ultimate Sliced frzn	⅔ cup	50	0	0	0	12	1	5

FOOD	PORTION	CALS	PROT	FAT	CHOL	CARB	FIBER	SOD
Chukar Cherries								
Dried	¼ cup	120	tr	0	0	29	2	0
Crunchies								
Freeze Dried	¼ cup (6 g)	20	0	0	0	5	1	0
Emily's								
Dark Chocolate Covered	6 (1.4 oz)	170	1	8	0	28	2	0
FruitziO								
Strawberries Freeze Dried	1 pkg (0.9 oz)	100	2	0	0	22	3	0
LiteHouse								
Glaze Sugar Free	3 tbsp	35	0	0	0	8	0	55
Marie's								
Glaze	2 tbsp	40	0	0	0	10	0	40
Polar								
Strawberries In Syrup	½ cup	90	1	0	0	21	1	10
Stoneridge Orchards								
Dried	⅓ cup (1.4 oz)	140	0	0	0	35	0	15
STUFFING/DRESSING								
Fresh Gourmet								
All Natural Multi-Grain w/ Cranberries not prep	⅓ cup (1 oz)	110	3	3	0	19	1	360
Organic Seasoned not prep	⅓ cup (1 oz)	110	3	3	0	19	1	350
Pepperidge Farm								
Corn Bread	¾ cup	170	4	2	0	33	2	480
Cube	¾ cup	140	4	1	0	28	2	530
Herb Seasoned	¾ cup (1.5 oz)	170	5	2	0	33	3	600
One Step Turkey	½ cup	170	4	7	0	23	1	540
TAKE-OUT								
bread	1 cup	352	6	17	0	44	2	1028
cornbread	½ cup	179	3	9	0	22	3	455
kishke stuffed derma	1 piece (1.3 oz)	166	2	12	13	13	1	145
oyster	1 cup	304	7	18	23	29	2	953
sausage	½ cup	292	8	11	12	40	1	258
STURGEON								
broiled	3 oz	115	18	4	65	0	0	59

FOOD	PORTION	CALS	PROT	FAT	CHOL	CARB	FIBER	SOD
roe raw	1 oz	59	7	3	–	tr	–	–
smoked	1 oz	49	9	1	23	0	0	210
TAKE-OUT								
breaded & fried	4 oz	252	19	15	85	9	1	416
SUCKER								
white baked	3 oz	101	18	3	45	0	0	44
SUGAR (*see also* FRUCTOSE, SYRUP)								
brown organic	1 tsp	17	0	0	0	4	0	0
brown packed	1 cup (7.7 oz)	828	0	0	0	214	–	86
brown unpacked	1 cup (5.1 oz)	547	0	0	0	141	0	57
cinnamon sugar	1 tsp	16	tr	tr	0	4	tr	0
cube	1 (2 g)	9	0	0	0	2	0	0
maple	1 piece (1 oz)	99	tr	tr	0	25	0	3
powdered	1 tbsp (0.3 oz)	31	0	0	0	8	–	0
powdered unsifted	1 cup (4.2 oz)	467	tr	tr	0	119	–	2
raw	1 pkg (5 g)	19	0	0	0	5	0	2
sugarcane stem	3 oz	54	1	0	0	14	3	–
white	1 packet (3 g)	12	0	0	0	3	0	0
white	1 tbsp (0.4 oz)	49	0	0	0	13	0	0
white	1 cup (7 oz)	773	0	0	0	200	–	3
white	1 tsp (4 g)	15	0	0	0	4	–	0
Bob's Red Mill								
Date Sugar	1 tsp	11	0	0	0	3	0	0
Turbinado	1 tsp	10	0	0	0	3	0	0
Domino								
Dark Brown	1 tsp (4 g)	15	0	0	0	4	–	0
Demerara Raw Cane	1 tsp	15	0	0	0	4	0	0
Equinox								
Organic Maple Flakes	2 tsp	15	0	0	0	4	–	0
Sugar In The Raw								
Turbinado Sugar	1 pkg (5 g)	20	0	0	0	5	–	0
Tree Of Life								
Date Sugar	1 tsp (4 g)	10	0	0	0	3	0	0

FOOD	PORTION	CALS	PROT	FAT	CHOL	CARB	FIBER	SOD
Organic Cane Juice Dehydrated	1 tsp (3.5 g)	15	0	0	0	3	0	10
Turbinado	1 tsp (4 g)	15	0	0	0	4	0	0
Wholesome Sweeteners								
Organic	1 tsp (4 g)	15	0	0	0	4	0	0
Organic Fair Trade Dark Brown Sugar	1 tsp (4 g)	15	0	0	0	4	0	0
Organic Fair Trade Powdered	¼ cup (1 oz)	120	0	0	0	30	0	0
Organic Fair Trade Sucanat	1 tsp (4 g)	15	0	0	0	4	0	0
Organic Turbinado	1 tsp (4 g)	15	0	0	0	4	0	0
SUGAR SUBSTITUTES								
Emerald City								
Erythritol	1 tsp (4 g)	0	0	0	0	4	0	0
Emerald Forest								
Xylitol	1 tsp (4 g)	10	0	0	0	4	0	0
Equal								
Packet	1 pkg	0	0	0	0	tr	–	0
Fibrelle								
Fiber-Rich Sweetener	1 tbsp (0.4 oz)	15	0	0	0	11	7	0
Fructevia								
All Natural	1 tsp (4 g)	5	0	0	0	2	0	0
Fruit Sweetness								
Sugar Substitute	1 serv (0.9 oz)	0	0	0	0	0	0	0
Nature's Family								
Sun Crystals	1 pkg (4.5 g)	4	0	0	0	1	–	0
Nevella								
No Calorie Sweetener	1 tsp (0.5 g)	0	0	0	0	tr	0	0
Neway								
Sweet Sensation	¼ tsp	0	0	0	0	tr	0	0
PureVia								
All Natural	1 pkg (2 g)	0	0	0	0	2	0	0
Splenda								
Brown Sugar Blend	½ tsp (2 g)	10	0	0	0	2	0	0
Cafe Sticks	1 pkg (1 g)	0	0	0	0	tr	0	0
Flavor Accents Sticks	1 pkg (1 g)	0	0	0	0	tr	0	0
Flavors For Coffee	1 pkg (1 g)	0	0	0	0	tr	0	0
No Calorie Granulated	1 tsp (0.5 g)	0	0	0	0	tr	0	0

FOOD	PORTION	CALS	PROT	FAT	CHOL	CARB	FIBER	SOD
No Calorie Sweetener w/ Fiber	1 pkg	0	0	0	0	2	1	0
Sugar Blends	½ tsp (2 g)	10	0	0	0	2	–	0
Steel's								
Nature Sweet Brown Crystals	1 tsp (3 g)	6	0	0	0	3	0	0
Nature Sweet Crystals	1 tsp (4 g)	8	0	0	0	4	0	0
Sugar Free Vanilla Flavor	1 tbsp (0.5 oz)	23	0	0	0	11	0	0
Stevia In The Raw								
100% Natural Sweetener	1 pkg (1 g)	0	0	0	0	0	0	0
Steviva								
Blend	1 tbsp (0.4 oz)	2	0	0	0	0	0	0
Sugar Twin								
Granulated Brown	1 tsp (0.4 g)	0	0	0	0	tr	0	0
Granulated White	1 tsp (0.4 g)	0	0	0	0	tr	0	0
Liquid	¼ tsp (1.3 g)	0	0	0	0	0	0	0
Packets	1 (0.8 g)	0	0	0	0	1	–	0
Sun Crystals								
Natural Sweetener	1 pkg (5 g)	5	0	0	0	1	–	0
Susta								
Natural Sweetener	1 pkg (2 g)	5	0	0	0	2	1	0
Suzanne								
Somersweet Baking Blend	1 tsp (4 g)	5	0	0	0	4	2	0
Sweet Fiber								
All Natural	1 pkg	0	0	0	0	tr	tr	0
Sweete								
Sugar Free	1 pkg	0	0	0	0	tr	0	10
Truvia								
Calorie Free Sweetener	1 pkg (3.5 g)	0	0	0	0	3	0	0
Whey Low								
Gold	1 tsp	4	0	0	0	4	0	0
Granular	1 tsp	4	0	0	0	4	0	0
Maple Buzz	¼ cup	57	0	0	0	57	0	0
Wholesome Sweeteners								
Organic Zero	1 pkg (6 g)	0	0	0	0	6	0	0
ZSweet								
All Natural	1 pkg (1 g)	0	0	0	0	tr	0	0

FOOD	PORTION	CALS	PROT	FAT	CHOL	CARB	FIBER	SOD
SUGAR-APPLE								
fresh	1	146	3	tr	0	37	–	15
fresh cut up	1 cup	236	5	1	0	59	–	24
SUNCHOKE								
fresh raw sliced	½ cup	57	2	tr	0	13	–	–
SUNFISH								
pumpkinseed baked	3 oz	97	21	1	73	0	0	87
SUNFLOWER								
seeds dry roasted w/ salt	¼ cup	186	6	16	0	8	3	131
seeds dry roasted w/o salt	¼ cup	186	6	16	0	8	4	1
seeds w/ hulls dried	¼ cup	66	3	6	0	2	1	0
Arrowhead Mills								
Organic Seeds	¼ cup	170	7	15	0	6	3	0
Bob's Red Mill								
Seeds Roasted & Salted	3 tbsp	186	6	15	0	6	5	104
Dakota Gourmet								
Seeds Honey Roasted	¼ cup (1 oz)	170	5	12	0	8	2	110
Lance								
Shelled Seeds	1 pkg (1.8 oz)	300	6	25	0	14	3	160
SunButter								
Creamy	2 tbsp	200	7	16	0	7	4	120
Organic	2 tbsp	203	8	16	0	7	3	100
SunGold								
Seeds Roasted Salted	1 oz	172	7	15	0	4	2	168
Tree Of Life								
Seeds Kernels Raw	¼ cup (1.3 oz)	210	8	18	0	7	2	15
SUSHI								
TAKE-OUT								
california roll	1 (1.2 oz)	48	1	1	17	8	tr	163
crabmeat mayonnaise	1 (1.2 oz)	60	2	2	3	10	tr	155
futomaki roll	1 (1.8 oz)	73	2	1	22	14	1	228
ikura salmon roe & cucumber	1 (1.1 oz)	50	3	1	22	7	1	141
inari	1 sm (1.2 oz)	46	1	1	0	9	0	79
kappa cucumber roll	1 (1.1 oz)	43	1	0	0	9	tr	106

FOOD	PORTION	CALS	PROT	FAT	CHOL	CARB	FIBER	SOD
kim bap	1 (1.2 oz)	56	2	2	10	8	0	68
nigiri	1 (0.7 oz)	27	1	0	6	5	0	30
prawn cooked	1 (1.1 oz)	36	1	0	0	8	1	105
preserved radish roll	1 (0.3 oz)	9	0	0	0	2	tr	45
saba raw mackerel	1 (0.8 oz)	33	1	1	2	5	tr	47
salmon slice	1 (1.2 oz)	59	2	1	3	10	tr	115
sashimi ahi	1 slice (0.3 oz)	10	2	0	4	0	0	3
scallop cooked	1 (1.1 oz)	43	2	tr	10	8	tr	130
seasoned baby octopus	1 (1.2 oz)	55	2	tr	19	10	tr	150
seasoned jellyfish	1 (1.2 oz)	58	2	1	1	11	tr	246
seaweed roll	1 (1.1 oz)	43	1	1	1	9	1	188
sweet beancurd	1 (1.2 oz)	64	2	2	0	10	1	147
tekka tuna maki	1 (0.6 oz)	25	1	0	0	5	0	24
torigai cockle	1 piece (1.1 oz)	41	3	0	0	7	tr	131
tuna roll	1 (0.6 oz)	19	1	0	0	4	tr	48
unagi grilled eel	1 (1 oz)	54	2	2	9	8	1	114
vegetable roll	1 (1.2 oz)	27	1	1	0	5	–	47
vinegared ginger	⅓ cup (1.6 oz)	48	1	tr	0	12	–	6
wasabi	2 tsp (0.3 oz)	5	tr	tr	0	1	–	124
yellowtail roll	1 (0.6 oz)	25	1	1	0	3	–	32
SWAMP CABBAGE								
chopped cooked w/o salt	1 cup	20	2	tr	0	4	2	120
SWEET POTATO (*see also* YAM)								
baked w/ skin w/o salt	1 lg (6.3 oz)	162	4	tr	0	37	6	65
baked w/ skin w/o salt	1 med (4 oz)	103	2	tr	0	24	4	41
canned in syrup	½ cup	106	1	tr	0	25	3	38
canned mashed	½ cup	129	3	tr	0	30	2	96
leaves cooked w/o salt	1 cup	22	1	tr	0	5	1	8
paste dulce de calabaza	1 oz	82	tr	tr	0	21	tr	2
Diner's Choice								
Mashed	⅔ cup	160	3	3	0	33	2	105
Dr. Praeger's								
Sweet Potato Bites	2 (2 oz)	110	3	3	0	20	1	180
Glory								
Casserole	½ cup	180	2	0	0	43	2	250

FOOD	PORTION	CALS	PROT	FAT	CHOL	CARB	FIBER	SOD
Cut Fresh	1 serv (5 oz)	140	2	0	0	36	4	50
Sweet Potatoes	⅔ cup	160	3	0	0	37	2	35
Green Giant								
Candied	¾ cup	240	2	7	0	41	3	430
Health Is Wealth								
Southern Style	½ pkg (5 oz)	190	2	5	15	36	2	260
Jake & Amos								
Sweet Potato Butter	1 tbsp (0.5 oz)	25	0	0	0	6	0	10
Mann's								
Fresh Cubes	1 serv (3 oz)	60	1	0	0	15	3	10
Fries Fresh	1 serv (3 oz)	60	1	0	0	15	3	10
Mrs. Paul's								
Candied	1 serv (5 oz)	300	1	1	0	73	3	130
Princella								
In Light Syrup	⅔ cup	160	0	0	0	39	3	35
Mashed	⅔ cup	120	1	0	0	28	3	30
Royal Prince								
Candied	½ cup	210	1	0	0	50	2	30
Trappey's								
Sugary Sam Cut Sweet	⅔ cup	160	0	0	0	39	3	35
Tree Of Life								
Organic Puree	½ cup (4.5 oz)	130	3	0	0	30	2	100
TAKE-OUT								
candied	1 serv (3.7 oz)	151	1	3	8	29	3	74
white fried batata blanca frita	1 serv (8 oz)	792	7	29	0	129	19	43
SWEETBREAD (PANCREAS)								
beef braised	3 oz	230	23	15	223	0	0	51
lamb braised	3 oz	199	19	13	340	0	0	44
pork braised	3 oz	186	24	9	268	0	0	36
veal braised	3 oz	218	25	12	–	0	0	58
Rumba								
Beef	4 oz	260	14	23	250	0	0	110
SWISS CHARD								
cooked	½ cup	18	2	tr	0	4	–	158
raw chopped	½ cup	3	tr	tr	0	1	–	38

FOOD	PORTION	CALS	PROT	FAT	CHOL	CARB	FIBER	SOD
SWORDFISH								
cooked	3 oz	132	22	4	43	0	0	98
raw	3 oz	103	17	3	33	0	0	76
SYRUP								
corn dark & light	¼ cup	240	0	tr	0	65	0	99
date syrup	1 tbsp	63	tr	tr	–	15	0	–
maple	1 tbsp	52	0	0	0	13	–	2
maple	1 cup (11.1 oz)	824	tr	1	0	212	–	27
raspberry	1 oz	76	tr	0	0	19	–	1
rose hip	1 oz	9	0	0	–	2	0	–
sorghum	1 cup (11.6 oz)	957	0	0	0	247	–	28
sorghum	1 tbsp (0.7 oz)	61	0	0	0	16	–	2
sugar syrup	¼ cup	76	0	0	0	20	0	1
Cary's								
Maple	¼ cup	210	0	0	0	53	–	5
Sugar Free	¼ cup	30	0	0	0	12	tr	115
Hershey's								
Caramel	2 tbsp (1.4 oz)	110	tr	0	0	27	–	125
Strawberry	2 tbsp (1.4 oz)	100	0	0	0	26	–	10
Strawberry Sugar Free	2 tbsp (1 oz)	10	0	0	0	4	–	55
Lundberg								
Organic Sweet Dreams Brown Rice	2 tbsp	110	1	0	0	31	0	30
Monin								
Acai	1 oz	90	0	0	0	23	–	0
Amaretto	1 oz	97	0	0	0	24	–	0
Banana	1 oz	98	0	0	0	24	–	0
Coconut	1 oz	100	0	0	0	25	–	0
Organic Vanilla	1 oz	100	0	0	0	24	–	0
Pure Cane	1 oz	101	0	0	0	25	–	0
Navitas Naturals								
Yacon	2 tbsp	90	0	0	0	22	0	25

FOOD	PORTION	CALS	PROT	FAT	CHOL	CARB	FIBER	SOD
Nesquik								
Strawberry Calcium Fortified	2 tbsp (1.4 oz)	110	0	0	0	27	0	0
Neway								
Sweet Sensation Luo Han Guo Syrup	1 tsp	8	0	0	0	2	0	0
Steel's								
Maple Flavor No Sugar Added	3 tbsp (1.6 oz)	64	0	0	0	16	0	10
Tree Of Life								
Maple Grade A	¼ cup	200	0	0	0	53	–	10
Wholesome Sweeteners								
Organic Blue Agave	1 tbsp (0.7 oz)	60	0	0	0	16	0	0
Organic Blue Agave Cinnamon	2 tbsp (1 oz)	120	0	0	0	16	0	0
Organic Blue Agave Maple	2 tbsp (1 oz)	120	0	0	0	16	0	0
Organic Corn Syrup	2 tbsp (1 oz)	120	0	0	0	30	0	30
TAHINI (*see* SESAME)								
TAMARIND								
dried sweetened pulpitas	½ cup	279	3	1	0	73	5	28
dried sweetened pulpitas	1 piece (0.8 oz)	56	1	tr	0	15	1	6
fresh	1 (2 g)	5	tr	tr	0	1	tr	1
fresh cut up	1 cup	143	2	tr	0	38	3	17
TAMARIND JUICE								
nectar	1 cup	143	tr	tr	0	37	1	18
TANGERINE								
CANNED								
in light syrup	1 cup	154	1	tr	0	41	2	15
juice pack	1 cup	92	2	tr	0	24	2	12
FRESH								
fresh	1 med (3.1 oz)	47	1	tr	0	12	2	2
fresh	1 lg (4.2 oz)	64	1	tr	0	16	2	2
fresh	1 sm (2.7 oz)	40	1	tr	0	10	1	2
sections	1 cup	103	2	1	0	26	4	4

FOOD	PORTION	CALS	PROT	FAT	CHOL	CARB	FIBER	SOD
Noble								
Florida Tangerines	1 (3.8 oz)	50	1	1	0	15	3	0
River Pride								
Sweet	1 (3.8 oz)	50	1	1	0	15	3	0
TANGERINE JUICE								
canned sweetened	1 cup	124	1	1	0	30	1	2
fresh	1 cup	106	1	tr	0	25	1	2
Natalie's Orchid Island Juice								
100% Juice	8 oz	106	1	0	0	25	0	2
Odwalla								
100% Juice	8 oz	110	1	0	0	25	0	0
Santa Cruz								
Organic Sparkling	8 oz	110	0	0	0	26	0	10
SSips								
Drink	1 box (7 oz)	120	0	0	0	31	–	10
TAPIOCA								
pearl dry	¼ cup (1.3 oz)	136	tr	tr	0	34	tr	0
starch	1 oz	98	17	tr	–	24	–	1
Let's Do Organic								
Granulated	1 tbsp	35	0	0	0	9	0	0
Starch	1 tbsp	0	0	0	0	9	0	0
Mon Chong Loong								
Starch	1 oz	110	0	0	0	26	0	0
TARO								
chips	10 (0.8 oz)	115	1	6	0	16	–	79
leaves cooked	½ cup	18	2	tr	0	3	–	2
raw sliced	½ cup	56	1	tr	0	14	–	6
shoots sliced cooked	½ cup	10	1	tr	0	2	–	1
sliced cooked	½ cup (2.3 oz)	94	tr	tr	0	23	–	10
tahitian sliced cooked	½ cup	30	3	tr	0	5	–	37
TARPON								
fresh	3 oz	87	17	2	–	0	0	70
TARRAGON								
dried crumbled	1 tsp	2	tr	tr	0	tr	0	0
ground	1 tsp	5	tr	tr	0	1	tr	1

FOOD	PORTION	CALS	PROT	FAT	CHOL	CARB	FIBER	SOD
TEA/HERBAL TEA (*see also* ICED TEA)								
HERBAL								
chamomile brewed	1 cup	2	0	tr	0	tr	0	2
Celestial Seasonings								
Chamomile as prep	1 cup	0	0	0	0	0	0	0
REGULAR								
brewed tea	1 cup (6 oz)	2	0	0	0	1	0	5
Daily Detox								
Original	1 tea bag	0	0	0	0	0	0	0
Hansen's								
Tea Stix Blackberry	½ pkg (2 g)	5	0	0	0	1	–	5
Lipton								
Black Tea as prep	8 oz	0	0	0	0	0	0	0
Oregon Chai								
Chai Tea Latte Original Caffeine Free Concentrate	½ cup	78	0	0	0	18	–	8
Chai Tea Latte Original Concentrate	½ cup	78	0	0	0	19	–	8
Chai Tea Latte Spiced Original Mix	1 pkg	100	2	1	5	20	–	135
Chai Tea Latte Vanilla Mix	1 pkg	120	2	2	5	25	–	130
Organic Chai Cider Concentrate	½ cup	110	0	0	0	26	–	10
Organic Chai Nog Concentrate	½ cup	90	0	0	0	15	–	15
Red Rose								
English Breakfast Tea Bag as prep	1 cup	0	0	0	0	0	0	0
Tastefully Simple								
Oh My! Itty Bitty Chai Mix as prep w/ water	1 pkg (1.2 oz)	140	2	3	0	25	0	60
TAKE-OUT								
chai spiced latte decaf	1 cup	130	2	3	0	23	0	45
TEMPEH								
tempeh	½ cup (2.9 oz)	160	15	9	0	8	–	7

FOOD	PORTION	CALS	PROT	FAT	CHOL	CARB	FIBER	SOD
White Wave								
Five Grain	⅓ block (2.7 oz)	160	12	6	0	15	7	10
WildWood								
Organic Nori Seaweed	3 oz	170	13	7	0	16	4	0
TESTICLES								
prairie oysters cooked	1 pair (6.8 oz)	241	44	6	673	0	0	739
THYME								
dried crumbled	1 tsp	3	tr	tr	0	1	tr	1
fresh	1 tsp	1	tr	tr	0	tr	tr	0
ground	1 tsp	4	tr	tr	0	1	1	1
TILAPIA								
Dr. Praeger's								
Fillets Lightly Breaded	1 (4.5 oz)	220	16	9	25	20	3	240
Gorton's								
Fillets Crunchy Breaded frzn	1 (3 oz)	80	14	3	50	tr	–	150
High Liner								
Loins	1 fillet (4 oz)	110	23	2	25	0	0	25
SeaPak								
Tenders	2 (4 oz)	280	14	14	25	24	1	460
Van de Kamp's								
Lightly Breaded Fillets	1 (4 oz)	240	16	11	35	17	1	280
TAKE-OUT								
battered & fried	1 fillet (4 oz)	206	21	9	109	8	tr	133
breaded & fried	1 fillet (4 oz)	300	26	14	142	16	1	708
broiled w/o fat	1 fillet (3.5 oz)	128	26	3	57	0	0	56
TILEFISH								
cooked	½ fillet (5.3 oz)	220	37	7	–	0	0	88
cooked	3 oz	125	21	4	–	0	0	50
raw	3 oz	81	15	2	–	0	0	45
TOFU								
firm	¼ block (3 oz)	118	13	7	0	3	1	11

FOOD	PORTION	CALS	PROT	FAT	CHOL	CARB	FIBER	SOD
firm	½ cup	183	20	11	0	5	2	17
fresh fried	1 piece (0.5 oz)	35	2	3	0	1	tr	2
fuyu salted & fermented	1 block (⅓ oz)	13	1	1	0	1	tr	316
koyadofu dried frozen	1 piece (½ oz)	82	8	5	0	2	tr	1
okara	½ cup	47	2	1	0	8	1	6
regular	½ cup	94	6	6	0	2	1	9
regular	¼ block (4 oz)	88	9	6	0	2	1	8
Amy's								
Organic Tofu Scramble w/ Hash Browns & Veggies	1 pkg (8.9 oz)	320	19	19	0	19	4	580
House								
Atsu-Age Cutlet	1 (2.5 oz)	100	11	5	0	2	5	10
Cut-Age Shredded Fried	1 serv (0.5 oz)	50	4	4	0	0	0	10
Ganmodoki Fritter Small	3 (1.6 oz)	120	7	9	0	2	0	105
Medium Firm	3 oz	60	7	3	0	1	tr	30
Organic Extra Firm	3 oz	90	11	5	0	0	0	20
Organic Firm	3 oz	60	8	3	0	0	0	20
Soft Silken	3 oz	50	5	3	0	2	tr	30
Steak Cajun	1 (3 oz)	40	12	1	0	1	tr	75
Steak Grilled	1 (3 oz)	90	9	5	0	2	0	15
Sukui	3 oz	45	5	2	0	2	0	30
Tokusen Kinugoshi	1 piece (5 oz)	90	10	4	0	3	tr	30
Yaki Broiled	3 oz	90	9	5	0	2	0	15
TofuTown								
Tofu Tenders Havana Black Bean	½ pkg (5 oz)	210	15	8	0	18	2	690
Tofu Tenders Mediterranean Tahini	½ pkg (5 oz)	240	15	13	0	16	3	640
Tofu Tenders Sesame Ginger Teriyaki	½ pkg (5 oz)	240	15	9	0	24	3	680
Tree Of Life								
Organic Firm	½ block (3.2 oz)	110	11	5	0	4	2	5

FOOD	PORTION	CALS	PROT	FAT	CHOL	CARB	FIBER	SOD
White Wave								
Baked Garlic Herb Italian	1 piece (2 oz)	90	9	5	0	2	1	240
Baked Sesame Peanut Thai	1 piece (2 oz)	90	9	5	0	2	1	280
Baked Zesty Lemon Pepper	1 piece (2 oz)	90	9	5	0	3	1	200
Extra Firm	⅕ block (3.2 oz)	110	11	6	0	3	1	5
Organic Extra Firm	⅕ block (3.2 oz)	110	11	6	0	3	1	5
Organic Firm	⅓ block (3.2 oz)	110	11	6	0	3	1	5
Organic Soft	⅕ block (3.2 oz)	110	10	6	0	3	1	5
Reduced Fat	⅕ block (3.2 oz)	90	10	4	0	4	2	5
WildWood								
Organic Baked Aloha	1 piece (3.5 oz)	180	20	5	0	15	3	239
Organic Calcium Rich Medium	3 oz	70	7	4	0	2	1	5
Organic Golden Pineapple Teriyaki	3 oz	160	13	12	0	5	1	230
Organic High Protein Super Firm	3 oz	100	14	4	0	5	1	45
Organic Smoked Mild Szechuan	3 oz	150	14	6	0	11	2	368
TAKE-OUT								
breaded deep fried w/ soy sauce japanese style	1 piece (0.4 oz)	15	0	1	1	1	tr	16
soy sauce marinated & grilled	1 serv (4 oz)	181	19	11	0	6	1	294
stir-fried w/ vegetables	1 cup (7.6 oz)	186	5	10	0	21	3	782
TOMATILLO								
fresh	1 (1.2 oz)	11	tr	tr	0	2	1	0
fresh chopped	½ cup (2.3 oz)	21	1	1	0	4	1	1

FOOD	PORTION	CALS	PROT	FAT	CHOL	CARB	FIBER	SOD
TOMATO								
CANNED								
green pickled	½ cup (2.5 oz)	26	1	tr	0	6	1	89
green whole pickled	1 (2.6 oz)	27	1	tr	0	6	1	92
paste	1 can (6 oz)	139	7	1	0	32	7	1343
paste	¼ cup (2.3 oz)	54	3	tr	0	12	3	517
paste no salt added	1 can (6 oz)	139	7	1	0	32	7	167
puree	1 can (28 oz)	312	14	2	0	74	16	3280
puree	1 cup (8.8 oz)	95	4	1	0	22	5	998
puree w/o salt	1 can (28 oz)	312	14	2	0	74	16	230
sauce	1 cup (8.6 oz)	59	3	tr	0	13	4	1284
sauce no salt added	1 cup (8.6 oz)	102	3	tr	0	21	4	27
stewed	1 cup (8.9 oz)	66	2	tr	0	16	3	564
Cento								
Paste	2 tbsp (1.2 oz)	30	1	0	0	7	2	25
Contadina								
Paste Italian Herbs	2 tbsp	35	1	1	0	7	1	290
Dei Fratelli								
Chopped Italian Tomatoes	½ cup (4.3 oz)	40	1	1	0	8	1	270
Del Monte								
Diced w/ Garlic & Onion	½ cup	40	2	1	0	8	tr	610
Organic Tomato Paste	2 tbsp	30	2	0	0	6	1	20
Petite Cut Garlic & Olive Oil	½ cup (4.4 oz)	40	1	1	0	9	1	450
Hunt's								
Diced w/ Basil Garlic & Oregano	½ cup	35	1	0	0	7	2	410
Paste No Salt Added	2 tbsp (1.2 oz)	30	1	0	0	6	2	15

FOOD	PORTION	CALS	PROT	FAT	CHOL	CARB	FIBER	SOD
Muir Glen								
Organic Chunky Tomato & Herb	½ cup	60	2	1	0	11	2	350
Organic Diced Fire Roasted	½ cup	30	1	0	0	6	1	290
Organic Diced w/ Basil & Garlic	½ cup	30	1	0	0	6	1	290
Polar								
Grape	½ cup	50	0	0	0	12	2	20
Pomi								
Chopped	½ cup	20	1	0	0	4	3	10
Progresso								
Crushed w/ Added Puree	¼ cup (2.1 oz)	20	1	0	0	4	1	95
Diced	½ cup (4.4 oz)	25	1	0	0	5	1	250
Puree	¼ cup (2.2 oz)	25	1	0	0	5	1	15
Whole Peeled w/ Basil	½ cup (4.2 oz)	20	1	0	0	4	1	260
Redpack								
Crushed In Puree	¼ cup	20	0	0	0	4	1	120
Diced In Juice	½ cup	25	1	0	0	5	1	220
Petite Diced Onion Celery & Green Pepper	½ cup	45	1	0	0	10	1	370
Rienzi								
Italian Cherry Tomatoes No Salt Added	⅓ can (4.5 oz)	30	1	0	0	6	1	60
S&W								
Crushed	¼ cup (2.1 oz)	20	1	0	0	4	1	125
Paste	2 tbsp (1.2 oz)	30	2	0	0	6	1	20
Petite Cut	½ cup (4.4 oz)	25	1	0	0	6	2	250
Puree	¼ cup (2.2 oz)	30	1	0	0	6	2	15
Ready-Cut Italian Recipe	½ cup (4.2 oz)	25	1	0	0	4	tr	190
Ready-Cut No Salt Added	½ cup (4.4 oz)	25	1	0	0	6	2	50

FOOD	PORTION	CALS	PROT	FAT	CHOL	CARB	FIBER	SOD
Stewed No Salt Added	½ cup (4.4 oz)	35	1	0	0	9	2	50
Stewed Original	½ cup (4.3 oz)	35	1	0	0	7	2	270
Whole Peeled	½ cup (4.4 oz)	25	1	0	0	6	2	250
DRIED								
sun dried	1 piece (2 g)	5	tr	tr	0	1	tr	42
sun dried	¼ cup (0.5 oz)	35	2	tr	0	8	2	283
sun dried in oil drained	¼ cup (1 oz)	59	1	4	0	6	2	73
sun dried in oil drained	1 piece (3 g)	6	tr	tr	0	1	tr	8
tomato powder	1 oz	85	4	tr	0	21	5	38
FRESH								
bruschetta	¼ cup	50	2	3	0	6	tr	360
cherry	½ cup (2.6 oz)	13	1	tr	0	3	1	1
cherry	1 (0.6 oz)	3	tr	tr	0	1	tr	1
grape tomatoes	20	30	1	0	0	6	1	0
green	1 sm (3.2 oz)	21	1	tr	0	5	1	12
green	1 med (4.3 oz)	28	1	tr	0	6	1	16
green	1 lg (6.4 oz)	42	2	tr	0	9	2	24
green chopped	1 cup (6.3 oz)	41	2	tr	0	9	2	23
orange	1 (4 oz)	18	1	tr	0	4	1	47
orange chopped	1 cup (5.5 oz)	25	2	tr	0	5	1	66
plum	1 (2.2 oz)	11	1	tr	0	2	1	3
red	1 sm (3.2 oz)	16	1	tr	0	4	1	5
red	1 med (4.3 oz)	22	1	tr	0	5	2	6
red	1 lg (6.4 oz)	33	2	tr	0	7	2	9
red chopped	½ cup (3.2 oz)	16	1	tr	0	4	1	4
red slice	1 lg (0.9 oz)	5	tr	tr	0	1	tr	4
roma	1 (2.2 oz)	11	1	tr	0	2	1	3
yellow	1 (7.4 oz)	32	2	1	0	6	2	49
yellow chopped	½ cup (2.4 oz)	10	1	tr	0	2	1	16

FOOD	PORTION	CALS	PROT	FAT	CHOL	CARB	FIBER	SOD
Earthbound Farms								
Organic Roma	1 med (5.2 oz)	35	1	1	0	7	1	5
Ready Pac								
Bruchetta	2 tbsp (1.6 oz)	70	0	7	0	3	1	250
TAKE-OUT								
aspic	½ cup (4 oz)	32	3	tr	0	6	tr	242
broiled slices	2 (2.9 oz)	18	1	tr	0	4	1	5
broiled whole	1 med (3.7 oz)	23	1	tr	0	5	2	6
bruschetta on toasted italian bread	1 slice	106	4	3	0	18	tr	355
fried slices	2 (2.5 oz)	122	2	9	17	8	1	127
scalloped	½ cup (4 oz)	99	2	5	0	12	1	611
stewed	½ cup (1.8 oz)	40	1	1	0	7	1	230
stuffed w/ rice	1 (5.2 oz)	110	2	3	0	20	2	396
stuffed w/ rice & meat	1 (5.2 oz)	142	7	6	18	15	2	437
TOMATO JUICE								
tomato juice	1 cup (8.5 oz)	41	2	tr	0	10	1	654
tomato juice w/o added salt	1 cup (8.5 oz)	41	2	tr	0	10	1	24
Campbell's								
Healthy Request	8 oz	50	2	0	0	10	2	480
Low Sodium	8 oz	50	2	0	0	10	2	140
Organic	8 oz	50	2	0	0	10	2	680
Dei Fratelli								
Tomato Juice	8 oz	40	2	0	0	10	1	450
Lakewood								
Organic	8 oz	35	1	0	0	7	1	140
Tree Of Life								
Organic 100% Juice	8 oz	50	1	0	0	10	–	480
TONGUE								
beef simmered	3 oz	241	16	19	112	0	0	55
lamb braised	3 oz	234	18	17	161	0	0	57
pork braised	3 oz	230	20	16	124	0	0	93
veal braised	3 oz	172	22	9	202	0	0	54

FOOD	PORTION	CALS	PROT	FAT	CHOL	CARB	FIBER	SOD
Rumba								
Beef	4 oz	250	17	18	95	4	0	75
TORTILLA								
corn	1 (6 in diam)	56	1	1	0	12	1	40
corn w/o salt	1 (6 in diam)	56	1	1	0	12	1	3
flour w/o salt	1 (8 in diam)	114	3	3	0	20	1	167
French Meadow Bakery								
Fat Flush	1 (1 oz)	100	5	1	0	18	3	105
Gluten Free	1 (1.5 oz)	120	1	1	0	24	1	290
Hemp	1 (1.1 oz)	90	5	3	0	12	3	130
La Tortilla Factory								
Carb Cutting Original	1 (1.3 oz)	60	5	2	0	11	7	150
Organic Yellow Corn	2 (2.4 oz)	120	3	2	0	25	2	0
Smart & Delicious Low Fat Low Sodium	1 (2.5 oz)	150	5	2	0	32	6	170
Rudi's Organic Bakery								
Spelt	1 (2 oz)	140	5	3	0	27	1	200
Salba Smart								
Whole Wheat Omega-3 Enriched	1 (1.5 oz)	120	4	3	0	21	2	360
Tumaro's								
Honey Wheat	1 (8 in)	110	3	2	0	23	2	135
Low In Carbs Garden Vegetable	1 (8 in)	100	7	3	0	12	8	115
Low In Carbs Green Onion	1 (8 in)	100	7	3	0	13	7	115
Low In Carbs Multi Grain	1 (8 in)	100	7	3	0	13	8	115
Low In Carbs Salsa	1 (8 in)	100	7	3	0	13	8	115
Pesto & Garlic	1 (8 in)	110	3	1	0	23	1	135
Premium White	1 (8 in)	120	3	2	0	23	tr	130
Soy-full Heart 8 Grain 'N Soy	1 (1.4 oz)	100	6	0	0	14	4	60
Soy-full Heart Apple 'N Cinnamon	1 (1.4 oz)	90	6	3	0	13	4	65
Soy-full Heart Wheat Soy & Flax	1 (1.4 oz)	90	6	3	0	13	4	65
Spinach & Vegetables	1 (8 in)	110	3	2	0	23	1	140

TORTILLA CHIPS (see CHIPS)

FOOD	PORTION	CALS	PROT	FAT	CHOL	CARB	FIBER	SOD
TRAIL MIX								
Back To Nature								
Bar Harbor Blend	1 oz	130	2	7	0	17	2	0
Harvest Blend	1 oz	150	5	10	0	12	3	5
Nantucket Blend	1 oz	130	3	7	0	15	3	25
Pacific Heights Blend	1 oz	160	4	11	0	13	3	40
Bear Naked								
Peak Chocolate Cherry	½ cup (1.1 oz)	120	2	5	0	21	2	0
Peak Pecan Apple Flax	½ cup (1.1 oz)	140	4	8	0	16	2	45
Craisins								
Cranberry & Chocolate	1 pkg (1.75 oz)	230	5	28	–	26	–	170
Fruit & Nuts	1 pkg (1.4 oz)	230	3	10	–	31	–	60
Enjoy Life								
Gluten Free Not Nuts! Beach Bash	1 oz	130	4	7	0	13	2	45
Gluten Free Not Nuts! Mountain Mambo	1 oz	140	5	8	0	12	2	45
Kopali								
Organic Mix	½ pkg (1 oz)	130	4	6	0	15	4	40
Mrs. May's								
Coconut Almond Crunch	1 oz	183	4	15	0	10	2	40
Navitas Naturals								
3 Berry Cacao Nibs & Cashews	1 oz	110	3	5	0	16	4	45
Goji Cacao Nibs & Cashews	1 oz	120	4	6	0	13	3	70
Goji Golden Berry & Mulberry	1 oz	90	3	0	0	19	2	65
Planters								
Berry Nut & Chocolate	3 tbsp (1 oz)	120	2	5	0	18	1	20
SunRidge Farms								
Cherry Pecan Vanilla Dream	¼ cup (1.4 oz)	200	5	12	0	20	3	10
Organic Deluxe	¼ cup (1 oz)	140	4	8	0	13	2	10
SunRise								
Honey Coated	3 tbsp (1 oz)	137	5	6	1	14	4	67
W/ Fruit	3 tbsp (1 oz)	130	4	6	0	16	2	50

FOOD	PORTION	CALS	PROT	FAT	CHOL	CARB	FIBER	SOD
TREE FERN								
chopped cooked	½ cup	28	tr	tr	0	8	–	3
TRIPE								
beef simmered	3 oz	80	10	3	133	2	0	58
Rumba								
Beef Tripe	4 oz	110	15	5	105	0	0	50
TAKE-OUT								
mondongo w/ potatoes	1 cup	300	24	11	148	26	6	1565
TRITICALE								
dry	½ cup (3.4 oz)	323	13	2	0	69	–	5
TROUT								
baked	3 oz	162	23	7	63	0	0	57
rainbow cooked	3 oz	129	22	4	62	0	0	29
seatrout baked	3 oz	113	18	4	90	0	0	63
TRUFFLES								
fresh	0.5 oz	4	2	tr	0	9	2	39
Aux Delices Des Bois								
Black Truffle Butter	0.5 oz	90	0	10	25	0	0	80
TUNA								
CANNED								
light in oil	1 can (6 oz)	399	50	14	30	0	0	606
light in oil	3 oz	169	25	7	15	0	0	301
light in water	1 can (5.8 oz)	192	42	1	49	0	0	558
light in water	3 oz	99	22	1	25	0	0	287
white in oil	1 can (6.2 oz)	331	47	14	55	0	0	704
white in oil	3 oz	158	23	7	26	0	0	336
white in water	3 oz	116	23	2	35	0	0	333
white in water	1 can (6 oz)	234	46	4	72	0	0	673
Bumble Bee								
Sensations Lemon & Pepper w/ Crackers	1 pkg (3.6 oz)	200	19	8	25	13	0	460
Solid White Albacore In Water	¼ cup (2 oz)	60	13	1	25	0	0	180

FOOD	PORTION	CALS	PROT	FAT	CHOL	CARB	FIBER	SOD
Chicken Of The Sea								
Albacore Solid In Water	2 oz	60	13	1	25	0	0	180
Chunk White Albacore In Water	¼ cup (2 oz)	50	11	1	25	0	0	250
Polar								
Albacore Solid White In Water	2 oz	70	18	1	30	0	0	250
Chunk Light In Water	2 oz	60	13	1	25	0	0	250
Progresso								
Albacore Solid White Olive Oil	¼ cup (2 oz)	90	16	3	20	0	0	330
Light Olive Oil drained	¼ cup (2 oz)	120	15	6	35	0	0	330
StarKist								
Chunk Light In Water	¼ cup (2 oz)	60	13	5	30	0	0	250
Chunk Light In Water Flavor Pouch	1 pkg (3 oz)	90	19	1	45	0	0	380
Low Sodium Chunk White In Water	¼ cup (2 oz)	60	15	1	25	0	0	100
Solid Light In Water	2 oz	60	13	1	30	0	0	250
Solid White Albacore In Water	2 oz	70	15	1	25	0	0	250
Tuna Creations Hickory Smoked Flavor Pouch	2 oz	60	13	1	20	0	0	–
Tonnino								
Fillets In Olive Oil	2 oz	90	16	3	26	tr	0	260
Fillets In Olive Oil w/ Jalapeno	2 oz	80	13	5	20	1	tr	115
Fillets In Olive Oil w/ Oregano	2 oz	90	15	4	25	0	0	220
Fillets In Spring Water Wild Caught	2 oz	50	14	1	16	1	0	200
Ventresca In Olive Oil	2 oz	110	13	6	25	2	tr	190
Tree Of Life								
Wild Light Tongol Chunk In Spring Water No Salt Added	¼ cup (2.4 oz)	50	12	0	45	0	0	50
Wild Planet								
Albacore Wild	2 oz	120	16	6	15	0	0	250
Albacore Wild Fillet	2 oz	120	16	6	15	0	0	250
Albacore Wild No Salt	2 oz	120	16	6	15	0	0	100

FOOD	PORTION	CALS	PROT	FAT	CHOL	CARB	FIBER	SOD
Albacore Wild Smoked Troll Caught	2 oz	90	12	5	20	0	0	540
Skipjack Wild Light	2 oz	69	13	2	22	0	0	268
FRESH								
bluefin cooked	3 oz	157	25	5	42	0	0	43
bluefin raw	3 oz	122	20	4	32	0	0	33
skipjack baked	3 oz	112	24	1	51	0	0	40
yellowfin baked	3 oz	118	25	1	49	0	0	40
FROZEN								
SeaPak								
Seasoned Ahi Steaks	1 (4.5 oz)	240	24	14	45	2	0	840
MIX								
StarKist								
Lunch To-Go Chunk Light	1 pkg	310	20	9	40	27	2	720
Tuna Helper								
Creamy Broccoli as prep	1 cup	310	6	11	12	39	2	912
Creamy Pasta as prep	1 cup	320	5	12	15	39	1	888
Tetrazzini as prep	1 cup	290	6	10	12	33	1	768
TAKE-OUT								
tuna salad	1 cup	383	33	19	27	19	–	824

TURBOT

FOOD	PORTION	CALS	PROT	FAT	CHOL	CARB	FIBER	SOD
european baked	3 oz	104	17	3	–	0	0	163

TURKEY (*see also* JERKY, TURKEY DISHES, TURKEY SUBSTITUTES)

FOOD	PORTION	CALS	PROT	FAT	CHOL	CARB	FIBER	SOD
CANNED								
w/ broth	1 cup	220	32	9	89	0	0	630
Hormel								
Chunk White & Dark	2 oz	70	11	3	45	0	0	270
Premium Chunk White	2 oz	60	11	2	35	0	0	230
FRESH								
breast roasted pre-basted w/ skin	3.5 oz	126	22	3	42	0	0	397
breast roasted w/ skin	4 oz	212	32	8	83	0	0	70
breast roasted w/o skin	4 oz	212	33	4	77	0	0	253
dark meat w/o skin roasted	3 oz	170	26	7	78	0	0	72
dark meat w/o skin roasted	1 cup (5 oz)	262	40	10	119	0	0	110
ground cooked	3 oz	193	22	11	84	0	0	88
leg w/ skin roasted	1 (19 oz)	1136	152	54	464	0	0	420
light meat w/ skin roasted half turkey	2.3 lbs	2069	87	87	794	0	0	658

FOOD	PORTION	CALS	PROT	FAT	CHOL	CARB	FIBER	SOD
light meat w/o skin roasted	4 oz	183	35	4	81	0	0	75
neck simmered	1 (5.3 oz)	274	41	11	186	0	0	84
skin roasted	1 oz	141	13	13	36	0	0	17
skin roasted from half turkey	8.7 oz	1096	49	98	281	0	0	132
tail cooked	1 (2 oz)	197	13	16	53	0	0	223
w/ skin roasted	1 serv (4.2 oz)	249	34	12	98	0	0	82
w/ skin roasted	½ turkey (4 lbs)	3857	522	181	1514	0	0	1269
w/o skin roasted	1 cup (5 oz)	238	41	7	107	0	0	99
w/o skin roasted	1 serv (3.7 oz)	177	31	5	80	0	0	74
wing w/ skin roasted	1 (6.5 oz)	426	51	23	151	0	0	114
wing w/o skin roasted	1 (5.2 oz)	237	45	5	147	0	0	584
Butterball								
Burger Patties	1 (4 oz)	150	22	8	80	0	0	330
Cutlets	4 oz	120	28	1	70	0	0	55
Drumstick	4 oz	170	22	8	70	0	0	70
Ground 7% Fat	4 oz	150	22	8	80	0	0	95
Ground White	4 oz	130	26	4	75	0	0	75
Strips	4 oz	120	28	1	70	0	0	55
Thighs	4 oz	170	22	8	70	0	0	80
Wings	1 (6.3 oz)	380	36	25	115	0	0	90
Empire								
Gound White	4 oz	160	23	8	65	0	0	125
Honeysuckle White								
85% Lean Ground	4 oz	240	20	17	85	0	0	70
93% Lean Patties	1 (4 oz)	160	22	8	80	0	0	200
97% Lean Ground White	4 oz	130	26	2	65	0	0	70
99% Fat Free Breast Cutlets	4 oz	120	28	1	70	0	0	55
99% Fat Free Breast Tenderloin	4 oz	120	28	1	70	0	0	55
Drumettes	4 oz	180	24	8	75	0	0	75
Marinated Strips Asian Grill	4 oz	160	17	7	55	8	0	490
Necks	4 oz	150	23	6	90	0	0	105
Tenderloins Creamy Dijon Mustard	4 oz	140	21	4	50	0	0	500
Tenderloins Homestyle	4 oz	130	21	4	55	0	0	440
Tenderloins Teriyaki	4 oz	140	21	4	50	5	0	530

FOOD	PORTION	CALS	PROT	FAT	CHOL	CARB	FIBER	SOD
Thighs	4 oz	190	21	11	75	0	0	75
Whole Honey Roasted	4 oz	180	20	9	70	5	0	250
Wings	4 oz	220	23	14	80	0	0	60
Perdue								
Breast Fillets Boneless Skinless cooked	3 oz	110	26	1	60	0	0	40
Drumsticks roasted	3 oz	140	21	7	125	0	0	250
Ground Breast cooked	3 oz	110	25	1	50	0	0	40
Patties cooked	1 (3 oz)	160	20	8	85	0	0	65
Whole Breast Bone-In Seasoned	4 oz	140	20	7	75	1	0	410
Whole Dark Meat cooked	3 oz	190	21	11	90	0	0	70
Whole White Meat roasted	3 oz	150	23	7	65	0	0	50
Shady Brook								
Breast Tenderloin Lemon Garlic	4 oz	130	21	4	55	4	0	460
Breast Tenderloin Rotisserie	4 oz	130	21	4	50	4	0	700
Tenderloin Zesty Italian Herb	4 oz	130	21	4	50	4	0	490
FROZEN								
roast boneless seasoned light & dark meat roasted	3.5 oz	155	21	6	53	3	0	680
sticks breaded fried	1 (2.2 oz)	179	9	11	41	11	–	536
Butterball								
Boneless Roast	4 oz	130	22	5	65	0	0	460
Breast Boneless Roast	4 oz	110	21	3	45	1	0	500
Breast Tenderloin Teriyaki	4 oz	110	21	1	55	4	–	780
Breast Whole	4 oz	110	21	3	45	1	0	500
Breast Whole Smoked Cooked	3 oz	120	18	5	45	1	0	650
Whole Turkey	1 serv (4 oz)	170	20	10	70	0	0	320
Whole Turkey Baked	3 oz	130	17	7	45	0	0	580
Honeysuckle White								
Breast Boneless Roast	4 oz	170	21	7	60	0	0	700
Jennie-O								
Burger	1 (4 oz)	160	19	9	100	0	0	90
Organic Prairie								
Whole Young	4 oz	90	23	10	70	0	0	70

FOOD	PORTION	CALS	PROT	FAT	CHOL	CARB	FIBER	SOD
READY-TO-EAT								
bologna	1 slice (1 oz)	59	3	4	21	1	tr	351
breast	1 slice (0.7 oz)	22	4	tr	9	1	tr	213
ham	1 slice (1 oz)	35	5	1	20	1	tr	312
pastrami	2 oz	70	9	2	39	2	tr	559
salami	1 slice (1 oz)	48	5	3	21	tr	0	281
Applegate Farms								
Organic Herb	2 oz	50	11	1	30	0	0	420
Butterball								
Breast Honey Roasted Thick Sliced	1 slice (1 oz)	35	5	1	15	2	0	280
Breast Oven Roasted Extra Thin Slice	7 slices (2 oz)	70	10	2	25	3	0	580
Breast Smoked Thin Sliced	4 slices (1.9 oz)	70	7	2	25	4	0	560
Breast Strips Oven Roasted	½ pkg (3 oz)	90	18	1	40	2	–	750
Deep Fried Original Thick Sliced	1 slice (1 oz)	30	5	1	15	1	0	260
Carl Buddig								
Honey Roasted Sliced	2 oz	90	9	5	–	2	–	–
Turkey Sliced	2 oz	90	9	5	–	tr	–	–
Healthy Ones								
Oven Roasted 97% Fat Free	7 slices (2 oz)	60	9	2	20	2	–	460
Honeysuckle White								
Simply Done Whole Breast	4 oz	160	21	7	60	2	0	500
Hormel								
Natural Choice Deli Turkey Honey	4 slices (2 oz)	60	10	1	25	3	0	440
Natural Choice Deli Turkey Oven Roasted	4 slices (2 oz)	60	10	1	25	3	0	440
Natural Choice Deli Turkey Smoked	4 slices (2 oz)	60	10	1	25	3	0	440
Oscar Mayer								
Breast Smoked Shaved	2 oz	50	8	1	20	2	0	570
Sara Lee								
Breast Cracked Pepper	4 slices (1.8 oz)	50	9	1	25	1	0	480

FOOD	PORTION	CALS	PROT	FAT	CHOL	CARB	FIBER	SOD
Breast Hardwood Smoked	4 slices (1.8 oz)	50	11	1	20	1	0	490
Tyson								
Breast Oven Roasted	2 slices (1.6 oz)	40	8	1	15	1	0	560
TURKEY DISHES								
FROZEN								
gravy & turkey	1 cup (8.4 oz)	160	14	6	–	11	–	1328
TAKE-OUT								
boneless breast w/ cranberry apple stuffing	1 serv (5 oz)	260	32	9	80	10	1	250
turkey a la king	1 cup (8.5 oz)	465	24	34	190	16	1	880
turkey creole w/o rice	1 cup	189	29	4	69	9	2	585
turkey croquette	1 (2 oz)	158	10	9	28	8	tr	226
turkey divan	1 cup	321	40	14	135	9	3	387
turkey fricassee	1 cup	322	29	18	85	8	tr	693
turkey meatloaf	1 lg slice (5 oz)	243	29	9	122	11	1	658
turkey salad	1 cup	417	29	32	100	3	1	288
turkey tetrazzini	1 cup	369	19	18	49	29	2	657
TURKEY SUBSTITUTES								
Worthington								
Turkee Slices	3 slices (3.3 oz)	180	14	12	0	5	0	530
Yves								
Meatless Deli Turkey Slices	4 slices	100	16	2	0	5	0	340
Meatless Ground Turkey	⅓ cup	60	12	1	0	8	2	330
TURMERIC								
ground	1 tsp	8	tr	tr	0	1	tr	1
TURNIPS								
canned greens	½ cup	17	2	tr	0	3	–	325
cooked mashed	½ cup (4.2 oz)	47	2	tr	0	10	–	25
cubed cooked	½ cup (3 oz)	33	1	tr	0	7	–	17

FOOD	PORTION	CALS	PROT	FAT	CHOL	CARB	FIBER	SOD
fresh greens chopped cooked	½ cup	15	1	tr	0	3	2	21
frzn greens cooked	½ cup	24	3	tr	0	4	2	12
greens raw chopped	½ cup	7	tr	tr	0	2	1	11
raw cubed	½ cup (2.4 oz)	25	1	tr	0	6	–	14
Allens								
Seasoned	½ cup	35	4	1	0	5	2	860
Glory								
Greens Fresh	2 cups	20	1	0	0	5	3	30
Greens Seasoned canned	½ cup	35	1	0	0	4	2	490
Root Cut Fresh	½ cup	20	1	0	0	4	1	45
Sensibly Seasoned Greens	½ cup	20	1	0	0	4	2	240
TURTLE								
raw	3.5 oz	85	18	1	–	0	0	–
TUSK FISH								
raw	3.5 oz	79	17	tr	–	0	0	113
VANILLA								
vanilla extract	1 tbsp (0.5 oz)	37	tr	tr	0	2	0	1
vanilla extract	1 tsp (4.2 g)	12	0	0	0	1	0	0
vanilla extract alcohol free	1 tsp (4.2 g)	2	0	0	0	1	0	0
Bob's Red Mill								
Organic Extract	1 tsp	0	0	0	0	0	0	0
VEAL (*see also* VEAL DISHES)								
breast braised	3 oz	226	23	14	96	0	0	55
chop breaded fried	1 med (6.5 oz)	290	35	12	142	13	tr	577
chop cooked	1 med (6.5 oz)	230	26	13	109	0	0	444
cubed braised	3 oz	160	30	4	123	0	0	79
cutlet cooked	3 oz	141	26	4	83	0	0	311
ground broiled	3 oz	146	21	6	88	0	0	71
leg roasted	3 oz	136	24	4	88	0	0	58
loin roasted	3 oz	184	21	10	88	0	0	79
patty breaded fried	1 (2.8 oz)	211	16	13	80	7	tr	329
shank braised	3 oz	162	27	5	105	0	0	79

FOOD	PORTION	CALS	PROT	FAT	CHOL	CARB	FIBER	SOD
VEAL DISHES								
TAKE-OUT								
marengo	1 serv (8.8 oz)	274	33	9	118	7	1	607
marsala	1 slice + sauce (3.4 oz)	268	12	19	69	6	tr	191
paprikash	1 serv (8.8 oz)	280	36	12	138	5	1	829
parmigiana	1 serv (6.4 oz)	362	27	21	146	15	2	790
picatta	1 piece + sauce (3.5 oz)	154	16	9	72	2	tr	546
scallopini	1 slice + sauce (3.4 oz)	238	18	17	64	2	tr	304
stew	1 serv (8.8 oz)	192	15	6	50	18	3	605
VEGETABLE JUICE								
low sodium tomato & vegetable juice	1 cup	53	1	tr	0	11	2	169
vegetable juice cocktail	8 oz	46	2	tr	0	11	2	653
Bolthouse Farms								
Vedge Tomato Carrot Celery	8 oz	60	3	0	0	11	2	440
Dei Fratelli								
Vegetable Juice	8 oz	45	2	2	0	11	1	600
Green To Go								
100% Natural Organic as prep	1 pkg (0.3 oz)	32	1	tr	0	6	tr	12
Lakewood								
Super Veggie	6 oz	40	2	0	0	9	4	135
Mott's								
100% Juice Veggie Blend	1 bottle (14 oz)	90	5	1	0	15	4	790
V8								
100% Vegetable Essential Antioxidants	8 oz	50	2	0	0	11	2	480

FOOD	PORTION	CALS	PROT	FAT	CHOL	CARB	FIBER	SOD
Calcium Enriched	8 oz	50	2	0	0	11	2	460
High Fiber	8 oz	60	2	0	0	13	5	480
Low Sodium	8 oz	50	2	0	0	10	2	140
Low Sodium Spicy Hot	8 oz	50	2	0	0	11	2	140
Vegetable Juice	8 oz	50	0	0	0	10	2	420
Walnut Acres								
Organic Incredible Vegetable	8 oz	50	2	0	0	12	1	580
VEGETABLES MIXED								
CANNED								
mixed vegetables	½ cup	39	2	tr	0	8	–	122
peas & carrots	½ cup (4.5 oz)	48	3	tr	0	11	3	332
peas & onions	½ cup (2.1 oz)	31	2	tr	0	5	1	265
succotash	½ cup	102	4	1	0	23	–	325
Del Monte								
Savory Sides Homestyle Vegetable Medley	½ cup	70	1	3	0	11	2	380
Savory Sides Rio Grande Vegetables	½ cup	70	2	0	0	14	2	470
McSweet								
Giardiniera	5 pieces (1 oz)	25	0	0	0	6	tr	240
S&W								
Mixed	½ cup (4.4 oz)	45	2	0	0	10	2	360
Peas & Pearl Onions	½ cup (4.3 oz)	40	3	0	0	11	3	530
The Gracious Gourmet								
Tapenade Fennel Blood Orange	2 tbsp (1 oz)	50	0	5	0	3	tr	190
Veg-All								
Original Mixed	½ cup	40	1	0	0	8	2	290
DRIED								
Crunchies								
Freeze Dried Power Veggies Buttered	½ cup (0.7 oz)	110	6	3	0	17	4	300

FOOD	PORTION	CALS	PROT	FAT	CHOL	CARB	FIBER	SOD
Freeze Dried Power Veggies Herb Spiced	½ cup (0.7 oz)	110	6	3	0	17	5	110
Freeze Dried Roasted Veggies	⅝ cup (1 oz)	100	4	1	0	21	2	35
Freeze Dried Roasted Veggies BBQ	½ cup (0.8 oz)	100	3	2	0	20	4	260
Fun-Yums								
Fresh Crispy Mixed Veggies	1 serv (0.9 oz)	114	1	4	–	18	1	48
FRESH								
Mann's								
Broccoli & Carrots	1 serv (3 oz)	25	2	0	0	5	2	25
Broccoli & Cauliflower	1 serv (3 oz)	25	2	0	0	4	2	25
California Stir Fry	1 serv (3 oz)	30	2	0	0	6	2	30
Low Mein Stir Fry	1 serv (3 oz)	80	3	1	0	14	2	250
Medley	1 serv (3 oz)	25	2	0	0	5	2	25
Ready Pac								
Carrots & Celery w/ Ranch Dressing	1 pkg (7 oz)	250	2	21	15	14	3	500
Ready Fixin's Chop Suey	1½ cups (3 oz)	15	1	0	0	2	1	45
FROZEN								
mixed vegetables cooked	½ cup	54	3	tr	0	12	2	32
peas & carrots cooked	½ cup (2.8 oz)	38	3	tr	0	8	3	54
peas & carrots creamed	½ cup (4.3 oz)	111	4	6	4	12	2	235
succotash cooked	½ cup	79	4	1	0	17	–	38
Birds Eye								
Asparagus Gold & White Corn & Baby Carrots	⅔ cup	70	2	1	0	13	1	15
Italian Herb Harvest Vegetables	1¼ cups	90	2	6	15	6	2	150
Spring Vegetables In Citrus Sauce	1¼ cups	70	2	4	10	8	2	280
Steamfresh Asian Medley	1 cup (3.3 oz)	50	2	2	0	6	2	310
Steamfresh Broccoli Cauliflower & Carrots	¾ cup	30	1	0	0	5	2	30

FOOD	PORTION	CALS	PROT	FAT	CHOL	CARB	FIBER	SOD
Steamfresh Broccoli & Cauliflower	1 cup	30	1	0	0	4	2	25
Steamfresh Broccoli Carrots Sugar Snap Peas & Water Chestnuts	¾ cup (2.9 oz)	35	1	0	0	6	2	25
Steamfresh Mixed Vegetables	⅔ cup (3.2 oz)	40	2	0	0	12	2	20
C&W								
Early Harvest Peas & Baby Carrots	⅔ cup	60	3	0	0	10	3	150
Petite Peas & Pearl Onions	⅔ cup	60	4	0	0	11	3	160
Cascadian Farm								
Organic Mixed Vegetables	⅔ cup	60	2	0	0	12	2	20
Organic Peas & Carrots	⅔ cup	50	2	0	0	10	3	75
French Meadow Bakery								
Vegetarian Sweet N' Spicy Cuban Style Veggies	1 pkg (12 oz)	250	6	9	0	39	7	450
Green Giant								
Garden Vegetable Medley as prep	½ cup	70	2	1	0	14	2	220
Mixed Vegetables as prep	½ cup	50	2	0	0	11	2	20
Southwestern Style as prep	½ cup	90	4	1	0	18	4	190
Steamers Basil Vegetable Medley as prep	¾ cup	45	2	1	0	10	2	270
Szechuan Vegetables as prep	½ cup	50	2	1	0	9	2	410
Health Is Wealth								
Veggie Munchees Vegan	6 (3 oz)	150	4	4	0	26	3	500
La Choy								
Chop Suey Vegetables	½ cup (2.2 oz)	15	tr	0	0	3	tr	640
Fancy Chinese Mixed Vegetables	½ cup (2.9 oz)	15	1	2	0	3	1	60
Stir Fry Vegetables	½ cup	15	tr	0	0	3	2	180
Melrose Made Gourmet								
Vegetable Souffle Fat Free	1 serv (4 oz)	70	12	0	0	5	3	530
Seapoint Farms								
Organic Veggie Blends w/ Edamame Eat Your Greens	¾ cup	60	5	2	0	7	3	30

FOOD	PORTION	CALS	PROT	FAT	CHOL	CARB	FIBER	SOD
Veggie Blends w/ Edamame Garden	¾ cup	60	4	2	0	7	3	25
Veggie Blends w/ Edamame Oriental	¾ cup	60	4	1	0	8	3	80
TAKE-OUT								
buddha's delight	1 serv (16 oz)	174	17	5	35	17	3	1368
fukujinzuke japanese pickled vegetables	1 tbsp (6 g)	8	0	0	0	2	0	180
pakoras	4 (1.7 oz)	57	2	2	0	7	2	530
ratatouille	1 serv (3.5 oz)	96	2	7	0	7	4	812
samosa	1 (2.4 oz)	206	4	11	12	22	2	311
stir fry mixed vegetables	1 serv (4 oz)	66	3	5	0	3	2	292
succotash	½ cup	111	5	1	0	23	–	16

VENISON (*see also* JERKY)

FOOD	PORTION	CALS	PROT	FAT	CHOL	CARB	FIBER	SOD
cubed stewed	1 cup (5 oz)	266	51	6	157	0	0	375
hamburger grilled	1 (3.3 oz)	174	25	8	91	0	0	73
loin steak lean only broiled	1 (2 oz)	81	16	1	43	0	0	31
shoulder lean only braised	3 oz	162	31	3	96	0	0	44
tenderloin roasted	3 oz	127	25	2	75	0	0	48
top round lean only broiled	3 oz	129	27	2	72	0	0	38
TAKE-OUT								
meatloaf	1 lg slice (5 oz)	238	27	10	125	9	1	576
stew w/ potatoes & vegetables	1 cup (8.8 oz)	179	19	2	48	22	4	544

VINEGAR

FOOD	PORTION	CALS	PROT	FAT	CHOL	CARB	FIBER	SOD
balsamic	1 tbsp	14	tr	0	0	3	–	4
cider	1 tbsp	3	0	0	0	tr	0	1
coconut	1 tbsp (0.5 oz)	1	0	tr	–	tr	–	–
red wine	1 tbsp	3	tr	0	0	tr	0	1
white	1 tbsp	3	0	0	0	tr	0	0
Barengo								
Balsamic	1 tbsp (0.5 oz)	15	0	0	0	4	–	0
Red Wine	1 tbsp (0.5 oz)	0	0	0	0	0	0	0

FOOD	PORTION	CALS	PROT	FAT	CHOL	CARB	FIBER	SOD
Carapelli								
Balsamic	1 tbsp	15	0	0	0	4	0	0
Red Wine	1 tbsp	5	0	0	0	0	0	0
White Wine	1 tbsp	5	0	0	0	0	0	0
Gedney								
Apple Cider	1 tbsp	3	0	0	0	0	0	0
Distilled White	1 tbsp	3	0	0	0	0	0	0
Gourme Mist								
Balsamic Of Modena	1 sec spray	1	0	0	0	0	0	0
Balsamic Vinegar + Raspberry	1 sec spray	1	0	0	0	0	0	0
Heinz								
Apple Cider	1 tbsp (0.5 oz)	0	0	0	0	0	0	0
Malt	1 (0.5 oz)	0	0	0	0	0	0	0
Red Wine	1 tbsp (1 oz)	0	0	0	0	0	0	0
Tarragon	1 tbsp (0.5 oz)	0	0	0	0	0	0	0
White	1 tbsp (0.5 oz)	0	0	0	0	0	0	0
Holland House								
Malt	1 tbsp (0.5 oz)	0	0	0	0	0	0	0
Red Wine	1 tbsp (0.5 oz)	0	0	0	0	0	0	0
Latino Chef								
Lulo	1 tbsp	35	1	3	0	1	–	0
Passion Fruit	1 tbsp	40	0	3	–	2	tr	0
Lucini								
Balsamic 10 Year Gran Reserve	1 tbsp (0.5 oz)	20	0	0	0	4	–	0
Balsamic Dark Cherry Infused	1 tbsp	30	0	0	0	7	–	3
Italian Wine Pinot Noir	1 tbsp (0.5 oz)	<1	0	0	0	0	0	2
Mitsukan								
Rice	1 tbsp (0.5 oz)	0	0	0	0	0	0	0
Rice Seasoned	1 tbsp (0.5 oz)	25	0	0	0	5	–	420

FOOD	PORTION	CALS	PROT	FAT	CHOL	CARB	FIBER	SOD
Nakano								
Natural Rice	1 tbsp (0.5 oz)	0	0	0	0	0	0	0
Red Wine Italian Herb Seasoned	1 tbsp (0.5 oz)	20	0	0	0	5	–	240
Rice Pesto Seasoned	1 tbsp (0.5 oz)	20	0	0	0	5	–	240
Rice Red Pepper Seasoned	1 tbsp (0.5 oz)	20	0	0	0	5	–	240
Progresso								
Balsamic	2 tbsp (0.5 oz)	10	0	0	0	2	–	0
Tree Of Life								
Organic Apple Cider Raw Unfiltered	1 tbsp	0	0	0	0	tr	–	0
WAFFLES								
FROZEN								
Aunt Jemima								
Blueberry	2 (2.5 oz)	190	4	5	5	32	1	450
Low Fat	2 (2.5 oz)	160	4	3	0	30	1	420
Kashi								
Heart To Heart Honey Oat	2 (3 oz)	160	6	3	0	31	3	370
Lifestream								
Organic Fig + Flax	2 (2.8 oz)	210	5	0	0	29	6	410
Organic Pomegran Plus	2 (2.8 oz)	190	5	5	0	31	5	370
Van's								
Belgian Multigrain	2 (2.7 oz)	190	4	8	0	25	4	310
Mini Homestyle	4 (2.8 oz)	210	4	8	0	32	1	470
Organic Flax	2 (2.7 oz)	190	4	9	0	24	3	390
Organic Homestyle	2 (2.7 oz)	200	4	9	0	25	2	430
Original 97% Fat Free	2 (2.7 oz)	140	4	2	0	26	3	320
Original Buttermilk	2 (2.7 oz)	220	4	9	0	31	1	450
Wheat Free Buckwheat	2 (3 oz)	230	2	9	0	36	2	370
Wheat Free Flax	2 (3 oz)	210	3	8	0	33	1	380
MIX								
plain as prep 7 in diam	1 (2.6 oz)	218	6	11	52	25	–	383
READY-TO-EAT								
Kashi								
GoLean Blueberry	2 (3 oz)	170	8	3	0	33	6	300
GoLean Original	2 (3 oz)	170	8	3	0	33	6	330

FOOD	PORTION	CALS	PROT	FAT	CHOL	CARB	FIBER	SOD
Unique Belgique								
Imported From Belgium	2 (2.3 oz)	230	4	12	55	27	1	300
TAKE-OUT								
belgian	1 (4.7 oz)	412	10	13	19	65	3	958
blueberry 9 in sq	1 (7 oz)	556	13	16	24	90	5	1232
round 10 in diam	1 (6.8 oz)	598	14	18	27	94	5	1390
square 9 in	1 (7 oz)	620	15	19	28	98	5	1440
whole wheat 9 in sq	1 (7 oz)	534	18	22	188	67	5	990
WALNUTS								
black chopped	¼ cup	193	8	18	0	3	2	1
english chopped	¼ cup	191	4	19	0	4	2	1
english ground	¼ cup	131	3	13	0	3	1	0
english halves	14 (1 oz)	185	4	18	0	4	2	1
english in shell	7 (1 oz)	183	4	18	0	4	2	1
honey roasted	¼ cup	172	4	16	0	7	2	5
Back To Nature								
Unroasted Unsalted	1 oz	190	4	18	0	4	2	0
Diamond								
Chopped	¼ cup	200	5	20	0	4	2	0
Planters								
NUT-rition Omega-3 Mix	¼ cup (1.1 oz)	160	3	10	0	15	2	0
WASABI (*see* HORSERADISH)								
WATER								
ice cubes	3	0	0	0	0	0	0	2
tap water	8 oz	0	0	0	0	0	0	7
Acquafibre								
Fiber Enhanced All Flavors	1 bottle (11.15 oz)	5	0	0	0	0	5	1
Adirondack								
Sparkling All Flavors	8 oz	0	0	0	0	0	0	0
Aloe Breeze								
Organic All Flavors	8 oz	0	0	0	0	0	0	10
Apple & Eve								
Water Fruits All Flavors	1 bottle (10 oz)	90	0	0	0	21	–	10
Aqua Pacific								
Water	1 liter	0	0	0	0	0	0	10

FOOD	PORTION	CALS	PROT	FAT	CHOL	CARB	FIBER	SOD
Aquafina								
Alive Wellness Berry Pomegranate	8 oz	10	0	0	0	2	0	65
Ayala's								
Herbal All Flavors	1 bottle	0	0	0	0	0	0	0
Bot								
Fortified All Flavors	1 bottle (12 oz)	40	0	0	0	10	0	0
Dasani								
Purified Water	8 oz	0	0	0	0	0	0	0
Dox								
Cardio Water	1 bottle (12 oz)	20	0	0	0	5	–	30
Evian								
Spring Water	1 liter	0	0	0	0	0	0	6
EX								
Aqua Vitamins Raspberry	1 bottle (16.9 oz)	110	0	0	0	27	–	5
Fiji								
Natural Artesian	1 liter	0	0	0	0	0	0	0
Gerolsteiner								
Sparkling Mineral	8 oz	0	0	0	0	0	0	30
H 10 O								
Citrus Sport For Men	1 bottle (15.9 oz)	0	0	0	0	0	0	20
Peach Mango Tea For Women	1 bottle (15.9 oz)	0	0	0	0	0	0	20
H2Odwalla								
Enhanced Tropical Orange	1 bottle (20 oz)	120	0	0	0	33	2	15
Organic Enhanced Blueberry Tea	1 bottle (20 oz)	120	0	0	0	29	–	20
Organic Enhanced Jasmine Lime	1 bottle (20 oz)	120	0	0	0	30	–	20
Hawaiian Springs								
Naturally Pure	1 liter	0	0	0	0	0	0	0
Highland Spring								
Spring Water	1 liter	0	0	0	0	0	0	9
IQ								
H2O Orange Mango	8 oz	40	0	0	0	10	–	0

FOOD	PORTION	CALS	PROT	FAT	CHOL	CARB	FIBER	SOD
Island Chill								
Artesian Water	1 liter	0	0	0	0	0	0	–
Jana								
Natural European Artesian	1 liter	0	0	0	0	0	0	0
Joint Juice								
Fitness Water All Flavors	1 bottle (18 oz)	10	0	0	0	1	–	55
Jones Soda								
24C Multi Vitamin Enhanced All Flavors	1 bottle	100	0	0	0	24	–	30
Klear Splash								
Mini Sip	1 pkg (4 oz)	0	0	0	0	0	0	0
Life Water								
B-Strong	1 bottle (20 oz)	100	0	0	0	42	–	55
Enlighten	1 bottle (20 oz)	100	0	0	0	41	–	55
Zingseng	1 bottle (20 oz)	100	0	0	0	41	–	55
Liquid Salvation								
Ultra Hydrating	1 bottle	0	0	0	0	0	0	0
Nui								
All Natural Kid Water	10 oz	90	0	0	0	21	3	10
O Water								
Hydrate Black Raspberry	8 oz	25	0	0	0	7	0	0
Replenish Lemon Lime	8 oz	25	0	0	0	7	0	0
Vitalize Peach Mango	8 oz	25	0	0	0	7	0	0
Propel								
Fitness Water All Flavors	1 bottle (24 oz)	30	0	0	0	6	–	220
R.W. Knudsen								
Organic Sparkling Essence Lemon	1 can (10.5 oz)	0	0	0	0	0	0	0
San Benedetto								
Sparkling Mineral Water	1 liter	0	0	0	0	0	0	7
Skinny Water								
Hi-Energy Acai Grape Blueberry	8 oz	0	0	0	0	0	0	10
Total-V Passionfruit Lemonade	8 oz	0	0	0	0	0	0	10

FOOD	PORTION	CALS	PROT	FAT	CHOL	CARB	FIBER	SOD
Snapple								
Antioxidant Water Awaken Dragonfruit	8 oz	50	0	0	0	12	–	0
Antioxidant Water Restore Agave Melon	8 oz	60	0	0	0	13	–	0
Lyte Water	8 oz	0	0	0	0	0	–	–
SoNu								
Organic 10 Calories All Flavors	8 oz	10	0	0	0	4	0	5
Organic All Flavors	8 oz	45	0	0	0	13	0	5
Sparkling Ice								
All Flavors	1 bottle (16 oz)	0	0	0	0	0	0	0
Special K2O								
Protein Water All Flavors	1 bottle (16.6 oz)	50	5	0	0	8	–	30
Trim Water								
Purified	1 bottle (20 oz)	10	0	0	0	3	0	65
Twist								
Organics All Flavors	8 oz	10	0	0	0	2	0	0
Vitamin + Fiber Water								
All Fruit Flavors	8 oz	50	0	0	0	13	3	10
VitaminWater								
XXX Acai Blueberry Pomegranate	8 oz	50	0	0	0	13	–	0
WaterPlus								
Antioxidants Acai Berry	8 oz	50	0	0	0	13	–	0
Electrolytes Fruit Punch	8 oz	50	0	0	0	13	–	0
Extra-C Orange Tangerine	8 oz	50	0	0	0	13	0	0
Vitamins Dragonfruit Kiwi	8 oz	50	0	0	0	13	–	0
WATER CHESTNUTS								
chinese sliced canned	½ cup	35	1	tr	0	9	–	6
fresh sliced	½ cup	66	1	tr	0	15	–	9
La Choy								
Sliced	½ cup	25	1	0	0	5	1	10
Polar								
Sliced	2 tbsp	10	1	0	0	3	1	15

FOOD	PORTION	CALS	PROT	FAT	CHOL	CARB	FIBER	SOD
WATERCRESS								
cooked w/o fat	1 cup	15	3	tr	0	2	1	427
raw chopped	1 cup	4	1	tr	0	tr	tr	14
WATERMELON								
cut up	1 cup	46	1	tr	0	12	1	2
seeds dried	¼ cup	150	8	13	0	4	–	27
wedge	1 lg (20 oz)	172	3	1	0	43	2	6
wedge	1 sm (2.5 oz)	21	tr	tr	0	5	tr	1
wedge	1 med (10 oz)	86	2	tr	0	22	1	3
whole melon	1 (9 lb)	1227	25	6	0	309	16	41
Jake & Amos								
Pickled Sweet Rind	2 tbsp (1 oz)	70	0	0	0	17	0	40
Mini Me								
Personal Seedless	2 cups (10 oz)	80	1	0	0	27	2	0
WATERMELON JUICE								
juice	8 oz	71	1	tr	0	18	1	2
EarthWise								
Watermelon Supreme	8 oz	100	0	0	0	26	0	10
WHALE								
beluga dried	1 oz	93	20	2	35	0	0	63
beluga raw	3.5 oz	111	27	1	80	0	0	78
WHEAT								
sprouted	1 cup (3.8 oz)	214	8	1	0	46	1	17
starch	3.5 oz	348	tr	tr	–	86	–	2
Amazing Grass								
Organic Wheat Grass	1 tbsp (0.3 oz)	35	2	0	0	4	2	2
Arrowhead Mills								
Whole Grain Wheat	¼ cup (1.6 oz)	150	7	1	0	31	5	0
Bob's Red Mill								
Vital Wheat Gluten	¼ cup	120	23	1	0	6	0	9
Near East								
Taboule Wheat Salad as prep	⅔ cup (3.5 oz)	120	3	3	0	24	5	270

FOOD	PORTION	CALS	PROT	FAT	CHOL	CARB	FIBER	SOD
White Wave								
Seitan Chicken Meat Of Wheat	3 oz	130	24	0	0	9	3	270
Seitan Traditional	3 oz	90	18	1	0	3	1	380
Seitan Vegetarian Stir Fry Strips	3 oz	110	22	2	0	2	1	420
WHEAT GERM								
plain	¼ cup	108	8	3	0	14	4	1
Bob's Red Mill								
Wheat Germ	2 tbsp	59	4	2	0	7	2	2
Kretschmer								
Original Toasted	¼ cup (0.6 oz)	35	3	1	0	10	7	0
Tree Of Life								
Toasted	3 tbsp (0.8 oz)	100	9	3	0	12	3	0
WHEY								
acid dry	1 tbsp	10	tr	tr	0	2	0	28
sweet dry	1 tbsp	26	1	tr	0	6	0	81
sweet fluid	½ cup	33	1	tr	2	6	0	66
whey cheese	1 oz	126	4	8	–	9	0	146
Action Whey								
Dream Shake All Flavors	1 scoop (0.8 oz)	90	15	3	40	3	1	50
Bob's Red Mill								
Protein Concentrate	¼ cup	80	16	1	30	1	0	40
Sweet Dairy	1 tbsp	30	1	0	1	6	0	70
Wellements								
Whey Protein Chocolate	1 scoop (1 oz)	120	22	2	42	4	0	55
Whey Protein Vanilla	1 scoop (1 oz)	120	22	2	39	4	0	55
WHIPPED TOPPINGS								
cream pressurized	1 tbsp (3 g)	8	tr	tr	2	tr	–	4
cream pressurized	1 cup (2.1 oz)	154	2	13	46	7	–	78
nondairy frzn	1 tbsp	13	tr	1	0	1	–	1

FOOD	PORTION	CALS	PROT	FAT	CHOL	CARB	FIBER	SOD
nondairy powdered as prep w/ whole milk	1 cup	151	3	10	8	13	–	53
nondairy pressurized	1 tbsp (4 g)	11	tr	1	0	1	–	2
nondairy pressurized	1 cup	184	1	16	0	11	–	43
Cool Whip								
Chocolate	2 tbsp	25	0	2	–	2	–	0
Free	2 tbsp	15	0	0	0	3	–	5
Regular	2 tbsp	25	0	2	–	2	–	0
Strawberry	2 tbsp	25	0	2	–	2	–	0
Soyatoo								
Rice Whip	2 tbsp (6 g)	10	0	1	0	1	0	0
Soy Whip	2 tbsp (6 g)	10	0	1	0	1	0	0
TruWhip								
Whipped Topping	2 tbsp (0.4 oz)	30	0	2	0	3	0	0
WHITE BEANS								
canned	1 cup	306	19	1	0	58	–	13
dried regular cooked	1 cup	249	17	1	0	45	–	11
dried small cooked	1 cup	253	16	1	0	46	–	4
WHITEFISH								
baked	3 oz	146	21	6	65	0	0	56
smoked	1 oz	39	7	tr	9	0	0	285
smoked	3 oz	92	20	1	28	0	0	866
WHITING								
broiled w/o fat	3 oz	99	20	1	71	0	0	112
fillet broiled w/o fat	1 (2.5 oz)	84	17	1	60	0	0	95
fillet steamed w/o fat	1 (2.6 oz)	84	17	1	63	0	0	61
hake raw	3.5 oz	84	17	1	–	0	0	101
TAKE-OUT								
fillet battered & fried	1 (3.1 oz)	157	15	7	66	6	tr	110
fillet breaded & fried	1 (3.1 oz)	191	17	10	75	7	tr	350
WILD RICE								
cooked	1 cup (5.8 oz)	166	7	1	0	35	3	5
Gourmet House								
Cracked as prep	1 cup	170	6	0	0	35	2	0
Quick Cooking not prep	½ cup	170	6	0	0	25	2	0
Thai Jasmine as prep	¾ cup	160	3	0	0	36	0	0

FOOD	PORTION	CALS	PROT	FAT	CHOL	CARB	FIBER	SOD
Lundberg								
Organic Quick not prep	¼ cup	150	6	1	0	33	2	0
WINE								
chianti	1 serv (5 oz)	125	tr	0	0	4	0	6
chinese cooking	1 bottle (15 oz)	559	0	0	0	3	0	43
cooking	¼ cup (2 oz)	29	tr	0	0	4	0	363
haiku	1 serv	93	tr	0	0	3	0	2
japanese plum	3 oz	139	tr	tr	0	16	0	–
japanese sake	2 oz	78	tr	0	0	3	0	1
kir	1 serv	78	tr	0	0	3	0	4
liebfraumilch	4 oz	86	–	–	–	–	–	–
madeira	3.5 oz	169	0	0	–	10	0	–
marsala	4 oz	80	–	–	–	–	–	–
merlot	4 oz	95	–	–	–	–	–	–
muscat	1 serv (5 oz)	123	tr	0	0	8	–	–
nonalcoholic	1 serv (5 oz)	9	1	0	0	2	0	10
port	1 serv (3.5 oz)	165	tr	0	0	14	0	9
red barbera	1 serv (5 oz)	125	tr	0	0	4	–	–
red burgundy	1 serv (5 oz)	127	tr	0	0	5	–	–
red cabernet franc	1 serv (5 oz)	122	tr	0	0	4	–	–
red claret	1 serv (5 oz)	122	tr	0	0	4	–	–
red gamay	1 serv (5 oz)	115	tr	0	0	4	–	–
red mouvedre	1 serv (5 oz)	129	tr	0	0	4	–	–
red pinot noir	1 serv (5 oz)	121	tr	0	0	3	–	–
red syrah	1 serv (5 oz)	122	tr	0	0	4	–	–
red zinfandel	1 serv (5 oz)	129	tr	0	0	4	–	–
sake screwdriver	1 serv	175	2	tr	0	23	tr	3
sangria	1 serv	88	tr	tr	0	6	tr	4
sangria blanco	1 serv	155	1	tr	0	24	3	13
sherry	2 oz	84	tr	0	0	5	–	–
vermouth dry	3.5 oz	105	–	0	0	1	–	–
vermouth sweet	3.5 oz	167	–	0	0	12	–	–
wassail wine	1 serv	142	1	tr	0	22	2	6
white	1 serv (5 oz)	121	tr	0	0	4	0	7
white fume blanc	1 serv (5 oz)	121	tr	0	0	3	–	–
white pinot blanc	1 serv (5 oz)	119	tr	0	0	3	–	–
white pinot grigio	1 serv (5 oz)	122	tr	0	0	3	–	–

FOOD	PORTION	CALS	PROT	FAT	CHOL	CARB	FIBER	SOD
white riesling	1 serv (5 oz)	118	tr	0	0	6	–	–
white sauvignon blanc	1 serv (5 oz)	119	tr	0	0	3	–	–
wine cooler	1 (7 oz)	116	tr	tr	0	14	0	15
wine spritzer	1 serv (7 oz)	73	tr	0	0	2	0	16
Almaden								
Merlot	5 oz	115	–	0	0	5	–	–
Bartles & Jaymes								
Wine Cooler Classic Original	1 bottle (12 oz)	190	–	0	0	29	–	–
Beringer								
Chardonnay	5 oz	125	–	0	0	0	–	–
Carlo Rossi								
Cabernet Sauvignon	5 oz	125	–	0	0	5	0	tr
Franzia Vinter								
Select Merlot	5 oz	105	–	0	0	0	–	–
Holland House								
Cooking Wine Marsala	2 tbsp (1 oz)	45	0	0	0	4	–	190
Cooking Wine Red	2 tbsp (1 oz)	20	0	0	0	1	–	190
Cooking Wine Sherry	2 tbsp (1 oz)	45	0	0	0	2	–	190
Cooking Wine Vermouth	2 tbsp (1 oz)	35	0	0	0	2	–	190
Cooking Wine White	2 tbsp (1 oz)	20	0	0	0	0	0	190
Twin Valley								
Cabernet Sauvignon	5 oz	120	–	0	0	5	–	–

WINGED BEANS

dried cooked w/o salt	1 cup	253	18	10	0	26	3	22

WRAPS (*see* BREAD, SANDWICHES)

YACON

Navitas Naturals								
Slices Dried	1 oz	90	1	0	0	22	1	10

YAM (*see also* SWEET POTATO)

CANNED

Glory								
Candied	½ cup	210	1	0	0	52	1	240
S&W								
Candied	½ cup (4.9 oz)	170	2	0	0	46	4	360

FOOD	PORTION	CALS	PROT	FAT	CHOL	CARB	FIBER	SOD
FRESH								
mountain yam hawaii cooked w/o salt	1 cup	119	3	tr	0	29	–	17
yam cooked w/o salt	1 cup	158	2	tr	0	38	5	11
Earthbound Farms								
Organic	1 med (4.6 oz)	130	2	0	0	33	4	45
House								
Black Ita Konnyaku Yam Cake	1 serv (2 oz)	5	0	0	0	1	tr	0
YARDLONG BEANS								
sliced cooked w/o salt	1 cup	49	3	tr	0	10	–	4
YAUTIA (*see* MALANGA)								
YEAST								
baker's compressed	1 cake (0.6 oz)	18	1	tr	0	3	1	5
baker's dry	1 tbsp	35	5	1	0	5	3	6
baker's dry	1 pkg (7 g)	21	3	tr	0	3	2	4
brewer's dry	1 tbsp	35	5	1	0	5	3	6
Bob's Red Mill								
Active Dry	1 tbsp	25	0	1	0	5	2	0
YELLOW BEANS								
fresh cooked w/o salt	1 cup	44	2	tr	0	10	4	4
fresh raw	1 cup	34	2	tr	0	8	4	7
YELLOWTAIL								
baked	4 oz	199	32	7	75	0	0	53
YOGURT (*see also* YOGURT DRINKS, YOGURT FROZEN)								
plain lowfat	8 oz	143	12	4	14	16	0	159
plain nonfat	8 oz	127	13	tr	5	17	0	175
plain whole milk	8 oz	138	8	7	30	11	0	104
tofu yogurt	1 cup	246	9	5	0	42	1	92
Better Whey								
All Fruit Flavors	1 pkg (6 oz)	145	15	1	5	23	3	80
Plain	1 pkg (6 oz)	130	17	1	5	17	3	95
Breyers								
Creme Savers All Flavors	1 pkg (6 oz)	160	6	2	10	31	0	170

FOOD	PORTION	CALS	PROT	FAT	CHOL	CARB	FIBER	SOD
Fruit On The Bottom Black Cherry	1 pkg (6 oz)	160	5	1	10	32	tr	80
Fruit On The Bottom Chocolate Raspberry	1 pkg (6 oz)	170	5	1	10	34	tr	75
Fruit On The Bottom Mixed Berry	1 pkg (6 oz)	160	5	1	10	31	tr	75
Fruit On The Bottom Peach Mango Orange	1 pkg (6 oz)	160	5	1	10	31	tr	75
Fruit On The Bottom Pineapple	1 pkg (6 oz)	150	5	1	10	31	tr	75
Fruit On The Bottom Strawberry	1 pkg (6 oz)	150	5	1	10	31	tr	70
Inspirations Cherry Chocolate Chip	1 pkg (4 oz)	140	4	3	5	23	0	65
Inspirations Mint Chocolate Chip	1 pkg (4 oz)	140	4	4	5	23	0	65
Inspirations Vanilla Bean	1 pkg (4 oz)	110	4	1	5	21	0	60
Light Blueberry	1 pkg (4 oz)	50	4	0	<5	8	tr	70
Smooth & Creamy Peaches 'N Cream	1 pkg (4 oz)	120	3	1	10	24	0	50
Smooth & Creamy Strawberry	1 pkg (4 oz)	110	3	1	10	23	0	50
Cabot								
Greek	1 pkg (6 oz)	210	7	17	55	9	0	80
Greek 2%	1 pkg (6 oz)	160	13	3	20	25	0	80
Non Fat Berry Banana	1 cup	130	8	0	5	24	0	115
Non Fat Black Cherry	1 cup	130	8	0	5	24	0	115
Non Fat French Vanilla	1 cup	130	8	0	5	24	–	115
Non Fat Plain	1 cup	100	10	0	5	19	0	135
Non Fat Raspberry	1 cup	130	8	0	5	24	0	115
Chobani								
Greek Yogurt Nonfat Blueberry	1 pkg (6 oz)	140	14	0	0	20	tr	65
Greek Yogurt Nonfat Caramel	1 pkg (6 oz)	140	16	0	0	13	0	75
Greek Yogurt Nonfat Honey	1 pkg (6 oz)	150	16	0	0	20	0	75
Greek Yogurt Nonfat Peach	1 pkg (6 oz)	140	14	0	0	20	tr	65
Greek Yogurt Nonfat Plain	1 pkg (6 oz)	100	18	0	0	7	0	80
Greek Yogurt Nonfat Pomegranate	1 pkg (6 oz)	140	14	0	0	21	0	75

FOOD	PORTION	CALS	PROT	FAT	CHOL	CARB	FIBER	SOD
Greek Yogurt Nonfat Raspberry	1 pkg (6 oz)	140	14	0	0	22	1	65
Greek Yogurt Nonfat Strawberry	1 pkg (6 oz)	140	14	0	0	20	tr	65
Greek Yogurt Nonfat Vanilla	1 pkg (6 oz)	120	16	0	0	13	0	75
Dannon								
Activia Blueberry	1 pkg (4 oz)	110	5	2	10	19	0	65
Activia Cherry	1 pkg (4 oz)	110	5	2	10	19	0	75
Activia Peach	1 pkg (4 oz)	110	5	2	10	19	0	70
Activia Prune	1 pkg (4 oz)	110	5	2	10	19	0	75
Activia Strawberry	1 pkg (4 oz)	110	5	2	5	19	0	75
Activia Strawberry Banana	1 pkg (4 oz)	110	4	2	5	19	0	75
Activia Vanilla	1 pkg (4 oz)	110	5	2	10	19	0	70
Activia Light Blueberry	1 pkg (4 oz)	70	4	0	<5	13	2	65
Activia Light Peach	1 pkg (4 oz)	70	4	0	<5	12	2	65
Activia Light Raspberry	1 pkg (4 oz)	70	4	0	<5	13	2	75
Activia Light Strawberry	1 pkg (4 oz)	70	4	0	<5	13	2	70
Activia Light Vanilla	1 pkg (4 oz)	70	5	0	<5	14	3	70
All Natural Coffee	1 pkg (6 oz)	150	7	3	10	25	0	100
All Natural Lemon	1 pkg (6 oz)	150	7	3	10	25	0	100
All Natural Plain	1 pkg (6 oz)	100	8	3	10	12	0	115
All Natural Vanilla	1 pkg (6 oz)	150	7	3	10	25	0	100
Fage								
Total Cherry	1 pkg (5.3 oz)	210	8	12	20	17	0	35
Total Classic	1 pkg (5.3 oz)	210	8	12	20	17	0	35
Total Classic With Honey	1 pkg (5.3 oz)	250	8	12	20	28	0	35
Total Peach	1 pkg (5.3 oz)	210	8	12	20	17	0	35
Total Strawberry	1 pkg (5.3 oz)	210	8	12	20	17	0	35
Fiber One								
Creamy Nonfat Vanilla	1 pkg (4 oz)	80	4	0	<5	19	5	65
Friendship								
Plain	1 cup	150	12	3	15	18	1	190
Horizon Organic								
Kids Strawberry	1 pkg (4 oz)	110	4	1	5	20	1	75
Lowfat Blended Blueberry	1 pkg (6 oz)	160	7	2	10	30	2	110

FOOD	PORTION	CALS	PROT	FAT	CHOL	CARB	FIBER	SOD
Tube Lowfat Blueberry	1 (2 oz)	70	2	1	5	12	0	40
Whole Milk Plain	1 cup	160	10	7	30	14	0	150
La Yogurt								
Lowfat Blueberries 'N' Cream	1 pkg (6 oz)	200	7	2	10	39	0	90
Lowfat Fruit On The Bottom Cherry	1 pkg (8 oz)	230	6	3	10	47	tr	85
Lowfat Fruit On The Bottom Probiotic Peach	1 pkg (6 oz)	160	6	2	5	31	0	100
Lowfat Fruit On The Bottom Strawberry	1 pkg (8 oz)	220	9	2	10	43	tr	140
Lowfat Peaches 'N' Cream	1 pkg (6 oz)	200	7	2	10	39	0	90
Lowfat Pina Colada	1 pkg (6 oz)	160	5	2	5	30	0	90
Lowfat Probiotic Pina Colada	1 pkg (6 oz)	160	5	2	5	30	0	90
Lowfat Probiotic Plain	1 pkg (6 oz)	100	9	2	10	12	0	130
Lowfat Probiotic Vanilla	1 pkg (6 oz)	150	8	2	10	26	0	120
Lowfat Vanilla 'N' Cream	1 pkg (6 oz)	200	7	2	10	39	0	90
Nonfat Banana Cream	1 pkg (6 oz)	100	6	0	0	18	0	90
Nonfat Probiotic Cherry	1 pkg (6 oz)	100	6	0	0	17	0	90
Nonfat Probiotic Peach	1 pkg (6 oz)	90	6	0	0	16	0	85
Nonfat Probiotic Raspberry	1 pkg (6 oz)	90	6	0	0	15	0	85
Nonfat Probiotic Vanilla	1 pkg (6 oz)	90	6	0	0	15	0	85
Sabor Latino Lowfat Dulce De Leche	1 pkg (6 oz)	190	7	2	10	36	0	105
Sabor Latino Lowfat Guava	1 pkg (6 oz)	190	7	2	10	37	0	110
Sabor Latino Lowfat Horchata	1 pkg (6 oz)	210	7	2	10	41	0	105
Sabor Latino Lowfat Papaya	1 pkg (6 oz)	190	7	2	10	37	0	105
Land O' Lakes								
Strawberry Light	1 pkg (8 oz)	80	8	0	0	38	0	135
Strawberry Lowfat	1 pkg (8 oz)	190	8	2	10	36	0	125
Liberte								
Plain Lowfat	1 pkg (6 oz)	110	9	4	15	10	0	110
Six Grains Peach	1 pkg (6 oz)	150	8	3	10	23	1	90
Six Grains Pear	1 pkg (6 oz)	160	8	3	10	23	1	90
Lowell								
Multi Grain Peach & Whole Grain	1 pkg (6 oz)	170	6	5	20	26	1	80

FOOD	PORTION	CALS	PROT	FAT	CHOL	CARB	FIBER	SOD
Mountain High								
Black Cherry Classic Lowfat	1 pkg (6 oz)	140	7	2	10	24	0	105
Blueberry Classic Lowfat	1 pkg (6 oz)	140	7	2	10	24	0	105
Lemon Lowfat	1 pkg (8 oz)	190	10	2	10	34	0	150
Mountain Berry Classic Lowfat	1 pkg (6 oz)	150	7	2	10	26	0	110
Plain Fat Free	1 pkg (8 oz)	120	12	0	5	18	0	180
Plain Lowfat	1 pkg (8 oz)	140	11	3	15	18	0	170
Plain Original	1 pkg (8 oz)	180	11	8	35	17	0	160
Strawberry Classic Lowfat	1 pkg (6 oz)	140	7	2	10	24	0	105
Vanilla Fat Free	1 pkg (8 oz)	160	11	0	<5	30	0	160
Vanilla Lowfat	1 pkg (8 oz)	180	10	3	15	29	0	160
Vanilla Original	1 pkg (8 oz)	210	10	7	30	28	0	150
Nancy's								
Lowfat Lemon	1 pkg (8 oz)	150	11	3	20	16	0	170
Lowfat Maple	1 pkg (8 oz)	180	10	3	15	26	0	160
Lowfat Peach	1 pkg (8 oz)	170	10	3	15	26	0	150
Lowfat Plain	1 pkg (8 oz)	150	11	3	20	16	0	170
Lowfat Vanilla	1 pkg (8 oz)	140	10	3	15	15	0	160
Organic Soy Kiwi Lime	1 pkg (6 oz)	160	5	3	0	31	4	20
Organic Soy Mango	1 (6 oz)	170	4	3	0	33	3	20
Organic Soy Plain	1 pkg (6 oz)	150	5	3	0	25	2	20
Organic Soy Vanilla	1 pkg (6 oz)	120	4	3	0	19	3	20
Organic Whole Milk Fruit On The Top Blackberry	1 pkg (8 oz)	220	8	5	20	38	2	110
Organic Whole Milk Fruit On The Top Cherry	1 pkg (8 oz)	220	8	6	20	36	1	110
Organic Whole Milk Fruit On The Top Peach	1 pkg (8 oz)	220	8	5	20	38	tr	110
Organic Whole Milk Honey	1 pkg (8 oz)	170	10	8	30	17	0	160
Organic Whole Milk Plain	1 pkg (8 oz)	130	8	6	25	11	0	125
Oikos								
Blueberry	1 pkg (5.3 oz)	120	13	0	0	16	0	70
Caramel	1 pkg (4 oz)	110	10	0	0	17	0	60
Chocolate	1 pkg (4 oz)	110	10	0	0	17	tr	55
Honey	1 pkg (5.3 oz)	120	13	0	0	18	0	50
Plain	1 pkg (5.3 oz)	80	15	0	0	6	0	60
Strawberry	1 pkg (5.3 oz)	110	13	0	0	16	0	80
Super Fruits	1 pkg (5.3 oz)	130	13	0	0	18	0	80
Vanilla	1 pkg (5.3 oz)	110	15	0	0	12	0	60

FOOD	PORTION	CALS	PROT	FAT	CHOL	CARB	FIBER	SOD
Rachel's								
Essence Berry Jasmine w/ Zinc	1 pkg (6 oz)	160	8	3	10	28	2	115
Essence Plum Honey Lavender	1 pkg (6 oz)	160	8	3	10	28	2	115
Essence Pomegranate Acai	1 pkg (6 oz)	170	8	3	10	29	2	125
Exotic Kiwi Passion Fruit Lime	1 pkg (6 oz)	160	8	3	10	28	2	135
Exotic Orange Strawberry Mango	1 pkg (6 oz)	160	8	3	10	28	2	120
Exotic Pomegranate Blueberry	1 pkg (6 oz)	170	8	3	10	29	2	135
Siggi's								
Icelandic Skyr Vanilla 0% Milkfat	1 pkg (6 oz)	120	16	0	5	12	0	65
Silk								
Live! Blueberry	1 pkg (6 oz)	150	4	2	0	29	1	25
Soy Blueberry	1 pkg (6 oz)	150	4	2	0	29	1	25
Soy Key Lime	1 pkg (6 oz)	150	4	2	0	30	1	25
Soy Plain	1 cup (8 oz)	150	6	4	0	22	1	30
Soy Vanilla	1 pkg (6 oz)	150	5	3	0	25	1	20
Strawberry	1 pkg (6 oz)	160	4	2	0	31	1	25
SoDelicious								
Coconut Milk Plain	1 pkg (6 oz)	130	1	7	0	16	3	10
Coconut Milk Vanilla	1 pkg (6 oz)	150	1	6	0	22	2	5
Dairy Free Cinnamon Bun	1 pkg (6 oz)	160	6	3	0	29	3	25
Dairy Free Raspberry	1 pkg (6 oz)	150	6	3	0	29	3	35
Stonyfield Farm								
Lowfat Cherry Vanilla	1 pkg (6 oz)	130	7	2	5	23	0	110
Lowfat Fruit On The Bottom Blueberry	1 pkg (6 oz)	120	6	2	5	21	tr	90
Lowfat Fruit On The Bottom Peach	1 pkg (6 oz)	130	6	2	5	22	0	110
Lowfat Fruit On The Bottom Strawberry	1 pkg (6 oz)	120	6	2	5	21	tr	120
Lowfat Plain	1 pkg (6 oz)	90	7	2	5	11	0	110
O'Soy Chocolate	1 pkg (6 oz)	160	8	3	0	25	2	35
O'Soy Fruit On The Bottom Peach	1 pkg (6 oz)	170	7	3	0	30	2	45

FOOD	PORTION	CALS	PROT	FAT	CHOL	CARB	FIBER	SOD
O'Soy Fruit On The Bottom Strawberry	1 pkg (6 oz)	170	7	3	0	29	2	55
O'Soy Vanilla	1 pkg (6 oz)	150	7	3	0	24	1	40
Whole Milk Cream Top French Vanilla	1 pkg (6 oz)	170	6	6	25	23	0	95
Whole Milk Cream Top White Chocolate Raspberry	1 pkg (6 oz)	170	6	6	25	23	0	105
Straus								
Organic Maple Nonfat	1 pkg (8 oz)	170	12	0	5	30	0	160
Organic Maple Whole Milk	1 pkg (8 oz)	210	10	6	35	28	0	120
Organic Plain Lowfat	1 pkg (8 oz)	150	14	2	15	21	0	410
Organic Plain Nonfat	1 pkg (8 oz)	110	12	0	5	16	0	160
Organic Plain Whole Milk	1 pkg (8 oz)	160	10	7	30	13	1	115
The Greek Gods								
Honey	1 pkg (6 oz)	250	6	14	40	23	0	95
Plain Nonfat	1 pkg (6 oz)	60	6	0	0	10	2	105
Plain Traditional	1 pkg (4 oz)	130	4	11	30	5	0	70
Pomegranate	1 pkg (6 oz)	230	6	17	65	14	0	95
Vanilla Cinnamon Orange Reduced Fat	1 pkg (6 oz)	170	7	6	25	24	0	320
Voskos								
Greek Yogurt Exotic Fig	1 pkg (8 oz)	160	11	0	0	28	0	65
Greek Yogurt Plain Low Fat	1 pkg (8 oz)	160	23	3	20	9	0	100
Greek Yogurt Plain Non Fat	1 pkg (8 oz)	140	24	0	0	9	0	90
Greek Yogurt Plain Original	1 pkg (8 oz)	280	9	20	80	15	0	100
Greek Yogurt Wild Blueberry	1 pkg (8 oz)	120	13	0	10	16	0	55
Organic Vanilla Bean	1 pkg (5.3 oz)	130	12	0	0	20	0	45
Wallaby								
Lowfat Banana Vanilla	1 pkg (6 oz)	140	6	3	15	24	0	75
Lowfat Lemon	1 pkg (6 oz)	140	6	3	15	23	0	75
Lowfat Maple	1 pkg (6 oz)	140	6	3	15	24	0	75
Lowfat Plain	1 pkg (8 oz)	140	11	4	25	15	0	120
Lowfat Raspberry	1 pkg (6 oz)	140	7	3	15	23	0	75
Lowfat Vanilla	1 pkg (6 oz)	140	6	3	15	24	0	75
Original Guava	1 pkg (6 oz)	170	5	2	10	33	0	80
WildWood								
Organic Soyogurt Low Fat Peach	1 pkg (6 oz)	160	5	3	0	29	5	40

FOOD	PORTION	CALS	PROT	FAT	CHOL	CARB	FIBER	SOD
Organic Soyogurt Low Fat Vanilla	1 pkg (6 oz)	160	5	3	0	30	5	40
Organic Soyogurt Plain Unsweetened	1 pkg (6 oz)	110	6	4	0	14	4	45
Yofarm								
YoSmooth Apricot	1 pkg	220	6	6	20	36	–	90
YoSmooth Peach	1 pkg	220	6	6	20	35	–	100
YoSmooth Raspberry	1 pkg	230	6	6	20	36	–	95
Yoplait								
Delights Chocolate Raspberry	1 pkg (4 oz)	100	5	2	5	18	0	90
Delights Lemon Torte	1 pkg (4 oz)	100	5	2	5	16	0	80
Delights Triple Berry Creme	1 pkg (4 oz)	100	5	2	5	16	0	80
Light Strawberry	1 pkg (4 oz)	50	4	0	<5	8	tr	70
Orginal Coconut Cream	1 pkg (6 oz)	190	5	3	10	34	0	85
Orginal PassionFruit	1 pkg (6 oz)	170	5	2	10	33	0	80
Original Lemon Burst	1 pkg (6 oz)	180	5	2	10	36	0	80
Original Pina Colada	1 pkg (6 oz)	170	5	2	10	33	0	95
Whips All Chocolate Flavors	1 pkg (6 oz)	160	5	4	10	26	0	105
Whips All Fruit Flavors	1 pkg (4 oz)	140	5	3	10	25	0	75
Yo Plus All Flavors	1 pkg (4 oz)	110	4	2	10	21	3	70

YOGURT DRINKS (*see also* SMOOTHIES)

FOOD	PORTION	CALS	PROT	FAT	CHOL	CARB	FIBER	SOD
lassi	7 oz	78	0	5	19	8	0	–
Dahlicious								
Lassi Green Tea	1 bottle	110	7	0	0	21	2	100
Lassi Mango	1 bottle	130	8	0	0	27	2	100
Lassi Plain	1 bottle	110	7	0	0	21	2	100
Dannon								
Activia Mixed Berry	1 bottle (6 oz)	160	6	3	10	27	1	60
Activia Peach	1 bottle (6 oz)	170	6	3	10	27	1	65
Activia Vanilla	1 bottle (6 oz)	160	6	3	10	27	1	60
Danactive Blueberry	1 bottle (3.1 oz)	80	3	2	5	14	0	40
Danactive Strawberry	1 bottle (3.1 oz)	80	3	2	5	14	0	40
Danactive Vanilla	1 bottle (3.1 oz)	80	3	2	5	14	0	40

FOOD	PORTION	CALS	PROT	FAT	CHOL	CARB	FIBER	SOD
Danimals Smoothies Rockin' Raspberry	1 bottle (3.1 oz)	70	2	1	<5	15	0	35
Danimals Smoothies Strawberry Explosion	1 bottle (3.1 oz)	70	2	1	<5	15	0	35
Danimals Smoothies Strikin' Strawberry Kiwi	1 bottle (3.1 oz)	70	2	1	<5	15	0	30
Light & Fit Smoothie Mixed Berry & Pomegranate	1 bottle (7 oz)	70	4	0	<5	13	0	70
Light & Fit Smoothie Peach	1 bottle (7 oz)	70	4	0	<5	13	0	90
Light & Fit Smoothie Strawberry Banana	1 bottle (7 oz)	70	4	0	<5	14	0	75
Lifeway								
Lassi Mango	8 oz	160	11	2	10	25	3	125
Lassi Strawberry	8 oz	160	11	2	10	25	3	125
Promise								
Activ All Flavors	1 bottle (3.5 oz)	70	1	4	0	9	tr	20
Yo On The Go								
All Flavors	1 box (8 oz)	180	6	3	0	31	0	80
Yo-Goat								
All Flavors	8 oz	160	7	8	30	11	0	115
Plain	8 oz	150	9	9	30	11	0	115
Yoplait								
Kids All Flavors	1 bottle (3.1 oz)	70	2	2	5	11	–	40

YOGURT FROZEN

FOOD	PORTION	CALS	PROT	FAT	CHOL	CARB	FIBER	SOD
chocolate soft serve	1 cup	230	6	9	7	36	3	141
vanilla soft serve	1 cup	236	6	8	3	35	0	125
Dippin' Dots								
Strawberry Cheesecake	½ cup	100	4	0	0	21	1	80
Haagen-Dazs								
Lowfat Coffee	½ cup (3.7 oz)	200	8	5	65	31	0	50
Lowfat Tart Natural	½ cup (3.6 oz)	180	9	3	45	30	0	45
Lowfat Vanilla	½ cup (3.7 oz)	200	9	5	65	31	0	55
Lowfat Wildberry	½ cup (3.7 oz)	180	7	2	35	34	0	40

FOOD	PORTION	CALS	PROT	FAT	CHOL	CARB	FIBER	SOD
Julie's								
Organic Blackberry	½ cup	190	3	12	70	20	1	45
Organic Peanut Butter Fudge	½ cup	260	4	17	70	24	tr	125
Organic Strawberry	½ cup	200	3	12	70	22	0	50
Organic Vanilla	½ cup	220	4	15	85	20	0	55
Stonyfield Farm								
Fat Free After Dark Chocolate	1 serv (4 oz)	100	4	0	<5	21	1	55
Fat Free Gotta Have Vanilla	1 serv (4 oz)	100	4	0	<5	20	0	65
Fat Free Vanilla Fudge Swirl	1 serv (4 oz)	120	4	0	<5	25	0	65
Low Fat Creme Caramel	1 serv (4 oz)	130	4	2	5	26	0	95
Lowfat Cookies 'N Cream	1 serv (4 oz)	130	4	2	<5	25	0	110
Turkey Hill								
Fudge Ripple	½ cup	100	3	0	0	21	0	65
Neapolitan	½ cup	90	3	0	0	19	1	55
Smoothie Orange Cream Swirl	½ cup	100	2	0	0	22	0	40
Smoothie Peach Mango	½ cup	90	2	0	0	21	0	50
Vanilla Bean	½ cup	100	3	0	0	19	0	60
YOUNGBERRY JUICE								
Ceres								
100% Juice	8 oz	120	0	0	0	30	0	10
ZUCCHINI								
baby raw	1 (0.5 oz)	3	tr	tr	0	1	tr	0
canned italian style	1 cup	66	2	tr	0	16	–	849
fresh	1 sm (4.1 oz)	19	1	tr	0	4	1	12
pickled	¼ cup	16	tr	tr	0	4	1	71
raw sliced	1 cup	19	1	tr	0	4	1	11
sliced cooked w/o salt	1 cup	29	1	tr	0	7	3	5
C&W								
Yellow & Green	⅔ cup	20	1	0	0	3	tr	5
TAKE-OUT								
breaded & fried	6 slices (3 oz)	141	2	11	2	10	1	105
indian pakora	1 serv	46	2	2	1	7	2	141
sticks breaded & fried	6 (2 oz)	90	1	7	2	6	1	67

PART TWO

Restaurant Chains

YOU SHOULD KNOW

Bigger Isn't Always Better

Supersizing, add-ons, toppings, extras, stuffed, doubles, and "buy one get one free," may cost little, but the extra calories, fat, cholesterol, sugar, and sodium you'll be tempted to eat are no bargain.

FOOD	PORTION	CALS	PROT	FAT	CHOL	CARB	FIBER	SOD
A&W								
BEVERAGES								
Coke	1 sm (11 oz)	145	0	0	0	37	0	23
Diet Coke	1 sm (11 oz)	0	0	0	0	0	0	25
Diet Root Beer	1 sm (15 oz)	0	0	0	0	0	0	40
Float Diet Root Beer	1 sm (14 oz)	170	2	5	40	30	0	100
Float Root Beer	1 sm (14 oz)	330	2	5	40	70	0	100
Milkshake Chocolate	1 med	700	11	29	125	100	2	200
Milkshake Strawberry	1 med	670	11	29	115	90	0	180
Milkshake Vanilla	1 med	720	12	31	135	97	0	210
Root Beer	1 sm (15 oz)	220	0	0	0	57	0	40
DESSERTS								
Cone Vanilla	1 med	260	1	7	25	41	1	145
Freeze A&W Root Beer	1 med	480	25	10	40	89	0	230
Polar Swirl M&M	1 med	710	15	25	55	107	2	290
Polar Swirl Oreo	1 med	690	14	24	50	107	3	570
Polar Swirl Reese's	1 med	740	18	31	55	97	3	380
Sundae Caramel	1 med	340	8	9	35	57	0	250
Sundae Chocolate	1 med	320	8	8	30	53	0	180
Sundae Hot Fudge	1 med	350	8	11	30	54	4	140
Sundae Strawberry	1 med	300	7	8	30	47	0	140
Sundae Vanilla	1 med	310	7	8	30	52	0	140
MAIN MENU SELECTIONS								
Cheese Curds	1 serv	570	27	40	105	27	2	1220
Cheese Dog	1	320	11	20	40	25	1	910
Cheeseburger Original Bacon	1	570	27	33	90	41	2	1200
Cheeseburger Original Bacon Double	1	800	45	48	165	47	2	1600
Cheeseburger Original Double	1	720	41	42	150	46	2	1370
Chicken Strips	3	500	28	29	55	32	7	1050
Chili Bowl	1 serv	190	12	6	20	22	5	640
Coney Chili Dog	1	310	13	18	40	24	2	870
Coney Chili Dog Cheese	1	350	13	21	45	27	2	1070
Fries	1 lg	430	5	18	0	61	6	640
Fries Cheese	1 serv	380	4	19	5	50	4	870
Fries Chili	1 serv	370	8	16	10	49	5	780
Fries Chili & Cheese	1 serv	400	8	19	10	51	5	990
Hot Dog Plain	1	280	11	17	35	22	1	710

FOOD	PORTION	CALS	PROT	FAT	CHOL	CARB	FIBER	SOD
Onion Rings	1 serv	350	5	18	0	45	2	710
Papa Burger	1	720	41	42	145	46	2	1390
Sandwich Crispy Chicken	1	590	31	29	65	54	3	1170
Sandwich Grilled Chicken	1	440	31	19	90	54	2	860
SAUCES								
Dipping Sauce BBQ	1 serv (1 oz)	40	0	0	0	10	0	230
Dipping Sauce Honey Mustard	1 serv (1 oz)	100	0	6	0	12	0	170
Dipping Sauce Ranch	1 serv (1 oz)	160	0	17	15	2	0	240
Dipping Sauce Sweet & Sour	1 serv (1 oz)	45	0	0	0	12	0	120

AU BON PAIN

FOOD	PORTION	CALS	PROT	FAT	CHOL	CARB	FIBER	SOD
BAKED SELECTIONS								
Bagel Asiago Cheese	1	360	15	4	10	64	3	590
Bagel Cinnamon Raisin	1	320	11	1	0	67	3	440
Bagel Everything	1	350	13	5	0	64	3	990
Bagel Honey 9 Grain	1	330	13	2	0	68	6	540
Bagel Jalapeno Double Cheddar	1	350	17	10	30	55	2	650
Bagel Onion Dill	1	350	13	1	0	72	4	530
Bagel Plain	1	290	11	1	0	59	2	440
Bagel Poppy Seed	1	290	11	1	0	59	2	440
Bagel Sesame Seed	1	330	12	5	0	61	3	440
Baguette Artisan Honey Multigrain Salad Size	1 (3.5 oz)	240	8	3	0	47	4	460
Baguette Artisan Honey Multigrain Sandwich Size	1 (4.7 oz)	310	10	3	0	62	6	610
Baguette Artisan Salad Size	1 (3.5 oz)	210	7	1	0	44	2	460
Baguette Artisan Sandwich Size	1 (4.7 oz)	290	10	1	0	59	2	610
Blondie	1	330	7	19	35	61	3	350
Bread Artisan Multigrain	1 serv (4 oz)	260	9	3	0	51	4	610
Bread Artisan Sundried Tomato	1 serv (4 oz)	240	8	1	0	49	2	570
Bread Cheese	1 serv (4.8 oz)	290	14	8	2	55	3	730
Bread Country White	1 serv (4 oz)	240	6	1	0	50	2	590
Bread Bowl	1 (9.24 oz)	640	28	3	0	127	6	1830

FOOD	PORTION	CALS	PROT	FAT	CHOL	CARB	FIBER	SOD
Bread Stick Rosemary Garlic	1 (2.3 oz)	200	6	5	0	33	2	1430
Brownie Chocolate Chip	1	380	5	17	75	62	1	390
Brownie Hazelnut Mocha	1	430	6	21	65	58	3	360
Brownie Rocky Road	1	410	6	17	70	62	2	430
Ciabatta	1 sm	180	7	1	0	37	2	380
Cinnamon Roll	1	350	7	12	40	53	2	240
Cookie Chocolate Chip	1 (2 oz)	260	2	12	25	37	1	220
Cookie Confetti	1 (2.4 oz)	310	3	14	25	42	1	290
Cookie English Toffee	1 (2 oz)	210	2	11	20	26	1	240
Cookie Gingerbread	1 (2.7 oz)	300	4	9	10	50	1	140
Cookie Hazelnut Fudge	1 (2.25 oz)	290	4	16	40	34	3	150
Cookie Oatmeal Raisin	1 (2 oz)	230	3	8	35	36	2	190
Cookie Shortbread	1 (2.3 oz)	310	3	9	25	34	1	270
Creme De Fleur	1 serv	550	12	26	110	71	1	540
Croissant Almond	1	560	12	36	110	52	4	270
Croissant Apple	1	230	4	10	25	31	2	230
Croissant Chocolate	1	330	6	17	30	42	3	180
Croissant Plain	1 (2.8 oz)	260	5	15	55	28	1	190
Croissant Raspberry Cheese	1	330	7	16	60	41	1	280
Croissant Sweet Cheese	1	320	4	16	60	39	1	280
Danish Cherry	1	370	7	19	85	44	1	290
Danish Sweet Cheese	1	380	7	20	90	44	1	300
Focaccia	1 piece (4.4 oz)	310	11	4	0	57	3	640
Lahvash	1 (4 oz)	320	15	1	0	62	2	190
Macaroon Chocolate Dipped Cranberry Almond	1	320	4	16	0	42	3	190
Mini Loaf Bacon & Cheese	1 (4.8 oz)	540	13	31	95	50	1	790
Muffin Blueberry	1	510	9	19	20	76	5	550
Muffin Carrot Walnut	1	520	8	25	55	66	4	800
Muffin Corn	1	460	9	16	60	69	2	550
Muffin Cranberry Walnut	1	500	10	24	20	61	5	460
Muffin Double Chocolate Chunk	1	590	10	20	25	83	5	480
Muffin Pumpkin	1	490	9	17	65	75	2	520
Muffin Raisin Bran	1	410	10	9	30	74	9	590
Muffin Low Fat Triple Berry	1	290	5	2	25	61	2	310
Pastry Hazelnut Creme	1	540	10	34	85	50	3	380

FOOD	PORTION	CALS	PROT	FAT	CHOL	CARB	FIBER	SOD
Poundcake Cappuccino	1 slice (5.2 oz)	530	3	26	85	68	1	490
Poundcake Chocolate	1 slice (4.7 oz)	500	7	29	100	58	3	580
Poundcake Lemon	1 slice (4.9 oz)	520	5	27	85	64	0	460
Poundcake Marble	1 slice (4.7 oz)	490	6	27	90	59	1	520
Roll Pecan	1	630	10	32	30	80	3	330
Roll Soft	1 (4.7 oz)	410	11	11	20	65	3	700
Scone Cinnamon	1	430	9	24	130	48	1	360
Scone Orange	1	410	9	20	130	51	2	370
Shortbread Chocolate Dipped	1	350	3	20	25	38	1	280
Toasts Basil Pesto Cheese	3 pieces (2 oz)	140	5	2	0	26	1	330
Tulip Blueberry	1	370	4	20	65	44	1	300
Tulip Chocolate Raspberry	1	430	5	21	70	55	1	410
Tulip Key Lime	1	440	5	22	70	55	1	360
BEVERAGES								
Blast Caramel	1 med (16 oz)	540	6	17	60	104	0	105
Blast Coffee	1 med (16 oz)	440	8	21	75	71	0	115
Blast Mocha	1 med (16 oz)	440	7	17	60	80	2	95
Blast Vanilla	1 med (12 oz)	540	6	17	60	104	0	100
Caffe Americano	1 sm (12 oz)	5	0	0	0	1	0	15
Cappuccino	1 sm (12 oz)	120	6	7	20	10	0	85
Caramel Macchiato	1 sm (12 oz)	350	10	10	30	53	0	160
Chocolate Milk	1 (12 oz)	320	10	9	25	54	3	100
Hot Chocolate	1 sm (12 oz)	350	12	11	30	58	3	125
Iced Caramel Macchiato	1 sm (12 oz)	290	7	7	25	49	0	125
Iced Tea Peach	1 med (22 oz)	120	0	0	0	30	0	35
Latte Caffe	1 sm (12 oz)	200	11	11	45	17	0	170
Latte Chai	1 sm (12 oz)	290	11	11	30	38	0	130
Latte Iced Caffe	1 sm (12 oz)	110	6	6	20	19	0	80
Latte Iced Chai	1 sm (12 oz)	190	5	5	15	31	0	65

FOOD	PORTION	CALS	PROT	FAT	CHOL	CARB	FIBER	SOD
Latte Iced Mocha	1 sm (12 oz)	210	6	11	35	27	1	70
Latte Iced Vanilla	1 sm (12 oz)	240	5	5	15	44	0	65
Latte Iced White Chocolate	1 sm (12 oz)	250	5	11	35	35	0	135
Latte Mocha	1 sm (12 oz)	300	11	16	60	35	1	160
Latte Vanilla	1 sm (12 oz)	320	9	9	30	50	0	120
Latte White Chocolate	1 sm (12 oz)	310	9	14	45	41	0	180
Lemonade	1 med (22 oz)	300	0	0	0	72	0	0
Orange Juice	1 (8 oz)	110	2	0	0	26	1	0
Smoothie Peach	1 med (16 oz)	310	4	1	10	69	4	115
Smoothie Strawberry	1 med (16 oz)	310	4	1	10	66	3	110
MAIN MENU SELECTIONS								
Fruit Cup	1 sm (6 oz)	70	1	0	0	16	1	10
Harvest Rice Bowl Cajun Shrimp	1 (20 oz)	520	16	17	145	69	2	1660
Harvest Rice Bowl Cajun Shrimp w/ Brown Rice	1 (20 oz)	560	14	20	145	73	5	1660
Harvest Rice Bowl Mayan Chicken	1 (19.25 oz)	490	25	14	70	67	4	1430
Harvest Rice Bowl Mayan Chicken w/ Brown Rice	1 (19.25 oz)	540	23	16	70	71	7	1430
Harvest Rice Bowl Steak Teriyaki	1 (19.25 oz)	530	30	15	60	72	2	1520
Harvest Rice Bowl Steak Teriyaki w/ Brown Rice	1 (19.25 oz)	570	28	18	60	76	5	1520
Macaroni & Cheese	1 med (12 oz)	440	19	26	95	31	2	1280
Stew Beef	1 med (12 oz)	300	18	16	55	25	3	1070
Stew Chicken Vegetable	1 med (12 oz)	290	11	17	40	26	3	930
SALAD DRESSINGS AND SPREADS								
Artichoke Aioli	1 serv (1 oz)	130	1	14	10	1	0	180
Basil Pesto	1 serv (1 oz)	140	2	15	5	1	0	160
Chili Dijon	1 serv (1 oz)	120	1	12	10	3	1	130
Cream Cheese Honey Pecan	1 serv (2 oz)	120	4	10	35	5	0	340

FOOD	PORTION	CALS	PROT	FAT	CHOL	CARB	FIBER	SOD
Cream Cheese Honey Walnut	1 serv (2 oz)	140	3	9	30	12	0	150
Cream Cheese Lite	1 serv (2 oz)	120	4	9	30	5	0	280
Cream Cheese Plain	1 serv (2 oz)	170	3	16	50	4	0	290
Cream Cheese Strawberry	1 serv (2 oz)	180	3	15	45	9	0	250
Cream Cheese Sundried Tomato	1 serv (2 oz)	120	4	10	35	5	0	340
Cream Cheese Vegetable	1 serv (2 oz)	170	3	16	45	3	0	270
Dressing Balsamic Vinaigrette	1 serv (2.25 oz)	190	9	16	0	11	0	430
Dressing Blue Cheese	1 serv (1.75 oz)	230	2	24	20	2	0	550
Dressing Caesar	1 serv (2 oz)	280	2	28	20	4	0	400
Dressing Fat Free Raspberry Vinaigrette	1 serv (2.25 oz)	70	0	0	0	17	0	150
Dressing Light Honey Mustard	1 serv (2.25 oz)	180	1	11	10	21	1	590
Dressing Light Olive Oil Vinaigrette	1 serv (2.25 oz)	130	0	10	0	9	0	630
Dressing Light Ranch	1 serv (2.25 oz)	150	2	15	15	3	0	470
Dressing Thai Peanut	1 serv (2.25 oz)	230	5	13	0	24	1	840
Guacamole	1 serv (1 oz)	60	1	6	0	2	2	125
Honey Mustard	1 serv (2.5 oz)	210	1	13	15	23	1	650
Hummus Roasted Red Pepper	1 serv (2 oz)	80	2	5	0	6	2	250
Mayonnaise	1 serv (1 oz)	200	0	22	20	0	0	150
Mayonnaise Herb	1 serv (1 oz)	210	0	23	20	1	0	210
Mayonnaise Jalapeno	1 serv (1 oz)	140	2	15	15	0	0	260
Mayonnaise Tarragon Sauce	1 serv (2 oz)	420	0	45	40	2	0	420
Mustard	1 tsp	0	0	0	0	0	0	70
Spread Herb Bagel	1 serv (2 oz)	130	4	11	35	5	0	470
Spread Sundried Tomato	1 serv (0.53 oz)	70	1	6	0	4	0	85
SALADS								
Caesar Asiago	1 serv	210	11	12	25	18	3	470

FOOD	PORTION	CALS	PROT	FAT	CHOL	CARB	FIBER	SOD
Caesar Asiago Grilled Chicken	1 (8.5 oz)	340	29	13	65	19	3	680
Caesar Asiago Side	1 (3.2 oz)	120	6	6	15	12	2	260
Chef's	1 serv	230	22	14	60	7	3	1090
Garden	1 (7 oz)	80	4	2	0	14	4	210
Garden Side	1 (3.6 oz)	50	2	1	0	10	3	70
Mediterranean Chicken	1 (9.75 oz)	330	24	16	60	12	2	1170
Riviera	1 (9.5 oz)	260	7	7	15	46	5	250
Thai Peanut Chicken	1 (11 oz)	250	22	8	40	22	4	290
Tuna Garden	1 (10.5 oz)	350	21	25	55	14	4	470
Turkey Medallion Cobb	1 (11 oz)	340	27	19	260	15	3	980
Turkey Spinach Sonoma	1 (12.3 oz)	310	29	13	65	22	5	1310
SANDWICHES								
Arizona Chicken	1 (12 oz)	750	49	29	120	61	4	1480
Baguette Turkey & Swiss	1 (12.3 oz)	770	41	38	95	65	3	2120
Baja Turkey	1 (13 oz)	700	41	32	90	61	4	1970
Breakfast Asiago Bagel Prosciutto & Egg	1 (9.6 oz)	660	40	25	185	67	3	1580
Breakfast Asiago Bagel Sausage Egg & Cheddar	1 (10.2 oz)	770	36	45	215	55	0	1450
Breakfast Bagel & Bacon	1 (4.2 oz)	340	15	6	15	56	0	630
Breakfast Egg On A Bagel	1 (6.8 oz)	370	21	4	115	62	2	790
Breakfast Egg On A Bagel w/ Bacon	1 (7.2 oz)	410	25	8	130	58	0	980
Breakfast Egg On A Bagel w/ Bacon Cheese	1 (7.9 oz)	500	30	15	150	59	0	1120
Breakfast Egg On A Bagel w/ Cheese	1 (7.6 oz)	450	26	10	135	62	2	920
Breakfast Onion Dill Bagel Smoked Salmon & Wasabi	1 (7.1 oz)	490	18	11	45	77	3	1250
Caprese	1 (11.8 oz)	700	28	35	65	65	4	1120
Chicken Mozzarella	1 (14.5 oz)	800	50	27	105	71	2	1360
Chicken Pesto	1 (12.5 oz)	700	44	23	80	62	2	1340
Chicken Tarragon	1 (11 oz)	720	40	29	85	61	1	1190
Ciabatta Bacon & Egg Melt	1 (7 oz)	400	26	15	155	40	2	1160
Ciabatta Ham & Cheddar	1 (12 oz)	650	40	20	95	80	4	2330
Club Smoked Turkey	1 (11.6 oz)	780	43	43	115	56	2	2330
Croissant Ham & Cheese	1 (4.2 oz)	350	14	18	60	34	1	550
Croissant Spinach & Cheese	1	250	8	14	35	25	2	280

FOOD	PORTION	CALS	PROT	FAT	CHOL	CARB	FIBER	SOD
Hot BBQ Chicken On Farmhouse Roll	1 (14.3 oz)	970	50	44	130	78	4	1630
Hot Eggplant & Mozzarella	1 (12.4 oz)	710	26	37	60	68	6	1440
Hot Steakhouse On Ciabatta	1 (13 oz)	800	43	41	100	70	4	1850
Melt Tuna	1 (12.5 oz)	760	40	41	100	60	4	1240
Melt Turkey	1 (12.2 oz)	890	45	47	120	70	3	2360
Portobello & Goat Cheese	1 (10 oz)	610	18	33	35	61	6	1290
Portobello Egg & Cheddar	1 (8.5 oz)	590	22	37	200	42	3	1050
Prosciutto Mozzarella	1 (12.7 oz)	880	40	49	110	71	4	2270
Spicy Tuna	1 (10.3 oz)	640	28	34	65	57	6	1100
The Montana	1 (12.5 oz)	560	40	23	105	62	4	1370
Turkey & Cranberry Chutney	1 (10.9 oz)	680	30	24	60	63	3	1970
Wrap Chicken Caesar Asiago	1	700	42	25	75	69	3	930
Wrap Chopped Turkey Club	1 (12 oz)	660	35	27	165	70	4	1200
Wrap Hot Cajun Shrimp	1 (14.9 oz)	700	20	24	90	95	4	1680
Wrap Hot Mayan Chicken	1 (13.5 oz)	630	24	19	40	92	5	1400
Wrap Hot Steak Teriyaki	1 (13.5 oz)	660	28	19	40	93	5	1780
Wrap Mediterranean	1 (12.8 oz)	670	24	28	20	80	7	1240
Wrap Southwest Tuna	1 (14 oz)	900	46	51	110	72	5	980
Wrap Thai Peanut Chicken	1 (14.5 oz)	660	38	19	40	84	4	770
Wrap Turkey Spinach Sonoma	1 (12 oz)	630	35	19	45	80	5	1070
SOUPS								
Baked Stuffed Potato	1 med (12 oz)	350	9	21	60	30	2	990
Broccoli Cheddar	1 med (12 oz)	310	11	21	50	20	2	1000
Carrot Ginger	1 med (12 oz)	130	7	5	0	21	3	920
Chicken Florentine	1 med (12 oz)	240	8	13	35	25	1	1030
Chicken & Dumplings	1 med (12 oz)	210	11	7	50	28	2	1280
Chicken Noodle	1 med (12 oz)	130	9	3	15	20	2	1000
Clam Chowder	1 med (12 oz)	320	9	18	55	27	1	1020

FOOD	PORTION	CALS	PROT	FAT	CHOL	CARB	FIBER	SOD
Corn & Green Chili Bisque	1 med (12 oz)	250	5	14	35	29	3	1540
Corn Chowder	1 med (12 oz)	350	9	18	50	40	3	1120
Curried Rice & Lentil	1 med (12 oz)	150	9	2	0	30	8	1260
French Moroccan Tomato Lentil	1 med (12 oz)	180	10	2	0	32	8	1050
French Onion	1 med (12 oz)	130	4	5	10	19	2	1310
Garden Vegetable	1 med (12 oz)	80	3	2	0	14	3	1010
Harvest Pumpkin	1 med (12 oz)	190	8	10	25	26	2	1110
Hearty Cabbage	1 med (12 oz)	110	4	5	10	14	3	910
Italian Wedding	1 med (12 oz)	170	8	7	15	10	2	1300
Jamaican Black Bean	1 med (12 oz)	180	16	1	0	45	25	460
Mediterranean Pepper	1 med (12 oz)	100	5	3	0	18	5	580
Old Fashioned Tomato Rice	1 med (12 oz)	120	4	1	0	24	3	340
Pasta E Fagioli	1 med (12 oz)	240	11	8	5	36	9	930
Portuguese Kale	1 med (12 oz)	120	5	5	5	15	3	1130
Potato Cheese	1 med (12 oz)	250	7	14	50	25	2	1340
Potato Leek	1 med (12 oz)	300	5	20	60	28	2	1000
Red Beans Italian Sausage & Rice	1 med (12 oz)	200	15	5	10	28	16	1140
Southern Black Eyed Pea	1 med (12 oz)	180	12	2	5	31	12	950
Southwest Tortilla	1 med (12 oz)	200	4	11	10	24	4	1290
Southwest Vegetable	1 med (12 oz)	160	4	3	0	17	3	370

FOOD	PORTION	CALS	PROT	FAT	CHOL	CARB	FIBER	SOD
Split Pea	1 med (12 oz)	210	18	2	5	42	15	1190
Thai Coconut Curry	1 med (12 oz)	150	3	7	0	20	2	1150
Tomato Basil Bisque	1 med (12 oz)	210	6	8	25	29	5	490
Tomato Cheddar	1 med (12 oz)	240	12	15	25	17	2	1040
Tomato Florentine	1 med (12 oz)	120	5	3	5	19	2	1390
Tuscan Vegetable	1 med (12 oz)	170	7	5	10	24	3	1170
Vegetable Beef Barley	1 med (12 oz)	140	9	3	20	21	4	1000
Vegetarian Chili	1 med (12 oz)	230	12	3	0	40	11	1000
Vegetarian Lentil	1 med (12 oz)	140	10	2	0	32	11	1260
Vegetarian Minestrone	1 med (12 oz)	120	5	2	0	21	4	1120
Wild Mushroom Bisque	1 med (12 oz)	190	5	9	10	23	2	1010
YOGURT								
Blueberry w/ Fruit	1 sm (7.5 oz)	220	6	2	10	44	0	120
Blueberry w/ Granola & Fruit	1 sm (8.5 oz)	310	10	6	10	56	2	130
Strawberry w/ Blueberries	1 sm (7.5 oz)	220	6	2	10	44	0	120
Strawberry w/ Granola & Blueberries	1 sm (8.5 oz)	310	10	6	10	56	2	130
Vanilla w/ Blueberries	1 sm (7.5 oz)	190	10	2	10	32	0	160
Vanilla w/ Granola & Blueberries	1 sm (8.5 oz)	310	10	6	10	56	2	130

AUNTIE ANNE'S

FOOD	PORTION	CALS	PROT	FAT	CHOL	CARB	FIBER	SOD
BEVERAGES								
Dutch Ice Blue Raspberry	1 (14 oz)	165	0	0	0	38	0	20
Dutch Ice Grape	1 (14 oz)	180	0	0	0	43	0	20

FOOD	PORTION	CALS	PROT	FAT	CHOL	CARB	FIBER	SOD
Dutch Ice Kiwi Banana	1 (14 oz)	190	0	0	0	44	0	30
Dutch Ice Lemonade	1 (14 oz)	315	0	0	0	77	0	0
Dutch Ice Lemonade Strawberry	1 (14 oz)	330	0	0	0	81	0	0
Dutch Ice Mocha	1 (14 oz)	400	0	10	0	74	0	100
Dutch Ice Orange Creme	1 (14 oz)	280	0	0	0	64	0	35
Dutch Ice Pina Colada	1 (14 oz)	220	0	0	0	53	0	15
Dutch Ice Strawberry	1 (14 oz)	220	0	0	0	50	0	40
Dutch Ice Watermelon	1 (14 oz)	200	0	0	0	50	0	35
Dutch Ice Wild Cherry	1 (14 oz)	210	0	0	0	48	0	25
Dutch Latte Caramel	1 (14 oz)	350	4	15	55	49	0	55
Dutch Latte Coffee	1 (14 oz)	290	4	14	50	38	0	135
Dutch Latte Mocha	1 (14 oz)	160	5	17	55	47	0	135
Dutch Shake Chocolate	1 (14 oz)	580	10	27	105	75	0	380
Dutch Shake Coffee	1 (14 oz)	590	10	27	105	77	0	304
Dutch Shake Strawberry	1 (14 oz)	610	10	27	105	78	0	304
Dutch Shake Vanilla	1 (14 oz)	510	10	27	105	58	0	300
Dutch Smoothie Blue Raspberry	1 (14 oz)	230	3	8	30	34	0	100
Dutch Smoothie Grape	1 (14 oz)	230	3	8	30	36	0	100
Dutch Smoothie Kiwi Banana	1 (14 oz)	240	3	8	30	38	0	100
Dutch Smoothie Lemonade	1 (14 oz)	300	3	8	30	53	0	80
Dutch Smoothie Mocha	1 (14 oz)	330	3	13	30	50	0	130
Dutch Smoothie Orange Creme	1 (14 oz)	280	3	8	30	46	0	100
Dutch Smoothie Pina Colada	1 (14 oz)	260	3	8	30	44	0	90
Dutch Smoothie Strawberry	1 (14 oz)	250	3	8	30	40	0	100
Dutch Smoothie Wild Cherry	1 (14 oz)	250	3	8	30	41	0	90
Lemonade	1 (22 oz)	180	0	0	0	43	0	0
Lemonade Strawberry	1 (22 oz)	190	0	0	0	48	0	0
DIPPING SAUCES								
Caramel Dip	1 serv (1.5 oz)	135	1	3	5	27	0	110
Cheese Sauce	1 serv (1.25 oz)	100	3	8	10	4	0	510

FOOD	PORTION	CALS	PROT	FAT	CHOL	CARB	FIBER	SOD
Cream Cheese Light	1 serv (1.25 oz)	70	3	6	25	1	0	140
Hot Salsa Cheese	1 serv (1.25 oz)	100	2	8	10	4	0	550
Marinara Sauce	1 serv (1.25 oz)	10	0	0	0	4	0	180
Sweet	1 serv (1.4 oz)	40	0	0	0	10	0	0
Sweet Mustard	1 serv (1.25 oz)	60	tr	2	40	8	0	120
PRETZELS								
Almond	1	400	9	8	20	72	2	400
Almond w/o Butter	1	350	9	2	0	72	2	390
Cinnamon Raisin w/o Butter	1	350	9	2	0	74	2	410
Cinnamon Sugar	1	450	8	9	25	83	3	430
Garlic	1	350	9	5	10	68	2	850
Garlic w/o Butter	1	320	9	1	0	66	2	830
Glazin' Raisin	1	510	11	4	10	107	4	480
Glazin' Raisin w/o Butter	1	470	11	1	0	104	3	460
Jalapeno	1	310	8	5	10	59	2	940
Jalapeno w/o Butter	1	270	8	1	0	58	2	780
Original	1	370	10	4	10	72	3	930
Original w/o Butter	1	340	10	1	0	72	3	900
Pretzel Dog	1	290	10	16	40	25	1	600
Sesame	1	410	12	12	15	64	7	860
Sesame w/o Butter	1	350	11	6	0	63	3	840
Sour Cream & Onion	1	340	9	5	10	66	2	930
Sour Cream & Onion w/o Butter	1	310	9	1	0	66	2	920
Stix	6	370	10	4	10	72	3	930
Stix w/o Butter	6	340	10	1	0	72	3	900
Whole Wheat	1	370	11	5	10	72	7	1120
Whole Wheat w/o Butter	1	350	11	2	0	72	7	1100
BAHAMA BREEZE								
BEVERAGES								
Beer Light	1 serv (12 oz)	103	–	0	0	6	–	14

FOOD	PORTION	CALS	PROT	FAT	CHOL	CARB	FIBER	SOD
Beer Regular	1 serv (12 oz)	153	–	0	0	13	–	14
Berries In Paradise	1 serv	110	–	0	0	24	–	15
Captain Berry Island	1 serv	110	–	0	0	24	–	15
Island Refresher	1 serv	370	–	7	–	73	–	30
Lemon Breeze	1 serv	410	–	0	0	103	–	0
Mango Beach	1 serv	300	–	8	–	56	–	20
Mango Mango Man	1 serv	300	–	8	–	56	–	20
Raspberry Surfer	1 serv	210	–	0	0	52	–	10
Shake Banana	1 serv	590	–	30	–	69	–	115
Shake Chocolate	1 serv	700	–	32	–	92	–	170
Shake Chocolate Banana	1 serv	760	–	31	–	108	–	70
Shake Mango	1 serv	450	–	25	–	47	–	115
Shake Raspberry	1 serv	560	–	29	–	64	–	170
Shake Strawberry	1 serv	530	–	32	–	50	–	190
Shake Strawberry Banana	1 serv	600	–	28	–	77	–	130
Shake Vanilla	1 serv	560	–	30	–	62	–	200
Slushies Kiwi	1 serv	120	–	0	0	29	–	30
Slushies Mango	1 serv	180	–	0	0	45	–	5
Slushies Strawberry	1 serv	240	–	0	0	58	–	40
Strawberry Beach	1 serv	370	–	7	–	74	–	30
Virgin Bahama Rita	1 serv	160	–	0	0	39	–	0
Virgin Ultimate Pina Colada	1 serv	340	–	9	–	65	–	20
Wine	1 serv (5 oz)	122	–	0	0	4	–	7
CHILDREN'S MENU SELECTIONS								
Bowtie Mac N' Cheese	1 serv	790	–	46	–	74	–	1100
Cheese Pizza	1 sm	750	–	23	–	101	–	1620
Crispy Chicken	1 serv	420	–	24	–	23	–	1580
French Fries	1 serv	265	–	13	–	34	–	470
Fresh Fruit Salad	1 serv	40	–	0	0	10	–	0
DESSERTS								
Bananas Supreme	1 serv	940	–	45	–	122	–	560
Chocolate Island	1 serv	1380	–	83	–	142	–	440
Dulce De Leche Cheesecake	1 serv	940	–	56	–	94	–	710
Rebecca's Key Lime Pie	1 serv	990	–	34	–	154	–	630
Warm Chocolate Pineapple Upside Down Cake	1 serv	1140	–	58	–	144	–	940

FOOD	PORTION	CALS	PROT	FAT	CHOL	CARB	FIBER	SOD
MAIN MENU SELECTIONS								
Bahamian Grilled Chicken Kabobs w/ Yellow Rice	1 serv	770	–	11	–	98	–	2480
Breeze Wood Grilled Chicken Breast w/ Citrus Butter Sauce	1 serv	680	–	39	–	18	–	2130
Breeze Wood Grilled Chicken Breast w/ Citrus Butter Sauce Lighter Portion	1 serv	390	–	23	–	11	–	1230
Broccoli	1 serv	120	–	9	–	6	–	125
Burger Wood Grilled Angus	1 serv	680	–	39	–	39	–	830
Chicken Santiago	1 serv	1180	–	58	–	85	–	4560
Chicken Santiago Lighter Portion	1 serv	1020	–	55	–	85	–	3680
Cinnamon Mashed Sweet Potatoes	1 serv	260	–	9	–	44	–	430
Coconut Shrimp Dinner	1 serv	794	–	50	–	60	–	347
Crab Claws St. Thomas	1 serv	710	–	64	–	13	–	1180
Crab Shrimp & Avocado Stack w/ Honey Red Pepper Drizzle	1 serv	250	–	6	–	20	–	840
Creole Baked Goat Cheese	1 serv	380	–	33	–	0	–	620
Crispy Yuca	1 serv	620	–	36	–	73	–	570
Filet Mignon w/ Onion Rings	1 serv	450	–	23	–	10	–	400
Fire Roasted Jerk Shrimp	1 serv	260	–	14	–	2	–	870
French Fries	1 serv	530	–	26	–	67	–	940
Garlic Mashed Potatoes	1 serv	290	–	20	–	24	–	780
Herb Cheese Toast	1 slice	120	–	5	–	15	–	180
Island Flatbread Grilled Chicken	1	515	–	22	–	43	–	1445
Island Flatbread Shrimp	1	480	–	20	–	43	–	1280
Island Flatbread Vine Ripened Tomato	1	430	–	20	–	43	–	1040
Island Onion Rings	1 serv	1910	–	116	–	186	–	2140
Jamaican Grilled Chicken Breast	1 serv	310	–	4	–	2	–	1900
Jamaican Grilled Chicken Breast Lighter Portion	1 serv	160	–	2	–	1	–	940

FOOD	PORTION	CALS	PROT	FAT	CHOL	CARB	FIBER	SOD
Linguine Calypso Shrimp Lighter Portion	1 serv	790	–	43	–	58	–	2430
Margarita Chicken w/ Roasted Corn Salsa	1 serv	470	–	6	–	30	–	1240
Margarita Chicken w/ Roasted Corn Salsa Lighter Portion	1 serv	310	–	5	–	24	–	790
Pasta Jerk Chicken	1 serv	1430	–	87	–	107	–	1500
Pasta Jerk Chicken Lighter Portion	1 serv	780	–	39	–	72	–	860
Pasta Lobster & Shrimp	1 serv	1080	–	42	–	82	–	2830
Pasta Pan-Seared Salmon	1 serv	1550	–	99	–	96	–	1860
Pasta Pan-Seared Salmon Lighter Portion	1 serv	910	–	55	–	68	–	1020
Plantains	1 serv	270	–	6	–	53	–	0
Quesadilla Fresh Vegetable	1	435	–	48	–	70	–	1910
Quesadilla Fresh Vegetable & Chicken	1	480	–	24	–	11	–	1490
Roasted Cuban Bread	1 serv	590	–	23	–	77	–	1030
Sandwich Cuban	1	1130	–	59	–	69	–	2450
Sandwich Oak Grilled Chicken	1	530	–	19	–	45	–	1330
Sandwich Sun Drenched Portobello & Veg	1	670	–	22	–	90	–	1170
Seafood Paella	1 serv	800	–	23	–	54	–	2910
Smothered Pork Tenderloin w/ Lemon Butter	1 serv	900	–	59	–	9	–	1970
Spinach Dip w/ Island Chips	1 serv	680	–	60	–	17	–	1180
Tacos Key West Fish	1 serv	550	–	26	–	30	–	1130
Tostones w/ Chicken	1 serv	1250	–	63	–	121	–	2400
West Indies Patties	1 serv	1150	–	68	–	102	–	1620
West Indies Ribs	1 serv	810	–	55	–	7	–	570
Wings Habanero	1 serv	920	–	53	–	11	–	2800
Wings Jamaican Grilled	1 serv	960	–	60	–	2	–	2570
Wood Grilled Top Sirloin w/ Cheese & Peppers	1 serv	440	–	21	–	4	–	570
Yellow Rice	1 serv	220	–	3	–	44	–	670
Yellow Rice & Black Beans	1 serv	280	–	3	–	55	–	1220
SALAD DRESSINGS AND TOPPINGS								
Citrus Mustard	1 serv	95	–	4	–	16	–	190

FOOD	PORTION	CALS	PROT	FAT	CHOL	CARB	FIBER	SOD
Dip Cilantro Vinaigrette	1 serv	110	–	6	–	12	–	840
Dipping Sauce Tangy	1 serv	50	–	1	–	12	–	190
Dressing Blue Cheese	1 serv	175	–	18	–	15	–	190
Dressing Caesar	1 serv	200	–	21	–	1	–	370
Dressing Ranch	1 serv	130	–	14	–	2	–	260
Dressing Tropical Island Vinaigrette	1 serv	60	–	4	–	15	–	600
Guava BBQ Sauce	1 serv	50	–	0	0	12	–	190
Homemade Croutons	12	500	–	29	–	47	–	740
Salsa Apple Mango	1 serv	20	–	0	0	5	–	15
Salsa Black Bean & Corn	1 serv	70	–	2	–	10	–	140
Salsa Mango Pineapple	1 serv	60	–	0	0	15	–	160
Salsa Tomato	1 serv	30	–	1	–	4	–	270
Sauce Chili Horseradish	1 serv	130	–	11	–	8	–	430
Sour Cream	1 serv	90	–	8	–	3	–	40
Sour Cream Ancho Chili	1 serv	70	–	6	–	4	–	290
SALADS								
Breeze No Dressing	1 serv	90	–	5	–	6	–	50
Caesar No Dressing	1 serv	70	–	3	–	6	–	210
Crispy Chicken Club w/ BBQ Drizzle	1 serv	880	–	52	–	47	–	3060
Fresh Fruit	1 serv	130	–	0	0	32	–	0
Grilled Chicken Caesar w/ Croutons w/o Dressing	1 serv	490	–	20	–	22	–	1520
Grilled Chicken Cobb	1 serv	600	–	38	–	4	–	1630
Grilled Fresh Salmon Tostada w/ Chimichurri Sauce w/o Dressing	1 serv	1045	–	57	–	52	–	1930
Tropical Fruit & Grilled Chicken On Greens w/o Dressing	1 serv	430	–	11	–	40	–	670
Vine Ripened Tomato	1 serv	60	–	1	–	12	–	490
SOUPS								
Bahamian Seafood Chowder	1 serv	600	–	47	–	27	–	1710
Chicken Tortilla	1 serv	290	–	12	–	26	–	1910
Cuban Black Bean	1 serv	320	–	4	–	52	–	1210

FOOD	PORTION	CALS	PROT	FAT	CHOL	CARB	FIBER	SOD
BAJA FRESH								
CHILDREN'S MENU SELECTIONS								
Kid's Mini Burrito Bean & Cheese	1 serv	540	18	14	25	84	11	1050
Kid's Mini Burrito Bean & Cheese w/ Chicken	1 serv	590	28	15	50	84	12	1200
Kid's Mini Quesadilla Cheese	1 serv	610	19	26	50	72	5	940
Kid's Mini Quesadilla Cheese w/ Chicken	1 serv	650	28	27	75	72	5	1090
Kid's Taquitos Chicken	1 serv	630	18	33	70	60	4	990
MAIN MENU SELECTIONS								
Black Beans	1 serv	360	23	3	5	61	26	1120
Burrito Baja Breaded Fish	1 serv	850	40	44	80	78	7	1900
Burrito Baja Carnitas	1 serv	830	45	45	115	67	8	2280
Burrito Baja Chicken	1 serv	790	52	38	120	65	8	2140
Burrito Baja Mahi Mahi	1 serv	780	51	38	115	66	7	1840
Burrito Baja Shrimp	1 serv	760	47	37	295	66	7	2230
Burrito Baja Steak	1 serv	850	49	46	125	67	7	2260
Burrito Bare Carnitas	1 serv	600	37	14	70	99	20	2480
Burrito Bare Chicken	1 serv	640	45	7	75	97	20	2330
Burrito Bare Steak	1 serv	700	41	15	80	99	19	2450
Burrito Bare Veggie & Cheese	1 serv	580	19	10	15	101	20	1950
Burrito Bean & Cheese Breaded Fish	1 serv	1030	54	41	95	108	20	1990
Burrito Bean & Cheese Carnitas	1 serv	1010	59	42	130	98	21	2370
Burrito Bean & Cheese Chicken	1 serv	970	67	35	135	96	21	2230
Burrito Bean & Cheese Mahi Mahi	1 serv	960	65	35	130	96	20	1930
Burrito Bean & Cheese No Meat	1 serv	840	39	33	65	96	20	1790
Burrito Bean & Cheese Shrimp	1 serv	950	61	34	310	96	20	2320
Burrito Bean & Cheese Steak	1 serv	1030	64	43	140	97	20	2350
Burrito Dos Manos Breaded Fish	1 serv	890	39	33	70	107	13	2025

FOOD	PORTION	CALS	PROT	FAT	CHOL	CARB	FIBER	SOD
Burrito Dos Manos Carnitas	1 serv	780	34	30	73	95	14	2115
Burrito Dos Manos Chicken	1 serv	760	38	26	75	94	14	2040
Burrito Dos Manos Mahi Mahi	1 serv	780	42	26	83	95	13	1915
Burrito Dos Manos Shrimp	1 serv	780	41	26	223	95	13	2220
Burrito Dos Manos Steak	1 serv	795	36	30	78	95	13	2105
Burrito Grilled Veggie	1 serv	506	32	33	65	94	16	1880
Burrito Mexicano Breaded Fish	1 serv	850	37	19	30	129	18	2040
Burrito Mexicano Carnitas	1 serv	830	42	20	70	119	19	2420
Burrito Mexicano Chicken	1 serv	790	50	13	75	117	20	2270
Burrito Mexicano Mahi Mahi	1 serv	790	49	13	70	117	18	1970
Burrito Mexicano Shrimp	1 serv	770	44	13	245	117	18	2370
Burrito Mexicano Steak	1 serv	860	47	21	118	118	18	2400
Burrito Ultimo Breaded Fish	1 serv	940	41	42	95	96	8	1950
Burrito Ultimo Carnitas	1 serv	920	46	44	130	86	9	2330
Burrito Ultimo Chicken	1 serv	880	54	36	140	84	9	2190
Burrito Ultimo Mahi Mahi	1 serv	880	52	36	130	84	8	1890
Burrito Ultimo Shrimp	1 serv	860	48	36	310	85	8	2280
Burrito Ultimo Steak	1 serv	950	50	44	140	85	8	2310
Chips & Guacamole	1 serv	1340	21	83	0	141	20	950
Chips & Salsa Baja	1 serv	810	13	37	0	98	14	1140
Fajitas Corn Tortillas Breaded Fish	1 serv	1060	51	37	85	130	22	2180
Fajitas Corn Tortillas Carnitas	1 serv	920	50	34	120	108	23	2610
Fajitas Corn Tortillas Chicken	1 serv	860	61	24	130	105	24	2400
Fajitas Corn Tortillas Mahi Mahi	1 serv	840	57	23	110	105	22	1960
Fajitas Corn Tortillas Shrimp	1 serv	840	55	23	390	106	22	2570
Fajitas Corn Tortillas Steak	1 serv	960	58	36	135	107	22	2600
Fajitas Flour Tortillas Breaded Fish	1 serv	1340	59	46	85	172	25	3020
Fajitas Flour Tortillas Carnitas	1 serv	1190	58	43	120	150	26	3450
Fajitas Flour Tortillas Chicken	1 serv	1140	69	33	130	147	27	3240

FOOD	PORTION	CALS	PROT	FAT	CHOL	CARB	FIBER	SOD
Fajitas Flour Tortillas Mahi Mahi	1 serv	1120	64	32	110	147	25	2800
Fajitas Flour Tortillas Shrimp	1 serv	1120	62	32	390	148	25	3410
Fajitas Flour Tortillas Steak	1 serv	960	58	36	135	170	22	2600
Guacamole Side	1 (3 oz)	110	2	13	0	5	2	270
Nachos Breaded Fish	1 serv	2090	78	116	185	176	31	2740
Nachos Carnitas	1 serv	2060	83	117	220	166	32	3120
Nachos Cheese	1 serv	1890	63	108	155	163	31	2530
Nachos Chicken	1 serv	2020	91	110	230	164	32	2980
Nachos Mahi Mahi	1 serv	2020	90	110	220	164	31	2600
Nachos Shrimp	1 serv	2000	85	110	395	164	31	3060
Nachos Steak	1 serv	2120	96	118	163	163	31	2990
Pico De Gallo Side	1 serv (8 oz)	50	2	1	0	12	3	890
Pinto Beans	1 serv	320	19	1	5	56	21	840
Pronto Guacamole Side	1 serv (6 oz)	560	9	34	0	60	8	370
Quesadilla Breaded Fish	1 serv	1400	62	86	170	96	8	2350
Quesadilla Carnitas	1 serv	1370	67	87	205	86	9	2730
Quesadilla Cheese	1 serv	1200	47	78	140	84	8	2140
Quesadilla Chicken	1 serv	1330	75	80	215	84	9	2590
Quesadilla Mahi Mahi	1 serv	1330	73	79	205	84	8	2290
Quesadilla Shrimp	1 serv	1310	69	79	385	84	8	2680
Quesadilla Steak	1 serv	1430	80	87	240	84	8	2600
Quesadilla Veggie	1 serv	1260	48	78	145	96	11	2310
Rice	1 serv	280	5	4	0	55	4	980
Rice & Beans Plate	1 serv	420	18	5	10	72	18	1320
Salsa Baja Side	1 serv (8 oz)	70	2	3	0	7	4	970
Salsa Roja Side	1 serv (8 oz)	70	3	1	0	13	4	1080
Salsa Verde Side	1 serv (8 oz)	50	2	0	0	11	3	1170
Soup Tortilla w/ Chicken	1 serv (13.6 oz)	320	17	14	40	29	4	2760
Soup Tortilla w/o Chicken	1 serv (12.4 oz)	270	8	14	45	29	4	2600
Taco Grilled Mahi Mahi	1 serv	230	12	9	20	26	4	300
Taco Baja Breaded Fish	1 serv	250	8	13	15	27	2	420
Taco Baja Chicken	1 serv	210	12	5	25	28	2	230
Taco Baja Shrimp	1 serv	200	11	5	90	28	2	280
Taco Baja Steak	1 serv	230	11	8	25	28	2	260
Taco Soft Breaded Fish	1 serv	240	10	11	20	23	2	490
Taco Soft Carnitas	1 serv	250	13	12	35	21	2	640

FOOD	PORTION	CALS	PROT	FAT	CHOL	CARB	FIBER	SOD
Taco Soft Chicken	1 serv	230	16	10	35	20	2	590
Taco Soft Mahi Mahi	1 serv	240	17	10	40	20	2	490
Taco Soft Shrimp	1 serv	230	15	10	105	21	2	640
Taco Soft Steak	1 serv	260	15	13	40	21	2	640
Taquitos Chicken w/ Beans	3	780	39	40	85	68	17	1810
Taquitos Chicken w/ Rice	3	740	30	40	85	66	8	1770
Veggie Mix	1 serv	110	3	0	0	24	6	330
SALAD DRESSINGS								
Chipotle Vinaigrette	1 serv (2.5 oz)	110	0	9	0	0	0	490
Fat Free Salsa Verde	1 serv (2.5 oz)	15	0	0	0	3	1	370
Olive Oil Vinaigrette	1 serv (2.5 oz)	290	0	31	0	2	0	290
Ranch	1 serv (2.5 oz)	260	2	26	50	4	0	470
SALADS								
Baja Ensalada Chicken	1 serv	310	46	7	18	18	7	1210
Baja Ensalada Shrimp	1 serv	230	28	6	250	18	6	1110
Baja Ensalada Steak	1 serv	450	54	18	150	18	6	1240
Chipotle w/ Carnitas	1 serv	640	38	30	95	56	10	1280
Chipotle w/ Chicken	1 serv	590	47	22	105	54	11	1110
Chipotle w/ Steak	1 serv	700	54	31	135	54	9	1140
Side By Side Carnitas	1 serv	570	46	40	140	16	8	1560
Side By Side Chicken	1 serv	500	60	27	150	12	9	1310
Side By Side Steak	1 serv	620	55	42	160	14	6	1550
Side Salad	1 (6.5 oz)	130	5	6	5	16	4	430
Tostada Breaded Fish	1 serv	1200	47	61	71	111	25	2140
Tostada Carnitas	1 serv	1180	52	62	100	100	26	2520
Tostada Chicken	1 serv	1140	60	55	115	98	27	2370
Tostada Mahi Mahi	1 serv	1130	59	55	105	99	25	2070
Tostada No Meat	1 serv	1010	32	53	40	98	25	1930
Tostada Shrimp	1 serv	1120	55	55	285	99	25	2460
Tostada Steak	1 serv	1230	65	63	140	98	25	2380

BASKIN-ROBBINS

FOOD	PORTION	CALS	PROT	FAT	CHOL	CARB	FIBER	SOD
BEVERAGES								
Cappuccino Blast w/ Whipped Cream	1 sm (16 oz)	330	6	14	55	48	0	110

FOOD	PORTION	CALS	PROT	FAT	CHOL	CARB	FIBER	SOD
Shake Chocolate Chip	1 sm (16 oz)	660	14	32	115	78	1	230
Shake Chocolate Chip Cookie Dough	1 sm (16 oz)	750	14	31	105	99	1	310
Shake Mint Chocolate Chip	1 sm (16 oz)	680	14	33	110	83	1	240
Shake Vanilla	1 sm (16 oz)	670	13	33	130	80	0	370
FROZEN YOGURT								
Cherries Jubilee	1 scoop (4 oz)	240	4	12	45	30	1	80
Vanilla Fat Free	1 scoop (4 oz)	150	6	0	0	32	0	105
ICE CREAM								
Butter Almond Crunch Reduced Fat No Sugar Added	1 scoop (4 oz)	220	7	11	25	31	4	140
Butter Pecan	1 scoop (4 oz)	280	5	18	50	24	1	95
Cabana Berry Banana Reduced Fat No Sugar Added	1 scoop (4 oz)	150	4	6	20	27	3	70
Chocolate	1 scoop (4 oz)	260	5	14	50	33	0	130
Chocolate Chip	1 scoop (4 oz)	270	5	16	55	28	1	95
Chocolate Chip Cookie Dough	1 scoop (4 oz)	310	5	15	50	36	0	135
Chocolate Overload Reduced Fat No Sugar Added	1 scoop (4 oz)	190	6	8	20	37	5	110
Gold Medal Ribbon	1 scoop (4 oz)	260	5	13	45	34	0	150
Mint Chocolate Chip	1 scoop (4 oz)	270	5	16	55	28	1	95
Nutty Coconut	1 scoop (4 oz)	300	6	20	45	28	1	90
Oreo Cookies 'N Cream	1 scoop (4 oz)	280	5	15	50	32	1	150
Peanut Butter 'N Chocolate	1 scoop (4 oz)	320	7	20	45	31	1	180

FOOD	PORTION	CALS	PROT	FAT	CHOL	CARB	FIBER	SOD
Pistachio Almond	1 scoop (4 oz)	290	7	19	50	25	1	85
Pralines 'N Cream	1 scoop (4 oz)	280	5	14	45	35	1	170
Reese's Peanut Butter Cup	1 scoop (4 oz)	300	6	18	50	31	1	130
Rocky Road	1 scoop (4 oz)	290	5	15	45	36	5	120
Sundae Caramel Soft Serve	1 (10 oz)	580	13	21	70	89	1	470
Sundae Hot Fudge Soft Serve	1 (10 oz)	610	14	25	65	86	1	430
Sundae Strawberry Soft Serve	1 (10 oz)	450	12	18	65	59	1	310
Tax Crunch	1 scoop (4 oz)	330	5	20	45	32	1	115
Vanilla	1 scoop (4 oz)	260	4	16	65	26	0	70
Vanilla Soft Serve	1 serv (6 oz)	280	8	11	40	37	0	200
Very Berry Strawberry	1 scoop (4 oz)	320	4	11	40	28	0	70
ICES								
Sherbet Rainbow	1 scoop (4 oz)	160	1	2	10	34	0	40
Sorbet Lemon	1 scoop (4 oz)	130	0	0	0	33	0	15
Sorbet Mango	1 scoop (4 oz)	120	0	0	0	32	0	10
Sorbet Strawberry	1 scoop (4 oz)	130	0	0	0	34	0	10

BEAR ROCK CAFE

FOOD	PORTION	CALS	PROT	FAT	CHOL	CARB	FIBER	SOD
SANDWICHES								
Colorado Turkey Club	1	855	38	37	126	95	5	2310
Coop's Chicken Salad Croissant	1	439	24	31	44	46	5	375
Garden Grill Ciabatta	1	406	12	25	33	55	4	907
Giant Panda Wrap	1	556	31	23	58	68	23	2045
Hoot Owl	1	641	34	42	92	32	2	1618
Rising Sunflower	1	596	35	35	86	35	2	1694

FOOD	PORTION	CALS	PROT	FAT	CHOL	CARB	FIBER	SOD
Roast Turkey & Bacon	1	522	32	30	71	31	2	1656
Rockslide Focaccia	1	958	43	62	129	57	3	2546
The Moose	1	976	54	54	142	64	7	2565
BEN & JERRY'S								
FROZEN YOGURT								
Low Fat Cherry Garcia	½ cup	170	4	3	20	32	tr	65
Low Fat Chocolate Fudge Brownie	½ cup	190	5	3	15	35	1	100
Low Fat Half Baked	½ cup	190	5	3	20	35	tr	100
Phish Food	½ cup	220	4	5	15	41	1	95
ICE CREAM								
Bar Cherry Garcia	1	270	4	19	35	29	1	45
Bar Half Baked	1	340	5	16	40	46	2	125
Bar Vanilla	1	300	4	20	45	26	1	60
Bar Vanilla Almond	1	340	5	23	65	30	2	135
Black & Tan	½ cup	230	4	13	50	24	1	55
Brownie Batter	½ cup	310	5	18	70	32	1	115
Butter Pecan	½ cup	280	4	21	65	20	1	105
Cherry Garcia	½ cup	250	4	14	60	26	tr	50
Chocolate	½ cup	260	4	16	50	25	2	50
Chocolate Chip Cookie Dough	½ cup	270	4	15	65	32	0	85
Chocolate Fudge Brownie	½ cup	260	5	13	35	32	2	80
Chubby Hubby	½ cup	330	7	20	55	31	1	150
Chunky Monkey	½ cup	300	5	18	55	30	1	45
Coffee	½ cup	240	4	15	75	21	0	60
Coffee Heath Bar Crunch	½ cup	290	4	18	65	29	0	–
Dave Matthews Band Magic Brownies	½ cup	250	4	13	60	29	0	75
Dublin Mudslide	½ cup	270	4	16	65	28	tr	80
Everything But The	½ cup	310	5	19	50	30	1	85
Fossil Fuel	½ cup	280	4	17	60	30	1	60
Fudge Central	½ cup	300	4	18	55	31	1	60
Half Baked	½ cup	280	5	14	50	34	tr	90
In A Crunch	½ cup	350	6	23	55	30	1	150
Karamel Sutra	½ cup	280	4	15	50	32	1	75
Marsha Marsha Marshmallow	½ cup	300	4	17	30	33	1	60
Mint Chocolate Cookie	½ cup	260	4	16	65	26	0	100

FOOD	PORTION	CALS	PROT	FAT	CHOL	CARB	FIBER	SOD
Neapolitan Dynamite	½ cup	250	4	13	45	29	1	70
New York Super Fudge Chunk	½ cup	310	5	20	40	29	2	55
Oatmeal Cookie Chunk	½ cup	270	4	15	55	31	tr	120
Organic Chocolate Fudge Brownie	½ cup	270	4	13	35	30	2	55
Organic Strawberry	½ cup	210	3	12	55	21	0	40
Organic Sweet Cream & Cookies	½ cup	250	4	15	60	24	0	95
Organic Vanilla	½ cup	220	3	14	65	18	0	50
Peanut Butter Cup	½ cup	360	7	26	60	27	1	125
Phish Food	½ cup	280	4	13	30	37	1	85
Pistachio Pistachio	½ cup	260	5	17	65	21	tr	55
Sandwich Wich Ice Cream Cookie	1	350	4	18	55	45	1	220
Strawberry	½ cup	230	4	13	65	26	0	50
The Godfather	½ cup	270	4	14	30	32	2	50
Turtle Soup	½ cup	280	4	15	60	30	1	100
Uncanny Cashew	½ cup	290	4	19	70	27	0	130
Vanilla Caramel Fudge	½ cup	280	4	15	70	31	0	105
Vanilla Heath Bar Crunch	½ cup	290	4	18	65	29	0	120
Vermonty Python	½ cup	310	4	19	60	30	1	90
SORBETS								
Berried Treasure	½ cup	110	0	0	0	29	1	5
Jamaican Me Crazy	½ cup	130	0	0	0	33	4	10
Strawberry Kiwi Swirl	½ cup	110	0	0	0	28	1	10

BILLY'S BURGER HUT

FOOD	PORTION	CALS	PROT	FAT	CHOL	CARB	FIBER	SOD
BEVERAGES								
Shake Chocolate	1 (20 oz)	420	9	10	30	63	0	260
Shake Vanilla	1 (20 oz)	320	8	10	25	49	0	157
MAIN MENU SELECTIONS								
Big Billy's Roast Beef Sub	1	843	51	54	151	62	3	2860
Billyburger	1	426	20	22	63	35	3	1076
Billyburger w/ Cheese	1	498	23	35	57	35	4	1276
Billy's Best Red Potato Salad	1 serv	190	2	9	80	12	3	650
Billy's Biggest Burger ½ Pounder w/ Everything	1	852	70	58	140	61	4	2229

FOOD	PORTION	CALS	PROT	FAT	CHOL	CARB	FIBER	SOD
Billy's Famous 7 Layer Salad	1 serv	558	10	49	119	18	2	680
Billy's Seafood Sandwich	1	399	21	18	42	43	3	890
Caesar Side Salad	1 serv	360	11	28	70	12	4	610
Chili w/ Cheese & Onion	1 serv	380	33	12	64	35	7	1004
Cowboy Cobb Salad	1 serv	735	29	45	239	25	9	1450
Cowboy Coleslaw	1 serv	180	1	9	10	11	3	250
French Fries	1 reg	230	5	12	0	25	1	253
Onion Rings	1 serv	250	2	10	0	37	1	955
Super Billy Burger w/ Bacon	1	663	35	41	98	39	4	1869
BLIMPIE								
DESSERTS								
Cookie Chocolate Chunk	1 (1.5 oz)	200	2	10	15	25	0	150
Cookie Oatmeal Raisin	1 (1.5 oz)	180	2	7	10	27	tr	150
Cookie Peanut Butter	1 (1.5 oz)	210	3	13	10	21	tr	170
Cookie Sugar	1 (2.5 oz)	320	3	16	35	42	0	240
Cookie White Chocolate Macadamia Nut	1 (1.5 oz)	200	2	11	15	25	0	110
SALAD DRESSINGS AND SAUCES								
Dressing Blue Cheese	1 serv (1.5 oz)	230	2	24	25	2	–	440
Dressing Buttermilk Ranch	1 serv (1.5 oz)	230	1	24	10	2	–	380
Dressing Buttermilk Ranch Light	1 serv (1.5 oz)	70	1	4	0	8	–	310
Dressing Creamy Caesar	1 serv (1.5 oz)	210	1	21	10	2	–	520
Dressing Creamy Italian	1 serv (1.5 oz)	180	0	18	0	4	0	420
Dressing Dijon Honey Mustard	1 serv (1.5 oz)	180	1	17	15	8	–	240
Dressing Italian Fat Free	1 serv (1.5 oz)	25	0	0	0	5	0	390
Dressing Italian Light	1 serv (1.5 oz)	20	0	1	0	2	–	770
Dressing Peppercorn	1 serv (1.5 oz)	240	1	26	20	1	0	450

FOOD	PORTION	CALS	PROT	FAT	CHOL	CARB	FIBER	SOD
Dressing Thousand Island	1 serv (1.5 oz)	210	0	20	15	6	0	350
Guacamole	1 serv (1 oz)	45	0	4	0	2	1	135
Mayonnaise	1 serv (1 oz)	200	0	22	20	0	0	200
Mustard Yellow Deli	1 serv (0.5 oz)	15	0	0	–	0	0	170
Oil Blend	1 serv (0.5 oz)	130	0	14	–	0	0	0
Sauce Blimpie Special	1 serv (0.5 oz)	40	0	5	0	0	–	0
Sauce Red Hot Original	1 serv (1 oz)	10	0	0	0	2	0	760
SALADS								
Antipasto	1 serv (11.6 oz)	254	20	14	60	12	4	1630
Buffalo Chicken	1 serv (7.7 oz)	220	25	9	60	10	4	840
Chicken Caesar	1 serv (9.4 oz)	190	25	8	65	6	3	460
Cole Slaw	1 side (4 oz)	160	1	9	5	20	2	240
Garden	1 serv (6.5 oz)	30	2	0	0	6	3	15
Macaroni	1 side (5 oz)	330	5	22	15	28	2	790
Northwest Potato	1 side (5 oz)	260	3	17	25	22	3	390
Potato	1 side (4.7 oz)	230	3	12	10	28	3	490
Tuna	1 serv (9.4 oz)	270	18	19	55	6	3	370
Ultimate Club	1 serv (10.1 oz)	280	23	14	65	10	3	1070
SANDWICHES								
6 Inch Sub Blimpie Best	1 (10.4 oz)	450	24	17	50	49	3	1330
6 Inch Sub Blimpie Best Super Stacked	1 (12.8 oz)	550	36	22	90	52	3	2090
6 Inch Sub Blimpie Trio Super Stacked	1 (13.5 oz)	510	40	15	90	51	3	1760
6 Inch Sub BLT	1 (7.2 oz)	430	15	22	25	43	2	960
6 Inch Sub BLT Super Stacked	1 (8.4 oz)	640	22	41	55	43	2	1440
6 Inch Sub Chicken Cheddar Bacon Ranch	1 (12.1 oz)	600	36	29	85	48	3	1570

FOOD	PORTION	CALS	PROT	FAT	CHOL	CARB	FIBER	SOD
6 Inch Sub Chicken Teriyaki	1 (8.7 oz)	450	33	12	65	52	2	1280
6 Inch Sub Club	1 (10.2 oz)	410	23	13	45	49	3	1050
6 Inch Sub Cuban	1 (8.2 oz)	410	29	11	65	43	1	1630
6 Inch Sub French Dip	1 (13.4 oz)	410	30	11	65	46	1	1650
6 Inch Sub Ham & Swiss	1 (10 oz)	420	23	14	45	49	3	1020
6 Inch Sub Hot Pastrami	1 (7.2 oz)	430	30	16	65	42	1	1350
6 Inch Sub Hot Pastrami Super Stacked	1 (10.1 oz)	570	46	23	110	43	1	2110
6 Inch Sub Meatball	1 (10 oz)	580	27	31	75	50	4	1960
6 Inch Sub Reuben	1 (9.2 oz)	530	34	20	70	52	3	1740
6 Inch Sub Roast Beef & Provolone	1 (10.8 oz)	430	28	14	55	46	3	980
6 Inch Sub Roast Beef & Provolone On Wheat	1 (11.3 oz)	430	32	16	60	44	6	1000
6 Inch Sub Tuna	1 (8.9 oz)	470	24	21	55	43	2	770
6 Inch Sub Turkey & Provolone	1 (10.8 oz)	410	24	13	40	49	3	1310
6 Inch Sub Turkey & Provolone On Wheat	1 (11.3 oz)	420	27	14	45	47	6	1350
6 Inch Sub VegiMax	1 (10.2 oz)	520	28	20	15	56	5	1270
Blimpie Burger	1 (6 oz)	460	21	24	70	42	1	1280
Blimpie Dog	1 (6.3 oz)	510	17	29	55	45	1	1420
Ciabatta Buffalo Chicken	1 (11.3 oz)	540	31	23	65	49	3	1970
Ciabatta French Dip	1 (13.8 oz)	430	31	11	65	49	2	1820
Ciabatta Grilled Chicken Caesar	1 (10.1 oz)	580	34	20	65	62	3	1480
Ciabatta Mediterranean	1 (10.1 oz)	450	26	8	35	65	3	1720
Ciabatta Roast Beef Turkey & Cheddar	1 (10 oz)	520	25	24	65	51	3	1780
Ciabatta Sicilian	1 (10 oz)	590	29	22	60	66	3	2170
Ciabatta Spicy Chicken & Pepperoni	1 (10.1 oz)	710	33	34	80	65	3	2070
Ciabatta Tuscan	1 (9.9 oz)	570	28	20	50	65	3	2030
Ciabatta Ultimate Club	1 (7.4 oz)	520	27	24	65	47	2	1600
Wrap Chicken Caesar	1 (9.7 oz)	220	30	8	60	56	4	1480
Wrap Southwestern	1 (10 oz)	530	23	22	55	61	4	1770
SOUPS								
Bean w/ Ham	1 serv (8.6 oz)	140	8	1	0	23	11	1070

FOOD	PORTION	CALS	PROT	FAT	CHOL	CARB	FIBER	SOD
Chicken Noodle	1 serv (8.6 oz)	130	7	4	30	18	2	1040
Chicken w/ White & Wild Rice	1 serv (8.6 oz)	250	14	10	30	15	4	1030
Cream Of Broccoli w/ Cheese	1 serv (8.6 oz)	250	7	19	55	13	tr	1040
Cream Of Potato	1 serv (8.6 oz)	190	5	9	<5	24	3	860
Garden Vegetable	1 serv (8.6 oz)	80	5	1	0	14	3	620
Grande Chili w/ Bean & Beef	1 serv (8.6 oz)	310	20	9	20	31	9	1440
Tomato Basil w/ Raviolini	1 serv (8.6 oz)	110	4	1	10	22	0	720
Vegetable Beef	1 serv (8.6 oz)	80	4	2	5	13	2	1010

BOB EVANS

BREAKFAST SELECTIONS

FOOD	PORTION	CALS	PROT	FAT	CHOL	CARB	FIBER	SOD
Bacon	1 piece	36	1	4	5	0	0	54
Benedict Ham & Cheese	1 serv	826	44	52	564	44	0	3137
Country Benedict Sausage	1 serv	936	44	66	536	40	0	2098
Country Benedict Spinach Bacon & Tomato	1 serv	729	30	48	494	42	1	1885
Country Biscuit Breakfast	1 serv	659	24	45	269	40	1	1703
Egg Beaters	1 serv	173	28	12	5	3	0	581
Egg Hardcooked	1	60	6	4	190	1	0	55
Egg Over Easy	1	101	7	8	229	1	0	68
Egg Scrambled	1 serv	255	20	17	723	2	0	213
French Toast	1 slice	131	3	2	25	13	1	175
French Toast Stuffed Plain	1 serv	599	11	20	99	53	3	689
Fruit & Yogurt Plate	1 serv	403	9	2	5	93	9	109
Grits	1 serv	178	3	7	9	28	2	172
Ham Smoked	1 slice	87	14	2	52	2	0	1131
Hotcake Blueberry	1	328	6	9	0	55	2	749
Hotcake Buttermilk	1	318	6	9	0	53	2	746
Hotcake Cinnamon	1	417	6	15	0	66	2	749
Hotcake Multigrain	1	322	7	10	0	52	3	773
Mush	1 serv	79	1	3	0	11	2	466
Oatmeal	1 serv	172	6	3	0	32	4	394

FOOD	PORTION	CALS	PROT	FAT	CHOL	CARB	FIBER	SOD
Omelette Bacon & Cheese	1 serv	825	40	66	826	6	1	1603
Omelette Border Scramble	1	756	42	58	846	15	3	1059
Omelette Egg Beaters Bacon & Cheese	1 serv	615	57	47	108	7	1	1972
Omelette Egg Beaters Border Scramble	1 serv	517	48	37	72	16	3	1411
Omelette Egg Beaters Farmer's Market	1 serv	569	49	41	92	14	2	2108
Omelette Egg Beaters Garden Harvest	1 serv	444	40	31	64	14	2	1610
Omelette Egg Beaters Ham & Cheddar	1 serv	426	51	29	80	5	1	1789
Omelette Egg Beaters Sausage & Cheddar	1 serv	502	49	40	73	4	1	1295
Omelette Egg Beaters Three Cheese	1 serv	435	43	34	78	5	1	1394
Omelette Farmer's Market	1	778	42	60	810	13	2	1739
Omelette Garden Harvest	1 serv	654	33	50	782	13	2	1241
Omelette Ham & Cheddar	1 serv	634	44	48	798	3	1	1419
Omelette Sausage & Cheddar	1 serv	741	42	61	847	3	1	942
Omelette Three Cheese	1 serv	645	35	52	796	4	1	1025
Omelette Western	1 serv	654	44	48	798	8	2	1420
Pot Roast Hash	1 serv	652	38	39	533	34	4	1084
Sausage Gravy Bowl	1 serv	268	7	17	17	21	0	1238
Sausage Link	1	125	5	11	14	0	0	184
Skillet Sunshine	1 serv	842	37	60	819	36	4	1474
Waffles Sweet Cream	1 serv	598	15	12	149	100	3	1288
CHILDREN'S MENU SELECTIONS								
Fruit & Yogurt Dippers	1 serv	275	7	2	5	61	5	95
Hotcakes	1 serv	501	9	17	0	79	2	1071
Kid's Macaroni & Cheese	1 serv	320	11	11	23	45	2	778
Kid's Pasta	1 serv	113	3	5	12	15	1	857
Mini Cheeseburgers	1 serv	306	12	19	40	21	1	525
Smiley Face Potatoes	1 serv	524	5	31	2	57	3	646
Sundae Fudge Blast	1 serv	244	3	11	25	33	0	81
Sundae Reese's I'm Smiling	1 serv	330	5	17	26	41	1	130
MAIN MENU SELECTIONS								
Seniors Chicken Parmesan	1 serv	522	38	26	127	33	3	2404

FOOD	PORTION	CALS	PROT	FAT	CHOL	CARB	FIBER	SOD
Seniors Garden Vegetable Alfredo	1 serv	363	11	23	36	29	5	1322
Seniors Garden Vegetable Alfredo Chicken	1 serv	452	26	26	74	29	5	1678
Seniors Steak Tips & Noodles	1 serv	422	33	22	101	23	2	2251
Seniors Stir-Fry Chicken	1 serv	368	21	13	37	44	5	1385
SOUPS								
Bean	1 cup	144	10	3	8	19	3	778
Cheddar Baked Potato	1 cup	294	10	20	34	19	1	1168
Sausage Chili	1 cup	268	16	17	42	18	7	687
Vegetable Beef	1 cup	135	6	5	14	17	3	370
BOJANGLES								
Biscuit	1	243	4	12	2	29	2	663
Biscuit Sandwich Bacon	1	290	8	17	10	26	1	810
Biscuit Sandwich Bacon Egg Cheese	1	550	17	42	160	27	1	1250
Biscuit Sandwich Cajun Filet	1	454	20	21	41	46	1	949
Biscuit Sandwich Country Ham	1	270	9	15	20	26	1	1010
Biscuit Sandwich Egg	1	400	8	30	120	26	1	630
Biscuit Sandwich Sausage	1	350	9	23	20	26	1	810
Biscuit Sandwich Smoked Sausage	1	380	10	26	20	27	1	940
Biscuit Sandwich Steak	1	649	14	49	34	37	1	1126
Botato Rounds	1 serv	235	3	11	13	31	3	328
Buffalo Bites	1 serv	180	27	5	105	5	0	720
Cajun Pintos	1 serv	110	6	0	0	18	6	480
Cajun Spiced Breast	1 serv	278	18	17	75	12	tr	565
Cajun Spiced Leg	1 serv	264	19	16	96	11	tr	530
Cajun Spiced Thigh	1 serv	310	15	23	67	11	tr	465
Cajun Spiced Wing	1 serv	355	21	25	94	11	tr	630
Chicken Supremes	1 serv	337	21	16	58	26	1	629
Corn On The Cob	1 serv	140	5	2	0	34	2	20
Dirty Rice	1 serv	166	5	6	10	24	1	762
Green Beans	1 serv	25	0	0	0	5	2	710
Macaroni & Cheese	1 serv	198	7	14	26	12	tr	418
Marinated Cole Slaw	1 serv	136	1	3	0	26	3	454

FOOD	PORTION	CALS	PROT	FAT	CHOL	CARB	FIBER	SOD
Potatoes w/o Gravy	1 serv	80	2	1	0	16	1	380
Sandwich Cajun Filet w/ Mayo	1	437	22	22	55	41	3	506
Sandwich Cajun Filet w/o Mayo	1	337	22	11	45	41	3	401
Sandwich Grilled Filet w/ Mayo	1	335	23	16	61	25	2	645
Sandwich Grilled Filet w/o Mayo	1	235	23	5	51	25	2	540
Seasoned Fries	1 serv	344	5	19	13	39	4	480
Southern Style Breast	1 serv	261	16	16	76	12	tr	702
Southern Style Leg	1 serv	254	19	15	94	11	tr	446
Southern Style Thigh	1 serv	308	16	21	78	14	tr	630
Southern Style Wing	1 serv	337	17	21	86	19	tr	684
Sweet Biscuit Bo Berry	1	320	4	18	tr	37	1	560
Sweet Biscuit Cinnamon	1	320	4	18	tr	37	1	560

BOSTON MARKET

DESSERTS

FOOD	PORTION	CALS	PROT	FAT	CHOL	CARB	FIBER	SOD
Apple Pie	1 slice	420	3	20	0	56	2	650
Brownie Chocolate Chip Fudge	1	580	9	23	90	81	3	390
Chocolate Cake	1 serv	600	5	32	65	75	2	210
Cookie Chocolate Chip	1	370	4	19	20	49	2	340
Cornbread	1 piece	180	2	5	10	31	0	320

MAIN MENU SELECTIONS

FOOD	PORTION	CALS	PROT	FAT	CHOL	CARB	FIBER	SOD
Broccoli w/ Garlic Butter	1 serv	80	3	6	0	6	3	230
Butternut Squash	1 serv	140	2	5	10	25	2	35
Carver Boston Chicken	1	700	44	29	90	68	3	1560
Carver Boston Meatloaf	1	940	49	45	155	96	6	2080
Carver Boston Sirloin Dip	1	1000	67	51	200	70	3	1690
Carver Boston Turkey	1	770	66	27	125	68	3	1810
Carver Boston Turkey Dip	1	770	66	27	125	67	3	1890
Cinnamon Apples	1 serv	210	0	3	0	47	3	15
Cranberry Walnut Relish	1 serv	140	1	2	0	30	2	0
Creamed Spinach	1 serv	280	9	23	70	12	4	580
Dip Spinach Artichoke	1 serv	100	3	8	15	3	1	220
Family Meals Boneless Turkey Breast	1 serv (5 oz)	180	38	3	70	0	0	620

FOOD	PORTION	CALS	PROT	FAT	CHOL	CARB	FIBER	SOD
Family Meals Roasted Turkey	1 serv (5 oz)	180	38	3	72	0	0	635
Family Meals Rotisserie Chicken	1 serv (6 oz)	290	39	14	175	4	0	710
Family Meals Spiral Sliced Ham	1 serv (8 oz)	450	40	26	140	13	0	2230
Family Meals Whole Turkey	1 serv (6.7 oz)	310	40	18	135	0	0	940
Fresh Vegetable Stuffing	1 serv	190	3	8	0	25	2	580
Garden Fresh Coleslaw	1 serv	170	2	9	10	21	2	270
Garlic Dill New Potatoes	1 serv	140	3	3	0	24	3	120
Green Bean Casserole	1 serv	60	2	2	5	9	2	620
Green Beans	1 serv	60	2	4	0	7	3	180
Individual Meals 1 Thigh & 1 Drumstick	1 serv	300	32	17	180	6	0	630
Individual Meals ¼ White Rotisserie Chicken	1 serv	290	45	11	170	4	0	780
Individual Meals ¼ White Rotisserie Chicken No Skin	1 serv	210	42	2	135	6	0	640
Individual Meals 3 Piece Dark	1 serv	380	45	19	250	7	0	880
Individual Meals 3 Piece Dark Skinless	1 serv	240	37	8	205	7	0	650
Individual Meals Award Winning Roasted Sirloin	1 serv	290	39	15	125	0	0	440
Individual Meals Meatloaf	1	480	29	33	125	23	2	970
Individual Meals Roasted Turkey	1 serv	180	38	3	72	0	0	635
Macaroni & Cheese	1 serv	330	14	12	30	39	1	1290
Mashed Potatoes	1 serv	210	4	9	25	29	3	660
Pot Pie Pastry Topped Chicken	1	780	29	47	125	60	4	930
Poultry Gravy	1 serv (4 oz)	15	1	1	0	4	0	570
Seasonal Fresh Fruit Salad	1 serv	60	1	0	0	15	1	20
Spinach w/ Garlic Butter Sauce	1 serv	130	5	9	20	9	5	200
Squash Casserole	1 serv	320	9	24	50	21	3	1380
Steamed Fresh Vegetables	1 serv	60	2	2	0	8	3	40
Sweet Corn	1 serv	170	6	4	0	37	2	95
Sweet Potato Casserole	1 serv	460	4	17	20	77	3	210

FOOD	PORTION	CALS	PROT	FAT	CHOL	CARB	FIBER	SOD
SALADS								
Entree Caesar	1	500	13	45	45	12	3	1190
Entree Caesar w/o Dressing	1	140	11	8	15	8	2	280
Entree Market Chopped	1	580	10	48	10	30	9	1990
Entree Market Chopped w/o Dressing	1	210	10	9	10	28	9	280
Side Caesar	1	400	5	40	30	7	2	980
Side Caesar w/o Dressing	1	40	3	2	5	3	1	75
Side Market Chopped	1	440	4	43	5	12	3	1790
Side Market Chopped w/o Dressing	1	80	3	4	5	10	3	85
SOUPS								
Chicken Noodle	1 serv	170	13	5	60	17	1	210
Chicken Tortilla w/ Toppings	1 serv	340	12	22	45	24	1	1310
Tortilla Soup w/o Toppings	1 serv	80	5	5	15	7	1	900

BOSTON PIZZA

FOOD	PORTION	CALS	PROT	FAT	CHOL	CARB	FIBER	SOD
CHILDREN'S MENU SELECTIONS								
Baked Salmon w/ Caesar Salad	1 serv	330	23	14	–	13	tr	330
Bug N' Cheese	1 serv	500	21	13	–	73	3	710
Chicken Fingers w/ Fries	1 serv	390	26	19	–	28	2	570
Pizza Pint Size	1	390	19	7	–	64	tr	520
Quesadilla Bacon Double Cheeseburger w/ Caesar Salad	1 serv	540	26	27	–	49	3	1660
Reduced Size Fruit Cup	1 serv	80	0	0	0	18	tr	0
Sandwich Grilled Chicken w/ Garden Greens	1 serv	600	10	38	–	45	3	1000
Super Spaghetti	1 serv	440	12	13	–	68	5	690
Wrap Ham & Cheese w/ Fries	1 serv	550	16	28	–	60	4	790
DESSERTS								
Blondie Maple	1	850	7	43	–	111	1	350
Blondie Maple Bite Size	1	430	4	21	–	58	tr	170
Brownie Chocolate Addiction	1	490	5	13	–	92	2	170
Brownie Chocolate Addiction Bite Size	1	200	2	7	–	35	1	90

FOOD	PORTION	CALS	PROT	FAT	CHOL	CARB	FIBER	SOD
Cheesecake New York	1 slice	620	11	33	–	80	0	440
Cheesecake Vanilla Bean	1 slice	770	9	52	–	70	1	320
Chocolate Explosion	1 serv	890	11	50	–	103	4	510
Tarte Au Sucre	1 serv	310	4	21	–	71	1	9500
MAIN MENU SELECTIONS								
Angus Beef Sirloin Steak w/ Spaghetti	1 serv	1260	72	70	–	83	8	1560
Baked 3 Cheese Penne	1 half order	460	21	14	–	62	4	1030
Baked Seven Cheese Ravioli	1 half order	310	17	14	–	28	2	1000
Baked Shrimp & Feta Penne	1 half order	480	28	19	–	54	4	690
Boston's Lasagna	1 half order	340	18	10	–	45	3	860
Boston's Smokey Mountain Spaghetti	1 order	1290	59	47	–	161	13	2650
Chicken & Mushroom Fettuccini	1 half order	710	23	38	–	72	4	680
Chicken Parmesan w/ Seasonal Vegetables	1 serv	1060	47	74	–	55	9	1190
Fries	1 serv	430	7	25	–	45	5	640
Garlic Mashed Potatoes	1 serv	730	6	60	–	42	5	1800
Garlic Toast	1 slice	150	3	6	–	20	1	330
Homestyle Lasagna	1 order	590	39	33	–	37	4	1910
Jambalaya Fettuccini	1 half order	860	33	51	–	71	6	2170
Lemon Baked Salmon w/ Fries	1 serv	1150	50	74	–	61	9	2330
Mama Meata Penne	1 half order	940	35	62	–	66	7	1890
Mushroom Chicken w/ Garlic Mashed Potatoes	1 serv	1030	68	62	–	53	9	1450
Pad Thai w/ Chicken	1 serv	2110	77	47	–	356	21	30
Pad Thai w/ Shrimp	1 serv	2090	77	45	–	358	22	390
Pollo Pomodoro Spaghetti	1 serv	520	26	14	–	73	7	1060
Salmon Filet Lemon Baked	1 serv	430	51	13	–	33	10	250
Scallop & Prawn Fettuccini	1 half order	710	21	41	–	67	5	660
Seasoned Vegetables	1 serv	70	0	0	–	10	4	760
Shrimp Skewers Lime & Parmesan	1 serv	190	15	7	–	20	3	1020
Sicilian Penne	1 half order	720	20	48	–	55	5	740
Sirloin Steak w/ Prawns & Fries	1 serv	1480	78	104	–	58	9	2140

FOOD	PORTION	CALS	PROT	FAT	CHOL	CARB	FIBER	SOD
Slow Roasted Pork Back Ribs w/ Fries	1 serv	1680	68	123	–	78	8	2080
Spaghetti w/ Alfredo Sauce	1 half order	440	15	11	–	70	3	710
Spaghetti w/ Bolognese	1 half order	400	15	5	–	73	5	670
Spaghetti w/ Creamy Tomato Sauce	1 half order	410	14	11	–	66	4	410
Spaghetti w/ Pomodoro Sauce	1 half order	450	13	14	–	68	5	720
Spicy Italian Penne	1 half order	980	30	61	–	81	5	1440
Starter Baked Raviolo Bites	1 serv	450	20	22	–	45	4	1410
Starter Basket Garlic Twist	1 serv	1140	32	39	–	165	tr	2910
Starter Basket Three Cheese Toast	1 serv	730	33	34	–	72	0	1580
Starter Boston's Poutine	1 serv	740	23	45	–	53	7	1860
Starter Bruschetta Sun Dried Tomato	1 serv	470	10	21	–	59	5	1130
Starter Cactus Cuts Potatoes & Dip	1 serv	1150	15	89	–	72	7	1430
Starter Chicken Fingers	1 serv	360	46	14	–	12	0	520
Starter Chicken Fingers Buffalo Style	1 serv	370	46	14	–	14	1	2080
Starter Cracked Pepper Dry Ribs	1 serv	380	69	41	–	3	1	1880
Starter Nachos Cactus w/ Cactus Dip	1 serv	1830	59	128	–	111	12	3160
Starter Nachos Spicy Chicken w/ Sour Cream & Salsa	1 serv	1430	73	72	–	126	12	2330
Starter Nachos Taco Beef w/ Sour Cream & Salsa	1 serv	1560	73	86	–	129	13	2180
Starter Nachos w/ Sour Cream & Salsa	1 serv	1320	53	71	–	126	12	1790
Starter Panzerotti Roll	1	820	41	32	–	94	3	1370
Starter Pizza Bread Bandera w/ Santa Fe Ranch Dip	1 serv	960	32	54	–	89	tr	1880
Starter Pizza Bread w/o Sauce	1 serv	500	15	12	–	84	0	660
Starter Potato Skins	1 serv	650	22	46	–	39	tr	1390

FOOD	PORTION	CALS	PROT	FAT	CHOL	CARB	FIBER	SOD
Starter Quesadilla Oven Roasted Chicken	1 serv	900	43	39	–	96	6	1850
Starter Quesadilla Southwest w/ Sour Cream & Salsa	1 serv	770	55	27	–	77	4	1740
Starter Shrimp Stuffed Mushroom Caps	1 serv	490	23	41	–	12	2	1150
Starter Team Platter w/ Dips & Sauces	1 serv	3030	153	205	–	144	12	3930
Starter Thai Chicken Bites	1 serv	540	46	15	–	55	2	1540
Starter Wings Breaded BBQ	1 serv	930	72	52	–	28	tr	3770
Starter Wings Breaded Honey Garlic	1 serv	940	72	52	–	31	0	3470
Starter Wings Breaded Mild	1 serv	880	72	52	–	17	0	3380
Starter Wings Breaded Teriyaki	1 serv	940	73	52	–	30	tr	3720
Starter Wings Breaded Thai	1 serv	1110	73	52	–	73	2	4720
Starter Wings Oven Roasted BBQ	1 serv	670	54	42	–	19	tr	410
Starter Wings Oven Roasted Honey Garlic	1 serv	700	54	42	–	26	2	125
Starter Wings Oven Roasted Hot	1 serv	620	53	42	–	9	tr	1060
Starter Wings Oven Roasted Teriyaki	1 serv	670	54	42	–	20	tr	360
Starter Wings Oven Roasted Thai Chili	1 serv	770	52	40	–	50	1	1030
The Ribber w/ Spaghetti	1 serv	970	49	43	–	96	5	1540
Tortellini w/ Alfredo Sauce	1 half order	340	12	15	–	37	1	880
Tortellini w/ Bolognese	1 half order	300	13	9	–	40	3	840
Tortellini w/ Creamy Tomato Sauce	1 half order	310	11	14	–	33	2	580
Tortellini w/ Pomodoro Sauce	1 half order	340	10	18	–	35	3	880
Veal Parmesan w/ Spaghetti	1 serv	1020	44	72	–	106	9	1920
PIZZA								
Bacon Double Cheeseburger Individual	1 pie	1140	73	54	–	94	2	2600
Bacon Double Cheeseburger Slice	1 med	280	18	12	–	25	tr	660

FOOD	PORTION	CALS	PROT	FAT	CHOL	CARB	FIBER	SOD
BBQ Chicken Individual	1 pie	730	37	24	–	93	1	1270
BBQ Chicken Slice	1 med	190	10	6	–	25	0	350
Boston Royal Individual	1 pie	840	53	27	–	98	3	1520
Boston Royal Slice	1 med	210	13	6	–	26	tr	410
Californian Slice	1 med	280	11	15	–	24	0	280
Clubhouse Individual	1 pie	1040	44	56	–	94	3	1070
Deluxe Individual	1 pie	850	55	29	–	94	2	1550
Deluxe Slice	1 med	220	14	7	–	25	tr	420
Great White North Slice	1 med	240	16	9	–	24	0	400
Hawaiian Individual	1 pie	780	49	20	–	101	2	1150
Hawaiian Slice	1 med	210	13	5	–	27	0	320
Indy California	1 (11.3 oz)	440	16	12	–	69	7	490
La Quebecoise Individual	1 pie	770	42	27	–	93	3	1650
La Quebecoise Slice	1 med	200	11	7	–	25	tr	460
Meateor Individual	1 pie	950	63	37	–	91	1	1640
Meateor Slice	1 med	260	17	10	–	25	0	460
Pepperoni Individual	1 pie	750	40	27	–	89	2	1650
Pepperoni Slice	1 med	200	10	7	–	24	0	450
Pepperoni & Mushroom Individual	1 pie	750	41	27	–	90	2	1650
Pepperoni & Mushroom Slice	1 med	200	10	7	–	24	tr	460
Popeye Individual	1 pie	720	41	22	–	93	2	1170
Popeye Slice	1 med	200	11	7	–	25	tr	320
Rustic Italian Individual	1 pie	950	49	39	–	102	3	4270
Rustic Italian Slice	1 med	260	13	10	–	28	tr	1250
Spicy Perogy Individual	1 pie	980	46	45	–	99	2	1090
Spicy Perogy Slice	1 med	280	13	13	–	28	0	330
Szechuan Individual	1 pie	750	39	17	–	99	1	800
Szechuan Slice	1 med	200	10	4	–	27	0	210
Tandoori Individual	1 pie	730	40	24	–	90	2	940
Tandoori Slice	1 med	200	11	6	–	25	tr	260
Thai Chicken Individual	1 pie	840	45	28	–	108	4	1090
Thai Chicken Slice	1 med	240	12	8	–	30	1	300
The Basic Individual	1 pie	620	34	16	–	88	1	1140
The Basic Slice	1 med	160	9	4	–	24	0	310
Tropical Chicken Individual	1 pie	970	59	39	–	97	tr	1690
Tropical Chicken Slice	1 med	260	15	10	–	26	0	450
Tuscan Individual	1 pie	940	50	37	–	106	5	1650
Tuscan Slice	1 med	250	13	10	–	29	1	460

FOOD	PORTION	CALS	PROT	FAT	CHOL	CARB	FIBER	SOD
Ultimate Pepperoni Individual	1 pie	870	46	37	–	89	2	2010
Ultimate Pepperoni Slice	1 med	230	12	9	–	24	tr	550
Vegetarian Individual	1 pie	680	37	16	–	101	4	1160
Vegetarian Slice	1 med	180	9	4	–	26	1	320
Zorba The Greek Individual	1 pie	800	43	29	–	97	4	1400
Zorba The Greek Slice	1 med	210	11	8	–	26	1	390
SALAD DRESSINGS AND TOPPINGS								
House Dressing	1 serv (2 oz)	270	1	28	–	4	tr	210
Ketchup	1 serv (2 oz)	60	1	1	–	15	tr	460
Salsa	1 serv (2 oz)	20	1	1	–	3	tr	350
Sour Cream	1 serv (2 oz)	100	2	9	–	3	0	0
SALADS								
Chipotle Chicken & Bacon	1 serv	630	28	41	–	40	6	1040
Crispy Chicken Pecan	1 serv	1100	62	86	–	25	6	1310
Entree Caesar	1 serv	500	13	38	–	29	4	920
Entree Spinach	1 serv	450	13	41	–	9	3	890
Garden Greens w/ House Dressing	1 serv	310	3	29	–	13	4	230
Garden Greens w/ Low Fat Raspberry Vinaigrette	1 serv	130	2	6	–	19	3	160
Side Caesar	1 serv	170	5	11	–	13	1	300
Starter Spinach	1 serv	250	9	22	–	6	2	510
Taco Salad Beef w/o Sour Cream & Salsa	1 serv	610	31	33	–	50	6	830
Taco Salad Chicken w/o Sour Cream & Salsa	1 serv	480	31	19	–	48	6	990
Thai Chicken Salad	1 serv	1060	61	40	–	117	12	1020
SANDWICHES								
Beef Dip w/ Fries & Au Jus	1 serv	1340	77	62	–	118	5	3330
Boston Brute w/ Caesar Salad & Au Jus	1 serv	820	40	30	–	99	4	2660
Boston Cheesesteak w/ Caesar Salad & Au Jus	1 serv	1300	86	66	–	90	3	3350
Buffalo Chicken w/ Fries	1 serv	1220	55	53	–	130	7	4200
Chicken Parmesan w/ Fries	1 serv	1370	53	81	–	107	7	1810
Ciabatta Chicken w/ Caesar Salad	1 serv	920	40	53	–	73	4	1130
New York Steak w/ Garden Greens & Au Jus	1 serv	660	43	39	–	32	2	870

FOOD	PORTION	CALS	PROT	FAT	CHOL	CARB	FIBER	SOD
Stromboli Bacon Double Cheeseburger w/ Caesar Salad	1 serv	910	34	38	–	111	3	4230
Stromboli Chicken Santa Fe w/ Caesar Salad	1 serv	750	33	22	–	106	4	940
Stromboli Smoked Ham & Chicken w/ Caesar Salad	1 serv	880	52	31	–	99	1	820
Wrap Thai Chicken	1	570	26	9	–	98	6	1260
SOUPS								
Baked French Onion	1 serv	330	17	14	–	40	3	2480
Clam Chowder	1 serv	260	9	14	–	18	0	910
BRUEGGER'S BAGELS								
BAGELS								
Asiago Parmesan	1	330	14	4	5	62	4	640
Baked Apple	1	370	12	3	0	77	5	660
Blueberry	1	330	11	2	0	67	4	530
Chocolate Chip	1	350	12	5	0	64	4	570
Cinnamon Sugar	1	330	11	2	0	69	4	510
Cranberry Orange	1	330	11	2	0	68	4	510
Everything	1	320	12	2	0	64	4	740
Garlic	1	320	12	2	0	65	4	560
Honey Grain	1	330	13	3	0	65	5	510
Jalapeno Bagel	1	320	12	2	0	64	4	560
Multi-Grain	1	350	12	4	0	68	6	540
Onion	1	320	12	2	0	64	4	560
Plain	1	320	12	2	0	64	4	560
Poppy	1	320	12	3	0	64	4	560
Pumpernickel	1	330	12	3	0	67	12	620
Pumpkin	1	330	11	2	0	68	6	500
Rosemary Olive Oil	1	350	12	7	0	64	4	540
Salt	1	320	12	2	0	64	4	1610
Sesame	1	360	13	3	0	68	4	660
Sourdough	1	340	13	2	0	68	4	640
Square Asiago Parmesan	1	360	15	5	5	66	4	740
Square Everything	1	320	12	2	0	64	4	740
Square Plain	1	350	13	3	0	70	4	670
Square Sesame	1	360	13	3	0	68	4	660
Sun Dried Tomato	1	320	12	2	0	64	4	640
Whole Wheat	1	390	16	6	0	73	9	680

FOOD	PORTION	CALS	PROT	FAT	CHOL	CARB	FIBER	SOD
DESSERTS								
Brownie Chocolate Chunk	1	330	4	18	55	40	2	150
Cake Lemon Pound	1 slice	320	5	13	75	48	tr	170
Cookie Chocolate Chip	1	500	5	22	40	71	3	300
Cookie Oatmeal Raisin	1	460	5	19	40	71	3	240
Cookie Peanut Butter	1	480	8	23	40	63	2	300
Cookie Triple Chocolate Chunk	1	560	6	28	35	71	3	350
Cookie White Chocolate Macadamia	1	580	6	31	35	70	1	360
Luscious Lemon Bar	1	300	3	16	95	36	0	120
Marshmallow Chew	1	280	2	6	10	55	0	330
Muffin Blueberry	1	450	8	19	65	64	3	290
Muffin Chocolate	1	460	6	24	30	57	3	250
Oreo Dream Bar	1	470	5	28	60	49	2	270
Pecan Chocolate Chunk	1 slice	310	3	19	40	32	1	160
Raspberry Sammies	1 slice	340	3	16	45	44	1	170
Seven Layer Bar	1	650	10	43	10	58	5	280
Toffee Almond Bar	1	400	4	19	50	53	1	340
SALADS								
Caesar w/ Dressing	1 serv	270	9	17	40	22	2	900
Tossed Chicken Caesar w/ Dressing	1 serv	370	27	20	85	23	2	1420
Tossed Mandarin Medley	1 serv	340	8	17	20	36	4	660
Tossed Sesame Chicken	1 serv	480	22	28	45	30	2	780
SANDWICHES								
BLT w/ Mayo	1	570	20	23	35	72	5	1060
Chicken Breast	1	660	47	11	95	87	5	780
Chicken Fajita	1	530	30	11	80	81	6	1040
Chicken Salad w/ Mayo	1	630	28	26	80	73	5	1080
Cranberry Gobbler	1	620	32	21	55	78	5	1430
Cuban Chicken	1	680	44	25	85	74	4	2180
Denver Egg	1	460	30	18	205	74	5	1150
Egg Cheese	1	420	23	18	195	71	4	1090
Egg Cheese Bacon	1	460	28	23	210	65	4	980
Egg Cheese Ham	1	460	31	18	210	73	4	1270
Egg Cheese Sausage	1	640	32	38	235	72	5	1130
Ham	1	460	27	7	30	76	5	2110
Herby Turkey	1	560	30	14	45	78	5	1310
Leonardo Da Veggie	1	480	21	12	30	74	5	870

FOOD	PORTION	CALS	PROT	FAT	CHOL	CARB	FIBER	SOD
Radishy Roast Beef	1	560	35	18	60	73	5	1270
Roadhouse Chicken	1	710	50	19	100	84	4	1600
Roast Beef	1	730	30	36	65	71	5	1280
Santa Fe Turkey	1	490	30	9	50	75	5	1450
Smoked Salmon	1	490	28	10	45	74	5	770
Softwich BLT w/ Mayo	1	600	22	25	40	73	5	1220
Softwich Chicken Breast	1	630	47	11	95	81	5	800
Softwich Chicken Fajita	1	570	39	10	20	81	6	1180
Softwich Chicken Salad	1	670	32	27	95	76	5	1220
Softwich Cranberry Gobbler	1	730	40	28	80	80	5	1750
Softwich Cuban Chicken	1	810	56	32	125	77	4	2740
Softwich Garden Veggie	1	380	15	3	0	76	6	680
Softwich Ham	1	510	29	6	40	85	5	1770
Softwich Herby Turkey	1	580	33	14	50	80	5	1490
Softwich Hummus	1	540	20	13	0	85	11	930
Softwich Leonardo Da Veggie	1	550	25	15	40	79	6	1160
Softwich Mediterranean	1	790	30	33	45	90	11	1280
Softwich Peanut Chicken	1	590	36	12	60	82	5	1810
Softwich Radishy Roast Beef	1	670	43	26	90	75	5	1540
Softwich Roadhouse Chicken	1	670	50	19	100	74	4	1620
Softwich Roast Beef	1	750	33	40	75	72	5	1350
Softwich Roasted Turkey	1	550	32	15	45	74	5	1450
Softwich Smoked Salmon	1	520	30	11	50	76	5	800
Softwich Supreme Club w/o Mayo	1	880	55	39	120	79	5	2780
Softwich Tuna Salad	1	720	26	34	45	76	5	1170
Softwich Western Wheat	1	820	30	58	225	76	8	1480
Supreme Club w/o Mayo	1	470	28	9	35	72	5	1460
Tuna Salad	1	620	23	27	35	73	5	990
Turkey	1	510	26	14	35	70	5	1290
Wrap Classic w/ Bacon	1	520	36	45	405	52	4	1120
Wrap Classic w/ Ham	1	510	40	41	420	54	4	1630
Wrap Classic w/ Sausage	1	660	38	60	435	52	4	1210
Wrap Rio Grande Bacon	1	560	34	49	415	55	4	1380
Wrap Rio Grande Ham	1	630	31	34	400	55	4	1450
Wrap Rio Grande Sausage	1	510	27	47	400	53	4	960

FOOD	PORTION	CALS	PROT	FAT	CHOL	CARB	FIBER	SOD
Wrap Sesame Chicken Salad	1	770	31	36	45	80	5	1100
Wrap Tossed Chicken Caesar	1	660	36	28	85	73	5	1740
Wrap Tossed Mandarin Medley Salad	1	630	17	25	20	87	7	980
SOUPS								
Chicken Pot Pie	1 cup	250	10	19	80	12	2	1100
Chicken Spaetzle	1 cup	120	9	5	25	12	1	1050
Chicken Wild Rice	1 cup	260	2	19	75	16	1	1170
Creamy Tomato	1 cup	150	5	9	15	16	3	820
Hearty Mushroom Barley	1 cup	110	5	2	0	18	4	790
Italian Wedding	1 cup	160	8	8	20	15	2	680
Minestrone	1 cup	120	7	2	0	21	5	780
Moroccan Stew	1 cup	140	4	3	0	26	4	330
New England Clam	1 cup	300	10	18	55	23	1	840
Sweet Potato Cheddar	1 cup	200	6	11	20	20	2	580
SPREADS								
Cream Cheese Bacon Scallion	1 scoop (1.5 oz)	140	3	12	40	5	0	150
Cream Cheese Cucumber Dill	1 scoop (1.5 oz)	140	3	13	35	3	0	120
Cream Cheese Garden Veggie	1 scoop (1.5 oz)	130	3	11	35	5	1	140
Cream Cheese Honey Walnut	1 scoop (1.5 oz)	150	3	12	35	8	tr	125
Cream Cheese Jalapeno	1 scoop (1.5 oz)	140	3	13	45	4	0	150
Cream Cheese Light Garden Veggie	1 scoop (1.5 oz)	90	6	6	25	3	0	105
Cream Cheese Light Herb Garlic	1 scoop (1.5 oz)	100	6	6	25	4	0	125
Cream Cheese Light Plain	1 scoop (1.5 oz)	100	3	6	25	4	tr	125
Cream Cheese Olive Pimento	1 scoop (1.5 oz)	140	3	13	45	3	0	130
Cream Cheese Onion & Chive	1 scoop (1.5 oz)	140	3	13	35	3	0	105
Cream Cheese Plain	1 scoop (1.5 oz)	130	3	11	40	6	tr	125

FOOD	PORTION	CALS	PROT	FAT	CHOL	CARB	FIBER	SOD
Cream Cheese Pumpkin	1 scoop (1.5 oz)	120	3	11	45	4	0	135
Cream Cheese Strawberry	1 scoop (1.5 oz)	140	3	13	30	4	0	100
Cream Cheese Wildberry	1 scoop (1.5 oz)	140	3	12	40	5	0	120
Hummus	1 scoop (2 oz)	110	5	6	0	10	0	120

BURGER KING

BEVERAGES

FOOD	PORTION	CALS	PROT	FAT	CHOL	CARB	FIBER	SOD
Apple Juice	1 (6.67 oz)	90	0	0	0	23	–	15
BK Joe Regular	1 sm	5	1	0	0	1	–	15
BK Joe Turbo	1 sm (12 oz)	10	1	0	0	1	–	20
Chocolate Milk 1% Low Fat	1 (9 oz)	180	9	3	15	31	1	140
Coke Classic	1 sm (16 oz)	140	0	0	0	39	–	0
Diet Coke	1 sm (16 oz)	0	0	0	0	0	0	15
Dr Pepper	1 sm (16 oz)	140	0	0	0	39	–	35
Iced Coffee Mocha BK Joe	1 (16 oz)	380	6	10	40	66	1	290
Icee Coco Cola	1 sm (16 oz)	110	0	0	0	31	–	10
Icee Minute Maid Cherry	1 sm (16 oz)	110	0	0	0	31	–	5
Milk 1% Low Fat	1	110	8	3	10	13	0	130
Minute Maid Orange Juice	8 oz	140	2	0	0	33	–	20
Shake Chocolate	1 sm (16 oz)	470	8	14	55	75	1	320
Shake Oreo Sundae Chocolate	1 sm (16 oz)	680	9	24	55	105	2	480
Shake Oreo Sundae Strawberry	1 sm (16 oz)	660	9	23	55	103	1	380
Shake Oreo Sundae Vanilla	1 sm (16 oz)	610	9	24	60	87	1	400
Shake Strawberry	1 sm (16 oz)	460	7	14	55	73	0	240
Shake Vanilla	1 sm (16 oz)	400	8	15	60	57	0	240
Sprite	1 sm (16 oz)	140	0	0	0	39	–	30
Water Nestle Pure Life	1 bottle (16 oz)	0	0	0	0	0	0	0

BREAKFAST SELECTIONS

FOOD	PORTION	CALS	PROT	FAT	CHOL	CARB	FIBER	SOD
Biscuit Bacon Egg & Cheese	1	410	16	25	150	31	1	1320
Biscuit Ham Egg &	1	390	16	22	145	31	1	1410
Biscuit Sausage	1	390	12	26	35	28	1	1020
Biscuit Sausage Egg & Cheese	1	530	20	37	175	31	1	1490

FOOD	PORTION	CALS	PROT	FAT	CHOL	CARB	FIBER	SOD
Croissan'wich Bacon Egg & Cheese	1	340	15	20	155	26	tr	890
Croissan'wich Double w/ Bacon Egg & Cheese	1	430	21	27	175	27	tr	1250
Croissan'wich Double w/ Ham Bacon Egg & Cheese	1	420	24	24	180	27	1	1600
Croissan'wich Double w/ Ham Egg & Cheese	1	420	27	23	185	27	1	2210
Croissan'wich Double w/ Ham Sausage Egg & Cheese	1	550	28	37	205	27	1	2040
Croissan'wich Double w/ Sausage Bacon Egg & Cheese	1	550	25	39	200	27	1	1420
Croissan'wich Double w/ Sausage Egg & Cheese	1	680	29	51	220	26	1	1590
Croissan'wich Egg & Cheese	1	300	12	17	145	26	tr	740
Croissan'wich Ham Egg & Cheese	1	340	18	18	160	26	1	1230
Croissan'wich Sausage & Cheese	1	370	14	25	50	23	tr	810
Croissan'wich Sausage Egg & Cheese	1	470	19	32	180	26	tr	1060
French Toast Sticks	3 pieces	240	4	13	0	26	1	260
Hash Browns	1 lg	620	5	40	0	60	6	1200
Hash Browns	1 sm	260	2	17	0	25	2	500
Omelet Sandwich Enormous	1	730	37	45	330	44	2	1940
Omelet Sandwich Ham	1	290	13	13	85	33	1	870
DESSERTS								
Cini-minis	1 serv	390	7	18	20	51	2	560
Dutch Apple Pie	1 serv	300	2	13	0	45	1	270
Hershey Sundae Pie	1	310	3	19	10	32	1	220
MAIN MENU SELECTIONS								
BK Chicken Fries	6 pieces	260	12	15	35	18	2	650
BK Stacker Double	1	610	34	39	125	32	1	1100
BK Stacker Quad	1	1000	62	68	240	34	1	1800
BK Stacker Triple	1	800	48	54	185	33	1	1450
BK Veggie Burger	1	420	23	16	10	46	7	1100

FOOD	PORTION	CALS	PROT	FAT	CHOL	CARB	FIBER	SOD
Cheeseburger	1	330	17	16	55	31	1	780
Cheeseburger Double	1	500	30	29	105	31	1	1030
Chicken Sandwich Original	1	660	24	40	70	52	4	1440
Chicken Sandwich Tendercrisp	1	790	33	44	70	68	5	1640
Chicken Sandwich Tendergrill	1	510	37	19	75	49	4	1180
Chicken Tenders	5 pieces	210	12	12	35	13	0	600
Chick'n Crisp Spicy Sandwich	1	480	15	31	45	36	1	870
Double Cheeseburger	1	410	25	21	85	30	1	600
French Fries No Salt Added	1 sm	230	2	13	0	26	2	240
French Fries Salted	1 lg	500	5	28	0	57	5	820
French Fries Salted	1 sm	230	2	13	0	26	2	380
Hamburger	1	290	15	12	40	30	1	560
Onion Rings	1 lg	440	6	22	0	53	5	620
Onion Rings	1 sm	140	2	7	0	18	2	210
Sandwich BK Big Fish	1	640	24	32	65	67	3	1450
The Angus Steak Burger	1	640	33	33	185	55	3	1260
Whopper	1	670	28	39	95	51	3	1020
Whopper w/ Cheese	1	760	33	47	115	52	3	1450
Whopper Double	1	900	47	57	175	51	3	1090
Whopper Double w/ Cheese	1	990	52	64	195	52	3	1520
Whopper Jr.	1	370	15	21	50	31	2	570
Whopper Jr. w/ Cheese	1	410	18	24	60	32	2	780
Whopper Triple	1	1130	67	74	255	51	3	1160
Whopper Triple w/ Cheese	1	1230	71	82	275	52	3	1590
SALAD DRESSINGS AND TOPPINGS								
Breakfast Syrup	1 serv (1 oz)	80	0	0	0	21	0	20
Croutons Garlic Parmesan	1 serv	60	1	2	0	9	0	120
Dipping Sauce Barbecue	1 serv (1 oz)	40	0	0	0	11	0	310
Dipping Sauce Honey Mustard	1 serv (1 oz)	90	0	6	10	8	0	180
Dipping Sauce Ranch	1 serv (1 oz)	140	1	15	5	1	0	95
Dipping Sauce Sweet And Sour	1 serv (1 oz)	40	0	0	0	11	0	55
Dressing Ken's Creamy Caesar	1 serv (2 oz)	210	3	21	25	4	0	610

FOOD	PORTION	CALS	PROT	FAT	CHOL	CARB	FIBER	SOD
Dressing Ken's Fat Free Ranch	1 serv (2 oz)	60	0	0	0	15	2	740
Dressing Ken's Honey Mustard	1 serv (2 oz)	270	1	23	20	15	0	520
Dressing Ken's Ranch	1 serv (2 oz)	190	1	20	20	2	0	560
Jam Grape	1 serv	30	0	0	0	7	0	0
Jam Strawberry	1 serv	30	0	0	0	7	0	0
Ketchup	1 pkg	10	0	0	0	3	0	125
Mayonnaise	1 pkg	80	0	9	10	1	0	75
SALADS								
Chicken Garden Tendercrisp	1	410	29	22	70	26	5	1080
Chicken Garden Tendergrill w/o Dressing or Croutons	1	240	33	9	80	8	4	720
Side Garden w/o Dressing	1	15	1	0	0	3	1	0
BURGERVILLE								
BEVERAGES								
Barq's Root Beer	1 (20 oz)	180	0	0	0	49	0	39
Coca Cola	1 (20 oz)	161	0	0	0	44	0	10
Diet Coke	1 (20 oz)	0	0	0	0	0	0	16
Hot Chocolate Ghirardelli	1 (12 oz)	230	4	0	10	38	2	190
House Coffee	1 (10 oz)	5	0	0	0	1	0	5
Iced Tea	1 (20 oz)	0	0	0	0	0	0	0
Iced Tea Nestea Raspberry	1 (20 oz)	127	0	0	0	34	0	15
Lemonade Odwalla	1 (20 oz)	240	0	0	0	65	0	120
Milk 2%	1 (8 oz)	121	8	5	18	12	0	122
Orange Juice Odwalla	1 (10 oz)	138	3	0	0	31	1	31
Pibb Xtra	1 (20 oz)	163	0	0	0	42	0	40
Sprite	1 (20 oz)	158	0	0	0	42	0	34
BREAKFAST SELECTIONS								
Bagel	1	310	12	1	0	63	2	700
Bagel Bacon And Egg	1	490	23	16	250	64	2	1070
Bagel Ham And Egg	1	490	28	13	260	65	2	1380
Bagel Sausage And Egg	1	640	27	31	280	64	2	1100
Breakfast Platter w/ Bacon	1 serv	730	25	49	460	55	1	1060
Breakfast Platter w/ Ham	1 serv	725	30	46	500	56	1	1570
Breakfast Platter w/ Sausage	1 serv	880	29	64	520	56	1	1090

FOOD	PORTION	CALS	PROT	FAT	CHOL	CARB	FIBER	SOD
Hash Browns	1 serv	230	2	15	0	22	0	410
Toaster Biscuit	1	320	5	9	0	31	1	210
Toaster Biscuit Bacon And Egg	1	450	16	29	580	32	1	580
Toaster Biscuit Ham And Egg	1	440	21	26	260	33	1	890
Toaster Biscuit Sausage And Egg	1	600	20	44	280	32	1	610
DESSERTS								
Cone Vanilla	1	250	5	11	50	32	0	100
Cone YoCream Frozen Yogurt	1	190	4	0	0	39	0	110
Cookie Chocolate Chunk	1	320	4	14	20	48	0	340
Cookie Oatmeal Raisin	1	290	4	8	30	50	1	270
Cookie Sugar	1	305	3	15	20	39	1	250
Cookie White Chocolate Macadamia	1	340	4	16	20	46	0	360
Strawberry Shortcake	1 serv	440	6	15	25	72	3	500
Sundae Caramel	1	380	6	15	65	56	0	160
Sundae Fresh Strawberry	1	340	6	14	60	48	1	110
Sundae Hot Fudge	1	380	7	18	60	51	0	160
Sundae Triple Berry	1	340	6	14	60	46	0	110
Sundae YoCream Caramel	1	260	4	1	5	56	0	150
Sundae YoCream Hot Fudge	1	260	5	4	0	51	0	150
Sundae YoCream Strawberry	1	220	4	0	0	48	1	100
Sundae YoCream Triple Berry	1	200	4	0	0	43	0	100
MAIN MENU SELECTIONS								
Apple Slices	1 serv	29	0	0	0	9	2	0
Cheeseburger	1	350	14	19	35	29	2	730
Cheeseburger Colossal	1	520	30	30	75	31	5	1160
Cheeseburger Double Beef	1	430	22	25	55	29	2	790
Cheeseburger Tillamook	1	630	34	40	105	31	5	1080
Cheeseburger Tillamook Pepper Bacon	1	690	39	46	120	28	5	1170
Chicken Strips	5	320	23	14	30	26	0	746
French Fries	1 serv	410	6	18	0	57	6	240

FOOD	PORTION	CALS	PROT	FAT	CHOL	CARB	FIBER	SOD
Gardenburger Spicy Black Bean	1	550	24	32	40	45	10	1140
Gardenburger The Original	1	450	18	19	30	52	8	1490
Halibut	3 pieces	320	21	16	10	24	0	720
Hamburger	1	300	12	15	25	29	2	510
Hamburger Burgerville Classic	1	510	27	30	65	30	5	910
Onion Rings Walla Walla	1 serv	810	12	48	0	83	1	1260
Sandwich Crispy Chicken	1	490	21	19	40	59	3	1300
Sandwich Deluxe Crispy Chicken	1	590	27	30	80	56	3	1430
Sandwich Halibut	1	480	18	27	20	41	2	880
Sandwich Low Fat Grilled Chicken	1	320	24	5	24	44	3	880
Sandwich Nine Grain Turkey Club	1	550	27	32	55	38	3	970
Sweet Potato Fries	1 serv	530	4	29	0	60	3	510
Turkey Burger Seasoned	1	540	36	29	60	33	5	900
Yukon Golds	1 serv	450	5	21	0	59	5	590
SALAD DRESSINGS AND TOPPINGS								
Burgerville Spread Cup	1	280	0	30	20	4	0	360
Cream Cheese	1 serv	100	2	10	30	1	0	100
Cream Cheese Light	1 serv	70	3	5	15	2	0	150
Dip BBQ Sauce	1 serv	60	1	1	0	13	0	560
Dressing Blue Cheese	1 serv	240	1	24	15	3	0	340
Dressing Caesar	1 serv	220	1	22	25	2	0	250
Dressing Honey Mustard	1 serv	210	0	20	15	6	0	200
Dressing Ranch	1 serv	195	0	21	15	2	0	315
Sauce Sweet And Sour	1 serv	90	0	4	0	12	0	120
Tartar Cup	1	260	0	28	0	2	0	360
Vinaigrette Honey Lime	1 serv	250	0	23	0	10	0	440
Vinaigrette Raspberry	1 serv	45	0	2	0	6	0	260
SALADS								
Grilled Chicken	1	430	32	27	75	16	7	650
Rogue River Smokey Blue	1	290	9	11	25	38	4	200
Side Salad	1	50	3	3	10	4	2	75
Wild Smoked Salmon & Hazelnuts	1	440	30	28	35	19	7	1000

FOOD	PORTION	CALS	PROT	FAT	CHOL	CARB	FIBER	SOD
CARL'S JR.								
BEVERAGES								
Malt Chocolate	1 (15 oz)	780	17	35	105	98	1	360
Malt Oreo Cookie	1 (15 oz)	790	18	39	105	91	1	420
Malt Strawberry	1 (15 oz)	770	17	35	105	97	0	310
Malt Vanilla	1 (15 oz)	760	17	35	105	99	0	300
Shake Chocolate	1 (14 oz)	710	14	33	100	85	1	290
Shake Oreo Cookie	1 (14 oz)	720	16	37	100	79	1	350
Shake Strawberry	1 (14 oz)	700	14	33	100	84	0	240
Shake Vanilla	1 (14 oz)	710	14	33	100	86	0	230
BREAKFAST SELECTIONS								
Breakfast Burger	1	830	37	47	275	65	3	1580
Burrito Bacon & Egg	1	570	30	33	515	37	1	990
Burrito Loaded Breakfast	1	820	38	51	595	52	2	1530
Burrito Steak & Egg	1	660	40	36	545	44	2	1690
French Toast Dips w/o Syrup	5	430	9	18	0	58	1	530
Hash Brown Nuggets	1 serv	330	3	21	0	32	3	460
Sandwich Sourdough Breakfast	1 serv	460	28	21	280	39	2	1050
Sunrise Croissant Sandwich	1	560	20	41	290	27	1	970
DESSERTS								
Cheesecake Strawberry Swirl	1 serv	290	6	17	55	30	0	230
Chocolate Cake	1 serv	300	3	12	30	48	1	350
Cookie Chocolate Chip	1	350	3	18	20	46	1	330
MAIN MENU SELECTIONS								
Burger Jalapeno	1	720	27	45	90	50	3	1320
Burger Teriyaki	1	660	28	34	80	61	3	1070
Cheeseburger Double Western Bacon	1	970	62	52	155	71	3	1820
Cheeseburger Western Bacon	1	710	32	33	85	70	3	1480
Chicken Breast Strips	3	420	23	25	50	28	1	1210
Chicken Stars	4	170	9	11	25	10	1	320
CrissCut Fries	1 serv	410	5	24	0	43	4	950
Famous Star w/ Cheese	1	660	27	39	85	53	3	1260
Fish & Chips	1 serv	630	26	28	10	68	3	990
French Fries	1 sm	290	5	14	0	37	3	180
Fried Zucchini	1 serv	320	6	19	0	31	0	850

FOOD	PORTION	CALS	PROT	FAT	CHOL	CARB	FIBER	SOD
Hamburger Big	1	470	24	17	60	54	3	1000
Hamburger Kid's	1	460	24	17	60	53	2	1060
Onion Rings	1 serv	430	6	21	0	53	2	550
Sandwich Bacon Swiss Crispy Chicken	1	720	35	35	85	64	3	1750
Sandwich Carl's Catch Fish	1	660	22	31	30	75	3	1290
Sandwich Charbroiled BBQ Chicken	1	360	34	5	60	48	4	1150
Sandwich Charbroiled Chicken Club	1	550	40	25	95	43	4	1410
Sandwich Charbroiled Santa Fe Chicken	1	610	37	32	100	43	4	1540
Sandwich Spicy Chicken	1	560	15	30	40	59	2	1480
Six Dollar Burger The Bacon Cheese	1	1070	46	76	170	50	3	1010
Six Dollar Burger The Guacamole Bacon	1	1140	43	86	160	54	6	2010
Six Dollar Burger The Jalapeno	1	1030	39	74	150	52	3	2050
Six Dollar Burger The Low Carb	1	490	33	37	130	6	2	1290
Six Dollar Burger The Original	1	1010	40	68	150	60	3	1980
Six Dollar Burger The Western Bacon	1	1130	47	66	150	83	4	2540
Super Star w/ Cheese	1	930	47	59	160	54	3	1600
SALAD DRESSINGS								
Blue Cheese	1 serv (2 oz)	320	2	34	20	1	0	410
House	1 serv (2 oz)	220	1	22	20	2	0	440
Italian Fat Free	1 serv (2 oz)	15	0	0	0	4	0	770
Low Fat Balsamic	1 serv (2 oz)	35	0	15	0	5	0	480
Thousand Island	1 serv (2 oz)	240	0	23	20	7	0	460
SALADS								
Charbroiled Chicken	1	260	34	7	75	16	5	710
Side	1	50	3	3	5	5	2	60

CARVEL

FOOD	PORTION	CALS	PROT	FAT	CHOL	CARB	FIBER	SOD
Brown Bonnet	1	370	3	21	55	40	0	105
Cake Ice Cream	1 slice	270	4	14	35	33	1	135
Carvelanche Cake Mix	1 reg (16 oz)	720	13	27	85	106	0	540

FOOD	PORTION	CALS	PROT	FAT	CHOL	CARB	FIBER	SOD
Carvelanche Cookies & Cream	1 reg (16 oz)	550	7	30	120	64	0	280
Carvelanche Triple Fudge Cake Mix	1 reg (16 oz)	900	16	41	65	134	4	300
Chipsters	1	330	4	16	40	44	4	220
Cone Cake Chocolate	1 lg	600	13	30	80	71	3	310
Cone Cake Chocolate	1 sm	260	6	13	35	32	1	135
Cone Cake Vanilla	1 lg	650	9	36	180	68	0	300
Cone Cake Vanilla	1 sm	280	4	16	75	31	0	135
Cone Sugar Chocolate	1 sm	300	7	13	40	40	1	160
Cone Sugar Vanilla	1 sm	320	5	15	75	39	0	160
Cone Waffle Chocolate	1 lg	660	15	30	80	86	3	340
Cone Waffle Chocolate	1 sm	330	7	13	47	47	2	160
Cone Waffle Vanilla	1 lg	710	10	36	180	83	1	330
Cone Waffle Vanilla	1 sm	350	5	16	75	46	1	160
Dashers Banana Barge	1	940	17	46	110	121	7	250
Dashers Bananas Foster	1	600	6	24	100	90	2	350
Dashers Fudge Brownie	1	810	9	42	120	98	4	400
Dashers Mint Chocolate Chip	1	720	8	39	110	85	2	350
Dashers Peanut Butter Cup	1	1090	20	63	55	97	4	630
Dashers Strawberry Shortcake	1	590	8	29	100	78	2	170
Flying Saucer 98% Fat Free Chocolate	1	180	5	3	0	34	1	160
Flying Saucer 98% Fat Free Vanilla	1	180	5	3	0	35	1	170
Flying Saucer Chocolate	1	230	4	10	20	33	1	125
Flying Saucer Deluxe Sprinkles	1	330	4	15	40	47	1	120
Flying Saucer Vanilla	1	240	4	11	45	33	1	170
Ice Cream Chocolate	1 sm (4 oz)	250	6	13	35	29	0	130
Ice Cream Vanilla	1 sm (4 oz)	240	3	14	70	25	0	115
Ice Cream No Fat Chocolate	1 sm (4 oz)	160	3	0	0	37	0	55
Ice Cream No Fat Vanilla	1 sm (4 oz)	160	5	0	0	33	0	75
Sherbet All Flavors	1 sm (4 oz)	180	1	2	5	39	0	70
Sinful Love Bar	1	460	4	29	25	47	5	220
Sprinkle Cup	1	230	2	15	45	28	1	75
Sundae Bittersweet Fudge	1 reg	690	8	38	77	77	1	280

FOOD	PORTION	CALS	PROT	FAT	CHOL	CARB	FIBER	SOD
Sundae Caramel	1 reg	670	8	34	145	81	0	360
Sundae Hot Fudge	1 reg	670	8	38	145	73	1	280
Sundae Strawberry	1 reg	580	7	33	145	63	1	210
Sundae Mini Chocolate Syrup	1	200	2	9	45	27	0	85
Thick Shake Chocolate	1 reg (16 oz)	650	14	27	70	93	2	320
Thick Shake Vanilla	1 reg (16 oz)	610	10	28	135	81	0	260
Thinny Thin Classic Sundae No Fat Fudge	1 reg	380	8	2	0	81	0	180
Thinny Thin Classic Sundae No Fat Strawberry	1 reg	320	8	0	0	69	1	150
Thinny Thin Miniature Sundae No Fat	1	190	4	0	0	45	0	95
Thinny Thin Miniature Sundae No Sugar Added	1	200	5	3	15	42	0	125
Thinny Thin No Fat Carvelanche Strawberry	1 (16 oz)	430	12	0	0	91	1	160
Thinny Thin No Fat Chocolate	1 sm	160	3	0	0	37	0	55
Thinny Thin No Fat Vanilla	1 sm	160	5	0	0	33	0	75
Thinny Thin No Sugar Added Vanilla	1 sm	180	7	3	20	34	0	115
Thinny Thin Parfait No Fat	1	190	4	0	0	42	0	95
Thinny Thin Shake No Fat Chocolate	1 (16 oz)	440	5	0	0	104	0	190
Thinny Thin Shake No Fat Mocha	1 (16 oz)	440	10	0	0	97	0	230
Thinny Thin Shake No Fat Vanilla	1 (16 oz)	300	9	0	0	62	0	135

CHICKEN OUT ROTISSERIE

MAIN MENU SELECTIONS

FOOD	PORTION	CALS	PROT	FAT	CHOL	CARB	FIBER	SOD
1/4 Dark Chicken w/ Skin	1 serv	337	36	18	125	5	1	903
1/4 Dark Chicken w/o Skin	1 serv	223	31	10	107	1	0	247
Apple Cornbread Stuffing	1 serv (7 oz)	453	9	21	38	58	2	1612
Baked Potato Wedges	1 serv (8 oz)	220	4	6	0	39	6	260
Chunky Cinnamon Applesauce	1 serv (7 oz)	241	1	4	9	52	5	36

FOOD	PORTION	CALS	PROT	FAT	CHOL	CARB	FIBER	SOD
Cranberry Relish	1 serv (7 oz)	285	1	2	45	69	3	64
Creamed Spinach	1 serv (6 oz)	320	9	25	75	16	3	1190
Edamame Beans In Sweet Pepper Sauce	1 serv (7 oz)	200	17	8	0	18	8	75
Farm Fresh Cole Slaw	1 serv (7 oz)	226	2	17	9	18	3	417
Fresh Fruit Salad	1 serv (7 oz)	110	1	0	0	29	3	10
Grilled Chicken Filet Skinless	1 (6 oz)	290	53	6	145	3	0	660
Half Sandwich BBQ & Cole Claw	1	340	30	7	75	41	2	1115
Half Sandwich Classic Grilled Chicken	1	405	67	33	175	55	1	1370
Half Sandwich Signature Chicken Salad	1	305	17	22	55	10	1	545
Just The Turkey Burger	1 (7 oz)	360	42	27	100	65	5	2000
Macaroni & Cheese	1 serv (7 oz)	290	10	72	10	46	6	640
Mashed Sweet Potatoes	1 serv (7 oz)	423	4	1	0	102	4	120
Pulled BBQ Chicken	1 serv (6 oz)	360	44	7	125	27	0	1860
Pulled Rotisserie Chicken Breast	1 serv (6 oz)	290	53	6	145	3	0	610
Red Skin Mashed Potatoes	1 serv (7 oz)	334	5	16	42	44	4	1317
Sandwich Hot Openfaced Pulled Chicken On Biscuit	1	1180	72	47	225	113	7	3470
Steamed Vegetable Medley	1 serv (7 oz)	30	2	0	0	6	2	25
Wrap Apricot Chicken Salad	½	412	24	19	51	37	3	835
Wrap Asian Chicken Salad	½	341	22	12	46	35	2	684
Wrap BBQ Chicken w/ Cole Slaw	½	395	32	9	73	43	2	1517
Wrap Chopped Veggie	½	315	23	7	48	40	4	630
Wrap Cobb Salad	½	430	27	21	125	32	3	950
Wrap Freshly Roasted Turkey w/ Cucumber Sauce	½	325	24	14	65	27	3	445
Wrap Garden Veggie & Cheese	½	352	16	18	36	32	3	842
Wrap Grilled Chicken	½	359	22	15	50	32	2	693
Wrap Grilled Chicken Caesar	½	386	24	18	54	31	2	711
Wrap Santa Fe	½	371	24	16	50	34	3	961

FOOD	PORTION	CALS	PROT	FAT	CHOL	CARB	FIBER	SOD
Wrap Spinach & Milan Cutlet	½	315	22	7	45	43	4	770
SALAD DRESSINGS								
Buttermilk Ranch	1 oz	110	0	11	10	1	0	280
Creamy Caesar	1 oz	181	1	20	9	0	0	237
Creamy Cole Slaw	1 oz	125	0	11	0	6	0	252
Honey Balsamic Vinaigrette	1 oz	161	0	16	2	4	0	58
Honey Mustard Fat Free	1 oz	50	0	0	0	11	0	150
Southwest	1 oz	146	0	16	7	2	1	222
SALADS								
Apricot Chicken Salad	1 serv (6 oz)	610	49	36	135	23	3	930
Asian Chicken w/o Dressing or Wontons	1 serv	325	41	9	96	21	7	441
Caesar Grilled Chicken w/o Dressing or Croutons	1 serv	310	45	10	111	10	5	556
Caesar w/o Dressing Croutons or Roll	1 serv	90	7	4	10	8	5	109
Chicken Cobb	1 serv	720	62	29	385	48	7	1760
Chopped Veggie & Chicken w/o Dressing or Croutons	1 serv	300	42	5	95	25	9	530
Freshly Roasted Turkey Breast	1 serv	320	45	10	100	13	7	260
Garden Grilled Chicken w/o Dressing or Croutons	1 serv	269	40	5	96	17	6	474
Green Leaf Fruit & Granola	1 serv	380	10	11	0	67	11	200
Milan Chicken Cutlet	1 serv	348	53	7	132	17	4	568
Santa Fe Chicken w/o Dressing or Tortilla Strips	1 serv	399	47	15	126	22	8	606
Signature Chicken Salad	1 serv (6 oz)	790	44	58	145	22	2	1440
Spinach w/ Milan Cutlet	1 serv	550	47	22	110	46	8	910
SOUPS								
Chicken Noodle	1 serv (13 oz)	211	30	6	80	9	1	396
Vegetable Primavera	1 serv (13 oz)	330	26	7	45	45	10	1580

CHIPOTLE

FOOD	PORTION	CALS	PROT	FAT	CHOL	CARB	FIBER	SOD
Barbacoa	1 serv (4 oz)	228	27	13	59	1	0	544
Black Beans	1 serv (4 oz)	130	9	1	0	22	12	318

FOOD	PORTION	CALS	PROT	FAT	CHOL	CARB	FIBER	SOD
Carnitas	1 serv (4 oz)	227	29	12	66	0	0	873
Cheese	1 serv (1 oz)	110	7	9	30	tr	0	180
Chicken	1 serv (4 oz)	219	29	11	96	0	0	431
Chips	1 serv (4 oz)	490	7	19	0	71	5	130
Crispy Taco Shells	3	180	3	7	0	26	2	30
Fajita Vegetables	1 serv (3 oz)	100	1	8	0	6	1	640
Flour Tortilla	1 (6 inch)	300	9	8	0	48	6	630
Flour Tortilla	1 (13 inch)	330	9	8	0	55	5	710
Guacamole	1 serv (4 oz)	170	2	15	0	8	5	370
Lettuce	1 serv (1 oz)	5	tr	0	0	tr	tr	0
Pinto Beans	1 serv (4 oz)	138	9	1	0	23	10	374
Rice	1 serv (3.5 oz)	168	3	5	0	28	tr	427
Salsa Corn	1 serv (4 oz)	100	3	1	0	22	3	540
Salsa Tomato	1 serv (4 oz)	25	1	0	0	6	1	560
Sour Cream	1 serv (2 oz)	120	2	10	40	2	0	30
Steak	1 serv (4 oz)	230	29	12	51	2	0	306
Tomatillo Green	1 serv (2 oz)	15	1	tr	0	3	1	227
Tomatillo Red	1 serv (2 oz)	28	1	1	0	4	1	493
Vinaigrette	1 serv (2 oz)	282	0	26	17	11	0	1525
CHURCH'S CHICKEN								
DESSERTS								
Pie Apple	1 pie (3 oz)	280	2	11	5	39	1	250
Pie Edward's Double Lemon	1 pie (3 oz)	300	5	14	25	39	0	160
Pie Edward's Strawberry Cream Cheese	1 pie (2.8 oz)	280	4	15	15	32	2	130
MAIN MENU SELECTIONS								
Biscuit Honey Butter	1	240	3	12	<5	28	1	540
Cajun Rice	1 reg	130	1	7	5	16	tr	260
Chicken Fried Steak w/ White Gravy	1 serv (7.5 oz)	610	24	43	70	31	2	1465
Cole Slaw	1 reg	150	1	10	5	15	2	170
Corn On The Cob	1 ear	140	4	3	0	24	9	15
Country Fried Steak w/ White Gravy	1 serv (5.8 oz)	470	21	28	65	36	1	1620
Crunchy Tenders	1 (2 oz)	120	12	6	35	6	tr	440
French Fries	1 reg	290	3	14	0	38	4	320
Jalapeno Cheese Bombers	4 (4 oz)	240	8	10	30	29	3	970

FOOD	PORTION	CALS	PROT	FAT	CHOL	CARB	FIBER	SOD
Macaroni & Cheese	1 reg	210	8	11	15	23	1	690
Mashed Potatoes & Gravy	1 reg	70	2	2	tr	12	1	480
Okra	1 reg	350	3	22	0	36	5	590
Original Breast	1	200	22	11	80	3	1	450
Original Leg	1	110	10	6	55	3	0	280
Original Thigh	1	330	21	23	110	8	1	680
Original Wing	1	300	27	19	120	7	3	540
Sandwich Bigger Better Chicken w/ Cheese	1	510	20	27	50	46	4	1070
Sandwich Country Fried Steak	1	490	13	32	30	38	2	880
Sandwich Spicy Fish	1	320	10	20	25	25	2	560
Spicy Breast	1	320	21	20	75	12	1	760
Spicy Crunchy Tenders	1 (2 oz)	135	11	7	25	7	4	480
Spicy Fish Fillet	1 piece (2.3 oz)	160	7	9	25	13	1	350
Spicy Leg	1	180	12	11	65	8	1	470
Spicy Thigh	1	480	22	35	135	20	2	1035
Spicy Wing	1	430	29	27	125	17	2	1020
Sweet Corn Nuggets	1 reg	600	7	29	0	72	5	1260
Whole Jalapeno Peppers	2	10	0	0	0	2	1	390
SAUCES								
BBQ	1 pkg	30	0	0	0	7	0	180
Creamy Jalapeno	1 pkg	100	0	11	10	1	0	140
Honey	1 pkg	27	0	0	0	7	0	0
Honey Mustard	1 pkg	110	0	11	10	4	0	130
Hot Sauce	1 pkg	0	0	0	0	0	0	210
Ketchup	1 pkg	18	0	0	0	5	0	190
Purple Pepper	1 pkg	45	0	0	0	12	0	26
Ranch	1 pkg	130	0	13	10	1	0	320
Sweet & Sour	1 pkg	30	0	0	0	8	0	120

CICI'S

FOOD	PORTION	CALS	PROT	FAT	CHOL	CARB	FIBER	SOD
EXTRAS								
Apple Pizza	1 slice	149	3	4	0	26	1	193
Brownie	1	143	1	6	0	22	1	96
Cinnamon Roll	1	139	2	6	0	20	1	99
Garlic Bread	1 slice	99	4	5	5	10	tr	120
PIZZA								
Buffet 12 Inch Alfredo	1 slice	139	8	5	10	18	1	199

FOOD	PORTION	CALS	PROT	FAT	CHOL	CARB	FIBER	SOD
Buffet 12 Inch Bacon Cheddar	1 slice	145	6	5	13	18	3	312
Buffet 12 Inch Bar-B-Que	1 slice	172	8	6	12	21	2	311
Buffet 12 Inch Beef	1 slice	170	9	7	20	18	1	281
Buffet 12 Inch Cheese	1 slice	152	7	5	9	20	1	305
Buffet 12 Inch Ham & Pineapple	1 slice	141	7	4	10	19	1	319
Buffet 12 Inch Ole	1 slice	108	5	4	7	13	2	261
Buffet 12 Inch Pepperoni	1 slice	175	8	7	13	21	2	384
Buffet 12 Inch Pepperoni & Jalapeno	1 slice	163	8	6	11	20	2	394
Buffet 12 Inch Sausage	1 slice	197	8	7	11	19	1	358
Buffet 12 Inch Spinach Alfredo	1 slice	151	7	5	11	20	2	215
Buffet 12 Inch Zesty Ham & Cheese	1 slice	153	6	6	9	18	1	271
Buffet 12 Inch Zesty Pepperoni	1 slice	157	6	7	7	18	1	302
Buffet 12 Inch Zesty Tomato Alfredo	1 slice	136	6	5	10	18	2	202
Buffet 12 Inch Zesty Veggie	1 slice	124	5	4	4	17	1	224
To-Go 15 Inch Bar-B-Que	1 slice	289	13	10	17	36	2	446
To-Go 15 Inch Cheese	1 slice	223	11	8	17	28	3	428
To-Go 15 Inch Ham & Pineapple	1 slice	225	11	8	21	27	2	394
To-Go 15 Inch Ole	1 slice	169	7	4	8	26	3	350
To-Go 15 Inch Pepperoni	1 slice	240	11	10	21	27	3	504
To-Go 15 Inch Spinach Alfredo	1 slice	243	11	8	18	32	3	347
To-Go 15 Inch Zesty Pepperoni	1 slice	246	10	12	12	26	2	475
To-Go 15 Inch Zesty Veggie	1 slice	213	9	9	7	25	2	394
CINNABON								
BAKED SELECTIONS								
Caramel Pecanbon	1	1100	16	56	63	141	8	600
Cinnabon Bites	6	520	8	16	10	78	2	530
Cinnabon Classic	1	813	15	32	67	117	4	801
Cinnabon Stix	1	379	6	21	16	41	1	413
Cinnamon Filled Churro	1	281	5	11	–	39	–	–

FOOD	PORTION	CALS	PROT	FAT	CHOL	CARB	FIBER	SOD
Minibon	1	339	6	13	27	49	2	337
BEVERAGES								
Caramelatta Chill	1 (16 oz)	520	12	19	75	76	0	250
Chillatta Cappuccino	1 (16 oz)	330	5	11	35	56	1	120
Chillatta Caramel	1 (16 oz)	480	8	18	65	72	0	270
Chillatta Chocolate Mocha	1 (16 oz)	460	8	14	45	72	3	270
Chillatta Mango	1 (16 oz)	340	6	11	40	57	0	105
Chillatta Strawberry	1 (16 oz)	330	5	11	40	54	0	105
Chillatta Strawberry Banana	1 (16 oz)	350	5	11	40	58	0	105
Chillatta Tropical Blast	1 (16 oz)	330	2	7	20	69	–	50
Mochalatta Chill	1 (16 oz)	450	11	18	60	66	1	310

CORNER BAKERY

FOOD	PORTION	CALS	PROT	FAT	CHOL	CARB	FIBER	SOD
BREAKFAST SELECTIONS								
Baked French Toast	1 serv	570	13	15	–	86	1	530
Buckhead Cheese Grits	1 serv	350	11	22	–	19	2	310
Fresh Berry Parfait	1 serv	330	–	–	–	–	–	–
Oatmeal	1 serv	280	12	7	–	41	3	320
Oatmeal Crunchy Honey Banana	1 serv	380	12	3	–	78	5	280
Oatmeal Swiss	1 serv	330	4	1	–	79	6	5
Panini Ham & Cheddar	1	720	42	34	–	57	2	1990
Panini Smoked Bacon & Cheddar	1	680	33	34	–	56	2	1990
Scrambler All American w/o Potatoes & Bread	1 serv	310	23	22	–	3	0	870
Scrambler Anaheim w/o Potatoes & Bread	1 serv	490	30	36	–	10	4	620
Scrambler Farmer's w/o Potatoes & Bread	1 serv	430	31	31	–	6	1	980
The Commuter Croissant	1	720	29	46	–	44	2	1390
PASTA								
Chicken Carbonara	1 serv	740	51	28	–	70	4	890
Half Moon Cheese Ravioli	1 serv	550	28	21	–	63	4	880
Penne w/ Marinara	1 serv	550	20	11	–	92	14	1080
Pesto Cavatappi	1 serv	930	52	40	–	93	13	830
SALAD DRESSINGS								
Caesar	1 serv	310	1	32	–	2	0	530
House	1 serv	280	0	27	–	8	0	680

FOOD	PORTION	CALS	PROT	FAT	CHOL	CARB	FIBER	SOD
Ranch	1 serv	160	2	16	–	2	0	440
Vinaigrette Balsamic	1 serv	300	0	31	–	4	0	10
SALADS								
Caesar	1 serv	520	11	44	–	19	5	970
Caesar w/ Roasted Chicken & Croutons	1 serv	640	27	49	–	8	5	1500
Chopped w/o Bread	1 serv	810	40	61	–	27	10	2340
Harvest	1 serv	860	19	68	–	53	10	930
Harvest w/ Roasted Chicken	1 serv	980	37	72	–	53	10	1460
Santa Fe Ranch	1 serv	680	19	44	–	56	10	1960
Santa Fe Ranch w/ Roasted Chicken	1 serv	800	37	49	–	56	10	1800
Side Cucumber Tomato	1 (6 oz)	120	1	9	–	9	2	170
Side Egg	1 (6 oz)	570	16	53	–	2	0	650
Side Roasted Potato Bacon	1 (6 oz)	370	8	23	–	29	3	1030
Side Seasonal Fruit Medley	1 (6 oz)	90	1	0	0	22	2	20
Side Tomato Mozzarella Pasta	1 (6 oz)	205	7	8	–	24	4	230
Side Tuna	1 (6 oz)	310	34	16	–	3	1	670
SANDWICHES								
Bavarian w/ Ham	1	720	40	25	–	78	4	3390
Bavarian w/ Turkey	1	690	39	22	–	78	4	3470
Chicken Pesto	1	840	41	41	–	75	5	2470
Panini California Grille	1	700	29	41	–	59	8	1480
Panini Chicken Pomodori	1	890	47	45	–	74	5	2230
Panini Club	1	900	50	48	–	72	4	2810
Panini Corned Beef Reuben	1	930	44	48	–	76	2	2500
Panini Grilled Ham & Swiss	1	880	45	44	–	75	4	2610
Southwest Roast Beef	1	840	44	37	–	78	5	2060
Tomato Mozzarella	1	670	28	26	–	73	5	1630
Tuna Salad On Olive Bread	1	450	29	16	–	42	3	1080
Turkey Derby	1	650	39	29	–	60	5	2620
Turkey Frisco	1	850	44	38	–	79	9	2920
Uptown Turkey	1	660	39	29	–	61	9	3020
SOUPS								
Big Al's Chili w/ Cheddar Cheese	1 (10 oz)	380	23	17	–	29	8	1450
Bread Bowl	1	420	12	30	–	21	2	1370
Cheddar	1 (10 oz)	310	9	23	–	16	2	1090

FOOD	PORTION	CALS	PROT	FAT	CHOL	CARB	FIBER	SOD
Chicken Wild Mushroom Brie Stew	1 (10 oz)	260	11	14	–	20	2	1110
Loaded Baked Potato w/ Garnish	1 (10 oz)	420	13	29	–	29	2	990
Mom's Chicken Noodle	1 (10 oz)	170	8	4	–	23	1	1440
Old Fashioned Beef Stew	1 (10 oz)	260	7	13	–	20	2	1050
Roasted Poblano Corn Chowder	1 (10 oz)	330	4	21	–	34	4	770
Roasted Tomato Basil w/o Garnish	1 (10 oz)	170	3	5	–	27	4	1220
Zesty Chicken Tortilla w/ Tortilla Strips	1 (10 oz)	230	8	11	–	26	5	1340

D'ANGELO'S

FOOD	PORTION	CALS	PROT	FAT	CHOL	CARB	FIBER	SOD
CHILDREN'S MENU SELECTIONS								
D'Lite Turkey	1	217	19	3	14	30	3	369
Sub Cheeseburger	1	294	15	13	43	28	3	459
Sub Ham & Cheese	1	227	14	5	30	32	1	997
Sub Kidz Tuna	1	438	15	29	18	30	1	614
Sub Meatball	1	330	15	15	37	37	4	812
SALAD DRESSINGS								
Bleu Cheese	1 serv	152	1	15	15	3	0	283
Caesar	1 serv	397	6	43	43	6	0	1191
Caesar Fat Free	1 serv	57	0	0	0	9	0	1673
Creamy Italian	1 serv	340	0	37	0	9	0	851
Greek w/ Feta Cheese	1 serv	227	0	26	14	6	0	765
Honey Mustard	1 serv	150	0	142	0	7	0	210
Olive Oil Vinaigrette	1 serv	170	0	17	0	9	0	652
Ranch Lite	1 serv	240	2	19	20	6	1	961
SALADS								
Antipasto	1 serv	284	16	18	40	17	6	1109
Caesar w/ Dressing	1 serv	474	15	39	40	25	4	1208
Chicken Caesar w/ Dressing	1 serv	533	35	38	99	19	4	1654
Chicken Stir Fry w/o Dressing	1 serv	168	25	3	59	11	4	590
Cobb w/o Dressing	1 serv	292	27	17	76	11	4	636
Greek	1 serv	290	11	23	50	17	4	1098
Lobster w/o Dressing	1 serv	376	26	26	86	12	4	589
Roast Beef w/o Dressing	1 serv	131	19	3	42	10	4	208
Steak Tip Caesar	1 serv	661	32	50	95	21	3	1627

FOOD	PORTION	CALS	PROT	FAT	CHOL	CARB	FIBER	SOD
Tossed Garden w/o Dressing	1 serv	49	3	1	0	11	4	22
Turkey w/o Dressing	1 serv	157	26	2	22	10	4	86
SANDWICHES								
D'Lite Chicken Caesar Salad	1	374	34	7	68	43	4	2002
D'Lite Chicken Stir Fry	1	426	37	6	73	57	7	1241
D'Lite Classic Veggie	1	362	15	7	13	63	8	839
D'Lite Fresh Veggie	1	348	13	7	13	62	7	651
D'Lite Grilled Chicken Breast	1	388	31	7	67	52	6	953
D'Lite Roast Beef	1	338	25	5	42	51	6	727
D'Lite Turkey	1	347	28	4	19	51	6	595
D'Lite Turkey Cranberry	1	444	28	4	19	75	6	595
Pokket Big Papi	1	469	39	11	84	53	3	2536
Pokket BLT & Cheese	1	397	22	17	50	38	3	1266
Pokket Caesar Salad	1	616	20	39	40	54	3	1518
Pokket Capicola & Cheese	1	362	26	13	60	35	2	1547
Pokket Cheese	1	519	29	27	74	41	2	1765
Pokket Cheeseburger	1	459	27	25	85	31	2	811
Pokket Chicken Caesar Salad	1	674	40	39	99	47	3	1964
Pokket Chicken Club	1	526	34	28	87	36	2	1088
Pokket Chicken Honey Dijon	1	508	41	20	111	40	2	1165
Pokket Chicken Salad	1	623	27	42	71	34	2	639
Pokket Chicken Stir Fry	1	380	35	9	79	39	2	1276
Pokket Classic Vegetable	1	368	19	13	33	46	4	934
Pokket Classic Veggie No Cheese	1	212	9	1	0	44	4	331
Pokket Greek	1	790	16	61	50	49	4	1892
Pokket Grilled Chicken	1	303	29	5	67	35	2	739
Pokket Ham	1	229	17	3	33	35	2	1050
Pokket Ham & Cheese	1	326	22	10	53	38	2	1493
Pokket Ham & Salami	1	386	23	17	56	34	12	1301
Pokket Hamburger	1	399	24	20	72	29	2	343
Pokket Italian	1	525	28	30	80	36	2	1678
Pokket Lobster	1	530	29	31	84	34	2	897
Pokket Meatball	1	574	26	31	73	52	4	1765
Pokket Mortadella & Cheese	1	410	21	21	56	35	2	1114

FOOD	PORTION	CALS	PROT	FAT	CHOL	CARB	FIBER	SOD
Pokket Number 9	1	407	31	18	76	31	2	685
Pokket Pastrami	1	438	24	25	91	33	1	1643
Pokket Pepperoni	1	407	21	20	47	35	3	1147
Pokket Roast Beef	1	247	23	3	42	33	2	511
Pokket Salad	1	196	8	1	0	40	4	340
Pokket Salami & Cheese	1	509	25	30	75	33	2	1590
Pokket Seafood Salad	1	449	14	22	11	50	3	1182
Pokket Steak	1	305	25	12	59	24	1	324
Pokket Steak & Cheese	1	377	29	17	74	26	1	665
Pokket Steak Bomb	1	631	43	32	102	44	3	1794
Pokket Steak Tip	1	452	27	16	54	45	2	1189
Pokket Tuna	1	664	24	49	32	33	2	825
Pokket Turkey	1	256	26	2	19	33	2	379
Pokket Turkey Club	1	332	34	7	54	32	2	610
Sub Big Papi	1 sm	525	40	15	83	60	7	2700
Sub BLT & Cheese	1 sm	463	23	19	50	51	6	1437
Sub Capicola & Cheese	1 sm	408	25	13	50	48	5	1482
Sub Cheese	1 sm	589	30	28	74	55	5	1939
Sub Cheeseburger	1 sm	526	29	26	86	44	5	774
Sub Chicken Club	1	593	35	29	87	49	5	1260
Sub Chicken Honey Dijon	1	575	42	22	111	53	5	1338
Sub Chicken Salad	1 sm	692	29	44	71	48	5	813
Sub Chicken Stir Fry	1 sm	449	37	11	79	53	6	1449
Sub Classic Veggie	1 sm	462	21	15	34	64	8	1162
Sub Grilled Chicken	1 sm	369	30	7	67	48	5	911
Sub Ham	1 sm	302	18	5	33	49	2	1226
Sub Ham & Cheese	1 sm	395	24	11	53	52	2	1667
Sub Ham & Salami	1 sm	456	25	19	56	48	2	1475
Sub Hamburger	1 sm	466	25	22	73	42	5	503
Sub Italian	1 sm	614	30	31	80	54	3	1893
Sub Lobster	1 sm	598	30	33	84	48	5	1089
Sub Meatball	1 sm	644	28	33	73	66	7	1939
Sub Meatballs & Cheese	1 sm	750	36	41	94	67	7	2204
Sub Mortadella & Cheese	1 sm	479	23	23	56	49	5	1288
Sub Number 9	1 sm	450	31	19	74	41	4	802
Sub Pastrami	1 sm	613	34	34	118	47	5	1875
Sub Pepperoni	1 sm	603	28	33	72	49	7	1836
Sub Roast Beef	1 sm	320	25	5	42	48	5	687
Sub Salad	1 sm	281	10	3	0	57	8	522
Sub Salami & Cheese	1 sm	579	27	32	75	47	5	1764

FOOD	PORTION	CALS	PROT	FAT	CHOL	CARB	FIBER	SOD
Sub Seafood Salad	1 sm	498	14	23	10	61	6	1208
Sub Steak	1 sm	373	27	14	59	37	4	491
Sub Steak & Cheese	1 sm	446	31	19	74	40	4	832
Sub Steak Bomb	1 sm	670	43	33	102	52	6	1904
Sub Steak Tip	1 sm	545	29	18	54	63	3	1413
Sub Tuna	1	685	24	46	29	47	2	952
Sub Turkey Club	1 sm	401	33	9	48	49	3	806
Sub Toasted Italian Bistro	1 sm	585	29	31	81	49	5	1912
Sub Toasted Pastrami Reuben	1 sm	750	30	47	104	55	7	2226
Sub Toasted Roast Beef & Cheddar	1 sm	564	35	26	88	51	5	1117
Sub Toasted Spicy Meatball	1 sm	933	61	57	102	71	9	2560
Sub Toasted Tuna & Swiss	1 sm	796	32	54	55	49	5	1027
Sub Toasted Turkey & Ham	1 sm	532	33	24	66	49	5	1507
Sub Toasted Turkey Thanksgiving	1 sm	705	32	20	21	80	6	1315
Wrap Big Papi	1	593	41	23	83	56	4	2859
Wrap BLT & Cheese	1	544	24	26	50	54	4	1542
Wrap Buffalo Chicken Salad	1	823	40	44	101	67	4	2917
Wrap Caesar Salad	1	711	20	44	40	65	5	1679
Wrap Capicola & Cheese	1	494	25	20	50	53	4	1589
Wrap Cheese	1	675	30	35	74	59	4	2046
Wrap Cheeseburger	1	609	30	33	86	48	3	879
Wrap Chicken Caesar Salad	1	830	42	47	99	65	5	2246
Wrap Chicken Cobb	1	931	36	55	102	71	6	1790
Wrap Chicken Filet & Bacon	1	639	38	28	87	58	2	1078
Wrap Chicken Honey Dijon	1	672	60	29	110	43	5	1466
Wrap Chicken Salad	1	782	29	51	71	53	4	922
Wrap Chicken Stir Fry	1	535	37	17	79	57	4	1557
Wrap Classic Veggie	1	486	24	13	34	68	5	936
Wrap Greek	1	765	15	61	50	44	4	1723
Wrap Grilled Chicken	1	422	34	6	67	59	4	733
Wrap Ham & Cheese	1	435	26	10	53	60	3	1481
Wrap Ham & Salami	1	513	30	18	63	57	3	1449
Wrap Hamburger	1	509	28	21	74	50	3	340
Wrap Italian	1	631	32	29	80	59	3	1667
Wrap Lobster	1	749	33	43	86	57	3	954
Wrap Meatball	1	687	31	31	73	75	5	1755
Wrap Mortadella & Cheese	1	522	25	21	56	58	3	1103

FOOD	PORTION	CALS	PROT	FAT	CHOL	CARB	FIBER	SOD
Wrap Number 9	1	517	32	24	74	44	3	885
Wrap Pastrami	1	550	28	25	91	55	2	1632
Wrap Peppercorn Steak	1	702	41	40	110	45	3	1745
Wrap Pepperoni	1	519	25	21	47	57	4	1136
Wrap Roast Beef	1	448	26	13	42	58	4	881
Wrap Salad	1	324	13	2	0	66	6	337
Wrap Salami & Cheese	1	605	29	29	72	56	3	1510
Wrap Seafood Salad	1	541	17	22	10	69	3	1024
Wrap Steak	1	392	28	13	59	41	2	316
Wrap Steak & Cheese	1	464	33	18	74	43	2	657
Wrap Steak Bomb	1	670	43	33	102	52	6	1904
Wrap Steak Tip	1	432	26	16	54	41	2	1029
Wrap Tuna	1	731	27	44	29	56	3	769
Wrap Turkey	1	369	30	3	19	55	3	369
Wrap Turkey Club	1	415	34	8	48	52	3	590
SOUPS								
Beef Stew	1 sm	220	12	8	30	23	2	819
Broccoli & Cheddar Cheese	1 sm	270	9	21	60	11	2	859
Chicken Noodle	1 sm	110	6	3	25	14	1	829
Hearty Vegetable	1 sm	40	2	0	0	7	2	270
Italian Wedding	1 sm	120	6	6	15	11	2	919
Lobster Bisque	1 sm	360	8	29	105	16	1	819
New England Clam Chowder	1 sm	320	9	18	60	31	1	699
Portuguese Kale	1 sm	130	8	4	10	16	3	629

DENNY'S

BEVERAGES

FOOD	PORTION	CALS	PROT	FAT	CHOL	CARB	FIBER	SOD
Apple Juice	1 sm (10 oz)	141	0	0	0	52	0	28
Cappuccino	1 (8 oz)	100	3	2	0	28	1	220
Chocolate Milk	1 sm (10 oz)	160	8	3	10	26	1	150
Hot Chocolate	1 (8 oz)	100	3	2	0	28	1	219
Iced Tea Raspberry	1 serv (16 oz)	78	0	0	0	21	0	0
Lemonade	1 serv (15 oz)	150	0	0	0	35	0	38
Milk	1 sm (10 oz)	130	8	5	20	12	0	100
Orange Juice	1 sm (10 oz)	140	2	0	0	34	0	0
Ruby Red Grapefruit	1 sm (10 oz)	164	1	0	0	40	0	41
Tomato Juice	1 sm (10 oz)	56	2	0	0	11	2	680

FOOD	PORTION	CALS	PROT	FAT	CHOL	CARB	FIBER	SOD
BREAKFAST SELECTIONS								
All American Slam w/o Choices	1 serv (10 oz)	800	40	68	775	5	1	1410
Bacon Strips	4	140	9	11	30	1	0	467
Bacon Turkey	4 slices	150	17	8	65	1	0	650
Banana	1	110	1	0	0	29	4	–
Egg	1 (2 oz)	120	6	11	210	0	0	125
Egg Whites	1 serv (4 oz)	50	11	1	0	1	0	180
English Muffin w/o Margarine	1	130	4	1	0	25	1	250
Grand Slam Slugger w/o Choices	1 serv (13 oz)	780	29	42	475	71	3	1930
Grapes	1 serv (3 oz)	55	1	0	0	29	4	0
Grits w/ Margarine	1 serv (12 oz)	220	5	3	0	44	3	15
Ham Slice Grilled Honey	1 (3 oz)	120	14	5	45	8	0	710
Hash Browns	1 serv	210	2	12	0	26	2	650
Hashed Browns Cheddar Cheese	1 serv (5 oz)	300	8	19	20	26	2	780
Hashed Browns Everything	1 serv (8 oz)	340	8	21	20	33	2	1010
Lumberjack Slam w/o Choices	1 serv (15 oz)	940	46	47	555	80	4	2900
Moon Over My Hammy Omelette w/ Hash Browns w/o Choices	1 serv (16 oz)	770	42	53	790	31	2	2590
Oatmeal w/ Milk	1 serv (16 oz)	290	12	8	20	39	4	300
Omelette Southern w/ Hash Browns w/o Bread	1 serv (18 oz)	1070	38	80	795	47	4	2500
Omelette Veggie Cheese w/o Choices	1 serv (13 oz)	460	28	33	740	9	2	680
Omelette w/ Hash Browns w/o Choices	1 serv (16 oz)	700	38	46	770	32	2	2180
Pancakes Buttermilk	2	330	8	4	0	67	2	1170
Platter Chocolate Chip Pancakes w/o Meat	1 serv (13 oz)	640	24	22	480	87	4	1480
Sausage Links	4 (3 oz)	370	9	34	70	4	3	660
Senior Omelette w/o Choices	1 serv (9 oz)	470	26	37	510	7	1	820

FOOD	PORTION	CALS	PROT	FAT	CHOL	CARB	FIBER	SOD
Senior Scrambled Eggs & Cheddar	1 serv (13 oz)	870	35	48	525	72	4	2200
Senior Slam Belgian Waffle w/ Egg w/o Choices	1 serv (8 oz)	450	15	31	455	29	0	640
Skillet Bananas Foster French Toast w/o Meat	1 serv (15 oz)	860	32	33	720	107	3	1270
Slam Belgian Waffle w/ Margarine w/o Syrup	1 serv (13 oz)	1030	30	77	715	50	2	1765
Slam Everyday Value w/ Bacon	1 serv (12 oz)	650	25	30	440	69	2	1660
Slam Everyday Value w/ Sausage	1 serv (13 oz)	760	25	42	460	70	3	1750
Slam French Toast	1 serv (15 oz)	940	42	55	850	66	3	1780
Ultimate Omelette w/o Choices	1 serv (12 oz)	620	36	48	740	8	2	1170
CHILDREN'S MENU SELECTIONS								
Jr Grand Slam	1 serv (5 oz)	380	15	19	235	39	2	1000
Oreo Blender Blaster	1 serv (12 oz)	680	12	33	90	88	3	450
Pancake Softball w/ Meat	1 serv (4 oz)	250	7	11	20	30	1	730
Pancakes Chocolate Chip-In	1 serv (7 oz)	450	11	18	25	61	3	1160
Pit Stop Pizza w/o Side	1 serv (8 oz)	590	23	26	35	70	5	890
Slam Dribblers	1 serv (6 oz)	410	9	11	10	74	2	750
Slap Shot Slider w/o Side	1 (4 oz)	310	20	15	60	22	1	470
Spaghetti Set Go w/o Side	1 serv (6 oz)	260	7	7	0	40	7	470
Track & Cheese w/o Side	1 serv (7 oz)	340	12	11	25	48	2	830
DESSERTS								
Apple Crisp A La Mode	1 serv (13 oz)	740	7	21	35	134	5	570
Blender Blaster Oreo	1 serv (14 oz)	890	15	44	105	113	3	580
Cake Carrot	1 serv (8 oz)	820	9	45	125	100	2	660
Cake Hershey's Chocolate	1 serv (5 oz)	580	6	28	40	75	2	400
Cheesecake New York Style	1 serv (7 oz)	640	9	41	195	58	0	350
Float Rootbeer or Cola	1 (16 oz)	430	6	17	65	69	0	120
Hot Fudge Brownie A La Mode	1 serv (9 oz)	830	9	37	65	122	4	520
Milkshake	1 (12 oz)	560	11	26	100	76	tr	272

FOOD	PORTION	CALS	PROT	FAT	CHOL	CARB	FIBER	SOD
Pie Apple	1 serv (7 oz)	480	4	22	0	67	3	580
Pie Chocolate Peanut Butter Silk	1 serv (6 oz)	680	8	47	70	59	4	400
Pie Coconut Cream	1 serv (7 oz)	630	6	39	0	65	1	370
Pie Cookies & Cream	1 serv (7 oz)	630	5	39	5	67	3	510
Pie French Silk	1 serv (5 oz)	770	6	57	105	59	2	400
Pie Key Lime	1 serv (7 oz)	560	9	20	25	87	0	320
Pie Lemon Merinque	1 serv (7 oz)	500	2	19	0	82	1	380
Pie Pecan	1 serv (7 oz)	730	7	36	110	98	2	740
Pie Pumpkin	1 serv (7 oz)	500	8	18	80	77	3	570
Sundae Oreo	1 (9 oz)	760	9	37	60	103	3	470
Sundae Single Scoop	1 (4 oz)	300	4	16	40	36	1	90
Topping Cherry	1 serv (2 oz)	57	0	0	0	14	0	3
Topping Chocolate	1 serv (2 oz)	133	2	1	0	34	1	109
Topping Fudge	1 serv (2 oz)	201	1	10	3	30	1	96
Topping Strawberry	1 serv (2 oz)	77	1	1	0	17	1	8
MAIN MENU SELECTIONS								
Basket Of Puppies w/o Syrup	10 pieces	520	11	11	0	94	3	1640
Burger Bacon Cheddar w/o Choices	1 (15 oz)	900	60	50	160	50	3	1850
Burger Classic & Fries	1 serv (19 oz)	1190	56	62	110	101	8	1190
Burger Fit Fare Veggie w/o Choice	1 (10 oz)	460	29	10	20	65	8	1040
Burger Mushroom Swiss w/o Choices	1 (18 oz)	880	50	49	130	56	4	1800
Burger Veggie w/ Dressing w/o Choices	1 (11 oz)	520	29	12	20	75	9	1250
Burger Western w/o Choice	1 (17 oz)	1120	51	61	130	73	6	1580
Cheeseburger Double w/o Choices	1 serv (23 oz)	1420	87	87	260	53	4	2720
Chicken Strips Sweet & Tangy BBQ w/o Dipping Sauce	1 serv (13 oz)	820	58	30	115	83	58	2160
Chicken Strips w/ Buffalo Sauce	1 serv (13 oz)	720	57	32	115	52	0	2780
Chicken Wings Sweet & Tangy BBQ	1 serv (8 oz)	450	35	18	185	40	1	1400

FOOD	PORTION	CALS	PROT	FAT	CHOL	CARB	FIBER	SOD
Chicken Wings w/ Buffalo Sauce	1 serv (8 oz)	330	34	20	185	3	1	1860
Chopped Steak Mushroom Swiss w/o Choices	1 serv (13 oz)	900	54	66	165	13	1	1890
Chopped Steak Spicy Cowboy w/o Choices	1 serv (15 oz)	1050	55	63	170	57	3	1700
Club Sandwich w/o Choices	1 (10 oz)	550	24	32	50	39	3	1530
Coleslaw	1 serv (5 oz)	260	2	22	35	15	3	520
Corn	1 serv (4 oz)	130	4	3	0	26	1	250
Cottage Cheese	1 serv (3 oz)	70	9	2	10	5	0	300
Country Fried Steak w/ Gravy	1 serv (13 oz)	990	52	65	75	54	6	2580
Dippable Veggies w/o Dressing	1 serv (2.5 oz)	30	0	0	0	5	1	70
Fiesta Corn	1 serv (4 oz)	100	3	0	0	21	3	45
Fit Fare Grilled Tilapia	1 serv (17 oz)	600	58	11	110	66	3	1560
Fit Fare Sweet & Tangy BBQ Chicken w/ Vegetables & Tomatoes	1 serv (13 oz)	640	75	14	180	56	2	1430
French Fries Salted	1 serv (5 oz)	430	5	23	0	50	5	95
Fried Shrimp Platter w/ Fries	1 serv (18 oz)	1050	27	59	150	109	13	2410
Garlic Dinner Bread	2 pieces	170	4	9	0	21	1	350
Green Beans	1 serv (3 oz)	25	1	0	0	4	2	10
Haddock Fillet w/o Bread	1 serv (20 oz)	1330	36	81	130	116	8	2100
Homestyle Meatloaf w/ Gravy	1 serv (7 oz)	600	4	46	200	14	0	1880
Lemon Pepper Tilapia w/o Choices	1 serv (13 oz)	640	55	27	160	39	2	1190
Mashed Potatoes Plain	1 serv (5 oz)	170	2	7	20	76	1	510
Mashed Potatoes Smoked Cheddar	1 serv (4 oz)	120	4	5	10	49	1	390
Mozzarella Sticks w/o Sauce	1 serv (8 oz)	560	38	20	185	58	2	2480
Onion Rings	1 serv (5 oz)	520	5	36	0	48	3	980
Quesadilla Cheese	1 (8 oz)	690	25	42	75	48	6	1300

FOOD	PORTION	CALS	PROT	FAT	CHOL	CARB	FIBER	SOD
Ranchero Tilapia w/o Bread	1 serv (19 oz)	450	54	15	120	56	4	1020
Sampler w/o Sauce	1 serv (17 oz)	1380	53	71	80	139	6	3710
Sandwich Bacon Lettuce & Tomato w/o Choices	1 (7 oz)	520	15	35	35	35	2	620
Sandwich Chicken Ranch Melt w/o Choices	1 serv (12 oz)	790	36	38	85	74	3	2640
Sandwich Fried Cheese Melt w/ Marinara Sauce w/o Choices	1 (12 oz)	830	36	40	75	82	3	2920
Sandwich Hickory Grilled Chicken w/o Choices	1 (15 oz)	1020	50	60	115	72	4	1530
Sandwich Patty Melt w/o Choices	1 (13 oz)	1040	50	73	160	41	4	2180
Sandwich Philly Melt Prime Rib w/o Choices	1 serv (13 oz)	670	35	36	75	52	3	1710
Sandwich Pulled BBQ Chicken w/ Coleslaw	1 serv (14 oz)	670	21	23	60	96	4	1680
Sandwich Smoked Chicken Melt w/o Choices	1 (12 oz)	840	38	45	105	72	3	1820
Sandwich Spicy Buffalo Chicken Melt w/o Choices	1 (15 oz)	860	32	48	70	76	3	3760
Sandwich The Super Bird w/o Choices	1 (11 oz)	620	35	31	65	52	4	2170
Seasoned Fries	1 serv (5 oz)	510	6	33	0	48	5	1010
Senior Country Fried Steak w/o Choices	1 serv (8 oz)	520	26	34	40	30	3	1460
Senior Grilled Chicken w/o Choices	1 serv (5 oz)	200	36	6	90	0	0	360
Senior Grilled Shrimp Skewer w/o Choices	1 serv (8 oz)	280	18	6	135	36	2	650
Senior Homestyle Meatloaf w/o Choices	1 serv (4 oz)	290	16	23	100	5	0	760
Senior Mini Burgers Bacon Cheddar w/o Choice	1 (11 oz)	720	41	39	115	46	2	1270
Senior Sandwich Club w/o Choices	1 (10 oz)	570	29	34	60	37	4	1340

FOOD	PORTION	CALS	PROT	FAT	CHOL	CARB	FIBER	SOD
Senior Sandwich Grilled Cheese Deluxe w/o Choices	1 (7 oz)	520	16	28	40	49	2	1430
Senior Slam French Toast w/ Egg	1 serv (5 oz)	300	13	14	280	29	1	550
Senior Starter w/o Choice	1 serv (3 oz)	210	9	19	230	1	1	290
Shrimp Breaded	6	190	9	8	70	20	2	750
Shrimp Grilled Skewer	1	90	14	4	135	1	0	160
Skillet Bacon Chipotle Chicken w/o Sides	1 serv (7 oz)	360	47	18	125	4	0	800
Skillet Prime Rib Premium	1 serv (21 oz)	850	41	46	540	64	7	2080
Skillet Santa Fe	1 serv (14 oz)	710	33	52	485	30	5	1490
Skillet Ultimate	1 serv (15 oz)	740	27	56	475	34	6	1470
Slamburger Bacon w/ Fries	1 serv (15 oz)	1030	57	59	350	61	2	1780
Smoothered Cheese Fries	1 serv (10 oz)	860	21	53	65	75	7	990
Spinach Sauteed	1 serv (2 oz)	70	1	6	0	5	2	125
Spinach w/ Pico De Gallo & Spinach	1 serv (3 oz)	110	3	8	5	6	2	260
T-Bone Steak w/o Choices	1 serv (12 oz)	640	59	42	135	6	0	1250
T-Bone Steak & Breaded Shrimp	1 serv (13 oz)	830	68	50	204	25	2	2000
T-Bone Steak & Shrimp Skewer	1 serv (12 oz)	730	73	46	270	6	0	1410
The Big Dipper w/ Salsa w/o Dipping Sauce	10 pieces	1230	50	50	85	145	14	1640
Three Dip & Chips	1 serv (12 oz)	560	19	25	70	72	7	1430
Tomato Slices	2	10	1	0	0	2	1	3
Tsing Tsing Chicken	1 serv (14 oz)	900	52	26	130	114	4	2760
Vegetable Rice Pilaf	1 serv (5 oz)	190	4	3	0	35	2	490
Wrap Buffalo Chicken	1 (14 oz)	830	40	28	65	108	8	2280
Zesty Nachos	1 serv (22 oz)	1340	62	61	210	140	12	2800

FOOD	PORTION	CALS	PROT	FAT	CHOL	CARB	FIBER	SOD
SALAD DRESSINGS AND TOPPINGS								
BBQ Sweet & Spicy	1 serv (1.5 oz)	110	0	0	0	30	1	470
Cherry Topping	1 serv (3 oz)	86	0	0	0	21	0	7
Croutons	1 serv (0.25 oz)	90	3	3	0	15	0	240
Dressing Bleu Cheese	1 serv (1 oz)	110	1	11	20	1	0	220
Dressing Caesar	1 serv (1 oz)	100	1	10	5	0	0	300
Dressing French	1 serv (1 oz)	74	0	5	7	8	0	248
Dressing Honey Mustard	1 serv (1 oz)	160	0	15	10	5	0	140
Dressing Italian Fat Free	1 serv (1 oz)	9	0	0	0	3	0	367
Dressing Ranch	1 serv (1 oz)	130	0	14	5	0	0	200
Dressing Ranch Fat Free	1 serv (1 oz)	25	0	0	0	5	1	230
Dressing Thousand Island	1 serv (1 oz)	107	0	10	14	5	0	275
Pico De Gallo	1 serv (3 oz)	21	1	0	0	5	1	125
Sour Cream	1 serv (1.5 oz)	91	1	9	19	2	0	23
Syrup Maple Flavored	3 tbsp (1.5 oz)	143	0	0	0	36	0	26
Syrup Sugar Free Maple	1 serv (1.5 oz)	23	0	0	0	9	0	71
Vinaigrette Balsamic Low Fat	1 serv (1 oz)	35	0	1	0	7	0	140
Whipped Margarine	1 tbsp	50	0	6	0	0	0	40
SALADS								
Cranberry Apple w/ Chicken w/o Dressing	1 serv (11 oz)	320	36	10	90	22	3	400
Deluxe Salad w/ Chicken Strips w/o Choices	1 serv (18 oz)	590	42	29	90	43	4	1180
Deluxe Salad w/ Grilled Chicken Breast w/o Choices	1 serv (17 oz)	340	44	13	110	13	4	530
Nacho	1 serv (20 oz)	850	48	52	165	48	9	2140
SOUPS								
Broccoli & Cheddar	1 serv (12 oz)	370	9	16	40	48	7	1650
Clam Chowder	1 serv (12 oz)	270	5	17	35	24	1	1840

FOOD	PORTION	CALS	PROT	FAT	CHOL	CARB	FIBER	SOD
Loaded Baked Potato	1 serv (12 oz)	310	5	23	45	22	2	1520
Vegetable Beef	1 serv (12 oz)	140	7	5	10	17	3	1290

DOMINO'S PIZZA

FOOD	PORTION	CALS	PROT	FAT	CHOL	CARB	FIBER	SOD
OTHER MENU SELECTIONS								
Breadsticks	8	870	17	50	0	89	3	780
Buffalo Chicken Kickers	1 serv	510	43	21	100	36	7	1410
Cheesy Bread	1 serv	930	28	51	50	91	3	1140
Chocolate Lava Crunch Cakes	2	690	8	34	130	93	3	340
Cinna Stix	8	940	16	49	0	109	4	690
PIZZA MEDIUM								
Deep Dish Marinara Cheese	1/8 pie	219	7	9	14	27	3	509
Hand Tossed Marinara Cheese	1/8 pie	190	7	7	16	25	1	405
Thin Crust Marinara Cheese	1/4 pie	141	5	12	16	14	1	271
TOPPINGS FOR 1 MEDIUM PIZZA								
Anchovies	1 serv	110	13	8	45	63	0	3310
Bacon	1 serv	340	20	26	80	6	0	1260
Banana Peppers	1 serv	15	1	0	0	3	2	270
Beef	1 serv	300	16	26	65	0	–	570
Cheddar Cheese	1 serv	230	14	19	60	1	0	350
Cheese American	1 serv	310	16	26	80	3	0	1530
Cheese Provolone	1 serv	200	12	16	60	1	0	470
Chicken	1 serv	140	22	5	60	3	0	730
Chorizo	1 serv	90	12	4	30	1	0	600
Feta Cheese	1 serv	90	7	6	15	1	0	380
Garlic	1 serv	40	2	0	0	9	1	0
Green Chile Pepper	1 serv	10	1	0	0	3	2	10
Green Pepper	1 serv	10	0	0	0	3	1	0
Ham	1 serv	90	11	5	35	0	0	1020
Jalapenos	1 serv	15	1	0	0	3	2	960
Mushroom	1 serv	20	3	0	0	2	1	25
Olives Black	1 serv	100	1	10	0	2	2	410
Olives Green	1 serv	100	1	10	0	2	2	1250
Onion	1 serv	15	1	0	0	4	1	0
Parmesan Shredded	1 serv	170	13	12	35	1	0	460

FOOD	PORTION	CALS	PROT	FAT	CHOL	CARB	FIBER	SOD
Pepperoni	1 serv	240	11	21	50	0	0	1020
Philly Steak	1 serv	90	12	3	30	2	0	500
Pineapple	1 serv	60	0	0	0	16	1	10
Red Pepper Roasted	1 serv	10	1	0	0	2	1	95
Salami	1 serv	220	13	18	55	1	0	950
Sausage Italian	1 serv	350	12	30	55	9	0	1030
Spinach	1 serv	10	1	0	0	2	1	35
Tomato	1 serv	20	1	0	0	5	2	310
Wing Sauce	1 serv	10	0	0	0	2	1	920

DONATOS PIZZA

PIZZA

FOOD	PORTION	CALS	PROT	FAT	CHOL	CARB	FIBER	SOD
Hand Tossed Chicken Bacon Club	2 slices	780	29	46	–	61	5	–
Hand Tossed Chicken Spinach Mozzarella	2 slices	587	27	25	–	61	4	–
Hand Tossed Chicken Vegy Medley	2 slices	517	24	17	–	63	5	–
Hand Tossed Classic Trio	2 slices	640	27	30	–	66	6	–
Hand Tossed Founder's Favorite	2 slices	678	30	31	–	66	5	–
Hand Tossed Fresh Mozzarella Trio	2 slices	690	30	34	–	66	6	–
Hand Tossed Hawaiian	2 slices	578	26	22	–	69	6	–
Hand Tossed Margherita	2 slices	583	24	27	–	60	4	–
Hand Tossed Mariachi Beef	2 slices	591	24	24	–	68	5	–
Hand Tossed Mariachi Chicken	2 slices	617	28	24	–	68	5	–
Hand Tossed Pepperoni	2 slices	499	23	27	–	65	5	–
Hand Tossed Pepperoni Zinger	2 slices	645	27	30	–	65	5	–
Hand Tossed Serious Cheese	2 slices	597	27	25	–	65	5	–
Hand Tossed Serious Meat	2 slices	735	35	37	–	66	5	–
Hand Tossed Vegy	2 slices	550	22	19	–	70	6	–
Hand Tossed Works	2 slices	669	28	31	–	68	6	–
Thicker Crust Chicken Vegy Medley Large	¼ pie	580	34	20	–	66	5	–
Thicker Crust Founder's Favorite Large	¼ pie	780	43	36	–	70	5	–

FOOD	PORTION	CALS	PROT	FAT	CHOL	CARB	FIBER	SOD
Thicker Crust Hawaiian Large	¼ pie	680	37	26	–	76	6	–
Thicker Crust Mariachi Beef Large	¼ pie	710	36	31	–	73	6	–
Thicker Crust Mariachi Chicken Large	¼ pie	710	40	28	–	74	5	–
Thicker Crust Serious Meat Large	¼ pie	850	48	42	–	71	5	–
Thicker Crust The Works Large	¼ pie	770	39	35	–	74	6	–
Thicker Crust Vegy Large	¼ pie	630	31	23	–	75	7	–
Thin Crust Chicken Medley Vegy Large	¼ pie	497	31	20	–	51	3	–
Thin Crust Classic Trio Large	¼ pie	674	35	37	–	52	3	–
Thin Crust Founder's Favorite Large	¼ pie	702	39	38	–	52	2	–
Thin Crust Hawaiian Large	¼ pie	588	32	27	–	56	4	–
Thin Crust Mariachi Beef Large	¼ pie	630	32	32	–	55	3	–
Thin Crust Mariachi Chicken Large	¼ pie	639	35	30	–	56	3	–
Thin Crust Pepperoni Large	¼ pie	627	32	34	–	50	2	–
Thin Crust Serious Cheese Large	¼ pie	710	38	31	–	69	5	–
Thin Crust Serious Meat Large	¼ pie	736	44	42	–	52	3	–
Thin Crust The Works	¼ pie	689	35	37	–	56	4	–
Thin Crust Vegy Large	¼ pie	544	26	24	–	57	4	–
SALAD DRESSINGS								
House Italian	1 serv (1.5 oz)	230	0	24	–	1	0	–
Italian Light	1 serv (1.5 oz)	20	0	1	–	2	0	–
Pizza Dip Chicken Bacon Ranch	1 serv (3 oz)	450	1	47	–	4	0	–
SALADS								
Chicken Harvest w/o Dressing Entree	1	540	32	32	–	32	6	–
Harvest Side	1 serv	81	1	3	–	13	2	–

FOOD	PORTION	CALS	PROT	FAT	CHOL	CARB	FIBER	SOD
Italian Chef w/o Dressing Entree	1	290	19	20	–	8	1	–
Italian Side w/o Dressing	1	110	7	7	–	3	1	–
SIDES AND SUBS								
3 Cheese Garlic Bread	2 pieces	174	8	9	–	16	1	–
Big Don White Italian	1	717	35	34	–	68	3	–
Breadsticks w/ Pizza Sauce	2	261	7	9	–	38	3	–
Buffalo Wings Hot	5	597	34	48	–	11	0	–
Buffalo Wings Mild	5	618	34	48	–	13	0	–
Fresh Vegy Wheat	1	532	22	19	–	71	8	–
Stromboli 3 Meat	1	689	34	31	–	67	5	–
Stromboli Cheese	1	693	35	31	–	66	5	–
Stromboli Deluxe	1	613	28	25	–	68	5	–
Stromboli Pepperoni	1	716	34	34	–	67	5	–
Stromboli Vegy	1	606	27	24	–	69	5	–

DUNKIN' DONUTS

FOOD	PORTION	CALS	PROT	FAT	CHOL	CARB	FIBER	SOD
BAGELS								
Blueberry	1	330	11	3	0	65	5	620
Cinnamon Raisin	1	330	11	4	0	65	5	450
Everything	1	350	13	5	0	66	5	660
Garlic	1	340	12	3	0	68	6	660
Multigrain	1	390	14	8	0	65	9	560
Onion	1	310	11	2	0	63	3	380
Plain	1	320	11	3	0	63	5	660
Poppy Seed	1	350	13	6	0	64	5	660
Salt	1	320	11	3	0	63	5	3420
Sesame	1	360	13	6	0	63	5	660
Wheat	1	320	12	4	0	61	5	550
BAKED SELECTIONS								
Apple Fritter	1	400	5	15	0	63	2	530
Biscuit	1	280	5	14	0	32	1	620
Bismark Chocolate Iced	1	350	4	14	0	53	1	460
Brownie	1	430	3	23	55	56	1	260
Coffee Roll	1	370	5	18	0	49	2	510
Coffee Roll Chocolate Frosted	1	380	5	19	0	50	2	530
Coffee Roll Maple Frosted	1	380	5	18	0	50	2	520
Coffee Roll Vanilla Frosted	1	380	5	18	0	50	2	520
Cookie Chocolate Chunk	1	540	7	23	50	80	3	550
Cookie Oatmeal Raisin	1	480	8	14	40	83	5	310

FOOD	PORTION	CALS	PROT	FAT	CHOL	CARB	FIBER	SOD
Croissant Plain	1	310	7	16	0	35	1	350
Danish Apple Cheese	1	330	4	16	0	41	1	270
Danish Cheese	1	330	5	17	5	39	1	270
Danish Strawberry Cheese	1	320	4	16	0	40	1	260
Donut Apple Crumb	1	460	4	14	0	80	2	330
Donut Apple N' Spice	1	240	3	11	0	32	1	320
Donut Bavarian Kreme	1	250	3	12	0	31	1	330
Donut Blueberry Cake	1	330	3	18	25	38	1	460
Donut Blueberry Crumb	1	470	4	14	0	84	2	330
Donut Boston Kreme	1	280	3	12	0	38	1	350
Donut Bow Tie	1	310	4	15	0	39	1	400
Donut Chocolate Coconut	1	340	3	18	0	42	2	400
Donut Chocolate Frosted	1	340	3	19	25	38	1	330
Donut Chocolate Glazed Cake	1	280	3	15	0	33	1	400
Donut Chocolate Kreme Filled	1	310	4	16	0	37	1	340
Donut Cinnamon	1	290	3	18	25	30	1	310
Donut Double Chocolate Cake	1	290	3	16	0	34	1	410
Donut Glazed	1	220	3	9	0	31	1	320
Donut Glazed Cake	1	320	3	18	25	37	1	310
Donut Jelly Filled	1	260	3	11	0	36	1	330
Donut Maple Frosted	1	230	3	10	0	33	1	330
Donut Marble Frosted	1	230	3	10	0	32	1	330
Donut Old Fashioned	1	280	3	18	25	27	1	310
Donut Powdered	1	300	3	18	25	30	1	310
Donut Strawberry Frosted	1	230	3	10	0	33	1	330
Donut Sugar Raised	1	190	3	9	0	22	1	320
Donut Triple Chocolate	1	420	4	27	0	41	2	410
Donut Vanilla Kreme Filled	1	320	3	17	0	37	1	340
Eclair	1	350	4	14	0	53	1	460
English Muffin	1	160	6	2	0	31	2	340
French Cruller	1	250	2	20	35	18	0	105
Fritter Glazed	1	400	5	15	0	63	2	530
Muffin Blueberry	1	510	6	16	15	87	2	490
Muffin Blueberry Reduced Fat	1	450	6	10	15	86	2	670
Muffin Chocolate Chip	1	630	8	23	20	98	3	520
Muffin Coffee Cake	1	660	7	26	20	98	1	530

FOOD	PORTION	CALS	PROT	FAT	CHOL	CARB	FIBER	SOD
Muffin Corn	1	510	6	17	20	84	1	860
Muffin Cranberry Orange Low Fat	1	390	7	3	55	83	4	540
Muffin Honey Bran Raisin	1	500	7	14	15	86	5	450
Muffin Triple Chocolate	1	660	7	33	10	84	4	460
Munchkin Glazed Cake	1	60	1	3	5	8	0	65
Munchkins Cinnamon Cake	1	60	1	3	5	6	0	60
Munchkins Glazed	1	50	1	3	0	7	0	65
Munchkins Glazed Chocolate Cake	1	60	1	3	0	8	0	90
Munchkins Jelly Filled	1	60	1	3	0	8	0	65
Munchkins Plain Cake	1	50	1	3	5	5	0	60
Munchkins Powdered Cake	1	60	1	4	5	6	0	60
Munchkins Sugar Raised	1	40	1	3	0	5	0	65
Stick Cinnamon Cake	1	310	3	20	25	30	1	300
Stick Glazed Cake	1	340	3	20	25	38	1	300
Stick Glazed Chocolate Cake	1	390	3	25	0	40	2	540
Stick Jelly	1	400	3	20	25	54	1	320
Stick Plain Cake	1	300	3	20	25	26	1	300
Stick Powdered Cake	1	320	3	20	25	31	1	300
BEVERAGES								
Cappuccino	1 sm (10 oz)	80	4	4	15	7	0	70
Cappuccino Frozen w/ Skim Milk	1 sm (16 oz)	280	5	0	0	62	0	105
Cappuccino Frozen w/ Whole Milk	1 sm (16 oz)	300	5	4	15	61	0	105
Cappuccino w/ Sugar	1 sm (10 oz)	140	4	4	15	24	0	70
Coffee Blueberry	1 sm (10 oz)	15	0	0	0	2	0	5
Coffee Caramel	1 sm (10 oz)	10	0	0	0	2	0	5
Coffee Cinnamon	1 sm (10 oz)	15	0	0	0	2	0	5
Coffee Coconut	1 sm (10 oz)	10	0	0	0	1	0	5
Coffee French Vanilla	1 sm (10 oz)	10	0	0	0	1	0	5
Coffee Hazelunt	1 sm (10 oz)	10	0	0	0	1	0	5
Coffee Mocha	1 sm (10 oz)	110	1	0	0	26	1	20
Coffee Mocha w/ Cream	1 sm (10 oz)	170	2	6	20	27	1	30
Coffee Raspberry	1 sm (10 oz)	15	0	0	0	2	0	5
Coffee Regular	1 med (14 oz)	10	1	0	0	1	0	10
Coffee Regular	1 extra lg	15	1	0	0	2	0	15
Coffee Regular	1 sm (10 oz)	5	0	0	0	1	0	5

FOOD	PORTION	CALS	PROT	FAT	CHOL	CARB	FIBER	SOD
Coffee Regular	1 lg (20 oz)	10	1	0	0	2	0	15
Coffee Toasted Almond	1 sm (10 oz)	10	0	0	0	1	0	5
Coffee White Chocolate	1 sm (10 oz)	110	1	0	0	25	0	75
Coffee White Chocolate w/ Cream	1 sm (10 oz)	160	2	6	20	26	0	85
Coffee w/ Cream	1 sm (10 oz)	60	1	6	20	2	0	20
Coffee w/ Cream & Sugar	1 sm (10 oz)	120	1	6	20	19	0	20
Coffee w/ Milk	1 sm (10 oz)	25	1	1	5	2	0	20
Coffee w/ Milk & Sugar	1 sm (10 oz)	80	1	1	5	20	0	20
Coffee w/ Skim Milk	1 sm (10 oz)	15	2	0	0	3	0	25
Coffee w/ Skim Milk & Splenda	1 sm (10 oz)	25	2	0	0	5	0	25
Coffee w/ Skim Milk & Sugar	1 sm (10 oz)	70	2	0	0	20	0	25
Coffee w/ Splenda	1 sm (10 oz)	15	0	0	0	3	0	5
Coffee w/ Sugar	1 sm (10 oz)	60	0	0	0	18	0	5
Coolatta Coffee w/ Cream	1 sm (16 oz)	400	3	23	80	49	0	75
Coolatta Coffee w/ Milk	1 sm (16 oz)	240	4	4	15	50	0	90
Coolatta Coffee w/ Skim Milk	1 sm (16 oz)	210	4	0	0	51	0	90
Coolatta Strawberry Fruit	1 sm (16 oz)	300	0	0	0	72	0	40
Coolatta Tropicana Orange	1 sm (16 oz)	220	1	0	0	52	0	35
Coolatta Vanilla Bean	1 sm (16 oz)	430	3	6	20	90	0	170
Dunkaccino	1 sm (10 oz)	230	2	11	10	35	1	190
Espresso	1 (1.75 oz)	0	0	0	0	0	0	0
Espresso w/ Sugar	1 (1.75 oz)	30	0	0	0	7	0	5
Hot Chocolate	1 sm (10 oz)	210	2	7	0	39	2	270
Iced Coffee	1 sm (16 oz)	10	1	0	0	2	0	5
Iced Coffee Mocha w/ Cream	1 sm (16 oz)	180	2	6	20	28	1	35
Iced Coffee White Chocolate w/ Cream	1 sm (16 oz)	170	2	6	20	27	1	85
Iced Coffee w/ Cream	1 sm (16 oz)	70	1	6	20	3	0	20
Iced Coffee w/ Cream & Sugar	1 sm (16 oz)	120	1	6	20	20	0	20
Iced Coffee w/ Milk	1 sm (16 oz)	30	2	1	5	3	0	20
Iced Coffee w/ Milk & Sugar	1 sm (16 oz)	90	2	1	5	21	0	20
Iced Coffee w/ Skim Milk	1 sm (16 oz)	20	2	0	0	2	0	25
Iced Coffee w/ Skim Milk & Sugar	1 sm (16 oz)	80	2	0	0	21	0	25

FOOD	PORTION	CALS	PROT	FAT	CHOL	CARB	FIBER	SOD
Iced Coffee w/ Sugar	1 sm (16 oz)	70	1	0	0	19	0	5
Iced Latte	1 sm (16 oz)	120	6	6	25	10	0	105
Iced Latte Caramel Swirl	1 sm (16 oz)	220	8	6	25	35	0	150
Iced Latte Caramel Swirl w/ Skim Milk	1 sm (16 oz)	180	9	0	0	36	0	150
Iced Latte Lite	1 med (24 oz)	120	10	0	0	19	0	170
Iced Latte Mocha Swirl	1 sm (16 oz)	220	7	6	25	35	1	115
Iced Latte Mocha Swirl w/ Skim Milk	1 sm (16 oz)	180	8	0	0	36	1	125
Iced Latte w/ Skim Milk	1 sm (16 oz)	70	7	0	0	11	0	110
Iced Latte w/ Skim Milk & Sugar	1 sm (16 oz)	130	7	0	0	28	0	110
Iced Latte w/ Sugar	1 sm (16 oz)	170	6	7	25	27	0	100
Latte	1 sm (10 oz)	120	6	6	25	10	0	105
Latte Caramel Swirl	1 sm (10 oz)	220	8	6	25	35	0	150
Latte Lite	1 sm (10 oz)	80	7	0	0	13	0	110
Latte Lite Vanilla	1 sm (10 oz)	90	7	0	0	14	0	110
Latte Mocha Raspberry	1 med (16 oz)	340	10	9	35	54	2	160
Latte Mocha Spice	1 med (16 oz)	330	10	9	35	53	2	140
Latte Mocha Swirl	1 sm (10 oz)	220	7	6	25	35	1	115
Latte w/ Sugar	1 sm (10 oz)	170	6	6	25	27	0	100
Latte White Chocolate	1 med (16 oz)	320	9	9	40	50	0	250
Tea Regular Or Decaffeinated	1 (10 oz)	0	0	0	0	0	0	5
Tea w/ Milk	1 (10 oz)	20	1	1	5	1	0	20
Tea w/ Milk & Sugar	1 (10 oz)	80	1	1	5	19	0	20
Tea w/ Skim Milk	1 (10 oz)	10	1	0	0	2	0	20
Tea w/ Skim Milk & Sugar	1 (10 oz)	70	1	0	0	19	0	20
Tea w/ Sugar	1 (10 oz)	60	0	0	0	17	0	5
Turbo Shot	1 sm (1.75 oz)	0	0	0	0	0	0	0
CREAM CHEESE								
Blueberry Reduced Fat	1 serv (1.75 oz)	150	2	9	25	15	0	210
Onion & Chive Reduced Fat	1 serv (1.75 oz)	130	3	11	35	6	0	250

FOOD	PORTION	CALS	PROT	FAT	CHOL	CARB	FIBER	SOD
Plain	1 serv (1.75 oz)	150	3	15	40	3	0	250
Plain Reduced Fat	1 serv (1.75 oz)	100	4	8	25	5	0	250
Salmon Reduced Fat	1 serv (1.75 oz)	140	4	11	35	6	0	260
Strawberry Reduced Fat	1 serv (1.75 oz)	150	2	10	30	15	0	200
Veggie Reduced Fat	1 serv (1.75 oz)	120	2	10	30	6	0	240
SANDWICHES								
Bagel Bacon Egg Cheese	1	510	23	17	195	66	5	1340
Bagel Egg Cheese	1	470	20	14	195	66	5	1160
Bagel Ham Egg Cheese	1	510	26	16	215	67	5	1470
Bagel Sausage Egg Cheese	1	640	27	29	240	67	5	1560
Biscuit Egg Cheese	1	430	13	26	195	36	1	1110
Biscuit Sausage Egg Cheese	1	610	20	40	240	36	1	1510
Croissant Bacon Egg Cheese	1	510	19	31	195	39	2	1030
Croissant Egg Cheese	1	470	15	28	195	39	2	850
Croissant Ham Egg Cheese	1	510	21	30	215	39	2	1150
Croissant Original Chicken	1	640	26	35	55	53	2	1200
English Muffin Bacon Egg Cheese	1	360	18	16	195	34	2	1020
English Muffin Egg Cheese	1	320	15	13	195	34	2	840
English Muffin Egg White & Cheese	1	270	16	5	10	34	2	850
English Muffin Ham Egg Cheese	1	360	21	15	215	35	2	1140
English Muffin Ham Egg White & Cheese	1	310	22	7	30	34	2	1150
English Muffin Sausage Egg Cheese	1	490	22	28	240	35	2	1240
English Muffin Wheat Egg White & Cheese	1	260	15	6	10	33	2	870
English Muffin Wheat Ham Egg White & Cheese	1	300	21	8	30	33	2	1180
Flatbread Egg White Turkey	1	280	19	6	20	37	3	820
Flatbread Egg White Veggie	1	290	11	9	20	39	3	680
Flatbread Grilled Cheese	1	380	16	18	45	35	1	850

FOOD	PORTION	CALS	PROT	FAT	CHOL	CARB	FIBER	SOD
Flatbread Ham & Cheese	1	320	20	11	40	34	1	960
Flatbread Turkey Cheddar & Bacon	1	410	21	20	50	36	1	1110
Pressed Cuban	1	680	46	33	120	50	2	2000
SOUPS								
Broccoli Cheddar	1 serv (8 oz)	190	10	11	35	14	2	990
Chicken Noodle	1 serv (8 oz)	130	7	3	45	19	1	970

EL POLLO LOCO

FOOD	PORTION	CALS	PROT	FAT	CHOL	CARB	FIBER	SOD
DESSERTS								
Caramel Flan	1 serv (5.5 oz)	290	5	12	50	41	0	135
Churros	2	300	3	18	25	32	2	210
Cone Vanilla	1	330	8	8	35	55	0	180
Soft Serve Vanilla	1 cup (5 oz)	300	8	8	35	48	0	170
MAIN MENU SELECTIONS								
BBQ Black Beans	1 serv (6 oz)	200	7	3	0	38	4	520
Bowl The Original Pollo	1 serv	540	37	4	70	85	11	1590
Burrito BRC	1 (7.5 oz)	390	14	10	15	61	6	880
Burrito Classic Chicken	1 (10.3 oz)	500	30	14	95	63	6	1230
Burrito Twice Grilled	1 (15 oz)	830	66	37	215	58	5	2230
Burrito Ultimate Grilled	1 (13.6 oz)	650	38	20	100	80	8	1690
Chicken Breast	1 (4.3 oz)	220	36	9	140	0	0	620
Chicken Breast Skinless	1 (4 oz)	180	35	4	0	0	0	580
Chicken Leg	1 (1.8 oz)	90	12	4	70	0	0	170
Chicken Thigh	1 (3.1 oz)	220	21	15	180	0	0	320
Chicken Wing	1 (1.3 oz)	90	11	5	60	0	0	290
Cole Slaw	1 serv (6 oz)	120	1	9	5	8	2	200
Corn Cobbette	1 (5 oz)	90	2	1	0	19	2	0
French Fries	1 serv (5.5 oz)	440	6	21	0	57	6	910
Fresh Vegetables w/ Margarine	1 serv (4.1 oz)	60	2	3	0	8	3	65
Fresh Vegetables w/o Margarine	1 serv (4 oz)	35	2	0	0	8	3	35
Gravy	1 serv (1 oz)	10	0	0	0	2	0	150
Loco Nachos	1 serv	170	3	14	10	7	1	210
Macaroni & Cheese	1 serv (5.5 oz)	280	11	17	55	28	6	770
Mashed Potatoes	1 serv (5 oz)	100	2	1	0	20	2	350

FOOD	PORTION	CALS	PROT	FAT	CHOL	CARB	FIBER	SOD
Pinto Beans	1 serv (6 oz)	140	9	0	0	25	7	330
Quesadilla Cheese	1 (4.5 oz)	420	19	23	60	35	2	810
Refried Beans w/ Cheese	1 serv (6.3 oz)	270	14	7	10	36	10	730
Skinless Breast Meal	1 serv	310	35	12	105	17	5	780
Soup Chicken Tortilla w/o Tortilla Strips	1 serv (10 oz)	140	15	6	50	8	2	1040
Spanish Rice	1 serv (4.5 oz)	160	3	1	0	34	1	420
Taco Al Carbon	1 (3.1 oz)	150	11	5	40	17	1	290
Taco Soft Chicken	1 (4.5 oz)	270	17	13	75	19	2	700
Taquito Chicken	1	190	10	9	25	18	1	330
Tortilla Chips	1 serv (1.5 oz)	210	3	10	0	28	3	300
Tortilla Corn 6 Inches	2	120	2	2	0	24	2	60
Tortilla Flour 6.5 Inches	2	210	5	7	0	30	2	370
SALAD DRESSINGS AND TOPPINGS								
Creamy Cilantro	1 serv (1.5 oz)	220	1	23	20	1	0	300
Creamy Cilantro Light	1 pkg	70	1	5	5	6	0	400
Guacamole	1 serv (1 oz)	45	tr	4	0	4	tr	135
Hot Sauce Jalapeno	1 pkg	5	0	0	0	1	0	110
Italian Light	1 pkg	20	0	1	0	2	0	770
Jack & Poblano Queso	1 serv (1.8 oz)	100	3	8	<5	4	0	340
Ketchup	1 pkg	10	0	0	0	2	0	100
Pico De Gallo Medium	1 serv (1 oz)	10	0	1	0	1	0	190
Ranch	1 pkg	230	1	24	10	2	0	390
Salsa Avocado Hot	1 serv (1 oz)	30	0	3	0	1	tr	200
Salsa Chipotle Hot	1 serv (1 oz)	5	0	0	0	1	0	180
Salsa House Mild	1 serv (1 oz)	5	0	0	0	1	0	105
Sour Cream	1 serv (1 oz)	60	1	5	20	1	0	15
Thousand Island	1 pkg	220	0	21	20	6	0	350
SALADS								
Caesar Pollo	1 (11.4 oz)	520	27	38	100	17	4	980
Caesar Pollo w/o Dressing	1 (9.4 oz)	220	25	7	75	15	4	580
Garden	1 (4.8 oz)	120	5	4	15	9	2	290
Tostada Chicken	1 (17.3 oz)	840	40	40	100	76	7	1390
Tostada Chicken w/o Shell	1 (14.7 oz)	410	33	11	100	42	5	1100

FOOD	PORTION	CALS	PROT	FAT	CHOL	CARB	FIBER	SOD
EMERALD CITY SMOOTHIE								
Apple Andie	1 (11 oz)	230	11	1	5	46	2	95
Berry Berry	1 (13 oz)	350	8	0	0	77	9	25
Blueberry Blast	1 (13 oz)	380	13	0	0	78	9	110
Coconut Passion	1 (11 oz)	600	24	23	5	80	11	135
Cranberry Delight	1 (10 oz)	550	11	1	5	127	2	95
Energizer	1 (10 oz)	350	18	1	5	62	7	115
Fruity Supreme	1 (9 oz)	280	12	1	5	59	6	100
Grape Escape	1 (10 oz)	480	11	1	5	109	2	100
Guava Sunrise	1 (13 oz)	366	12	1	0	80	6	50
Kiwi Kic	1 (11 oz)	400	13	1	0	88	2	105
Lean Body	1 (11 oz)	330	40	8	80	24	8	460
Lean Out	1 (11 oz)	600	56	26	55	35	5	360
Low Carb	1 (10 oz)	350	54	2	65	27	2	250
Mango Mania	1 (8 oz)	370	11	0	0	82	2	105
Marionberry Fuel	1 (13 oz)	380	14	0	0	81	10	105
Mega Mass	1 (14 oz)	610	29	10	45	103	7	220
Mini Mass	1 (13 oz)	520	27	11	65	79	6	180
Mocha Bliss	1 (10 oz)	550	34	8	30	63	1	370
Nutty Banana	1 (11 oz)	720	27	25	5	97	9	290
Orange Twister	1 (10 oz)	140	3	0	0	31	2	5
Pacific Splash	1 (12 oz)	240	2	0	0	58	6	0
PB&J	1 (14 oz)	630	22	25	0	77	12	210
Peach Pleasure	1 (12 oz)	270	12	0	0	54	5	95
Peanut Passion	1 (11 oz)	580	22	25	0	61	10	210
Pineapple Bliss	1 (12 oz)	210	6	1	0	45	4	30
Power Fuel	1 (11 oz)	450	39	3	45	66	6	120
Quick Start	1 (10 oz)	280	17	0	5	46	4	260
Raspberry Dream	1 (13 oz)	410	18	1	5	80	10	115
Rejuvenator	1 (10 oz)	340	17	1	5	62	7	110
Sambazon	1 (15 oz)	410	14	6	0	92	8	95
Slim N Fit	1 (10 oz)	350	25	1	25	60	6	125
The Builder	1 (18 oz)	1270	67	46	85	144	10	630
Zesty Lemon	1 (14 oz)	430	19	9	40	67	5	170
Zip Zip	1 (10 oz)	240	18	3	5	35	3	95
Zone Zinger	1 (14 oz)	430	25	3	30	76	4	60
EVOS								
BEVERAGES								
Shake Mango Guava	1 reg (16 oz)	180	0	0	0	48	2	0

FOOD	PORTION	CALS	PROT	FAT	CHOL	CARB	FIBER	SOD
Shake Multi-Berry	1 reg (20 oz)	200	1	1	0	52	1	10
Shake Organic Cappuccino	1 reg (16 oz)	230	5	3	10	47	0	75
Shake Organic Vanilla	1 reg (16 oz)	180	6	3	10	30	0	55
Shake Strawberry Banana	1 reg (16 oz)	190	1	1	0	47	1	10
CHILDREN'S MENU SELECTIONS								
Kids Champion Burger	1	400	29	12	0	48	7	800
Kids Chicken Strips	1 serv	130	14	3	35	13	0	710
Kids Freerange Steakburger	1	390	27	15	70	39	2	480
Kids Good Corn Dog	1	150	7	4	0	27	3	500
MAIN MENU SELECTIONS								
Airbaked Chicken Strips	1 serv	260	28	6	70	26	0	1420
Airfries	1 reg	230	4	8	0	35	3	390
American Champion	1	420	30	12	0	53	6	1130
American DeLite	1	330	22	6	0	53	7	1040
Burger Bun	1	190	7	2	0	39	2	410
Cheddar Cheese Slice	1	80	5	7	20	0	0	135
Crispy Mesquite Chicken	1 serv	330	21	5	35	53	2	1120
Freerange Steakburger	1	400	27	15	70	42	3	810
Fresh Fruit Bowl	1 serv	200	2	1	0	52	4	20
Good Corn Dog	1	150	7	4	0	22	3	500
Herb Crusted Trout	1 serv	440	21	25	13	62	3	1300
Honey Mesquite Chicken	1 serv	290	26	3	45	41	2	770
Spicy Chipotle Turkey	1 serv	370	31	9	70	42	3	1050
Veggie Chili	1 reg	110	7	2	0	20	5	930
Veggie Garden Grill Italian	1	350	24	5	0	54	8	930
Wraps Avocado Turkey	1	480	32	15	70	51	4	1200
Wraps Crispy Buffalo Chicken	1	440	23	11	35	64	5	1280
Wraps Crispy Thai Trout	1	660	25	20	25	96	5	1570
Wraps Freerange Beef Taco	1	600	34	28	90	53	5	770
Wraps Honey Wheat	1	300	8	8	0	49	4	560
Wraps Southwest Soy Taco	1	500	35	25	20	58	10	1090
Wraps Spicy Thai Chicken	1	510	30	10	45	76	4	1290
Wraps Spinach Herb	1	310	9	8	0	52	3	840
Wraps Tomato Basil Chicken	1	520	25	11	35	82	4	1560
SALAD DRESSINGS AND TOPPINGS								
Balsamic Vinegar	1 serv (0.5 oz)	5	0	0	0	2	0	0
Crispy Noodles	1 serv (7 g)	35	1	1	0	5	0	90
Croutons Multi-Grain	1 serv (7 g)	30	1	2	0	4	0	70

FOOD	PORTION	CALS	PROT	FAT	CHOL	CARB	FIBER	SOD
Dressing Avocado	1 serv (3 oz)	190	3	21	10	5	2	200
Dressing Caesar	1 serv (1.7 oz)	300	2	32	35	2	0	510
Dressing Fat Free Vinaigrette	1 serv (1 oz)	5	0	0	0	2	0	250
Dressing Raspberry	1 serv (2 oz)	50	0	0	0	14	0	340
Dressing Spicy Thai	1 serv (1.4 oz)	150	0	9	0	15	0	470
Extra Virgin Olive Oil	1 serv (1 oz)	250	0	28	0	0	0	0
Herb Spread	1 serv (0.7 oz)	30	0	3	0	2	0	160
Ketchup Cayenne Firewalker	1 serv (1.2 oz)	35	1	0	0	9	0	380
Ketchup Garlic Gravity	1 serv (1.2 oz)	35	1	0	0	9	0	380
Ketchup Mesquite Magic	1 serv (1.2 oz)	35	1	0	0	9	0	420
Mustard	1 serv (0.5 oz)	10	1	0	0	1	0	170
Mustard Mesquite Honey	1 serv (0.7 oz)	80	0	8	5	3	0	180
Southwest Sour Cream	1 serv (1.4 oz)	60	2	35	15	4	0	160
Spicy Chipotle Mayo	1 serv (0.7 oz)	30	0	2	0	2	0	170
Tomato Basil Sauce	1 serv (1.4 oz)	150	2	15	5	5	0	150
SALADS								
Bordeaux Bistro w/o Dressing	1	260	13	22	40	7	3	510
For Salads Chicken Strips	1 serv (3 oz)	130	14	3	35	13	0	710
For Salads Grilled Chicken	1 serv (3 oz)	90	19	1	50	1	0	360
Mediterranean Summer w/o Dressing	1	200	13	8	25	22	6	920
Santa Ana Caesar w/o Dressing	1	20	2	0	0	4	2	30
Side Salad w/o Dressing	1	35	2	0	0	8	2	30
Spicy Thai w/o Dressing	1	35	2	0	0	7	2	30
SUPPLEMENTS								
Fat Burner	1 serv (5 g)	16	0	0	0	4	0	0

FOOD	PORTION	CALS	PROT	FAT	CHOL	CARB	FIBER	SOD
Go Energy	1 serv (5 g)	15	0	0	0	4	0	0
Mega Protein	1 serv (0.5 oz)	45	12	0	0	0	0	0
Multi-Vitamin	1 serv (5 g)	10	0	0	0	3	0	0
FAZOLI'S								
BEVERAGES								
Lemon Ice All Flavors	1	360	0	0	0	90	0	20
Lemon Ice Original	1 reg	180	0	0	0	45	0	15
Lemon Ice Strawberry	1	320	0	0	0	81	0	60
CHILDREN'S MENU SELECTIONS								
Fettuccine Alfredo	1 serv	290	9	5	5	50	2	420
Meat Lasagna	1 serv	260	14	13	35	21	2	880
Ravioli w/ Marinara	1 serv	290	13	7	30	43	3	580
Spaghetti w/ Meatballs	1 serv	350	14	7	20	55	4	620
Ziti w/ Meat Sauce	1 serv	190	9	6	15	25	3	710
DESSERTS								
Cheesecake Original	1 slice	290	6	22	95	17	0	220
Cheesecake Turtle	1 slice	450	6	28	75	43	2	340
Cookie Chocolate Chunk	1	510	5	26	75	68	3	350
MAIN MENU SELECTIONS								
Breadstick	1	100	3	2	0	20	0	160
Breadstick Garlic	1	150	3	7	0	20	1	290
Fettuccine Alfredo	1 sm	520	16	12	15	83	4	1060
Fettuccine w/ Marinara	1 serv	450	15	3	0	88	7	770
Fettuccine w/ Meat Sauce	1 serv	500	20	7	10	87	7	1020
Oven Baked Chicken Parmesan	1 serv	960	56	33	115	117	9	2350
Oven Baked Meat Lasagna	1 serv	510	27	25	70	43	5	1710
Oven Baked Rigatoni Romano	1 serv	1090	11	54	135	101	11	3180
Oven Baked Spaghetti	1 serv	680	32	22	65	90	7	1480
Oven Baked Spaghetti w/ Meatballs	1 serv	940	46	40	120	100	9	2370
Panini Four Cheese & Tomato	1	510	28	22	60	53	3	960
Panini Grilled Chicken	1	540	35	18	80	56	3	1360
Panini Smoked Turkey	1	620	35	29	95	54	3	2110
Penne w/ Alfredo	1 serv	520	16	12	15	83	4	1060
Penne w/ Marinara	1 serv	450	15	3	0	88	7	770

FOOD	PORTION	CALS	PROT	FAT	CHOL	CARB	FIBER	SOD
Penne w/ Meat Sauce	1 serv	500	20	7	10	87	7	1020
Pizza Slice Cheese	1	270	13	11	25	31	2	700
Pizza Slice Pepperoni	1	310	14	14	30	31	2	850
Platter Classic Sampler	1	810	34	25	55	110	8	2130
Platter Ultimate Sampler	1	980	43	29	70	134	11	2780
Ravioli w/ Marinara	1 serv	500	22	15	80	71	7	1210
Ravioli w/ Meat Sauce	1 serv	550	26	20	90	71	7	1460
Spaghetti w/ Alfredo	1 serv	520	16	12	15	83	4	1060
Spaghetti w/ Marinara	1 sm	450	15	3	0	88	7	770
Spaghetti w/ Meat Sauce	1 sm	500	20	7	10	87	7	1020
Submarinos Club	half	973	37	34	75	65	3	2870
Submarinos Ham n'Swiss	1	680	34	30	60	65	3	2440
Submarinos Italian Beef	half	660	46	24	90	68	3	2320
Submarinos Original	half	940	35	58	95	68	4	3040
Topping Broccoli	1 serv	25	3	0	0	5	3	10
Topping Broccoli & Tomatoes	1 serv	30	3	0	0	6	3	10
Topping Garlic Shrimp	1 serv	160	10	12	45	3	1	440
Topping Italian Sausage	1 serv	240	10	21	45	3	1	770
Topping Meatballs	1 serv	160	13	18	55	6	1	700
Topping Peppery Chicken	1 serv	70	14	1	35	1	0	330
Ziti w/ Meat Sauce	1 serv	480	23	15	40	65	6	1430
SALAD DRESSINGS								
Caesar	1 serv	220	1	25	45	1	0	350
Fat Free Honey Mustard	1 serv	60	0	0	0	15	1	350
Fat Free Italian	1 serv	25	0	0	0	6	0	390
Honey French	1 serv	220	0	18	0	14	0	310
Italian	1 serv	160	0	14	0	7	0	760
Ranch	1 serv	220	1	24	10	2	0	470
Ranch Lite	1 serv	120	1	12	5	2	0	350
SALADS								
Chicken & Fruit	1	220	23	2	55	28	4	700
Chicken & Pasta Caesar	1	440	35	15	65	41	4	1320
Chicken BLT Ranch	1	270	31	10	80	13	4	1060
Parmesan Chicken	1	360	31	15	65	31	4	850
Side Caesar	1	40	4	2	5	4	2	70
Side Garden	1	25	2	0	0	4	3	30
Side Pasta	1	320	11	12	5	41	1	620

FOOD	PORTION	CALS	PROT	FAT	CHOL	CARB	FIBER	SOD
FIVE GUYS BURGERS AND FRIES								
MAIN MENU SELECTIONS								
Bacon Burger	1 (9.8 oz)	780	43	50	140	39	2	690
Bacon Cheese Dog	1 (7 oz)	695	26	48	96	41	2	1700
Bacon Dog	1 (6.4 oz)	625	22	42	76	40	2	1390
Cheese Dog	1 (6.5 oz)	615	22	41	81	41	2	1440
Cheeseburger	1 (10.6 oz)	840	47	55	165	40	2	1050
Cheeseburger Bacon	1 (11 oz)	920	51	62	180	40	2	1310
Fries	1 reg (8.6 oz)	620	10	30	–	78	6	90
Fries	1 lg (16 oz)	1464	24	71	–	184	14	213
Grilled Cheese	1 (4 oz)	430	11	26	35	41	3	715
Hamburger	1 (9.3 oz)	700	39	43	125	39	2	430
Hot Dog	1 (5.9 oz)	545	18	35	61	40	2	1130
Little Burgers Bacon Burger	1 (6.5 oz)	560	27	33	80	39	2	640
Little Burgers Cheeseburger	1 (6.7 oz)	550	27	32	85	40	2	690
Little Burgers Cheeseburger Bacon	1 (7.2 oz)	630	31	39	100	40	2	950
Little Burgers Hamburger	1 (6 oz)	480	23	26	65	39	2	380
Veggie Sandwich	1 (7.3 oz)	440	16	15	25	60	2	1040
TOPPINGS								
A1 Steak Sauce	1 tbsp (0.6 oz)	15	0	0	0	3	0	280
Bacon	2 slices (0.5 oz)	80	4	7	15	0	0	260
BBQ Sauce	1 tbsp (0.6 oz)	60	0	8	0	16	0	400
Cheese	1 slice (0.7 oz)	70	4	6	20	tr	0	310
Green Peppers	1 serv (0.8 oz)	5	0	0	0	2	tr	1
Hot Sauce	1 tsp (5 g)	0	0	0	0	0	0	0
Jalapenos	1 serv (0.4 oz)	3	0	0	0	tr	0	184
Ketchup	1 tbsp (0.6 oz)	15	0	0	0	4	0	190
Lettuce	1 serv (1 oz)	4	0	0	0	1	tr	3
Mayonnaise	1 serv (0.5 oz)	100	0	11	10	0	0	75
Mushrooms	1 serv (0.9 oz)	10	1	0	–	1	tr	100
Mustard	1 tbsp (0.6 oz)	0	0	0	0	0	0	55

FOOD	PORTION	CALS	PROT	FAT	CHOL	CARB	FIBER	SOD
Onions	1 serv (0.9 oz)	10	0	0	0	3	tr	1
Pickle Chips	6 (1 oz)	5	0	0	0	1	0	265
Relish	1 serv (0.5 oz)	15	0	0	0	4	0	85
Tomatoes	1 serv (1.8 oz)	9	tr	0	0	2	tr	3
FRIENDLY'S								
BEVERAGES								
Milkshake Double Thick Vanilla	1	770	15	32	110	106	0	270
MAIN MENU SELECTIONS								
Apple Slices	1 serv	100	1	0	0	26	5	0
Applesauce	1 serv	110	0	0	0	27	1	0
Broccoli	1 serv	80	3	6	0	5	3	80
Burger All American	1	1190	43	68	120	103	8	1170
Burger BBQ Fronion	1	1560	55	91	160	134	8	2020
Burger Mushroom Swiss Bacon	1	1570	61	100	190	109	7	2040
Burger Soft Pretzel Bacon	1	1420	58	79	190	119	7	1360
Burger The Vermonter	1	1420	59	87	190	102	7	1530
Burger Ultimate Bacon Cheese	1	1400	55	86	170	103	7	2040
Burgermelt Deluxe Cheese Set-Up	1	1180	44	75	140	83	7	1310
Burgermelt Swiss Patty	1	1360	56	78	150	110	8	1220
Burgermelt Ultimate Grilled Cheese	1	1500	54	97	180	101	9	2090
Burgermelt Zesty Questo	1	1380	53	79	140	117	7	2410
Carrot & Celery Sticks w/ Ranch Dressing	1 serv	100	2	7	10	6	2	260
Chicken Strips Basket w/o Dipping Sauce	5 pieces	1030	37	58	90	93	8	1330
Chicken Strips Honey BBQ w/o Dipping Sauce	5 pieces	1560	38	74	110	188	0	2240
Chicken Strips Kickin' Buffalo w/o Dipping Sauce	5 pieces	1530	40	109	150	97	8	2860
Clamboat Basket	1 serv	1710	28	102	90	170	11	3340
Coleslaw	1 serv	160	1	12	10	13	2	260
Corn	1 serv	160	4	7	0	20	4	70

FOOD	PORTION	CALS	PROT	FAT	CHOL	CARB	FIBER	SOD
Fishamajig	1	970	30	51	70	99	7	1570
Friendly Frank	1	750	15	44	30	73	5	1070
Friendly's BTL	1	990	21	57	40	99	7	1110
Fronions Jumbo	1 serv	1430	14	90	30	140	7	2970
Garlic Bread	1 serv	330	4	14	0	48	4	160
Grilled Cheese	1	790	20	37	30	96	6	1280
Grilled Flounder	1 serv	980	38	48	80	100	7	3070
Mandarin Oranges	1 serv	80	0	0	0	20	0	10
Mashed Potatoes Homestyle	1 serv	240	4	12	30	29	2	160
Mini Mozzarella Cheese Sticks	1 serv	680	23	40	60	55	3	1870
Mixed Vegetables	1 serv	110	3	6	0	13	4	110
New England Fish 'N Chips	1 serv	1150	25	70	80	106	9	2120
Quesadillas Chicken	1 serv	1330	29	82	210	97	4	3350
Quesadillas Chicken Fajita	1 serv	1540	74	91	210	106	7	3870
Rice	1 serv	210	3	3	0	41	0	900
Shrimp Basket	1 serv	1090	27	60	180	110	9	3290
Sirloin Steak Tips	1 serv	1140	77	51	200	92	13	3350
Sliders Cheeseburger	1 serv	500	20	21	50	57	6	1440
Sliders Chicken	1 serv	740	23	42	60	69	7	1210
Spanish Rice	1 serv	330	7	15	0	41	0	1200
Supermelt Bruschetta Mozzarella	1	1140	57	54	140	105	7	1870
Supermelt Cheddar Jack Chicken	1	1070	56	49	140	98	6	2270
Supermelt Grilled Chicken Pesto	1	1360	59	82	160	98	6	2060
Supermelt Honey BBQ Chicken	1	1400	49	75	110	134	8	2160
Supermelt Kickin Buffalo Chicken	1	1430	45	86	100	118	7	2520
Supermelt Reuben	1	1130	54	56	100	105	6	2910
Supermelt Steak 'N Mushroom	1	1150	44	61	90	108	7	2120
Supermelt Tuna	1	1140	39	66	80	98	7	1700
Supermelt Turkey Club	1	990	44	46	80	102	7	2220
Tuna Roll	1	920	28	57	60	73	6	1080
Waffle Fries	1 serv	590	7	33	0	67	5	1430
Waffle Fries Loaded	1 serv	920	17	64	60	67	4	2510

FOOD	PORTION	CALS	PROT	FAT	CHOL	CARB	FIBER	SOD
Wrap Buffalo Chicken	1	1510	42	94	130	123	9	2640
Wrap Crispy Chicken	1	1140	31	54	60	132	10	1610
Wrap Crispy Chicken Caesar	1	1500	43	94	160	123	9	2300
Wrap Grilled Chicken Deluxe	1	1000	43	45	90	108	8	1810
SALAD DRESSINGS AND TOPPINGS								
Dressing Bleu Cheese	1 serv	470	6	48	60	3	0	720
Dressing Honey Mustard	1 serv	360	0	30	30	24	0	420
Dressing Italian	1 serv	410	0	42	0	6	0	690
Dressing Italian Fat Free	1 serv	30	0	0	0	8	0	420
Dressing Peppercorn Parmesan Lite	1 serv	230	3	21	20	6	0	630
Dressing Ranch	1 serv	330	3	33	30	3	0	750
Dressing Salsa Ranch	1 serv	170	2	17	20	5	1	620
Dressing Sesame Oriental	1 serv	270	0	14	0	36	0	960
Dressing Thousand Island	1 serv	390	0	36	20	15	0	840
Dressing Vinaigrette Dijon Low Fat	1 serv	110	0	3	0	21	0	1560
Sauce BBQ	1 serv	90	0	0	0	20	0	410
Sauce Honey Mustard	1 serv	180	0	16	20	12	0	210
Vinaigrette Balsamic	1 serv	180	0	15	0	9	0	1230
SALADS								
Apple Walnut Chicken w/o Dressing	1 serv	390	38	18	110	22	5	1140
Asian Chicken w/o Dressing	1 serv	490	36	20	80	41	6	1200
Chicken Caesar	1 serv	1030	47	84	220	32	3	2010
Chipotle Chicken w/o Dressing	1 serv	550	37	22	80	50	8	1440
Crispy Chicken w/o Dressing	1 serv	630	35	38	260	38	6	820
Kickin Buffalo Chicken w/o Dressing	1 serv	710	29	47	90	42	7	1370
Side w/o Dressing	1 serv	60	2	1	0	10	2	110
Steak & Bleu Cheese w/o Dressing	1 serv	640	44	34	120	41	8	1240
SOUPS								
Broccoli Cheddar	1 cup	200	7	13	40	14	1	780
Chili	1 cup	270	14	16	40	18	3	910
Chunky Chicken Noodle	1 cup	280	10	10	70	31	2	1970

FOOD	PORTION	CALS	PROT	FAT	CHOL	CARB	FIBER	SOD
Homestyle Clam Chowder	1 cup	270	11	18	60	17	1	890
Minestrone	1 cup	90	4	1	0	15	2	620
GREAT STEAK & POTATO								
BEVERAGES								
Great Steak Lemonade	1 sm (12 oz)	180	03	0	0	48	0	0
Orange Juice	1 (12 oz)	118	0	0	0	30	0	31
BREAKFAST SELECTIONS								
Potatoes Deluxe Home	1 serv (12 oz)	390	4	23	0	44	7	1460
Potatoes Fresh Cut Home	1 serv (10.6 oz)	380	3	23	0	42	6	1460
Sandwich Bacon Egg Cheese	1 (7.6 oz)	600	29	36	440	39	2	1300
Sandwich Egg Cheese	1 (7 oz)	500	23	29	425	39	2	890
Sandwich Ham Cheese	1 (5.5 oz)	430	18	22	40	41	2	1400
Sandwich Ham Egg Cheese	1 (9 oz)	570	31	32	450	42	2	1540
Sandwich Sausage Egg Cheese	1 (9 oz)	700	30	47	465	39	2	1300
Sandwich Steak Egg Cheese	1 (10 oz)	600	34	34	455	40	2	990
CHILDREN'S MENU SELECTIONS								
Grilled Cheese w/ Fry	1 serv (8.8 oz)	530	15	28	10	57	6	1290
Kid's Great Fry	1 (6.1 oz)	270	4	13	0	36	4	680
Kids Nuggets	1 serv (2.7 oz)	165	11	9	37	10	1	403
Slider Chicken w/ Fry	1 serv (11.5 oz)	570	23	25	50	60	6	1560
Slider Steak w/ Fry	1 serv (11.8 oz)	580	24	28	55	60	6	1530
MAIN MENU SELECTIONS								
Baked Potato Broccoli & Cheese	1 (8.9 oz)	400	13	24	45	35	4	1070
Baked Potato Cheese & Bacon	1 (7.8 oz)	530	25	35	85	29	3	840
Baked Potato Plain	1 (6 oz)	160	4	0	0	36	4	15
Baked Potato Sour Cream & Chive	1 (7.3 oz)	350	5	23	25	32	3	160
Baked Potato The King	1 (8.8 oz)	590	26	41	95	31	3	860
Cheeseburger	1 (10.2 oz)	640	40	35	105	41	3	730

FOOD	PORTION	CALS	PROT	FAT	CHOL	CARB	FIBER	SOD
Chicagoland Cheesesteak 7 Inch	1 (13.3 oz)	680	43	29	85	63	5	2480
Coney Island Fry	1 reg (12.7 oz)	570	18	30	45	61	12	2030
Great Fry	1 reg (10.2 oz)	440	7	20	0	60	7	1130
Great Steak Cheesesteak 7 Inch	1 (13.6 oz)	740	41	37	95	62	5	1270
Great Steak Cheesesteak Wrap	1 (13.7 oz)	820	40	43	95	67	5	1400
Gyro	1 (12 oz)	580	29	30	60	52	5	1550
Ham Delight 7 Inch	1 (13.1 oz)	710	36	33	85	71	5	2190
Ham Explosion 7 Inch	1 (14 oz)	710	37	34	85	70	6	2200
Hamburger	1 (9.7 oz)	590	37	30	105	40	3	480
Kansas City BBQ Cheesesteak 7 Inch	1 (12 oz)	680	40	26	65	71	5	1740
King Fry	1 reg (11.4 oz)	630	20	39	70	52	5	1970
Nacho Fry	1 reg (11.8 oz)	510	12	27	30	53	5	2570
Pastrami 7 Inch	1 (13.3 oz)	790	43	41	110	65	5	1850
Philly Buffalo Chicken 7 Inch	1 (13.8 oz)	660	37	24	60	65	5	2420
Philly Burger	1 (14.2 oz)	820	46	50	135	47	4	820
Philly Chicken Slider	1 (5.4 oz)	300	19	13	50	24	2	880
Philly Original Cheesesteak 7 Inch	1 (11.8 oz)	650	40	26	95	62	5	2570
Philly Original Chicken 7 Inch	1 (11 oz)	620	37	22	85	62	5	1670
Philly Original Chicken Wrap	1 (11.3 oz)	700	36	28	85	67	4	1800
Philly Steak Slider	1 (5.6 oz)	310	20	15	55	24	2	850
Philly Teriyaki Chicken	1 (14 oz)	290	40	32	85	65	5	2280
Philly Turkey 7 Inch	1 (13 oz)	670	38	30	75	64	5	1650
Philly Ultimate Chicken	1 (14.6 oz)	730	38	33	65	64	6	1590
Philly Ultimate Chicken Wrap	1 (14.7 oz)	810	36	39	65	69	5	1720
Potato Skins	1 serv (6.4 oz)	390	17	26	65	24	2	1070
Reuben 7 Inch	1 (12 oz)	690	37	33	95	61	5	2550

FOOD	PORTION	CALS	PROT	FAT	CHOL	CARB	FIBER	SOD
Super Steak Wrap Cheesesteak	1 (15.7 oz)	930	41	54	105	69	5	1500
The Great Potato Chicken	1 (13 oz)	600	32	33	100	37	4	1420
The Great Potato Ham	1 (12.8 oz)	520	29	28	95	43	4	2470
The Great Potato Steak	1 (13.5 oz)	620	35	38	105	37	4	1360
The Great Potato Turkey	1 (12.8 oz)	490	31	25	85	39	4	1930
Veggi Delight 7 Inch	1 (12.2 oz)	610	20	31	30	66	6	2040
Wacker Fry	1 reg (9.8 oz)	490	12	27	30	51	5	1600
Wisconsin Inside-Out 7 Inch	1 (6.2 oz)	560	24	27	20	57	4	1360
SALAD DRESSINGS AND SAUCES								
Dressing Ranch	1 oz	170	1	18	10	1	0	160
Dressing Thousand Island	1 oz	130	0	12	10	4	0	280
Mayonnaise	1 oz	200	0	22	20	0	0	200
Mayonnaise Dijon	1 oz	110	0	11	10	3	0	420
Oil	1 serv (0.3 oz)	60	0	7	0	0	0	0
Sauce Buffalo	1 oz	10	0	0	0	2	0	855
Sauce Marinara Dipping	2 oz	15	1	0	0	3	0	260
Sauce Teriyaki	1 oz	25	2	0	0	3	0	960
Sauce Tzatziki	1 oz	50	0	4	0	2	0	80
SALADS								
Chef w/o Dressing	1 (16.1 oz)	260	28	11	70	15	4	1320
Garden w/o Dressing	1 (12 oz)	60	3	1	0	13	5	40
Great Salad Grilled Chicken	1 (18.8 oz)	380	31	18	80	18	5	460
Great Salad Grilled Ham	1 (18.8 oz)	360	24	20	75	28	5	1520
Great Salad Grilled Steak	1 (19.3 oz)	400	33	23	85	18	5	590
Great Salad Grilled Turkey	1 (18.8 oz)	330	30	17	65	20	5	970
Side w/o Dressing	1 (6 oz)	30	2	0	0	6	2	20
Wedge Grilled Chicken	1 (14.8 oz)	270	24	12	60	11	3	610
Wedge Grilled Steak	1 (15.3 oz)	290	28	16	70	11	3	550

HUNGRY HOWIE'S PIZZA

OTHER MENU SELECTIONS								
Cajun Bread	¼ bread	300	9	9	2	46	1	239
Chicken Tenders	2	140	13	5	30	11	0	460
Cinnamon Bread	¼ bread	313	9	9	2	59	1	239
Howie Bread	¼ bread	300	9	9	2	46	1	239
Howie Wings	5	180	14	13	60	0	0	760

FOOD	PORTION	CALS	PROT	FAT	CHOL	CARB	FIBER	SOD
Sub Deluxe Italian	½ sub	506	24	18	44	61	2	1005
Sub Ham & Cheese	½ sub	475	26	15	44	61	2	1020
Sub Pizza	½ sub	689	30	34	86	67	3	1722
Sub Pizza Special	½ sub	606	29	24	65	68	3	1584
Sub Steak & Cheese	½ sub	491	27	15	47	64	2	914
Sub Turkey	½ sub	466	25	13	38	63	2	1108
Sub Turkey Club	½ sub	556	42	15	42	63	2	1065
Sub Vegetarian	½ sub	530	22	21	39	64	3	895
Three Cheeser Bread	¼ bread	370	15	14	17	47	1	384
PIZZA								
Cheese Slice	1 sm	161	10	4	11	20	1	370
Cheese Slice	1 lg	208	12	5	13	25	1	464
Cheese Slice	1 med	191	11	6	11	23	1	437
Cheese Slice	1 extra lg	395	23	9	25	42	2	882
Cheese Slice Thin	1 med	111	7	5	11	10	tr	256
Cheese Slice Thin	1 lg	124	8	6	13	11	1	323
Medium Topping Anchovies	1 serv	44	7	3	16	0	0	736
Medium Topping Bacon	1 serv	32	6	1	1	tr	0	–
Medium Topping Banana Peppers	1 serv	6	tr	0	0	1	0	162
Medium Topping Beef	1 serv	30	2	2	6	tr	tr	96
Medium Topping Black Olives	1 serv	7	0	tr	2	tr	tr	47
Medium Topping Ham	1 serv	7	1	tr	4	0	0	81
Medium Topping Mushrooms	1 serv	2	tr	0	0	tr	tr	0
Medium Topping Pepperoni	1 serv	22	1	2	6	0	0	75
Medium Topping Pineapple	1 serv	5	1	0	0	2	1	0
Medium Topping Sausage	1 serv	27	2	2	4	tr	tr	121
SALAD DRESSINGS AND SAUCES								
Dressing Blue Cheese	1 serv (1 oz)	150	1	16	20	1	0	300
Dressing Creamy Italian	1 serv (1 oz)	120	0	12	0	2	0	210
Dressing Fat Free Italian	1 serv (1.5 oz)	25	0	0	0	5	0	390
Dressing Fat Free Ranch	1 serv (1.5 oz)	45	0	0	0	10	1	540
Dressing French Style	1 serv (1 oz)	30	0	0	0	7	0	170
Dressing Greek	1 serv (1 oz)	110	0	11	0	2	0	70
Dressing Italian	1 serv (1 oz)	80	0	8	0	2	0	560
Dressing Ranch	1 serv (1 oz)	180	0	19	3	1	0	250

FOOD	PORTION	CALS	PROT	FAT	CHOL	CARB	FIBER	SOD
Dressing Thousand Island	1 serv (1 oz)	140	0	14	20	4	0	240
Sauce Dipping	1 serv (3 oz)	45	3	1	0	9	1	380
SALADS								
Antipasto	1 sm	115	9	7	28	3	2	554
Chef	1 sm	114	9	7	28	4	2	396
Garden	1 sm	20	1	tr	0	3	2	10
Greek	1 sm	126	7	7	29	8	2	581

IHOP

FOOD	PORTION	CALS	PROT	FAT	CHOL	CARB	FIBER	SOD
Pancake Buttermilk	5	770	22	25	115	115	7	2640
Pancake Buttermilk Short Stack	3	490	13	18	80	69	4	1610
Pancake Chocolate Chip	4	720	20	24	80	112	8	2070
Pancake Double Blueberry	4	800	19	17	80	144	11	2150
Pancake Harvest Grain 'N Nut	4	920	25	49	125	95	10	1810
Pancake New York Cheesecake	4	1100	26	44	190	152	8	2430
Pancake Strawberry Banana	4	760	20	17	80	137	10	2070

IVAR'S SEAFOOD BARS

FOOD	PORTION	CALS	PROT	FAT	CHOL	CARB	FIBER	SOD
Chicken	3 pieces (4.5 oz)	250	22	11	–	14	–	6
Chowder Salmon	1 cup	220	4	13	–	22	2	510
Chowder White	1 cup	330	17	19	–	24	4	1115
Clams	1 serv (5 oz)	400	17	21	–	33	1	–
Cocktail Sauce	¼ cup	50	1	0	0	12	1	730
Fish	3 pieces	220	22	9	–	12	1	7
French Fries	1 serv (3.5 oz)	300	4	16	–	34	2	1
Oysters	5	290	17	14	–	22	1	–
Prawns	1 serv (5 oz)	290	20	15	–	18	tr	17
Salmon Fried	3 pieces (4.5 oz)	210	24	9	–	9	1	–
Scallops	1 serv (5 oz)	240	22	9	–	14	tr	–
Tartar Sauce	2 tbsp	140	0	15	–	1	0	250

FOOD	PORTION	CALS	PROT	FAT	CHOL	CARB	FIBER	SOD
JACK IN THE BOX								
BEVERAGES								
Barq's Root Beer	1 (20 oz)	180	0	0	0	50	0	40
Chug Chocolate Milk Low Fat	1 (3.5 oz)	200	11	3	5	34	1	230
Chug Reduced Fat Milk	1 (3.5 oz)	130	10	5	25	13	0	130
Coca Cola Classic	1 (20 oz)	170	0	0	0	46	0	0
Coffee Regular & Decaf	1 (11 oz)	5	0	0	0	1	0	5
Diet Coke	1 (20 oz)	0	0	0	0	0	0	15
Dr Pepper	1 (20 oz)	150	0	0	0	42	0	50
Fanta Orange	1 (20 oz)	150	0	0	0	41	0	50
Fanta Strawberry	1 (20 oz)	150	0	0	0	41	0	10
Iced Tea	1 (20 oz)	5	0	0	0	2	0	20
Lemonade	1 (20 oz)	160	0	0	0	42	0	65
Orange Juice	1 (10 oz)	140	2	0	0	32	2	25
Shake Chocolate	1 (16 oz)	880	14	45	135	107	1	330
Shake Oreo	1 (16 oz)	910	14	49	135	102	1	420
Shake Strawberry	1 (16 oz)	880	13	44	135	105	0	290
Shake Vanilla	1 (16 oz)	790	13	44	135	83	0	280
Sprite	1 (20 oz)	160	0	0	0	42	0	40
BREAKFAST SELECTIONS								
Biscuit Bacon Egg Cheese	1	430	17	25	220	34	1	1100
Biscuit Chicken	1	450	15	24	30	42	2	980
Biscuit Sausage	1	440	12	29	35	32	2	870
Biscuit Sausage Egg Cheese	1	740	27	55	280	35	2	1430
Biscuit Spicy Chicken	1	460	21	22	40	44	2	1020
Breakfast Jack	1	290	17	12	220	39	1	760
Breakfast Jack Bacon	1	300	16	14	215	29	1	730
Breakfast Jack Sausage	1	450	20	28	245	29	1	840
Breakfast Sandwich Ciabatta	1	710	36	30	440	63	3	1730
Breakfast Sandwich Ultimate	1	570	34	27	445	49	2	1700
Burrito Hearty Breakfast	1	480	25	29	350	29	2	1210
Burrito Sirloin Steak & Egg w/o Salsa	1	790	37	48	450	52	6	1320
Croissant Sausage	1	580	21	39	255	37	2	770
Croissant Supreme	1	450	20	25	235	36	1	860
French Toast Sticks	4 (4.2 oz)	470	7	23	25	58	4	450

FOOD	PORTION	CALS	PROT	FAT	CHOL	CARB	FIBER	SOD
French Toast Sticks Blueberry	4	450	8	20	0	59	3	550
Hash Browns	1 serv	150	1	10	0	13	2	230
Sandwich Extreme Sausage	1	670	29	48	290	31	2	1300
DESSERTS								
Cake Chocolate Overload	1 serv (3.2 oz)	300	4	7	40	57	2	350
Cheesecake	1 serv (3.6 oz)	310	7	16	55	34	0	220
MAIN MENU SELECTIONS								
Bacon Cheddar Potato Wedges	1 serv (9 oz)	720	21	48	45	52	4	1360
Cheeseburger Bacon Ultimate	1	1090	46	77	140	53	2	2040
Cheeseburger Junior Bacon	1	430	20	25	60	30	1	820
Cheeseburger Sourdough Ultimate	1	950	38	73	125	36	2	1360
Cheeseburger Ultimate	1	1010	40	71	125	53	2	1580
Chicken Fajita Pita	1	280	21	9	60	30	2	1110
Chicken Sandwich	1	400	15	21	35	38	2	730
Chicken Strips Crispy	4	500	35	25	80	36	3	1260
Chicken Strips Grilled	4 (5 oz)	180	37	2	125	3	0	700
Ciabatta Burger Bacon 'N' Cheese	1	1120	45	76	135	66	4	1670
Ciabatta Burger Single Bacon 'N' Cheese	1	870	31	54	90	66	4	1550
Ciabatta Chipotle w/ Grilled Chicken	1	690	44	28	105	65	4	1850
Ciabatta Chipotle w/ Spicy Crispy Chicken	1	750	37	34	80	75	5	1650
Ciabatta Sirloin Steak 'N' Cheddar	1	770	43	38	110	65	4	1310
Club Sourdough Grilled Chicken	1	530	36	28	85	34	3	1430
Curly Fries Seasoned	1 sm (3 oz)	270	4	15	0	30	3	590
Egg Rolls	1	130	5	6	5	15	2	310
Fish & Chips	1 serv (7.6 oz)	570	17	30	35	58	4	1100
Fries Natural Cut	1 sm	340	5	17	0	41	5	620
Fruit Cup	1 serv	90	1	0	0	22	2	20

FOOD	PORTION	CALS	PROT	FAT	CHOL	CARB	FIBER	SOD
Hamburger	1	310	16	14	40	30	1	600
Hamburger Deluxe	1	370	17	21	45	31	2	560
Hamburger Deluxe w/ Cheese	1	460	21	28	70	33	2	930
Hamburger w/ Cheese	1	350	18	17	50	31	1	790
Jack's Spicy Chicken	1 serv	620	25	31	50	61	4	1100
Jack's Spicy Chicken w/ Cheese	1	700	29	37	70	62	4	1410
Jumbo Jack	1	600	21	35	45	51	3	940
Jumbo Jack w/ Cheese	1	690	25	42	70	54	3	1310
Mozzarella Cheese Sticks	3	240	11	12	25	21	1	420
Onion Rings	8 (4.2 oz)	500	6	30	0	51	3	420
Sampler Trio	1 serv	750	35	39	85	65	5	1760
Sandwich Bacon Chicken	1	440	19	24	40	39	2	970
Sirloin Burger w/ American Cheese & Red Onion	1	1120	54	73	190	63	4	2620
Sirloin Burger w/ Swiss & Grilled Onions	1	1070	53	71	180	61	4	1850
Sirloin Steak Melt	1	640	36	40	100	34	2	1490
Sourdough Jack	1	710	27	51	75	36	3	1230
Spicy Chicken Bites	1 serv	290	18	14	45	21	3	660
Stuffed Jalapeno	3 (2.5 oz)	230	7	13	20	22	2	690
Taco Monster Beef	1	240	8	14	20	20	3	390
Taco Regular Beef	1	160	5	8	15	15	2	270
SALAD DRESSINGS AND TOPPINGS								
Asian Sesame	1 serv (2.5 oz)	230	1	17	0	20	0	780
Bacon Ranch	1 serv (2.5 oz)	320	2	33	35	4	0	810
Creamy Southwest	1 serv (2.5 oz)	270	1	27	30	4	0	1060
Dipping Sauce Barbeque	1 serv (1 oz)	45	0	0	0	11	0	330
Dipping Sauce Buttermilk House	1 serv (0.9 oz)	130	0	13	10	3	0	210
Dipping Sauce Frank's Red Hot Buffalo	1 serv (1 oz)	10	0	0	0	2	0	840
Dipping Sauce Sweet & Sour	1 serv (1 oz)	45	0	0	0	11	0	160
Dipping Sauce Teriyaki	1 serv (1 oz)	60	1	0	0	13	0	460

FOOD	PORTION	CALS	PROT	FAT	CHOL	CARB	FIBER	SOD
Dipping Sauce Zesty Marinara	1 serv (0.8 oz)	15	0	0	0	4	0	200
Low Fat Balsamic	1 serv (2.5 oz)	40	0	2	0	6	0	600
Mayo Onion Sauce	1 serv (0.5 oz)	90	1	10	5	4	0	590
Ranch	1 serv (2.5 oz)	390	1	41	30	4	0	590
Ranch Lite	1 serv (2.5 oz)	190	1	18	25	3	0	700
Soy Sauce	1 serv (0.3 oz)	5	1	0	0	1	0	480
Syrup Log Cabin	1 serv (2 oz)	190	0	0	0	49	0	35
Taco Sauce	1 serv (0.3 oz)	0	0	0	0	0	0	80
Tartar Sauce	1 serv (1.5 oz)	210	0	22	20	2	0	370
SALADS								
Asian w/ Crispy Chicken w/o Dressing	1 (13.8 oz)	330	21	13	40	34	7	650
Asian w/ Grilled Chicken w/o Dressing	1 (12.8 oz)	160	22	2	65	18	5	380
Chicken Club w/ Crispy Chicken w/o Dressing	1 (14 oz)	480	33	27	80	26	6	1060
Chicken Club w/ Grilled Chicken w/o Dressing	1 (13 oz)	320	34	16	105	11	4	780
Side w/o Dressing	1 (4.3 oz)	50	3	3	10	5	2	60
Southwest w/ Crispy Chicken w/o Dressing	1 (16 oz)	480	30	23	70	44	9	1040
Southwest w/ Grilled Chicken w/o Dressing	1 (15 oz)	320	31	12	90	27	7	760

JAMBA JUICE

FOOD	PORTION	CALS	PROT	FAT	CHOL	CARB	FIBER	SOD
BEVERAGES								
Acai Super Antioxidant	1 (16 oz)	290	4	5	5	59	4	50
Acai Topper	1 (12 oz)	440	8	9	0	86	9	40
Aloha Pineapple	1 (16 oz)	300	5	1	5	70	3	15
Banana Berry	1 (16 oz)	300	3	1	5	72	3	65
Berry Fulfilling	1 (16 oz)	160	7	1	5	34	4	230
Berry Topper	1 (12 oz)	420	11	9	5	80	9	80
Blackberry Bliss	1 (16 oz)	260	1	1	0	61	4	25
Boost 3G Charger Super	1 (3 g)	5	0	0	0	2	2	–

FOOD	PORTION	CALS	PROT	FAT	CHOL	CARB	FIBER	SOD
Boost Antioxidant Power Super	1 (2.8 g)	0	–	–	–	–	–	–
Boost Calcium	1	0	–	–	–	–	–	–
Boost Daily Vitamin	1 (4.36 g)	0	–	–	–	–	–	–
Boost Energy	½ tsp (1.1 g)	0	–	–	–	–	–	–
Boost Flax & Fiber	1 (0.4 oz)	30	1	2	–	7	7	–
Boost Heart Happy	1 (0.75 g)	0	–	–	–	–	–	–
Boost Immunity	1 tsp (2.5 g)	0	–	–	–	–	–	–
Boost Soy Protein	1 (8.9 g)	30	8	0	–	0	0	–
Boost Weight Burner Super	1 (3.5 g)	30	0	3	0	0	0	–
Boost Whey Protein Super	1 (12 g)	45	10	0	5	1	–	20
Caribbean Passion	1 (16 oz)	270	2	1	5	63	3	35
Carrot Juice	1 (16 oz)	100	3	1	0	22	0	170
Chocolate Moo'd	1 (16 oz)	460	12	6	20	93	2	270
Chunky Strawberry Topper	1 (12 oz)	480	13	15	5	74	8	120
Coldbuster	1 (16 oz)	270	3	2	5	63	3	20
Mango Mantra	1 (16 oz)	170	7	1	5	36	3	230
Mango Metabolizer	1 (16 oz)	290	2	4	0	63	4	20
Mango Peach Topper	1 (12 oz)	450	11	9	5	86	8	80
Mango-A-Go-Go	1 (16 oz)	310	2	1	5	72	2	35
Matcha Green Tea Blast	1 (16 oz)	290	8	0	0	62	1	160
Mega Mango	1 (16 oz)	250	3	1	0	62	4	5
Orange Dream Machine	1 (16 oz)	350	8	2	5	75	tr	150
Orange Juice	1 (16 oz)	220	3	1	0	52	tr	0
Peach Perfection	1 (16 oz)	230	2	0	0	57	4	20
Peach Pleasure	1 (16 oz)	290	2	1	5	68	3	35
Peanut Butter Moo'd	1 (16 oz)	490	13	11	10	85	3	310
Pomegranate Heart Happy	1 (16 oz)	300	4	1	0	72	3	105
Pomegranate Paradise	1 (16 oz)	260	2	1	0	64	4	25
Pomegranate Pick-Me-Up	1 (16 oz)	280	2	2	5	67	3	40
Protein Berry Workout w/ Soy Protein	1 (16 oz)	290	15	1	0	55	4	180
Protein Berry Workout w/ Whey	1 (16 oz)	300	17	0	5	56	4	115
Razzmatazz	1 (16 oz)	300	2	1	5	70	3	40
Shot Matcha Energy Orange Juice	1 (4 oz)	60	1	0	0	13	tr	0
Shot Matcha Energy Soymilk	1 (4 oz)	70	3	0	0	14	0	45
Shot Wheatgrass Detox	1 oz	5	tr	0	0	tr	0	0

FOOD	PORTION	CALS	PROT	FAT	CHOL	CARB	FIBER	SOD
Strawberries Wild	1 (16 oz)	280	3	0	0	66	3	100
Strawberry Energizer	1 (16 oz)	300	2	1	5	71	3	25
Strawberry Nirvana	1 (16 oz)	170	7	0	5	36	3	230
Strawberry Surf Rider	1 (16 oz)	330	2	1	5	80	3	10
Strawberry Whirl	1 (16 oz)	240	1	1	0	59	5	20
FOOD								
Cheddar Tomato Twist	1 (3.2 oz)	240	8	5	15	41	2	430
Cookie Omega-3 Chocolate Brownie	1 (1.5 oz)	150	3	4	0	30	2	15
Cookie Omega-3 Oatmeal	1 (1.5 oz)	150	2	6	5	26	3	85
Loaf Reduced Fat Blueberry Lemon	1 (3 oz)	290	2	8	–	53	2	–
Loaf Reduced Fat Cranberry Orange	1 (3 oz)	310	6	9	20	52	4	200
Loaf Zucchini Walnut	1 (3 oz)	270	5	9	20	43	4	250
Oatcake Blueberry	1 (3.25 oz)	280	6	9	0	46	6	220
Oatmeal Apple Cinnamon	1 serv (9.1 oz)	290	8	4	5	60	5	25
Oatmeal Blueberry & Blackberry	1 serv (8.9 oz)	290	8	4	0	59	6	30
Oatmeal Fresh Banana	1 serv (9.6 oz)	280	9	4	0	57	6	20
Oatmeal w/ Brown Sugar	1 serv (7.6 oz)	220	8	4	0	44	5	20
Pretzel Apple Cinnamon	1 (5.2 oz)	380	11	4	0	76	4	250
Pretzel Sourdough Parmesan	1 (5 oz)	410	14	10	5	67	3	640

JIMMY JOHN'S

FOOD	PORTION	CALS	PROT	FAT	CHOL	CARB	FIBER	SOD
BEVERAGES								
Coke	1 sm	248	0	0	0	68	0	15
Diet Coke	1 sm	0	0	0	0	0	0	25
Iced Tea	1 sm	3	0	0	0	1	0	35
Iced Tea Raspberry	1 sm	195	0	0	0	53	0	23
Lemonade	1 sm	243	0	0	0	65	0	103
Lemonade Light	1 sm	13	0	0	0	3	0	13
Sprite	1 sm	243	0	0	0	65	0	55
SANDWICHES								
Giant Club Beach	1	798	37	37	73	78	2	1873
Giant Club Billy	1	867	48	40	99	77	1	2533

FOOD	PORTION	CALS	PROT	FAT	CHOL	CARB	FIBER	SOD
Giant Club Bootlegger	1	720	40	28	77	74	1	2152
Giant Club Country	1	840	47	38	107	75	1	2478
Giant Club Gourmet Smoked Ham	1	851	45	40	105	76	1	2553
Giant Club Gourmet Veggie	1	856	33	46	60	77	2	1500
Giant Club Hunter's	1	854	49	38	93	76	1	2387
Giant Club Italian Night	1	975	47	52	115	77	1	2763
Giant Club Lulu	1	790	42	34	76	74	1	2050
Giant Club Tuna	1	719	34	29	53	77	2	1578
Giant Club Ultimate Porker	1	843	40	41	74	73	6	1919
Slim Double Provolone	1	588	32	19	49	71	0	1225
Slim Ham & Cheese	1	534	34	12	59	72	0	1673
Slim Salami Capicola Cheese	1	624	35	21	68	72	0	1821
Slim Tuna Salad	1	577	24	19	29	72	1	1327
Slim Turkey Breast	1	407	27	1	37	70	0	1355
Sub Big John	1	564	24	27	40	54	1	1333
Sub J.J.B.L.T.	1	662	29	35	45	54	1	1332
Sub Pepe	1	684	30	37	70	55	1	1659
Sub Totally Tuna	1	502	21	20	29	57	2	1131
Sub Turkey Tom	1	555	24	26	48	54	1	1342
Sub Vegetarian	1	640	21	36	36	57	2	1054
Sub Vito	1	579	32	25	68	56	1	1685
The J.J. Gargantuan	1	1008	69	55	180	60	1	3783
Unwich Hunter's Club	1	520	35	38	93	8	2	1655
Unwich The J.J. Gargantuan	1	769	57	55	180	11	2	3255
SIDES								
Cookie Chocolate Chunk	1	421	5	18	51	62	1	427
Cookie Raisin Oatmeal	1	421	7	16	66	65	4	471
Jimmy Chips	1 pkg	160	2	8	0	18	0	80
Jimmy Chips BBQ	1 pkg	160	2	9	0	17	0	90
Jimmy Chips Jalapeno	1 pkg	150	2	7	0	18	0	290
Jimmy Chips Sea Salt & Vinegar	1 pkg	140	2	8	0	16	0	280
Pickle Spear	1	4	0	0	0	1	tr	355
Pickle Whole	1	15	0	0	0	3	1	1420

FOOD	PORTION	CALS	PROT	FAT	CHOL	CARB	FIBER	SOD
KENTUCKY FRIED CHICKEN								
BEVERAGES								
Diet Pepsi	1 med (14 oz)	0	0	0	0	0	0	45
Mt. Dew	1 med (14 oz)	190	0	0	0	54	0	90
Pepsi	1 med (14 oz)	180	0	0	0	47	0	45
DESSERTS								
Cake Double Chocolate Chip	1 slice	330	4	16	50	41	1	260
Cookie Sweet Life Chocolate Chip	1 (1.2 oz)	160	2	7	10	23	1	95
Cookie Sweet Life Oatmeal Raisin	1 (1.2 oz)	150	2	5	5	24	1	135
Cookie Sweet Life Sugar	1 (1.2 oz)	160	2	6	5	23	0	120
Lil' Bucket Chocolate Cream	1	280	3	13	0	38	3	230
Lil' Bucket Lemon Creme	1 serv	410	7	15	0	61	2	270
Lil' Bucket Strawberry Short Cake	1 serv	210	2	7	10	33	1	125
Pie Mini's Apple	3 (4 oz)	370	2	20	0	44	2	260
Teddy Graham Cinnamon Snacks	1 serv	90	1	3	0	15	1	95
MAIN MENU SELECTIONS								
Baked Beans	1 serv	220	8	1	0	45	7	730
Biscuit	1 (2 oz)	220	4	11	0	24	1	640
Bowl Chicken & Biscuit	1	870	29	44	60	88	7	2420
Bowl Mashed Potato w/ Gravy	1	740	27	36	60	80	7	2350
Bowl Rice w/ Gravy	1	620	26	28	60	67	6	2150
Chicken Pot Pie	1 (15 oz)	770	33	40	115	70	5	1680
Cole Slaw	1 serv	180	1	10	5	22	3	270
Corn On The Cob	1 ear (3 inch)	70	2	2	0	13	3	5
Crispy Strips	2 (3.5 oz)	240	20	13	50	11	0	800
Extra Crispy Breast	1 (5.7 oz)	440	34	27	105	15	0	970
Extra Crispy Drumstick	1 (2 oz)	160	12	10	55	6	0	370
Extra Crispy Thigh	1 (4 oz)	370	18	28	85	12	0	850
Extra Crispy Whole Wing	1 (1.8 oz)	170	13	11	55	6	1	350
Green Beans	1 serv	50	2	2	5	7	2	570
KFC Snacker	1	290	15	13	30	29	2	680

FOOD	PORTION	CALS	PROT	FAT	CHOL	CARB	FIBER	SOD
KFC Snacker Buffalo	1	260	15	8	25	31	1	860
KFC Snacker Fish	1	330	17	15	60	31	1	710
KFC Snacker Fish w/o Sauce	1	290	17	12	60	29	1	610
KFC Snacker Honey BBQ	1	210	14	3	40	32	2	530
KFC Snacker Ultimate Cheese	1	280	15	11	25	30	1	780
Macaroni & Cheese	1 serv	180	8	8	15	18	0	800
Mashed Potatoes w/ Gravy	1 serv	140	2	5	0	20	1	560
Mashed Potatoes w/o Gravy	1 serv	110	2	4	0	17	1	320
Original Recipe Breast	1 (5.6 oz)	360	37	21	115	7	0	1020
Original Recipe Breast w/o Skin Or Breading	1 (3.8 oz)	140	29	2	65	1	0	520
Original Recipe Drumstick	1 (2 oz)	130	12	8	65	2	0	350
Original Recipe Thigh	1 (4.4 oz)	330	20	24	110	8	0	870
Original Recipe Whole Wing	1 (1.6 oz)	130	11	8	50	4	0	350
Popcorn Chicken	1 reg (4 oz)	400	21	26	60	22	3	1160
Potato Salad	1 serv	180	2	9	5	22	2	470
Potato Wedges	1 serv	260	4	13	0	33	3	740
Sandwich Crispy Twister	1	550	26	28	55	49	3	1500
Sandwich Double Crunch	1	470	27	23	55	38	2	1190
Sandwich Honey BBQ	1	280	22	4	60	40	3	780
Sandwich Tender Roast	1	380	37	13	80	29	2	1180
Sandwich Tender Roast w/o Sauce	1	300	37	5	70	28	2	1060
Seasoned Rice	1 serv	180	4	1	0	32	2	630
Twister Oven Roasted	1	420	28	17	60	40	3	1250
Twister Oven Roasted w/o Sauce	1	330	28	7	50	39	3	1120
Wings Boneless Fiery Buffalo	5	420	28	20	65	33	3	2260
Wings Boneless Honey BBQ	5	450	28	20	65	41	4	1880
Wings Boneless Sweet & Spicy	5	440	27	19	65	38	3	1700
Wings Boneless Teriyaki	5	500	28	21	65	50	3	1730
Wings Fiery Buffalo	5	380	21	24	105	19	2	1480
Wings Honey BBQ	5	390	21	24	105	23	3	930

FOOD	PORTION	CALS	PROT	FAT	CHOL	CARB	FIBER	SOD
Wings Hot	5	350	20	24	105	14	2	740
Wings Hot & Spicy	5	400	21	24	105	24	2	760
Wings Teriyaki	5	480	22	25	105	40	2	830
SALAD DRESSINGS								
Creamy Parmesan Caesar	1 serv (2 oz)	260	2	26	15	4	0	540
Golden Italian Light	1 serv (1.5 oz)	45	0	3	0	6	0	660
Ranch	1 serv (2 oz)	200	1	20	25	3	0	470
Ranch Fat Free	1 serv (1.5 oz)	35	1	0	0	8	0	410
SALADS								
Crispy BLT w/o Dressing	1 (12 oz)	330	28	17	65	18	4	1130
Crispy Caesar w/o Dressing & Croutons	1 (11 oz)	350	29	19	70	16	3	1080
Croutons Parmesan Garlic	1 pkg	60	2	3	0	8	0	135
Roasted BLT w/o Dressing	1 (12 oz)	200	29	6	65	8	4	880
Roasted Caesar w/o Dressing & Croutons	1 (11 oz)	220	30	8	70	6	3	830
Side Caesar w/o Dressing & Croutons	1 (3 oz)	50	4	3	10	2	1	135
Side House w/o Dressing	1 (3 oz)	15	1	0	0	2	1	10

KOO-KOO-ROO

MAIN MENU SELECTIONS

FOOD	PORTION	CALS	PROT	FAT	CHOL	CARB	FIBER	SOD
Baked Yam	1 serv (6 oz)	197	3	tr	0	47	7	14
Black Beans	1 serv (6 oz)	125	8	3	0	23	6	487
Buffalo Wings	6	606	44	28	119	42	2	875
Burrito California Chicken	1	810	46	41	115	60	4	2182
Burrito Fajita Chicken	1	750	40	33	94	70	4	2995
Burrito Original Chicken	1	709	41	28	94	71	5	2926
Butternut Squash	1 serv (6 oz)	66	2	tr	0	17	3	3
Chicken Bowl Chargrilled w/o Sauce	1	569	41	19	132	57	4	1757
Chicken Bowl Spicy Garlic Ginger w/o Sauce	1	485	42	6	96	63	2	842
Creamed Spinach	1 serv (8 oz)	100	4	6	7	10	3	573
Italian Vegetable	1 serv (5.5 oz)	47	1	2	5	9	2	132

FOOD	PORTION	CALS	PROT	FAT	CHOL	CARB	FIBER	SOD
Kernel Corn	1 serv (4.5 oz)	105	4	1	0	26	3	162
Mashed Potatoes	1 serv (6.5 oz)	188	4	5	15	32	3	428
Original Breast	1 (4.1 oz)	187	34	6	117	tr	0	422
Original Chicken Dark	3 pieces (5 oz)	320	39	16	101	5	0	659
Roasted Garlic Potatoes	1 serv (5 oz)	133	2	5	5	21	2	247
Rotisserie Chicken Breast & Wing	1 serv (6.5 oz)	355	49	16	140	1	tr	675
Rotisserie Chicken Leg & Thigh	1 serv (4.8 oz)	300	31	18	114	1	tr	513
Rotisserie Half Chicken	1 serv (11.3 oz)	655	80	34	254	2	tr	1188
Sandwich BBQ Chicken	1	562	45	12	113	71	3	1398
Sandwich Chicken Caesar	1	781	56	36	138	63	2	1775
Sandwich Original Chicken	1	661	41	29	116	63	3	1144
Sandwich Turkey Hand Carved	1	599	46	32	122	31	5	786
Southwestern Bowl w/o Sauce	1	570	37	19	95	67	8	2798
Tostada Bowl w/o Sauce w/o Shell	1	528	40	22	99	45	7	2144
Traditional Turkey Dinner	1 serv	692	42	29	127	67	8	3719
Turkey Breast Sliced	1 serv	182	25	8	76	0	0	66
Turkey Pot Pie	1	883	37	44	98	83	6	1287
Wrap Caesar Chicken	1	757	42	39	97	59	4	1890
Wrap Chipotle Chicken	1	924	42	43	123	89	6	2449
SALADS								
BBQ Chicken w/o Dressing	1	365	38	14	104	22	6	897
Cantaloupe & Honeydew	1 serv (5 oz)	50	1	tr	0	12	1	14
Chicken Caesar w/o Dressing	1	286	34	11	80	13	4	967
Chinese Chicken w/o Dressing	1	550	40	29	72	39	10	853
Creamy Coleslaw	1 serv (5 oz)	238	1	20	28	14	2	639
Cucumber	1 serv (4.5 oz)	41	1	tr	0	9	2	190
House	1	113	6	4	4	16	5	206

FOOD	PORTION	CALS	PROT	FAT	CHOL	CARB	FIBER	SOD
Tangy Tomato	1 serv (4.5 oz)	60	1	4	0	6	1	173
Tossed w/ Dressing	1 serv (3 oz)	16	1	tr	0	3	1	9
SOUPS								
Chicken Noodle	1 serv (5 oz)	71	6	3	19	4	tr	426
Chicken Tortilla	1 serv (5 oz)	112	8	6	24	7	1	684
Ten Vegetable	1 serv (5 oz)	94	3	2	0	16	4	435
KRISPY KREME								
BEVERAGES								
Chillers Fruity Orange You Glad	1 (12 oz)	180	0	0	0	43	0	10
Chillers Fruity Very Berry	1 (12 oz)	170	0	0	0	43	0	10
Chillers Kremey Berries & Kreme	1 (12 oz)	620	3	28	30	92	tr	220
Chillers Kremey Chocolate Chocolate	1 (12 oz)	970	4	29	30	104	2	320
Chillers Kremey Lemon Sherbert	1 (12 oz)	630	3	28	30	95	tr	220
Chillers Kremey Lotta Latte	1 (12 oz)	670	4	28	30	49	tr	380
Chillers Kremey Mocha Dream	1 (12 oz)	670	3	28	30	105	1	320
Chillers Kremey Oranges & Kreme	1 (12 oz)	630	3	28	30	92	tr	220
DOUGHNUTS								
Apple Fritter	1	380	4	20	5	47	2	220
Caramel Kreme Crunch	1	380	4	19	10	40	tr	170
Chocolate Iced Cake	1	280	3	14	20	36	tr	320
Chocolate Iced Custard Filled	1	300	3	17	5	36	tr	150
Chocolate Iced Glazed	1	250	3	12	5	33	tr	100
Chocolate Iced Kreme Filled	1	350	3	20	5	39	tr	140
Chocolate Iced w/ Sprinkles	1	270	3	12	5	38	tr	100
Cinnamon Apple Filled	1	290	3	16	5	32	tr	150
Cinnamon Bun	1	260	3	16	5	28	tr	125
Cinnamon Twist	1	240	3	15	5	23	tr	130
Dulce De Leche	1	300	3	18	5	31	tr	160
Glazed Chocolate Cake	1	300	3	15	20	42	2	250
Glazed Cinnamon	1	210	2	12	5	24	tr	100

FOOD	PORTION	CALS	PROT	FAT	CHOL	CARB	FIBER	SOD
Glazed Creme Filled	1	340	3	20	5	39	tr	140
Glazed Cruller	1	240	2	14	15	26	tr	240
Glazed Cruller Chocolate	1	290	2	15	15	37	tr	240
Glazed Lemon Filled	1	290	3	16	5	36	tr	135
Glazed Maple Iced	1	240	2	12	5	32	tr	100
Glazed Original	1	200	2	12	5	22	tr	95
Glazed Pumpkin Spice	1	300	2	14	20	42	tr	250
Glazed Raspberry Filled	1	300	3	16	5	36	tr	125
Glazed Sour Cream	1	300	2	13	20	43	tr	250
Holes Glazed Blueberry	4	220	3	12	20	27	tr	280
Holes Glazed Cake	4	210	2	10	15	29	tr	240
Holes Glazed Chocolate Cake	4	210	2	10	15	29	tr	240
Holes Glazed Original	4	200	2	11	5	25	tr	90
Holes Glazed Pumpkin Spice	4	210	2	10	15	29	tr	240
New York Cheesecake	1	340	4	20	15	34	tr	200
Powdered Cake	1	290	3	14	20	37	tr	320
Powdered Strawberry Filled	1	290	3	16	5	33	tr	135
Sugar	1	200	2	12	5	21	0	95
Traditional Cake	1	230	3	13	20	25	tr	320
KRYSTAL								
BEVERAGES								
Coca Cola Classic	1 sm (16 oz)	129	0	0	0	40	0	9
Coco Cola Classic frzn	1 (16 oz)	130	0	0	0	36	0	12
Diet Coke	1 sm (16 oz)	tr	0	0	0	tr	0	15
Sprite	1 sm (16 oz)	126	0	0	0	39	0	33
BREAKFAST SELECTIONS								
4 Carb Scrambler Bacon	1 serv	370	24	29	595	4	1	830
4 Carb Scrambler Sausage	1 serv	600	32	51	600	3	2	1040
Biscuit & Gravy	1	280	5	14	0	34	0	710
Biscuit Bacon Egg Cheese	1	390	11	23	40	33	0	1090
Biscuit Chik	1	360	13	15	20	40	0	1030
Biscuit Plain	1	270	5	13	0	33	0	660
Biscuit Sausage	1	480	12	33	40	33	0	980
Country Breakfast	1 serv	660	24	42	590	46	8	1450
Kryspers	1 serv	190	1	13	10	17	2	340
Krystal Sunriser	1	240	12	14	255	14	2	460
Scrambler	1 serv	440	20	26	255	33	3	840

FOOD	PORTION	CALS	PROT	FAT	CHOL	CARB	FIBER	SOD
DESSERTS								
Fried Apple Turnover	1	220	3	10	<5	31	2	300
Lemon Icebox Pie	1 serv	260	5	9	25	41	2	180
MAIN MENU SELECTIONS								
BA Burger	1	470	22	27	55	39	2	760
BA Burger Cheese	1	530	25	32	55	40	2	1020
BA Burger Double Bacon Cheese	1	800	44	53	115	41	2	1600
Chik'n Bites	1 sm	310	17	19	55	16	1	790
Chik'n Bites Salad	1 serv	290	20	20	66	12	4	490
Fries	1 reg	470	4	20	20	53	7	90
Fries Chili Cheese	1 serv	540	13	28	45	59	6	800
Krystal	1	160	7	7	20	17	1	260
Krystal Bacon Cheese	1	190	10	10	25	16	2	430
Krystal Cheese	1	180	9	9	25	17	2	430
Krystal Chik	1	240	11	11	25	24	2	640
Krystal Chili	1 serv	200	13	7	25	22	7	1130
Krystal Double	1	260	13	13	40	24	2	550
Krystal Double Cheese	1	310	16	16	65	26	tr	800
Pup Chili Cheese	1	210	9	12	40	17	2	510
Pup Corn	1	260	5	19	50	19	1	480
Pup Plain	1	170	6	9	25	15	1	500

LITTLE CAESARS

FOOD	PORTION	CALS	PROT	FAT	CHOL	CARB	FIBER	SOD
DIPS AND SAUCES								
Crazy Sauce	1 serv (4 oz)	45	2	0	0	10	1	260
Dip Buffalo	1 serv (1.5 oz)	130	0	14	0	4	0	940
Dip Buffalo Ranch	1 serv (1.5 oz)	220	0	24	15	3	0	520
Dip Buttery Garlic	1 serv (1.5 oz)	380	0	42	0	0	0	420
Dip Cheezy	1 serv (1.5 oz)	210	1	21	15	3	0	450
Dip Chipotle	1 serv (1.5 oz)	220	0	24	15	2	0	560
Dip Ranch	1 serv (1.5 oz)	250	0	26	15	3	0	380
MAIN MENU SELECTIONS								
Cheese Bread Italian	1 (1.6 oz)	130	6	7	10	13	0	230

FOOD	PORTION	CALS	PROT	FAT	CHOL	CARB	FIBER	SOD
Cheese Bread Pepperoni	1 (1.7 oz)	150	7	8	15	13	0	280
Crazy Bread	1 (1.3 oz)	100	3	3	0	15	1	150
Pizza 3 Meat Treat	1/8 pie (4.8 oz)	350	17	18	40	30	1	730
Pizza Baby Pan!Pan! Cheese & Pepperoni	1 pie (4.9 oz)	360	16	18	35	33	1	610
Pizza Baby Pan!Pan! Just Cheese	1 pie (4.7 oz)	320	14	15	25	33	1	500
Pizza Deep Dish Just Cheese	1/8 pie (4.8 oz)	320	14	13	25	38	1	490
Pizza Deep Dish Pepperoni	1/8 pie (5 oz)	360	16	16	30	38	1	610
Pizza Hot-N-Ready Just Cheese	1/8 pie (4 oz)	240	12	9	20	30	1	410
Pizza Hot-N-Ready Pepperoni	1/8 pie (4.2 oz)	280	14	11	25	30	1	520
Pizza Hulu Hawaiian Pineapple & Canadian Bacon	1/8 pie (5.2 oz)	280	15	9	25	34	1	640
Pizza Hulu Hawaiian Pineapple & Ham	1/8 pie (5.3 oz)	270	15	9	25	33	1	600
Pizza Ultimate Supreme	1/8 pie (5.3 oz)	310	15	14	30	31	2	640
Pizza Ultimate Supreme Vegetarian	1/8 pie (5.4 oz)	270	13	10	20	32	2	530
Wings Barbecue	1 (1.2 oz)	70	4	4	20	3	0	220
Wings Hot	1 (1.2 oz)	60	4	5	20	1	0	430
Wings Mild	1 (1 oz)	60	4	4	20	1	0	290
Wings Oven Roasted	1 (0.9 oz)	50	4	4	20	0	0	150

MAGGIE MOO'S

BEVERAGES

FOOD	PORTION	CALS	PROT	FAT	CHOL	CARB	FIBER	SOD
Shake Caramel Cowpuccino	1 (15 oz)	740	12	43	170	79	0	190
Shake Cinnamoo Swirl	1 (16 oz)	780	11	44	165	87	1	210
Shake Cookies 'N' Cream	1 (15 oz)	740	12	44	165	77	0	230
Shake Moocha Cowpuccino	1 (15 oz)	710	11	41	165	78	0	160
Shake Peanut Butter S'Moo	1 (16 oz)	780	16	46	155	82	4	400
Shake Strawberries 'N' Cream	1 (15 oz)	620	10	37	150	66	1	140

FOOD	PORTION	CALS	PROT	FAT	CHOL	CARB	FIBER	SOD
Zoomer Caramel Coffee	1 (15 oz)	380	1	13	0	65	0	400
Zoomer Creamy Mango	1 (17 oz)	400	1	3	0	96	1	100
Zoomer Mocha Coffee	1 (17 oz)	460	2	11	0	90	0	400
Zoomer Raspberry Pomegranate	1 (17 oz)	460	2	0	0	141	3	25
Zoomer Strawberry Banana	1 (18 oz)	350	2	10	0	69	3	300
Zoomer Triple Berry Pomegranate	1 (17 oz)	460	2	1	0	115	3	20
CONES								
Dark Chocolate	1 (1.5 oz)	200	2	7	5	30	1	15
Dark Chocolate w/ Butterfinger	1 (2 oz)	260	3	10	5	41	1	45
Dark Chocolate w/ Heath Bar	1 (2 oz)	280	3	12	10	39	1	65
Dark Chocolate w/ Peanuts	1 (2 oz)	280	6	15	5	33	2	15
Plain	1 (1 oz)	120	2	3	5	22	0	0
White Chocolate	1 (1.5 oz)	200	2	7	10	31	0	15
White Chocolate w/ Sprinkles	1 (2 oz)	210	2	7	10	34	0	15
ICE CREAM								
Amooretto Cream	1 serv (6 oz)	380	6	23	95	38	0	85
Apple Strudel	1 serv (6 oz)	380	6	21	85	44	0	85
Banana Pudding	1 serv (6 oz)	330	5	18	75	39	1	70
Black Cherry	1 serv (6 oz)	380	6	23	95	39	0	85
Blueberry Muffin	1 serv (6 oz)	390	6	20	75	48	1	65
Brownie Batter	1 serv (6 oz)	420	6	21	85	52	1	170
Butter Pecan	1 serv (6 oz)	380	6	21	85	44	0	140
Cake 6 inch Better Batter	1/8 cake (5.7 oz)	480	5	24	55	62	1	170
Cake 6 inch Chocolate Cream	1/8 cake (6.4 oz)	580	7	33	80	69	3	110
Cake 8 inch Caramel Drizzle	1/14 cake (6 oz)	530	6	33	65	55	11	125
Cake 8 inch Chocolate Espresso	1/14 cake (5.6 oz)	460	5	25	150	58	1	190
Cake 8 inch Chocolate Heaven	1/14 cake (5 oz)	400	6	22	60	45	2	150
Cake 8 inch Cookie Dreams	1/14 cake (5.3 oz)	440	5	22	55	57	1	150

FOOD	PORTION	CALS	PROT	FAT	CHOL	CARB	FIBER	SOD
Cake 8 inch Cookies 'N' Cream	1/14 cake (5.3 oz)	430	5	24	65	50	1	180
Cake 8 inch Cotton Candy Carnival	1/14 cake (5.9 oz)	490	6	25	65	65	1	95
Cake 8 inch Fudge Fantasy	1/14 cake (5.4 oz)	410	5	22	60	49	0	100
Cake 8 inch Maggie S'Mores	1/14 cake (7 oz)	610	8	23	55	94	2	440
Cake 8 inch Maggie's Mud	1/14 cake (5.3 oz)	440	7	25	60	49	2	210
Cake 8 inch Pecan Perfection	1/14 cake (5.6 oz)	500	7	33	60	50	3	150
Cake 8 inch Sprinkle	1/14 cake (5.7 oz)	370	4	19	55	46	0	65
Cake 8 inch Strawberry Cheesecream	1/14 cake (6.3 oz)	530	7	23	55	74	1	320
Cake 8 inch Truffle Dream	1/14 cake (5.8 oz)	500	6	28	75	58	2	95
Cake 8 inch Turtle	1/14 cake (6.3 oz)	590	7	40	65	54	2	115
Cappuccino	1 serv (6 oz)	380	3	22	90	41	0	85
Caramel Apple	1 serv (6 oz)	400	6	21	85	47	0	105
Carrot Cake	1 serv (6 oz)	420	6	21	80	51	0	200
Cheesecake	1 serv (6 oz)	380	6	21	85	43	0	80
Choco Mallo	1 serv (6 oz)	360	6	19	75	43	1	160
Chocolate	1 serv (6 oz)	390	7	22	80	44	2	200
Chocolate Banana	1 serv (6 oz)	370	7	20	80	43	2	160
Chocolate Better Batter	1 serv (6 oz)	420	7	21	50	54	1	160
Chocolate Peanut Butter	1 serv (6 oz)	450	9	28	80	42	2	220
Chocolate Raspberry	1 serv (6 oz)	380	6	20	80	46	2	180
Cinnamoo	1 serv (6 oz)	380	6	23	95	39	0	85
Cinnamoo Bunn	1 serv (6 oz)	530	7	23	60	74	1	250
Cocoa Amooretto	1 serv (6 oz)	390	7	23	90	42	1	160
Cool Mint	1 serv (6 oz)	380	6	23	95	38	0	85
Cotton Candy	1 serv (6 oz)	300	6	23	95	38	0	90
Creamy Coconut	1 serv (6 oz)	380	6	23	95	38	0	85
Cupcake Better Batter	1	430	5	21	45	58	1	55
Cupcake Caramel Pumpkin Pie	1	500	4	26	50	62	1	210
Cupcake Cherry Chocolate	1	280	5	13	50	39	1	75

FOOD	PORTION	CALS	PROT	FAT	CHOL	CARB	FIBER	SOD
Cupcake Chocolate	1	400	5	22	65	51	2	95
Cupcake Chocolate Heaven	1	340	5	18	45	41	1	105
Cupcake Cool Swirl	1	370	4	19	45	47	0	50
Cupcake Cotton Candy Carnival	1	330	4	18	50	40	0	50
Cupcake Maggie O	1	360	6	18	55	45	1	260
Cupcake Pecan Pie	1	440	4	28	45	43	1	150
Cupcake Snowcap Blush	1	360	4	18	45	45	1	45
Cupcake Sprinkle	1	340	4	18	50	42	0	50
Dark Chocolate	1 serv	390	7	23	90	42	2	170
Egg Nog	1 serv (6 oz)	390	6	22	90	45	0	80
Espresso Bean	1 serv (6 oz)	380	6	22	90	41	0	85
French Vanilla	1 serv	390	6	22	90	43	0	85
Fresh Banana	1 serv (6 oz)	340	6	19	80	38	1	70
Key Lime	1 serv	380	5	18	70	54	0	65
Maggie's Fudge	1 serv	630	8	34	120	74	0	170
Mint Chocolate	1 serv (6 oz)	390	7	23	80	43	1	180
Mocha	1 serv (6 oz)	390	6	23	850	42	1	135
Peanut Butter	1 serv (6 oz)	480	10	33	80	38	1	170
Pina Cowlada	1 serv (6 oz)	360	6	21	85	37	0	75
Pink Bubblegum	1 serv (6 oz)	380	6	23	95	39	0	85
Pink Peppermint Stick	1 serv (6 oz)	420	6	21	85	51	0	75
Pistachio	1 serv (6 oz)	380	6	23	95	39	0	85
Pizza 10 inch Cheese	1/10 pie (5.4 oz)	340	6	18	65	40	0	55
Pizza 10 inch Chocolate Lover's	1/10 pie	390	6	20	70	48	1	65
Pizza 10 inch Supreme	1/10 pie (6.1 oz)	450	7	24	70	53	1	100
Pumpkin Pie	1 serv (6 oz)	370	6	21	850	41	0	95
Raspberry	1 serv (6 oz)	370	6	21	85	42	0	100
Red Velvet Cake	1 serv (6 oz)	420	7	21	75	54	1	150
Rum Raisin	1 serv (6 oz)	380	6	23	95	39	0	90
Southern Peaches	1 serv (6 oz)	330	5	16	65	44	0	75
Strawberry	1 serv	350	6	21	85	37	0	75
Strawberry Banana No Sugar Added	1 serv (6 oz)	170	0	6	0	42	0	30
Udderly Cream	1 serv (6 oz)	380	6	23	95	38	0	85
Vanilla	1 serv (6 oz)	380	6	23	95	39	0	85

FOOD	PORTION	CALS	PROT	FAT	CHOL	CARB	FIBER	SOD
Vanilla Low Fat Lactose Free	1 serv (6 oz)	130	0	5	0	23	0	150
Very Yellow Marshmallow	1 serv (6 oz)	350	5	20	80	38	0	90
MARBLE SLAB CREAMERY								
Cone Honey Wheat	1	130	3	3	15	24	tr	10
Cone Sugar	1	130	2	3	15	23	0	10
Cone Vanilla Cinnamon	1	130	2	3	15	24	tr	10
Frozen Yogurt Nonfat	½ cup	100	3	tr	0	22	tr	55
Frozen Yogurt Nonfat No Sugar Added	½ cup	90	4	tr	0	17	tr	85
Ice Cream Reduced Fat	1 serv (6.75 oz)	390	6	20	80	47	0	130
Ice Cream Superpremium	1 serv (6.75 oz)	450	8	28	115	44	0	135
Sorbet	½ cup	90	0	0	0	22	0	5
MARCO'S PIZZA								
OTHER MENU SELECTIONS								
Cheezybread Bran	1 piece	80	3	2	5	11	0	105
Chicken Tumblers BBQ	1	67	4	2	9	7	0	164
Chicken Tumblers Hot & Spicy	1	57	4	2	9	5	0	157
Chicken Tumblers Naked	1	57	4	2	9	5	0	120
Chicken Wings BBQ	1	71	5	4	29	3	0	174
Chicken Wings Hot & Spicy	1	60	5	4	29	0	0	167
Chicken Wings Naked	1	60	5	4	29	0	0	130
Cinnasquares	1 piece	60	1	2	0	9	0	60
Salad Chicken Ranch	1 serv	240	22	13	60	10	3	1220
Salad Italian	1 serv	230	12	17	35	11	3	930
Sub Chicken Club	½	385	28	16	50	34	2	1150
Sub Ham & Cheese	½	400	21	21	43	33	1	865
Sub Italian	½	430	24	23	53	35	2	1175
Sub Steak & Cheese	½	380	29	15	60	33	1	605
Sub Veggie	½	355	16	16	33	39	3	1135
PIZZA								
Cheese Large	1 slice	280	14	8	20	33	2	510
Cheese Medium	1 slice	210	11	6	15	24	1	390
Cheese Small	1 slice	200	11	6	15	23	1	370
Chicken Fresco Large	1 slice	350	20	13	35	35	2	900
Chicken Fresco Medium	1 slice	260	15	10	25	26	1	670

FOOD	PORTION	CALS	PROT	FAT	CHOL	CARB	FIBER	SOD
Chicken Fresco Small	1 slice	180	11	7	20	19	1	480
Deep Pan Cheese	1 slice	290	15	8	20	36	2	530
Deep Pan Pepperoni	1 slice	330	16	12	25	36	2	650
Deluxe Uno Large	1 slice	380	20	16	40	35	2	700
Deluxe Uno Medium	1 slice	280	15	12	30	26	1	520
Deluxe Uno Small	1 slice	200	10	9	20	18	1	360
Garden Large	1 slice	310	16	10	20	36	2	740
Garden Medium	1 slice	230	12	8	15	26	2	530
Garden Small	1 slice	160	8	5	10	19	1	360
Hawaiian Chicken Large	1 slice	380	22	15	35	35	2	890
Hawaiian Chicken Medium	1 slice	260	15	10	25	26	1	620
Hawaiian Chicken Small	1 slice	180	10	6	15	18	1	430
Meat Supremo Large	1 slice	430	23	21	45	34	2	900
Meat Supremo Medium	1 slice	300	15	15	30	25	1	640
Meat Supremo Small	1 slice	210	11	10	20	18	1	430
Pepperoni Large	1 slice	310	15	11	25	33	2	640
Pepperoni Medium	1 slice	230	11	9	20	24	1	470
Pepperoni Small	1 slice	210	10	8	20	23	1	440
White Cheezy Large	1 slice	340	17	15	25	33	2	730
White Cheezy Medium	1 slice	260	13	11	20	24	1	550
White Cheezy Small	1 slice	170	9	7	10	17	1	360
MAUI WOWI								
SMOOTHIES								
Fresh Fruit Banana Banana	1 (12 oz)	210	2	1	0	50	2	55
Fresh Fruit Black Raspberry	1 (12 oz)	240	2	0	0	59	0	40
Fresh Fruit Kiwi Lemon Lime	1 (12 oz)	180	3	0	0	42	0	35
Fresh Fruit Lemon Wave	1 (12 oz)	415	tr	tr	0	108	tr	1
Fresh Fruit Mango Orange Banana	1 (12 oz)	240	3	1	0	57	tr	35
Fresh Fruit Passion Papaya	1 (12 oz)	220	2	1	0	54	tr	50
Fresh Fruit Pina Colada	1 (12 oz)	240	3	3	0	57	0	70
MAX & ERMA'S								
Black Bean Roll Up	1 serv	577	29	10	14	95	10	1203
Caribbean Chicken Lunch Portion	1 serv	536	28	20	97	59	3	1151
Fruit Smoothie	1	124	1	tr	0	29	1	4
Garlic Breadstick	1	156	4	6	0	21	0	293

FOOD	PORTION	CALS	PROT	FAT	CHOL	CARB	FIBER	SOD
Hula Bowl w/ Fat Free Honey Mustard Dressing w/o Breadsticks	1 serv	823	46	7	131	79	6	1554
Salad Baby Greens w/o Breadstick	1 serv	119	1	11	0	6	2	259
Salad Shrimp Stack	1 serv	322	20	12	178	116	3	823
Salad Dressing Bleu Cheese	2 tbsp	201	1	21	19	tr	0	169
Salad Dressing French Fat Free	2 tbsp	126	tr	tr	0	31	2	1034
Salad Dressing Honey Mustard Fat Free	2 tbsp	60	0	0	0	14	0	360
Salad Dressing Italian	2 tbsp	110	0	12	0	1	0	180
Salad Dressing Ranch	2 tbsp	120	1	13	11	1	0	90
Salad Dressing Tex Mex Low Fat	2 tbsp	23	3	tr	2	2	tr	129
McALISTER'S DELI								
CHILDREN'S MENU SELECTIONS								
Kid's Nacho	1 serv	734	12	43	17	74	3	679
Mac's Dog	1	307	10	19	35	24	1	827
Pita Pizza	1	503	24	21	46	54	3	887
Sandwich Ham & Cheese	1	455	26	22	75	39	4	1819
Sandwich PB&J	1	714	23	32	0	86	7	644
Sandwich Toasted Cheese	1	620	30	38	107	40	4	2031
Sandwich Turkey & Cheese	1	451	26	21	79	39	4	1670
DESSERTS								
Brownie Chocolate	1 (3.5 oz)	424	6	18	0	59	3	311
Brownie Delight	1 (11 oz)	917	13	48	108	111	4	519
Chocolate Loving Spoon Cake	1 (4 oz)	538	6	35	69	54	2	486
Ice Cream Vanilla Bean	1 scoop (5 oz)	160	3	10	40	19	0	70
Kentucky Pie	1 slice (12 oz)	807	14	64	211	110	1	393
New York Cheesecake	1 slice (5 oz)	505	7	35	92	37	2	239
Sundae Topping Caramel	2 tbsp	100	1	0	0	20	0	110
Sundae Topping Chocolate	1 tbsp	110	1	0	0	21	0	20
MAIN MENU SELECTIONS								
Appetizers Chips & Salsa	1 serv (5 oz)	87	3	5	0	9	0	128

FOOD	PORTION	CALS	PROT	FAT	CHOL	CARB	FIBER	SOD
Appetizers Dip Cheese & Chili	1 serv (5 oz)	572	10	35	17	54	3	598
Appetizers Dip Cheese & Veggie Chili	1 serv (5 oz)	552	9	31	9	58	5	583
Appetizers Nacho Basket	1 serv (6 oz)	579	10	33	17	61	3	832
Appetizers Nacho Chili	1 serv (6 oz)	564	12	37	26	46	4	713
Appetizers Nacho Veggie Chili	1 serv (6 oz)	537	11	31	14	52	6	693
Chicken Cordon Bleu	1 serv	810	59	39	156	53	2	2862
Chili Vegetarian	1 serv (8 oz)	133	8	1	0	28	15	987
Cole Slaw	1 serv (4 oz)	190	1	15	15	14	7	215
Fruit Cup	1 serv (4 oz)	98	1	0	0	12	2	12
Giant Spud Cheese	1 (27 oz)	930	55	48	60	139	19	60
Giant Spud Grilled Chicken	1 (27 oz)	839	52	25	–	99	19	88
Giant Spud Just A Spud	1 (26 oz)	604	20	4	0	123	18	63
Giant Spud Ole	1 (30 oz)	1252	68	60	120	110	18	770
Giant Spud Ole w/ Chili	1 (33 oz)	1512	69	78	99	134	21	1255
Giant Spud Ole w/ Veggie Chili	1 (33 oz)	1457	67	67	76	146	24	1214
Giant Spud Veggie	1 (28 oz)	668	29	18	0	99	18	347
Macaroni & Cheese	1 serv (4 oz)	200	8	7	20	17	1	580
Mashed Potatoes	1 serv (4 oz)	136	2	8	2	19	2	347
Meatloaf w/ Gravy	1 serv	340	40	37	189	21	1	752
Open-Faced Roast Beef	1 serv	751	55	21	87	88	6	3099
Pot Roast Spud	1 serv	906	38	30	72	121	17	125
Potato Salad	1 serv (4 oz)	200	3	11	1	22	3	161
Salmon Filet	1 serv	235	46	4	152	3	1	269
Steamed Vegetables	1 serv (4 oz)	43	1	0	0	7	3	52
SALAD DRESSINGS AND SAUCES								
Au Jus	1 serv (4 oz)	10	0	0	0	2	0	60
Comeback Gravy	1 serv (4 oz)	37	1	2	1	6	0	450
Dressing Blue Cheese	2 tbsp	140	0	15	10	1	0	290
Dressing Greek	2 tbsp	90	0	9	0	2	0	250
Dressing Lite Olive Oil Vinaigrette	2 tbsp	60	0	6	0	3	0	230
Dressing Lite Ranch	2 tbsp	100	0	10	10	1	0	290
Dressing Low Calorie Italian	2 tbsp	25	0	2	0	2	0	410
Dressing Parmesan Peppercorn	2 tbsp	150	0	16	2	2	0	310

FOOD	PORTION	CALS	PROT	FAT	CHOL	CARB	FIBER	SOD
Dressing Ranch	2 tbsp	100	0	11	10	1	0	290
Dressing Tomato Basil	2 tbsp	30	0	0	0	6	0	230
SALADS								
Caesar w/ Salmon	1 (17 oz)	800	34	53	109	42	5	1680
Chicken Fiesta	1 (20 oz)	493	38	22	92	34	8	991
Chicken Grill	1 (21 oz)	840	57	15	131	47	4	3164
Garden	1 (15 oz)	264	17	17	38	21	4	1312
Garden w/ Chicken Salad	1 (18 oz)	537	30	45	34	14	5	1333
Garden w/ Salmon	1 (17 oz)	315	28	10	76	28	6	883
Garden w/ Tuna Salad	1 (18 oz)	373	31	18	15	21	5	1361
Greek Chicken	1 (19 oz)	584	38	32	65	32	7	2161
Side Caesar	1 (6 oz)	328	5	24	16	19	1	679
Side Garden	1 (8 oz)	138	8	9	19	11	2	867
Taco	1 (26 oz)	641	38	40	86	33	11	1680
Taco w/ Veggie Chili	1 (26 oz)	641	38	40	64	33	15	1639
SANDWICHES								
BLT	1	654	28	38	56	50	6	2015
Chicken Salad	1	677	15	43	59	58	2	967
Deli Corned Beef On Wheat	1	369	34	9	76	39	4	1879
Deli Ham On Wheat	1	350	24	9	43	43	5	1854
Deli Pastrami On Wheat	1	371	33	10	75	36	4	1385
Deli Roast Beef On Wheat	1	398	27	12	29	49	5	1937
Deli Salami On Wheat	1	565	27	32	100	43	5	2465
Deli Turkey On Wheat	1	342	24	9	51	43	5	1556
French Dip	1	676	44	34	118	50	2	1889
Grilled Chicken Breast	1	751	50	36	120	56	2	1772
Grilled Chicken Club	1	1234	76	64	193	87	7	2733
Ham Melt	1	700	49	34	114	52	4	2303
McAlister's Club	1	1225	66	69	195	86	7	2845
Meatloaf Parmesan	1	708	47	36	140	49	5	1046
Memphian	1	585	41	26	85	48	4	2237
Muffuletta	¼ (8 oz)	615	36	35	67	40	2	2015
New Yorker	1	628	50	25	127	50	4	2119
Orange Cranberry Club	1	954	63	52	171	62	6	2230
Reuben On Rye	1	492	25	30	71	35	2	2175
Roast Beef Melt	1	635	40	32	102	48	4	2170
Salmon	1	608	37	21	76	66	3	1006
Submarine	1	833	50	48	130	53	3	2866
Sweetberry Chicken On Wheatberry	1	701	53	24	102	67	5	1618

FOOD	PORTION	CALS	PROT	FAT	CHOL	CARB	FIBER	SOD
Tuna Salad On Wheat	1	452	25	19	15	47	5	941
Turkey Melt	1	700	45	35	124	52	4	2262
Veggie On Pita	1	522	15	36	41	33	2	950
Wrap Greek Chicken	1	630	48	25	53	57	14	2813
Wrap Grilled Chicken Caesar	1	533	42	25	40	46	13	2023
SOUPS								
Asiago Cheese Bisque	1 (8 oz)	240	5	17	47	17	0	720
Broccoli Cheddar	1 (8 oz)	213	8	15	47	13	0	947
Cheddar Potato	1 (8 oz)	213	5	13	40	19	1	773
Cheesy Chicken Tortilla	1 (8 oz)	150	10	6	30	13	0	1470
Chicken & Sausage Gumbo	1 (8 oz)	150	8	5	20	17	2	1040
Clam Chowder	1 (8 oz)	200	8	11	40	09	0	960
Country Potato	1 (8 oz)	173	4	8	20	23	0	760
Country Vegetable	1 (8 oz)	93	3	1	0	17	3	973
French Onion	1 (8 oz)	80	1	1	7	11	1	144
Red Beans & Rice	1 (8 oz)	107	9	3	7	25	11	760
Southwest Roasted Corn	1 (8 oz)	90	4	4	0	20	3	893

McDONALD'S

FOOD	PORTION	CALS	PROT	FAT	CHOL	CARB	FIBER	SOD
BEVERAGES								
Apple Juice	1 box (6.8 oz)	90	0	0	0	23	0	15
Chocolate Milk 1% Low Fat	8 oz	170	9	3	5	26	1	150
Coca Cola Classic	1 sm (16 oz)	150	0	0	0	40	0	10
Coffee	1 sm (12 oz)	0	0	0	0	0	0	0
Diet Coke	1 sm (16 oz)	0	0	0	0	0	0	20
Half & Half Creamer	1 pkg	20	0	2	10	0	0	1
Hi-C Orange Lavaburst	1 sm (16 oz)	160	0	0	0	44	0	5
Iced Coffee Caramel	1 sm (16 oz)	130	1	5	20	21	1	80
Iced Coffee Hazelnut	1 sm (16 oz)	130	1	5	20	21	0	40
Iced Coffee Regular	1 sm (16 oz)	140	1	5	20	22	0	40
Iced Coffee Vanilla	1 sm (16 oz)	130	1	5	20	21	0	40
Iced Tea	1 sm (16 oz)	0	0	0	0	0	0	10
Milk Lowfat 1%	1 pkg	100	8	3	10	12	0	125
Orange Juice	1 sm (12 oz)	140	2	0	0	33	0	5
Powerade Mountain Blast	1 sm (16 oz)	100	0	0	0	27	0	85
Shake Triple Thick Chocolate	1 sm (12 oz)	440	10	10	40	76	1	190

FOOD	PORTION	CALS	PROT	FAT	CHOL	CARB	FIBER	SOD
Shake Triple Thick Strawberry	1 sm (12 oz)	420	10	10	40	73	0	130
Shake Triple Thick Vanilla	1 sm (16 oz)	420	9	10	40	72	0	140
Sprite	1 sm (16 oz)	150	0	0	0	39	0	40
BREAKFAST SELECTIONS								
Big Breakfast Regular Biscuit	1 serv	720	27	46	555	49	3	1500
Biscuit	1 reg	250	4	11	0	32	2	700
Biscuit Regular Bacon Egg Cheese	1	450	18	25	245	36	2	1360
Biscuit Regular Sausage	1	410	11	27	30	33	2	1040
Biscuit Regular Sausage w/ Egg	1	500	17	32	250	35	2	1130
Burrito Sausage	1	300	12	16	130	26	1	830
Deluxe Breakfast Regular Biscuit w/o Syrup & Margarine	1 serv	1070	36	55	575	109	6	2090
English Muffin	1	160	5	3	0	27	2	280
Hash Browns	1 serv	140	1	8	0	15	2	290
Hotcake Syrup	1 pkg (2 oz)	180	0	0	0	45	0	20
Hotcakes & Sausage w/o Syrup & Margarine	1 serv	520	15	24	50	61	3	930
Hotcakes w/o Syrup & Margarine	1 serv	350	8	9	20	60	3	590
McGriddles Bacon Egg Cheese	1	460	19	21	245	48	2	1360
McGriddles Sausage	1	420	11	22	35	44	2	1030
McGriddles Sausage Egg & Cheese	1	560	20	32	265	48	2	1360
McMuffin Sausage	1	370	14	22	45	29	2	850
McMuffin Sausage w/ Egg	1	250	21	27	285	30	2	920
McSkillet Burrito w/ Sausage	1	610	27	36	410	44	3	1390
McSkillet Burrito w/ Steak	1	570	32	30	430	44	3	1470
Sausage Patty	1	170	7	15	30	1	0	340
Scrambled Eggs	2	170	15	11	520	1	0	180
DESSERTS								
Apple Dippers	1 pkg	35	0	0	0	8	0	0
Apple Pie Baked	1	270	3	12	0	36	4	190
Cinnamon Melts	1 serv	460	6	19	15	66	3	370

FOOD	PORTION	CALS	PROT	FAT	CHOL	CARB	FIBER	SOD
Cookie Chocolate Chip	1	180	2	7	10	22	1	90
Cookie Oatmeal	1 (1.1 oz)	150	2	6	10	22	1	135
Cookie Sugar	1 (1.1 oz)	150	2	6	5	21	0	110
Cookies McDonaldland	1 pkg (2 oz)	250	4	8	0	42	1	270
Cookies McDonaldland Chocolate Chip	1 pkg	270	3	11	35	39	1	170
Fruit 'n Yogurt Parfait	1 serv	160	4	2	5	31	1	85
Ice Cream Cone Reduced Fat Vanilla	1	150	4	4	15	24	0	60
Kiddie Cone	1	45	1	1	5	8	0	20
McFlurry Oreo	1 (12 oz)	560	14	16	50	88	0	250
McFlurry w/ M&M's	1 (12 oz)	620	14	20	55	96	1	190
Peanuts For Sundae	1 serv	45	2	4	0	2	1	0
Sundae Hot Caramel	1	340	7	7	30	60	1	160
Sundae Hot Fudge	1	330	8	10	25	54	2	180
Sundae Strawberry	1	280	6	6	25	49	1	95
MAIN MENU SELECTIONS								
Apple Sauce Strawberry	1 serv	90	0	0	0	23	tr	0
Big Mac	1	540	25	29	75	45	3	1040
Big N' Tasty	1	460	24	24	70	37	3	720
Big N' Tasty w/ Cheese	1	510	27	28	85	38	3	960
Cheeseburger	1	300	15	12	40	33	2	750
Cheeseburger Double	1	440	25	23	80	34	2	1150
Cheesy Tots	6 pieces	210	7	12	20	20	2	650
Chicken McNuggets	4 pieces	170	10	10	25	10	0	450
Chicken Selects	3 pieces	380	23	20	55	28	0	930
Filet-O-Fish	1	380	15	18	35	38	2	660
French Fries	1 sm	250	2	13	0	30	3	140
French Fries	1 lg	570	6	30	0	70	7	330
Hamburger	1	250	12	9	25	31	2	520
McChicken	1	360	14	16	40	40	1	790
McRib	1	500	22	26	70	44	3	980
Onion Rings	1 sm	140	2	7	0	18	2	210
Quarter Pounder	1	410	24	19	65	37	3	730
Quarter Pounder Double w/ Cheese	1	740	48	42	155	40	3	1380
Quarter Pounder w/ Cheese	1	510	29	26	90	40	3	1190
Sandwich Chicken Classic Crispy	1	500	27	17	50	61	3	1330

FOOD	PORTION	CALS	PROT	FAT	CHOL	CARB	FIBER	SOD
Sandwich Chicken Classic Grilled	1	420	32	10	70	51	3	1190
Sandwich Club Chicken Crispy	1	660	39	28	80	63	4	1860
Sandwich Club Chicken Grilled	1	570	44	21	100	52	4	1720
Sandwich Ranch BLT Chicken Crispy	1	600	35	23	70	64	3	1900
Sandwich Ranch BLT Chicken Grilled	1	520	40	16	90	53	3	1760
Snack Wrap Grilled w/ Chipotle BBQ	1	260	18	8	45	28	1	820
Snack Wrap Grilled w/ Honey Mustard	1	260	18	9	45	27	1	800
Snack Wrap Grilled w/ Ranch	1	270	18	10	45	26	1	830
Snack Wrap w/ Chipotle BBQ	1	320	14	14	25	35	2	780
Snack Wrap w/ Honey Mustard	1	320	14	15	30	34	1	750
Snack Wrap w/ Ranch	1	140	14	16	30	32	2	780
SALAD DRESSINGS AND SAUCES								
Caramel Dip Low Fat	1 pkg	70	0	1	5	15	0	35
Dipping Sauce Buffalo	1 serv (1 oz)	80	0	8	5	2	0	350
Dipping Sauce Zesty Onion Ring	1 serv (1 oz)	150	0	15	15	3	tr	210
Dressing Ken's Light Italian	1 pkg (2 oz)	120	0	11	0	5	0	440
Dressing Newman's Own Creamy Caesar	1 pkg (2 oz)	170	2	18	20	4	0	500
Dressing Newman's Own Creamy Southwest	1 pkg (1.5 oz)	100	1	6	20	11	0	340
Dressing Newman's Own Low Fat Balsamic Vinaigrette	1 pkg (1.5 oz)	40	0	3	0	4	0	730
Dressing Newman's Own Low Fat Family Recipe Italian	1 pkg (1.5 oz)	60	1	3	0	8	0	730
Dressing Newman's Own Low Fat Sesame Ginger	1 pkg (1.5 oz)	90	1	3	0	15	0	740

FOOD	PORTION	CALS	PROT	FAT	CHOL	CARB	FIBER	SOD
Dressing Newman's Own Ranch	1 pkg (2 oz)	170	1	15	20	9	0	530
Honey	1 pkg (0.5 oz)	50	0	0	0	12	0	0
Ketchup	1 pkg	15	0	0	0	3	0	110
Sauce Barbecue	1 pkg (1 oz)	50	0	0	0	12	0	260
Sauce Creamy Ranch	1 pkg (1.5 oz)	200	0	22	10	2	0	320
Sauce Hot Mustard	1 pkg (1 oz)	60	1	3	5	9	2	250
Sauce Southwestern Chipotle Barbeque	1 pkg (1.5 oz)	70	0	0	0	18	1	260
Sauce Spicy Buffalo	1 pkg (1.5 oz)	60	0	7	0	1	2	960
Sauce Sweet'N Sour	1 pkg (1 oz)	50	0	0	0	12	0	150
Sauce Tangy Honey Mustard	1 pkg (1.5 oz)	70	1	3	5	13	0	170
SALADS								
Asian w/ Crispy Chicken w/o Dressing	1 serv	380	27	17	45	33	5	1030
Asian w/ Grilled Chicken w/o Dressing	1 serv	300	32	10	65	23	5	890
Asian w/o Chicken & Dressing	1 serv	150	8	7	0	15	5	35
Bacon Ranch w/ Crispy Chicken	1 serv	350	28	16	70	23	3	1150
Bacon Ranch w/ Grilled Chicken w/o Dressing	1 serv	260	33	9	90	12	3	1010
Bacon Ranch w/o Chicken	1 serv	140	9	7	25	10	3	300
Caesar w/ Crispy Chicken	1 serv	300	25	13	55	22	3	1020
Caesar w/ Grilled Chicken	1 serv	220	30	6	75	12	3	890
Caesar w/o Chicken	1 serv	90	7	4	10	9	3	180
Croutons Butter Garlic	1 pkg	60	2	2	0	10	1	140
Fruit & Walnut Snack Size	1 serv	210	4	8	5	31	2	60
Side Salad	1 serv	20	1	0	0	4	1	10
Southwest w/ Crispy Chicken w/o Dressing	1 serv	400	25	16	50	41	7	1110
Southwest w/ Grilled Chicken	1 serv	320	30	9	70	30	7	970
Southwest w/o Chicken & Dressing	1 serv	140	6	5	10	20	6	150

FOOD	PORTION	CALS	PROT	FAT	CHOL	CARB	FIBER	SOD
MIMI'S CAFE								
BEVERAGES								
Cappuccino	1 serv	86	4	5	17	7	0	72
Cappuccino Iced	1 serv	86	4	5	17	7	0	72
Espresso	1 serv	8	0	0	0	1	0	13
Hot Chocolate w/ Whipped Cream	1 serv	986	8	17	3	193	8	800
Mocha Iced	1 serv	376	6	11	17	70	2	102
Mocha Latte	1 serv	376	6	11	17	70	2	146
CHILDREN'S MENU SELECTIONS								
Chicken Fingers	1 serv	408	30	21	67	21	1	686
Grilled Cheese	1 serv	273	13	19	50	14	0	499
Macaroni & Cheese	1 serv	353	12	13	19	48	2	652
Mini Burger	1 serv	554	25	28	66	48	3	686
Mini Corn Dogs	1 serv	460	7	32	35	35	0	672
Pancakes Chocolate Chip	1 serv	563	11	29	73	71	3	747
Pancakes Mimi Mouse	1 serv	477	11	18	63	69	1	985
PB&J Soldiers	1 serv	730	18	40	0	78	4	728
Pepperoni Pizzadillas	1 serv	617	31	38	86	39	3	1600
Scrambled Eggs & Bacon	1 serv	216	18	16	441	1	0	449
Spaghetti	1 serv	343	13	5	–	62	5	711
Turkey Dinner	1 serv	337	11	16	69	25	3	1110
DESSERTS								
Apple Crisp Cinnamon	1 serv	898	7	37	25	141	4	427
Bread Pudding	1 serv	819	18	55	329	69	1	730
Brownie Triple Chocolate	1 serv	1950	25	87	303	280	6	1073
Cheesecake New York Style	1 serv	1075	19	42	373	85	4	744
Pie Banana Foster Mud	1 serv	1245	14	73	218	138	4	477
Pie Pecan Chocolate Chip	1 serv	1879	21	111	231	220	12	1064
MAIN MENU SELECTIONS								
Appetizer Dip Spinach & Artichoke	1 serv	2459	90	138	262	191	11	4320
Appetizer Fried Chicken Tenders	1 serv	800	60	33	134	60	3	1730
Appetizer Fried Dill Pickles	1 serv	972	16	42	12	132	12	3740
Appetizer Jazz Fest	1 serv	1252	43	72	122	108	8	2085
Appetizer Zucchini Parmesan	1 serv	626	22	28	26	73	7	1111
Blackened Sole w/ Shrimp Creole	1 serv	852	78	34	334	59	9	2312

FOOD	PORTION	CALS	PROT	FAT	CHOL	CARB	FIBER	SOD
Broiled Flat Iron Steak	1 serv	1026	68	58	164	58	9	1751
Burger Half Pound	1	684	42	34	132	48	3	668
Cafe Fish & Chips	1 serv	1290	69	57	121	119	10	2166
Cajun Blackened Salmon	1 serv	919	57	55	220	55	9	1915
Cheeseburger BBQ Ranch	1	999	58	57	192	62	3	1433
Cheeseburger Half Pound	1	855	53	48	177	49	3	932
Chicken Cordon Bleu	1 serv	1360	100	81	306	51	5	3007
Chicken Feta Penne	1 serv	1879	57	99	253	158	12	1756
Ciabatta Chicken	1	1251	70	72	213	81	4	1846
Ciabatta Meatloaf	1	1036	41	61	171	83	3	2017
Ciabatta Turkey Pesto	1	1248	45	73	172	83	6	1672
Club Cafe	1	1132	42	63	175	73	4	1438
Country Fried Steak	1 serv	1061	42	56	156	107	9	1418
Crab Cake Dinner	1 serv	1662	59	100	646	129	9	3732
Diablo Center Cut Pork Chops	1 serv	1094	54	73	219	55	8	2179
Dip Classic Beef	1	521	49	15	108	43	5	3928
Fillet Of Soul	1 serv	636	45	26	163	56	7	1316
French Quarter	1	1480	66	105	214	68	7	1917
Garlic Shrimp Spaghettini	1 serv	860	37	20	261	109	7	1073
Grilled Beef Liver	1 serv	1003	75	45	937	75	10	1457
Grilled Chicken Tuscan Style	1 serv	880	58	36	181	80	12	1529
Hibachi Salmon	1 serv	846	49	40	119	75	8	274
Mimi's Meatloaf	1 serv	910	43	53	291	68	8	2650
Mimi's Pot Roast	1 serv	1291	88	78	323	57	8	2252
Original Patty Melt	1	976	56	56	177	62	6	1261
Parmesan Crusted Chicken Breast	1 serv	1820	91	54	194	211	15	1466
Pasta Jambalaya	1 serv	1223	74	44	295	113	8	1727
Pot Pie Chicken	1 serv	1403	70	87	388	86	11	2416
Reuben West Coast	1	2015	62	138	226	120	11	3798
Sandwich 5 Way Grilled Cheese	1	703	39	39	92	49	2	1150
Sandwich Albacore & Avocado	1	993	33	71	94	58	9	960
Sandwich Bacon Lettuce & Tomato	1	586	24	34	56	48	7	1545
Sandwich Fresh Roasted Turkey Breast	1	532	20	27	134	28	1	546

FOOD	PORTION	CALS	PROT	FAT	CHOL	CARB	FIBER	SOD
Sandwich Turkey Walnut Salad On Raisin Bread	1	549	7	42	54	36	3	447
Sandwich Veggie Stack	1	836	27	43	48	93	6	1807
Slow Roasted Turkey Breast	1 serv	851	25	41	154	72	11	2086
Small Bites Black & Blue Quesadilla	1 serv	1241	73	80	216	60	7	2403
Small Bites Chicken & Fruit	1 serv	460	73	9	193	21	3	192
Small Bites Citrus Salmon	1 serv	699	44	43	119	37	10	368
Small Bites Crab Cakes	1 serv	412	18	25	212	27	2	1089
Small Bites Smokey Chicken Enchiladas	1 serv	1154	61	72	179	68	8	1922
Small Bites Sweet & Sour Coconut Shrimp	1 serv	608	22	50	120	79	4	767
Small Bites Thai Chicken Wrap	1 serv	1004	51	41	96	106	7	1522
Top Sirloin 12 oz	1 serv	947	79	48	237	49	7	1076
SALAD DRESSINGS								
Balsamic Vinaigrette	1 serv	316	0	32	0	8	0	337
Blue Cheese	1 serv	298	2	31	30	1	0	241
Caesar	1 serv	273	1	29	22	2	0	451
Chinese Sesame	1 serv	263	0	25	0	11	0	307
Dijon Vinaigrette	1 serv	296	0	32	0	3	0	335
Honey Mustard	1 serv	243	1	22	10	11	0	423
Non Fat French	1 serv	65	1	0	0	16	1	222
Ranch	1 serv	194	1	20	18	2	0	321
Thousand Island	1 serv	232	0	23	19	6	0	439
SALADS								
Asian Chopped	1 serv	751	81	22	193	55	14	347
Blue Cheese & Walnut	1 serv	728	26	53	53	45	10	1097
Caesar Blackened Chicken	1 serv	570	59	17	132	41	6	1565
Chopped Cobb	1 serv	524	35	32	329	18	4	1516
Fried Chicken	1 serv	764	23	67	272	16	3	469
Zesty Chicken Tostada	1 serv	1046	47	57	134	89	15	1184
SOUPS								
Broccoli Cheddar	1 serv	270	12	10	51	18	2	916
Chicken Gumbo	1 serv	235	7	12	17	25	2	1112
Clam Chowder	1 serv	240	10	14	49	21	2	657
Corn Chowder	1 serv	196	3	9	20	28	3	722
Cream Of Chicken	1 serv	337	0	29	32	19	1	1083
French Market Onion	1 serv	207	10	12	16	16	2	1269

FOOD	PORTION	CALS	PROT	FAT	CHOL	CARB	FIBER	SOD
Red Bean & Andouille Sausage	1 serv	256	13	10	29	30	5	706
Split Pea	1 serv	194	14	3	11	29	11	636
Vegetarian Vegetable	1 serv	60	2	0	0	12	2	1561
MR. HERO								
DESSERTS								
Eli's Cheesecake Oreo Cookie	1 slice (2.5 oz)	260	4	17	65	24	1	250
Eli's Cheesecake Original Plain	1 slice (2.6 oz)	280	4	19	80	22	0	260
Eli's Cheesecake Snickers	1 slice (2.3 oz)	270	4	18	65	23	1	220
Eli's Cheesecake Strawberry Swirl	1 slice (2.6 oz)	280	4	19	80	22	0	260
SALADS								
Garden Side	1 serv (7.3 oz)	32	1	0	0	7	2	11
Grilled Chicken	1 serv (13.4 oz)	166	23	3	55	13	3	588
Tuna Delight	1 serv (14.4 oz)	403	13	48	84	10	3	507
SANDWICHES								
Cheeseburger	1 (10.4 oz)	776	26	55	73	47	3	1122
Cheesesteak Hot Buttered	1 (9.4 oz)	669	28	42	80	45	3	1132
Chicken Grilled Philly	1 (9.1 oz)	421	34	10	75	48	4	1533
Deli Subs Original Italian	1 (9.5 oz)	641	22	39	58	47	3	1781
Deli Subs Tuna 'N Cheese	1 (9.7 oz)	724	21	54	83	44	3	1140
Deli Subs Turkey	1 (9.8 oz)	468	30	20	63	46	3	1574
Deli Subs Ultimate Italian	1 (10.3 oz)	675	27	40	78	46	3	2067
Romanburger	1 (11.3 oz)	861	30	62	90	48	3	1530
Steak Tuscan	1 (10.6 oz)	625	40	31	129	42	2	2259
Steak Zesty Bacon & Swiss	1 (9.8 oz)	616	38	32	112	42	3	1714
Subs Meatball	1 (9.3 oz)	724	30	47	75	47	4	1729
Taste Buddies Cheeseburger Bacon	1 (5.9 oz)	264	15	30	490	33	2	758
Taste Buddies Grilled Italiano	1 (5.3 oz)	440	00	32	48	32	2	901
Taste Buddies Italian Sausage	1 (5.4 oz)	368	19	22	53	34	1	1159

FOOD	PORTION	CALS	PROT	FAT	CHOL	CARB	FIBER	SOD
Taste Buddies Tuna 'N Cheese	1 (6 oz)	483	12	38	52	31	2	688
SIDES								
Breadsticks	2 (6 oz)	446	10	17	0	64	3	994
Jalapeno Poppers	1 serv (4.5 oz)	432	9	28	13	37	3	1156
Mozzarella Sticks	1 serv (8.7 oz)	565	31	43	60	12	1	961
Onion Petals	1 serv (5.7 oz)	597	6	37	0	56	2	1060
Potato Babycakes	1 serv (5.9 oz)	477	2	37	0	34	4	880
Potato Waffle Fries w/ Cheese Sauce	1 serv (7.2 oz)	482	4	34	0	42	3	954

MRS. FIELDS

FOOD	PORTION	CALS	PROT	FAT	CHOL	CARB	FIBER	SOD
Bites Double Fudge	3 (1.6 oz)	200	2	10	45	27	1	75
Brownie Butterscotch Blondie	1 (2.1 oz)	260	3	10	50	38	0	20
Brownie Double Fudge	1 (2.1 oz)	260	3	13	60	34	1	95
Brownie Pecan Fudge	1 (2.1 oz)	270	3	15	55	32	2	95
Brownie Special Walnut Fudge & Blondie	1 (2.2 oz)	260	3	13	55	35	1	55
Brownie Toffee Fudge	1 (2.1 oz)	260	3	14	60	34	1	110
Brownie Walnut Fudge	1 (2.1 oz)	270	3	15	55	32	2	95
Cake Chocolate Chip	1 piece (2.9 oz)	350	4	17	50	45	tr	330
Coffee Cake Chocolate Chip	1 sm piece (2.2 oz)	240	3	11	30	30	1	320
Coffee Cake Chocolate Chip	1 lg (2.4 oz)	250	3	12	30	32	1	340
Cookie Butter	1 (1.5 oz)	200	2	8	20	29	tr	180
Cookie Chocolate Covered Peanut Butter	1 (2.5 oz)	340	5	19	20	37	1	230
Cookie Chocolate Covered Semi-Sweet	1 (2.5 oz)	380	5	23	15	40	1	65
Cookie Chocolate Covered White Chunk Macadamia	1 (2.4 oz)	330	3	19	15	39	1	170
Cookie Cinnamon Sugar	1 (1.8 oz)	210	2	8	20	31	0	210
Cookie Cut Out	1 (2.4 oz)	280	2	11	2	44	0	180

FOOD	PORTION	CALS	PROT	FAT	CHOL	CARB	FIBER	SOD
Cookie Frosted Cinnamon Sugar	1 (2.1 oz)	270	2	11	20	39	0	210
Cookie Oatmeal Raisins & Walnuts	1 (1.7 oz)	200	3	9	15	27	1	180
Cookie Semi-Sweet Chocolate	1 (1.7 oz)	210	2	10	15	29	1	170
Cookie Semi-Sweet Chocolate w/ Walnuts	1 (1.7 oz)	220	2	11	15	28	1	160
Cookie Triple Chocolate	1 (1.7 oz)	210	2	10	15	28	1	170
Cookie White Chunk Macadamia	1 (1.7 oz)	230	2	12	15	28	0	170
Jelly Bellys	1 pkg (1.4 oz)	140	0	0	0	37	0	15
Mixed Nuts	1 pkg (2 oz)	350	9	32	0	13	3	5
Muffin Blueberry	1 (1.9 oz)	190	3	9	25	24	1	280
Muffin Chocolate Chip	1 (1.9 oz)	200	3	10	25	26	1	270
Nibbler Cinnamon Sugar	3 (1.4 oz)	180	2	8	10	25	0	210
Nibbler Debra's Special	3 (1.3 oz)	160	2	7	10	22	1	160
Nibbler Peanut Butter	3 (1.8 oz)	170	3	9	10	19	1	180
Nibbler Semi-Sweet Chocolate	3 (1.8 oz)	170	2	8	10	23	1	140
Nibbler Triple Chocolate	3 (1.8 oz)	160	2	8	10	22	1	150
Nibbler White Chunk Macadamia	3 (1.8 oz)	180	2	9	10	22	0	140
Taffy	1 pkg (2.4 oz)	160	0	2	0	38	0	65
NAKED PIZZA								
10 Inch Pie Original Crust	1 slice	81	4	5	–	8	3	161
10 Inch Pie Thin Crust	1 slice	64	4	5	–	5	2	143
12 Inch Pie Original Crust	1 slice	132	6	6	–	16	6	225
12 Inch Pie Thin Crust	1 slice	91	4	5	–	10	3	183
14 Inch Pie Original Crust	1 slice	161	7	7	–	20	7	259
14 Inch Pie Thin Crust	1 slice	114	5	5	–	11	4	153
NOAH'S BAGELS								
BAGELS AND BREADS								
Bagel Asiago Cheese Topped	1 (4.2 oz)	330	16	6	15	57	2	750
Bagel Blueberry	1 (3.7 oz)	270	10	1	0	59	3	520
Bagel Candy Cane	1 (3.7 oz)	270	9	3	5	54	2	540

FOOD	PORTION	CALS	PROT	FAT	CHOL	CARB	FIBER	SOD
Bagel Cheddar Stick	1 (4.2 oz)	330	14	6	15	57	2	670
Bagel Chocolate Chip	1 (3.7 oz)	290	9	4	0	60	3	510
Bagel Chopped Garlic	1 (3.9 oz)	290	11	3	0	58	2	580
Bagel Cinnamon Raisin	1 (3.7 oz)	270	9	1	0	58	3	510
Bagel Cinnamon Sugar	1 (4.1 oz)	310	10	3	0	64	2	600
Bagel Cracked Pepper	1 (3.7 oz)	280	9	4	0	55	2	520
Bagel Cranberry Orange	1 (3.5 oz)	250	9	1	0	54	3	520
Bagel Dutch Apple	1 (5 oz)	340	10	3	0	72	3	600
Bagel Egg	1 (3.7 oz)	290	12	3	75	57	2	590
Bagel Everything	1 (3.9 oz)	280	10	2	0	57	2	730
Bagel Good Grains	1 (3.9 oz)	280	12	2	0	58	4	560
Bagel Jalapeno Cheddar	1 (4.9 oz)	350	15	7	20	58	2	940
Bagel Onion	1 (3.7 oz)	270	10	2	0	57	3	540
Bagel Plain	1 (3.7 oz)	270	10	1	0	57	2	580
Bagel Poppyseed	1 (3.9 oz)	290	11	3	0	57	2	580
Bagel Power	1 (4 oz)	310	11	5	0	61	4	280
Bagel Pumpernickel	1 (3.7 oz)	260	10	2	0	57	3	530
Bagel Sesame Seed	1 (3.9 oz)	290	11	3	0	57	2	580
Bagel Six Cheese	1 (4.5 oz)	340	16	6	15	57	2	770
Bagel Spinach Florentine	1 (4.9 oz)	350	16	8	20	58	2	700
Bagel Sun Dried Tomato	1 (3.7 oz)	270	10	2	0	57	3	680
Bagel Whole Wheat	1 (3.7 oz)	260	11	1	0	57	4	560
Bagel Whole Wheat Sesame & Sunflower Seeds	1 (4.4 oz)	370	15	11	0	61	6	560
Bialy	1 (5.3 oz)	380	11	4	0	77	4	700
Bread Ciabatta	1 serv (4.25 oz)	290	10	3	0	60	2	640
Bread Corn Meal Rye	1 slice (2 oz)	150	6	2	0	31	2	410
Bread Harvest Grain	1 slice (2.3 oz)	180	7	2	0	36	4	220
Bread Marble Rye	1 slice (1.7 oz)	160	5	1	0	30	1	370
Bread Potato	1 slice (1.7 oz)	140	4	2	0	28	1	250
Challah Braided	1 serv (2 oz)	160	6	3	20	29	1	180
Challah Roll	1 (3 oz)	230	8	4	0	44	2	340
Pizza Bagel Artichoke Tomato & Red Onion	1 (11.1 oz)	550	31	20	55	67	5	1430
Pizza Bagel Artichoke & Spinach	1 (12 oz)	670	31	32	55	70	5	1870

FOOD	PORTION	CALS	PROT	FAT	CHOL	CARB	FIBER	SOD
Pizza Bagel Cheese	1 (6.2 oz)	420	23	11	35	60	3	1060
Pizza Bagel Cheesy Garlic & Herb	1 (6.2 oz)	500	24	19	55	62	2	1090
Pizza Bagel Pepperoni	1 (6.8 oz)	500	26	19	50	60	3	1360
Pizza Bagel Spinach & Mushroom	1 (9.5 oz)	580	27	25	55	68	4	1340
Pizza Bagel Tomato & Rosemary	1 (8.7 oz)	540	30	20	55	63	4	1240
BEVERAGES AND EXTRAS								
Cafe Latte Low Fat	1 reg (12 oz)	160	10	7	25	17	0	180
Cafe Latte Nonfat	1 reg (12 oz)	110	11	0	5	17	0	180
Cafe Latte Whole	1 reg (12 oz)	200	10	10	30	16	0	140
Cappuccino Low Fat	1 reg (12 oz)	120	7	5	20	13	0	130
Cappuccino Nonfat	1 reg (12 oz)	90	8	0	5	13	0	135
Cappuccino Whole	1 reg (12 oz)	150	7	8	25	13	0	110
Chai Tea Low Fat Milk	1 reg (12 oz)	220	3	2	5	47	0	65
Chai Tea Nonfat Milk	1 reg (12 oz)	210	3	0	0	47	0	65
Chai Tea Whole Milk	1 reg (12 oz)	230	3	3	10	47	0	55
Coca Cola	8 oz	99	0	0	0	27	0	6
Coca Cola Cherry	8 oz	104	0	0	0	28	0	4
Coffee Iced Americano	8 oz	0	0	0	0	0	0	0
Coffee Regular & Decaf	1 (12 oz)	0	0	0	0	0	0	0
Diet Coke	8 oz	1	0	0	0	0	0	10
Espresso	1 reg (2 oz)	0	0	0	0	0	0	0
Fanta Orange	8 oz	106	0	0	0	29	0	0
Frozen Drinks Cafe Caramel	1 (18 oz)	620	8	9	45	100	0	140
Frozen Drinks Cafe Mocha	1 (18 oz)	510	7	8	40	102	0	160
Frozen Drinks Strawberry Cream	1 (18 oz)	450	6	19	65	75	3	95
Frozen Drinks Wild Berry Fat Free	1 (18 oz)	270	4	0	5	62	5	75
Half & Half Creamer	1 oz	40	1	3	15	1	0	25
Hi-C Fruit Punch	8 oz	104	0	0	0	28	0	9
Hot Chocolate Nonfat	1 reg (12 oz)	220	12	2	5	37	1	330
Hot Chocolate Whole	1 reg (12 oz)	290	10	11	30	35	1	280
Iced Cappuccino Nonfat	1 reg (12 oz)	90	8	0	5	13	0	135

FOOD	PORTION	CALS	PROT	FAT	CHOL	CARB	FIBER	SOD
Iced Mocha Low Fat	1 reg (12 oz)	230	8	5	20	39	0	170
Iced Tea Raspberry	8 oz	78	0	0	0	21	0	9
Iced Tea Unsweetened	8 oz	1	0	0	0	0	0	14
Lemonade	1 (16 oz)	200	1	0	0	24	0	0
Lemonade Blackberry	1 (16 oz)	310	2	0	0	74	0	5
Macchiato Nonfat	1 reg (12 oz)	230	10	0	5	49	0	210
Macchiato Whole	1 reg (12 oz)	290	8	8	25	47	0	170
Milk Low Fat	8 oz	120	8	5	20	12	0	125
Milk Skim	8 oz	80	7	0	5	15	0	140
Milk Whole	8 oz	150	8	8	25	11	0	100
Mocha Low Fat	1 reg (12 oz)	230	8	5	20	39	0	170
Mocha Nonfat	1 reg (12 oz)	190	9	0	5	39	0	180
Mocha Whole	1 reg (12 oz)	270	8	9	25	38	0	150
Mr. Pibb	8 oz	97	0	0	0	26	0	14
On Top Reduced Fat Topping	2 tbsp (0.3 oz)	20	0	2	0	2	0	5
Orange Juice	1 (10 oz)	143	1	0	0	34	2	71
Sprite	8 oz	97	0	0	0	26	0	22
Syrup Blackberry	2 tbsp (1 oz)	100	0	0	0	25	0	0
Syrup Caramel	2 tbsp (1 oz)	70	0	0	0	18	0	0
Syrup Hazelnut	2 tbsp (1 oz)	100	0	0	0	25	0	0
Syrup Vanilla	2 tbsp (1 oz)	100	0	0	0	25	0	0
Syrup Vanilla Sugar Free	2 tbsp (1 oz)	116	0	0	0	0	0	0
Tea Hamey & Sons All Flavors	8 oz	0	0	0	0	0	0	0
Whipped Cream Light	2 tbsp (1 oz)	36	0	3	5	2	0	0
CREAM CHEESE AND SPREADS								
Butter	1 tbsp (0.5 oz)	110	0	11	30	0	0	80
Cream Cheese Whipped Onion & Chive	2 tbsp (0.7 oz)	70	1	6	20	3	0	60
Cream Cheese Whipped Plain	2 tbsp (0.7 oz)	70	1	7	20	1	0	65

FOOD	PORTION	CALS	PROT	FAT	CHOL	CARB	FIBER	SOD
Cream Cheese Whipped Reduced Fat Blueberry	2 tbsp (0.7 oz)	70	1	5	15	6	0	50
Cream Cheese Whipped Reduced Fat Garden Vegetable	2 tbsp (0.7 oz)	60	1	5	15	3	0	100
Cream Cheese Whipped Reduced Fat Garlic Herb	2 tbsp (0.7 oz)	60	1	5	15	3	0	100
Cream Cheese Whipped Reduced Fat Honey Almond	2 tbsp (0.7 oz)	70	1	5	15	6	0	45
Cream Cheese Whipped Reduced Fat Jalapeno Salsa	2 tbsp (0.7 oz)	60	1	5	15	3	0	105
Cream Cheese Whipped Reduced Fat Plain	2 tbsp (0.7 oz)	60	1	5	15	2	0	100
Cream Cheese Whipped Reduced Fat Strawberry	2 tbsp (0.7 oz)	60	1	5	15	2	0	100
Cream Cheese Whipped Reduced Fat Sun Dried Tomato & Basil	2 tbsp (0.7 oz)	60	1	5	15	2	0	100
Cream Cheese Whipped Smoked Salmon	2 tbsp (0.7 oz)	60	1	6	20	2	0	120
Deli Mustard	1 tsp (5 g)	0	0	0	0	0	0	65
Garlic Mayo	1 serv (1.5 oz)	270	0	27	20	8	0	320
Grape Jam	1 serv (1 oz)	110	0	0	0	28	0	0
Honey	1 serv (1 oz)	90	0	0	0	23	0	0
Hummus	1 serv (2 oz)	90	3	4	0	11	2	200
Mayo	1 tbsp (0.5 oz)	110	0	12	10	0	0	70
DESSERTS								
Cinnamon Twists	1 serv (3.8 oz)	370	5	21	0	41	2	125
Coffee Cake Apple Cinnamon	1 serv (6.6 oz)	700	5	28	5	108	1	280
Coffee Cake Chocolate Chip	1 serv (6.1 oz)	760	6	34	5	110	2	270
Coffee Cake Mixed Berry	1 serv (6.9 oz)	710	5	29	5	110	2	270
Cookie Chocolate Chip	1 (2.8 oz)	360	4	18	15	48	2	290

FOOD	PORTION	CALS	PROT	FAT	CHOL	CARB	FIBER	SOD
Cookie Chocolate Mudslide	1 (2.75 oz)	320	4	17	60	46	1	75
Cookie Iced Sugar	1 (3.7 oz)	480	4	15	25	76	1	260
Cookie Mini Chocolate Mudslide	1 (1.38 oz)	160	2	8	30	23	1	40
Cookie Mini Chocolate Chip	1 (1.38 oz)	180	2	9	5	24	1	150
Cookie Mini Iced Sugar	1 (1.87 oz)	230	2	7	15	39	1	130
Cookie Mini Oatmeal Raisin	1 (1.38 oz)	160	2	5	10	27	1	160
Cookie Oatmeal Raisin	1 (2.8 oz)	320	5	11	25	54	2	310
Cookie Snickerdoodle	1 (2.8 oz)	400	3	18	30	56	1	360
Marshmallow Crispy Treat	1 (3.9 oz)	410	5	7	0	86	0	125
Muffin Blueberry	1 (5 oz)	480	6	22	105	65	2	480
Muffin Cranberry Orange	1 (4.6 oz)	460	9	22	95	63	2	480
Muffin Strawberry White Chocolate	1 (5.5 oz)	550	7	25	105	78	1	510
Strudel Cinnamon Walnut	1 serv (5.4 oz)	630	9	42	35	56	4	360
SALAD DRESSINGS								
Caesar	2 tbsp (1 oz)	150	1	16	10	1	0	350
Harvest Chicken Salad	2 tbsp (1 oz)	90	0	8	2	3	0	410
Raspberry Vinaigrette	2 tbsp	160	0	14	0	8	0	0
SALADS								
Caesar	1 (10.5 oz)	600	13	53	50	23	6	1360
Caesar Chicken	1 (14 oz)	720	34	54	120	23	4	1840
Caesar Side	1 (4.5 oz)	280	6	27	20	7	2	680
City	1 (11.5 oz)	830	14	68	25	39	7	460
City w/ Chicken	1 (15 oz)	950	36	71	105	40	8	820
Southwestern Chicken	1 (15.2 oz)	710	35	41	95	54	10	1940
SANDWICHES								
Bagel & Lox	1 (11.2 oz)	520	25	21	50	65	4	1400
Bagel Dog Asiago	1 (7.1 oz)	510	23	21	60	59	2	1350
Bagel Dog Everything	1 (7.1 oz)	510	22	20	55	59	2	1460
Bagel Dog Original	1 (6.9 oz)	490	22	20	55	59	2	1310
Bagel Plain w/ Peanut Butter & Jelly	1 (6.2 oz)	550	17	15	0	90	4	580
Breakfast Wrap Santa Fe	1 (14.5 oz)	750	34	34	410	77	9	1410
Breakfast Wrap Veggie	1 (15.6 oz)	810	35	41	400	77	10	1330
California Chicken	1 (9.9 oz)	360	31	7	80	49	3	840
Club Blackened Chicken	1 (10.4 oz)	630	30	33	130	53	2	1500
Club Deli Pesto Turkey	1 (10.9 oz)	670	27	39	100	47	2	1310
Deli Chicken Salad	1 (11 oz)	1150	17	95	90	61	5	1190

FOOD	PORTION	CALS	PROT	FAT	CHOL	CARB	FIBER	SOD
Deli Cornbeef	1 (14 oz)	740	44	34	105	61	4	2820
Deli Egg Salad Kosher	1 (11.5 oz)	650	26	6	450	68	5	1280
Deli Melts Hummus	1 (10.2 oz)	570	28	19	40	76	6	1280
Deli Melts Pastrami	1 (9.6 oz)	530	38	17	85	61	3	1840
Deli Melts Roast Beef	1 (9.6 oz)	530	36	17	80	60	3	2190
Deli Melts Tuna	1 (11.6 oz)	700	42	33	90	82	3	1490
Deli Melts Turkey	1 (9.6 oz)	500	29	14	55	60	3	1420
Deli Melts Veggie	1 (12.3 oz)	590	25	25	50	70	5	1430
Deli Pastrami	1 (14 oz)	750	44	34	105	62	5	3180
Deli Roast Beef	1 (14 oz)	730	43	34	100	60	4	3750
Deli Tuna Salad	1 (13 oz)	740	28	45	55	53	5	1440
Deli Turkey	1 (14.5 oz)	720	29	29	55	67	5	2480
Deli Whitefish	1 (12.2 oz)	850	25	55	95	68	6	1470
Egg Mit Artichoke & Tomato	1 (12 oz)	620	28	28	390	67	4	1120
Egg Mit Bacon & Cheddar	1 (9.2 oz)	620	33	28	390	61	2	1210
Egg Mit Cheese & Tomato	1 (10 oz)	530	27	21	365	61	3	880
Egg Mit Lox & Chives	1 (8.8 oz)	490	28	17	355	59	2	890
Egg Mit Plain	1 (7.9 oz)	450	22	14	350	59	2	760
Egg Mit Spinach Mushroom & Swiss	1 (9.8 oz)	530	28	20	370	61	3	850
Egg Mit Turkey Sausage	1 (9.9 oz)	590	34	24	395	61	2	1060
Egg Mit w/ Cheese	1 (8.5 oz)	520	28	20	365	60	2	880
Kosher Vegetarian On Plain Bagel	1 (13.9 oz)	860	49	41	435	79	4	1510
Panini Albacore Tuna	1 (13.6 oz)	750	32	38	85	62	6	1560
Panini Egg Spinach Bacon	1 (11.8 oz)	790	27	43	405	65	5	1500
Panini Egg Vegetarian Omelet	1 (13.8 oz)	670	23	31	380	66	6	1100
Panini Italian Chicken	1 (12.5 oz)	810	47	40	125	67	5	2490
Panini Mediterranean	1 (10.6 oz)	550	11	18	20	77	9	1140
Panini Tomato Mozzarella	1 (7.9 oz)	440	7	16	20	59	6	960
Panini Turkey Club	1 (12.3 oz)	610	23	21	60	64	6	1820
Sandwich Rachel	1 (13.9 oz)	1030	51	68	170	53	2	3520
Sandwich Reuben	1 (13.9 oz)	770	51	41	150	47	3	3400
Sandwich Veg Out	1 (10.1 oz)	490	19	14	30	75	4	960
Wrap Albacore Tuna	1 (12.3 oz)	600	29	28	50	57	8	1030
Wrap Chicken Caesar	1 (12.6 oz)	790	37	46	130	62	7	1640
Wrap Southwestern Turkey	1 (13.5 oz)	750	25	37	60	74	9	1890
Wrap Veggie	1 (9.8 oz)	460	12	17	20	64	9	610

FOOD	PORTION	CALS	PROT	FAT	CHOL	CARB	FIBER	SOD
SIDES								
Cole Slaw	1 serv (3 oz)	120	1	6	5	15	2	180
Egg Salad	1 serv (5 oz)	330	13	29	450	3	0	450
Fresh Fruit Cup	1 (11 oz)	140	2	0	0	36	3	35
Fruit & Yogurt Parfait	1 (12 oz)	220	13	1	10	43	3	135
Kosher Pickle	1	5	0	0	0	1	0	650
Macaroni & Cheese	1 serv (6 oz)	340	15	17	27	32	1	606
Redskin Potato Salad	1 serv (3 oz)	160	1	12	10	13	1	360
Tuna Salad	1 serv (5 oz)	280	20	20	50	3	1	660
SOUPS								
Broccoli Cheese	1 cup (8.7 oz)	290	14	20	45	16	2	990
Chicken Noodle	1 cup (8.7 oz)	110	5	4	25	13	1	750
Italian Wedding	1 cup (8.7 oz)	160	11	6	20	15	2	1060
Tortilla	1 cup (8.7 oz)	300	13	19	40	19	3	920
Turkey Chili	1 cup (8.7 oz)	220	20	7	35	24	5	930

NOODLES & COMPANY

MAIN MENU SELECTIONS

FOOD	PORTION	CALS	PROT	FAT	CHOL	CARB	FIBER	SOD
Bangkok Curry	1 sm	250	5	6	0	42	3	430
Bangkok Curry	1 reg	490	9	13	0	85	7	860
Beef Braised	1 serv	190	28	10	75	0	0	370
Beef Sauteed	1 serv	210	25	12	75	0	0	480
Buttered Noodles	1 sm	310	17	8	20	42	4	790
Buttered Noodles	1 reg	620	33	16	40	84	7	1590
Chicken Breast Seasoned	1 serv	130	22	3	75	0	0	720
Chicken Parmesan Crusted	1 serv	190	17	8	50	17	0	620
Ciabatta Roll	1	160	6	2	0	31	2	430
Flatbread	1 serv	210	7	4	0	37	2	370
House Marinara	1 reg	650	27	12	20	107	7	730
House Marinara	1 sm	330	13	6	10	53	3	360
Mushroom Stroganoff	1 sm	390	14	15	65	50	5	490
Mushroom Stroganoff	1 reg	780	28	31	135	100	10	980
Organic Tofu	1 serv	180	16	11	0	4	0	220
Pad Thai	1 reg	700	11	20	120	117	5	1840
Pad Thai	1 sm	350	6	10	60	59	3	920
Pasta Fresca	1 reg	780	27	22	20	111	6	770

FOOD	PORTION	CALS	PROT	FAT	CHOL	CARB	FIBER	SOD
Pasta Fresca	1 sm	420	15	12	10	56	3	450
Penne Rosa	1 reg	810	24	26	0	119	15	1100
Penne Rosa	1 sm	420	12	13	0	60	8	550
Pesto Cavatappi	1 sm	510	18	21	60	62	4	630
Pesto Cavatappi	1 reg	910	36	30	85	124	8	1240
Potstickers	3	200	5	5	15	31	2	1150
Shrimp Sauteed	1 serv	35	8	0	75	0	0	190
Whole Grain Tuscan Linguine	1 sm	450	15	20	60	54	10	750
Whole Grain Tuscan Linguine	1 reg	770	26	26	50	108	20	1370
Wisconsin Mac & Cheese	1 sm	450	18	16	40	60	7	550
Wisconsin Mac & Cheese	1 reg	900	36	31	75	119	13	1100
SALADS								
Caesar	1 reg	320	11	28	35	11	2	780
Caesar	1 sm	160	5	14	15	5	1	390
Chinese Chopped	1 sm	150	3	7	0	11	3	180
Chinese Chopped	1 reg	310	6	15	0	23	6	370
Cucumber Tomato Side Salad	1	80	2	0	0	18	2	190
The Med	1 sm	150	5	6	10	19	2	480
The Med	1 reg	310	10	13	20	39	4	960
Tossed Green	1	60	1	6	0	3	1	140
SOUPS								
Chicken Noodle	1 reg	300	20	4	70	44	10	2290
Chicken Noodle	1 sm	150	10	2	35	22	5	1150
Thai Curry	1 reg	480	0	19	0	70	3	1580
Thai Curry	1 sm	240	0	10	0	35	2	790
Tomato Basil	1 sm	210	0	12	35	23	7	1760
Tomato Basil	1 reg	420	0	23	65	45	13	3530

PACIUGO GELATO

FOOD	PORTION	CALS	PROT	FAT	CHOL	CARB	FIBER	SOD
Milk Base Amarena Black Cherry Swirl	1 scoop (3.5 oz)	160	4	4	15	30	tr	50
Milk Base Banana Creme Pie	1 scoop (3.5 oz)	80	2	2	13	14	tr	35
Milk Base Cheesecake	1 scoop (3.5 oz)	90	3	4	18	12	tr	55
Milk Base Chocolate	1 scoop (3.5 oz)	80	3	3	8	14	tr	48

FOOD	PORTION	CALS	PROT	FAT	CHOL	CARB	FIBER	SOD
Milk Base Chocolate Cookies'N Milk	1 scoop (3.5 oz)	90	3	3	8	16	tr	63
Milk Base Coconut	1 scoop (3.5 oz)	80	2	3	8	13	tr	30
Milk Base Coffee	1 scoop (3.5 oz)	75	2	3	8	12	tr	30
Milk Base Fiordilatte	1 scoop (3.5 oz)	75	2	2	8	13	tr	30
Milk Base French Vanilla Bean	1 scoop (3.5 oz)	80	2	3	20	13	tr	30
Milk Base Green Tea	1 scoop (3.5 oz)	70	2	2	8	12	tr	30
Milk Base Hazelnut	1 scoop (3.5 oz)	85	3	4	8	11	tr	30
Milk Base Lemon Custard	1 scoop (3.5 oz)	75	3	3	30	12	tr	30
Milk Base Mascarpone Chocolate Rum	1 scoop (3.5 oz)	95	3	5	15	11	tr	35
Milk Base Pannacotta Wedding Cake	1 scoop (3.5 oz)	75	2	2	8	13	tr	28
Milk Base Peppermint	1 scoop (3.5 oz)	75	2	2	8	14	1	30
Milk Base Rose	1 scoop (3.5 oz)	70	8	2	8	12	tr	30
Milk Base Tiramisu	1 scoop (3.5 oz)	80	2	3	28	12	tr	30
Milk Base Zabajone	1 scoop (3.5 oz)	80	3	3	30	12	tr	30
No Sugar Added Chocolate	1 scoop (3.5 oz)	28	2	1	3	9	1	33
No Sugar Added Mint	1 scoop (3.5 oz)	25	1	1	3	9	1	23
No Sugar Added Mocha	1 scoop (3.5 oz)	28	2	1	3	9	1	22
No Sugar Added Strawberry Milk	1 scoop (3.5 oz)	23	1	1	1	8	1	19
Soy Banana	1 scoop (3.5 oz)	40	tr	2	0	6	1	3
Soy Blueberry	1 scoop (3.5 oz)	40	tr	2	0	6	1	3

FOOD	PORTION	CALS	PROT	FAT	CHOL	CARB	FIBER	SOD
Soy Chocolate	1 scoop (3.5 oz)	38	tr	2	0	5	1	9
Soy Coffee	1 scoop (3.5 oz)	35	tr	2	0	5	1	3
Soy Hazelnut	1 scoop (3.5 oz)	35	tr	2	0	5	1	3
Soy Strawberry	1 scoop (3.5 oz)	38	tr	2	0	6	1	3
Soy Wild Berries	1 scoop (3.5 oz)	40	tr	2	0	6	1	3
Water Base Blackberry	1 scoop (3.5 oz)	28	0	0	0	7	tr	0
Water Base Ginger Lemon	1 scoop (3.5 oz)	25	0	0	0	7	tr	0
Water Base Green Apple	1 scoop (3.5 oz)	28	0	0	0	7	tr	0
Water Base Lemon Sage	1 scoop (3.5 oz)	25	0	0	0	7	tr	0
Water Base Lychee	1 scoop (3.5 oz)	25	0	0	0	6	tr	0
Water Base Orange Vidalia	1 scoop (3.5 oz)	25	0	0	0	7	0	0
Water Base Passion Fruit	1 scoop (3.5 oz)	23	0	0	0	6	0	0
Water Base Pineapple	1 scoop (3.5 oz)	28	0	0	0	7	tr	0
Water Base Strawberry Port	1 scoop (3.5 oz)	25	0	0	0	6	tr	0
Water Base Watermelon	1 scoop (3.5 oz)	25	0	0	0	7	tr	0
PAPA JOHN'S								
DESSERTS								
Applepie	4 (6.7 oz)	480	8	10	0	90	2	520
Cinnamon Sweetsticks	4 (6.7 oz)	580	11	16	0	98	3	740
Cinnapie	4 (5.9 oz)	560	8	19	0	90	2	540
OTHER MENU SELECTIONS								
Breadsticks	2 (4 oz)	290	8	5	0	54	2	540
Breadsticks Garlic Parmesan	2 (4.4 oz)	340	9	10	0	54	2	720

FOOD	PORTION	CALS	PROT	FAT	CHOL	CARB	FIBER	SOD
Cheesesticks	4 (4.8 oz)	370	14	16	35	41	2	860
Chickenstrips	2 (2.3 oz)	130	12	5	25	10	0	430
Wings BBQ	2 (2.8 oz)	190	12	12	50	6	0	760
Wings Buffalo	2 (2.8 oz)	170	12	13	50	3	0	1070
Wings Honey Chipotle	2 (2.8 oz)	190	12	12	50	8	0	730
PIZZA								
BBQ Chicken & Bacon 12 inch	⅛ pie (3.8 oz)	250	11	8	25	32	1	730
BBQ Chicken & Bacon 16 inch	⅒ pie (5.6 oz)	370	16	12	35	48	2	1080
BBQ Chicken & Bacon 8 inch	¼ pie (3.5 oz)	230	10	7	20	30	1	670
Cheese 12 inch	⅛ pie (3.2 oz)	210	8	8	20	26	1	530
Garden Fresh 12 inch	⅛ pie (3.9 oz)	200	8	7	15	27	2	500
Garden Fresh 16 inch	⅒ pie (6 oz)	300	11	10	20	42	6	740
Garden Fresh 8 inch	¼ pie (3.6 oz)	180	6	5	10	26	1	440
Hawaiian BBQ Chicken 12 inch	⅛ pie (4.1 oz)	250	11	8	25	33	1	730
Hawaiian BBQ Chicken 16 inch	⅒ pie (6 oz)	370	16	12	35	49	2	1080
Original 16 inch	⅒ pie (4.6 oz)	300	11	10	25	40	2	740
Pepperoni 12 inch	⅛ pie (3.2 oz)	230	9	10	20	26	1	610
Pepperoni 16 inch	⅒ pie (4.8 oz)	340	13	14	30	40	2	900
Pepperoni 8 inch	¼ pie (3 oz)	210	8	9	15	25	1	560
Sausage 12 inch	⅛ pie (3.3 oz)	240	8	11	20	26	1	600
Sausage 16 inch	⅒ pie (4.9 oz)	350	12	15	30	40	2	860
Sausage 8 inch	¼ pie (3.1 oz)	220	7	9	15	25	1	540
Spicy Italian 12 inch	⅛ pie (3.6 oz)	270	10	13	25	27	1	690

FOOD	PORTION	CALS	PROT	FAT	CHOL	CARB	FIBER	SOD
Spicy Italian 16 inch	1/10 pie (5.5 oz)	400	15	20	40	41	2	1040
Spicy Italian 8 inch	1/4 pie (3.4 oz)	240	9	12	20	25	1	630
Spinach Alfredo 12 inch	1/8 pie (2.9 oz)	210	8	8	20	25	1	470
Spinach Alfredo 16 inch	1/10 pie (4.4 oz)	310	11	12	30	39	2	680
Spinach Alfredo 8 inch	1/4 pie (2.8 oz)	190	6	8	20	24	1	420
The Meats 12 inch	1/8 pie (3.6 oz)	250	11	12	25	26	1	710
The Meats 16 inch	1/10 pie (5.5 oz)	400	16	19	40	40	2	1100
The Meats 8 inch	1/4 pie (3.4 oz)	240	10	11	25	25	1	690
The Works 12 inch	1/8 pie (3.9 oz)	230	9	9	20	27	1	650
The Works 16 inch	1/10 pie (5.9 oz)	350	14	14	30	42	2	980
The Works 8 inch	1/4 pie (3.6 oz)	210	8	9	20	26	1	600
Tuscan Six Cheese 12 inch	1/8 pie (3.3 oz)	230	10	9	25	26	1	580
Tuscan Six Cheese 16 inch	1/10 pie (4.9 oz)	340	15	13	30	40	2	840
Tuscan Six Cheese 8 inch	1/4 pie (3 oz)	210	9	8	20	25	1	520
SAUCES AND SEASONINGS								
Crushed Red Pepper	1 pkg (1 g)	5	0	0	0	1	0	0
Parmesan Cheese	1 pkg (3.5 g)	15	–	1	5	0	0	45
Sauce Barbeque	1 serv (1 oz)	45	0	0	0	11	0	240
Sauce Blue Cheese	1 serv (1 oz)	160	1	16	20	1	0	250
Sauce Buffalo	1 serv (1 oz)	15	0	1	0	2	0	1030
Sauce Cheese	1 serv (1 oz)	40	1	4	5	1	0	160
Sauce Honey Mustard	1 serv (1 oz)	150	0	15	10	5	0	120
Sauce Pizza	1 serv (1 oz)	20	0	1	0	3	0	230
Sauce Ranch	1 serv (1 oz)	100	1	10	10	1	0	240
Sauce Special Garlic	1 serv (1 oz)	150	0	17	0	0	0	310
Special Seasoning	1 pkg (3 g)	5	0	0	0	1	0	410

FOOD	PORTION	CALS	PROT	FAT	CHOL	CARB	FIBER	SOD
PAPA MURPHY'S								
PIZZA								
DeLite Thin Crust Large All Meat	1/10 pie	190	11	11	35	13	0	430
DeLite Thin Crust Large Cheese	1/10 pie	140	8	7	20	13	0	230
DeLite Thin Crust Large Hawaiian	1/10 pie	160	9	7	25	15	0	290
DeLite Thin Crust Large Pepperoni	1/10 pie	170	9	9	30	13	0	320
DeLite Thin Crust Large Veggie	1/10 pie	160	8	9	20	13	tr	250
Original Crust Family Size All Meat	1/12 pie	360	19	18	55	31	0	900
Original Crust Family Size Cheese	1/12 pie	270	13	11	30	30	0	560
Original Crust Family Size Cowboy	1/12 pie	350	17	18	45	32	tr	900
Original Crust Family Size Hawaiian	1/12 pie	290	15	11	35	33	tr	670
Original Crust Family Size Murphy's Combo	1/12 pie	360	18	18	50	33	tr	940
Original Crust Family Size Papa's Favorite	1/12 pie	360	18	18	50	33	tr	910
Original Crust Family Size Pepperoni	1/12 pie	320	15	15	40	31	0	710
Original Crust Family Size Rancher	1/12 pie	330	17	16	45	31	tr	790
Original Crust Family Size Specialty Of The House	1/12 pie	320	16	15	40	32	tr	800
Original Crust Family Size Veggie Mediterranean	1/12 pie	310	13	14	30	34	3	610
Original Crust Family Size Veggie Combo	1/12 pie	300	14	13	30	33	tr	670
Original Crust Medium Cheese	1/8 pie	230	11	9	25	25	0	460
Stuffed Family Size 5 Meat	1/16 pie	370	18	16	45	39	0	910
Stuffed Family Size Big Murphy	1/16 pie	370	17	16	40	40	tr	890

FOOD	PORTION	CALS	PROT	FAT	CHOL	CARB	FIBER	SOD
Stuffed Family Size Chicago Style	1/16 pie	370	17	16	45	40	tr	850
Stuffed Family Size Chicken & Bacon	1/16 pie	370	20	15	50	39	0	820
Stuffed Large 5 Meat	1/12 pie	370	18	16	45	38	0	900
Stuffed Large Big Murphy	1/12 pie	360	17	15	40	39	tr	870
SALADS								
Club w/o Dressing & Croutons	½ serv (6.6 oz)	140	13	8	30	6	3	480
Garden w/o Dressing & Croutons	1 serv (7.2 oz)	100	6	6	10	8	3	260
Italian w/o Dressing & Croutons	½ serv (6.5 oz)	140	7	10	20	7	3	400

PEI WEI ASIAN DINER

FOOD	PORTION	CALS	PROT	FAT	CHOL	CARB	FIBER	SOD
CHILDREN'S MENU SELECTIONS								
Kid's Wei Honey Seared Chicken w/o Noodles Or Rice	1 serv	290	16	17	–	19	0	–
Kid's Wei Lo Mein Chicken w/o Noodles Or Rice	1 serv	180	20	7	–	7	0	–
Kid's Wei Teriyaki Chicken w/o Noodles Or Rice	1 serv	240	23	5	–	20	0	–
DESSERTS								
Cookie Chocolate Chip	1	342	5	14	–	53	2	–
Cookie Fortune	1	30	0	0	0	7	0	–
MAIN MENU SELECTIONS								
Bowl w/ Brown Rice Japanese Teriyaki Beef	1 serv	580	33	17	–	66	4	–
Bowl w/ Brown Rice Japanese Teriyaki Chicken	1 serv	460	28	7	–	64	4	–
Bowl w/ Brown Rice Japanese Teriyaki Shrimp	1 serv	410	20	5	–	64	4	–
Bowl w/ Brown Rice Japanese Teriyaki Vegetables & Tofu	1 serv	410	13	6	–	71	7	–
Bowl w/ White Rice Japanese Teriyaki Beef	1 serv	560	32	16	–	62	3	–

FOOD	PORTION	CALS	PROT	FAT	CHOL	CARB	FIBER	SOD
Bowl w/ White Rice Japanese Teriyaki Chicken	1 serv	440	28	6	–	60	3	–
Bowl w/ White Rice Japanese Teriyaki Shrimp	1 serv	390	20	5	–	61	3	–
Bowl w/ White Rice Japanese Teriyaki Vegetables & Tofu	1 serv	390	13	5	–	68	5	–
Crispy Potstickers	4	130	6	7	–	10	0	–
Edamame	1 serv	156	14	8	–	12	5	–
Fried Rice Beef	1 serv	630	37	21	–	68	3	–
Fried Rice Chicken	1 serv	525	32	11	–	68	3	–
Fried Rice Shrimp	1 serv	475	24	10	–	67	3	–
Fried Rice Vegetables & Tofu	1 serv	440	17	7	–	73	5	–
Ginger Broccoli Beef	1 serv	450	37	22	–	19	2	–
Ginger Broccoli Chicken	1 serv	300	31	9	–	19	2	–
Ginger Broccoli Shrimp	1 serv	230	22	7	–	18	2	–
Ginger Broccoli Vegetables & Tofu	1 serv	170	10	4	–	23	4	–
Honey Seared Chicken	1 serv	420	21	15	–	45	0	–
Honey Seared Shrimp	1 serv	370	14	14	–	43	0	–
Hot & Sour Soup	1 cup	150	7	9	–	11	2	–
Lemon Pepper Beef	1 serv	550	38	31	–	32	2	–
Lemon Pepper Chicken	1 serv	440	31	20	–	34	2	–
Lemon Pepper Shrimp	1 serv	380	22	18	–	34	2	–
Lemon Pepper Vegetables & Tofu	1 serv	230	10	10	–	29	4	–
Mandarin Kung Pao Beef	1 serv	610	40	34	–	31	3	–
Mandarin Kung Pao Chicken	1 serv	450	34	21	–	28	3	–
Mandarin Kung Pao Shrimp	1 serv	400	25	19	–	28	3	–
Mandarin Kung Pao Vegetables & Tofu	1 serv	290	13	15	–	23	4	–
Minced Chicken w/ Cool Lettuce Wraps w/o Rice Sticks	1 serv	250	22	4	–	31	3	–
Mongolian Beef	1 serv	420	36	22	–	14	1	–
Mongolian Chicken	1 serv	280	10	9	–	14	1	–

FOOD	PORTION	CALS	PROT	FAT	CHOL	CARB	FIBER	SOD
Mongolian Shrimp	1 serv	210	21	6	–	12	1	–
Mongolian Vegetables & Tofu	1 serv	180	10	6	–	19	3	–
Noodles Dan Dan Chicken	1 serv	390	26	7	–	54	3	–
Noodles Lo Mein Beef	1 serv	570	36	21	–	61	5	–
Noodles Lo Mein Chicken	1 serv	460	31	11	–	61	5	–
Noodles Lo Mein Shrimp	1 serv	400	23	8	–	60	5	–
Noodles Lo Mein Vegetables & Tofu	1 serv	400	16	8	–	66	7	–
Noodles Thai Blazing Beef	1 serv	630	28	32	–	55	4	–
Noodles Thai Blazing Chicken	1 serv	520	24	22	–	55	4	–
Noodles Thai Blazing Shrimp	1 serv	482	16	22	–	55	4	–
Noodles Thai Blazing Vegetables & Tofu	1 serv	430	10	18	–	59	6	–
Noodles Egg	1 serv	210	7	3	–	39	2	–
Noodles Rice	1 serv	130	0	0	0	32	0	–
Orange Peel Beef	1 serv	660	42	31	–	52	3	–
Orange Peel Chicken	1 serv	520	6	18	–	52	3	–
Orange Peel Shrimp	1 serv	460	27	16	–	51	3	–
Orange Peel Vegetables & Tofu	1 serv	330	14	10	–	46	4	–
Pad Thai Beef	1 serv	670	40	30	–	63	2	–
Pad Thai Chicken	1 serv	560	35	20	–	61	2	–
Pad Thai Shrimp	1 serv	490	27	17	–	60	2	–
Pei Wei Spicy Beef	1 serv	480	34	26	–	25	2	–
Pei Wei Spicy Chicken	1 serv	330	28	13	–	25	2	–
Pei Wei Spicy Shrimp	1 serv	300	19	11	–	29	2	–
Rice Brown	1 serv	170	4	2	–	37	3	–
Rice Fried	1 serv	260	9	5	–	44	2	–
Rice Sticks	1 cup	130	0	0	0	33	0	–
Rice White	1 serv	200	4	0	0	44	1	–
Spicy Korean Beef	1 serv	490	41	24	–	26	3	–
Spicy Korean Chicken	1 serv	350	15	11	–	26	3	–
Spicy Korean Shrimp	1 serv	280	26	9	–	24	3	–
Spicy Korean Vegetables & Tofu	1 serv	240	15	9	–	27	4	–
Spring Rolls	2	90	2	5	–	11	1	–

FOOD	PORTION	CALS	PROT	FAT	CHOL	CARB	FIBER	SOD
Sweet & Sour Chicken	1 serv	440	21	13	–	61	2	–
Sweet & Sour Shrimp	1 serv	390	14	11	–	59	2	–
Thai Coconut Curry Beef	1 serv	550	36	37	–	20	2	–
Thai Coconut Curry Chicken	1 serv	380	30	19	–	23	2	–
Thai Coconut Curry Shrimp	1 serv	300	21	17	–	18	2	–
Thai Coconut Curry Vegetables & Tofu	1 serv	220	8	14	–	19	2	–
Thai Dynamite Chicken	1 serv	390	33	19	–	20	2	–
Thai Dynamite Shrimp	1 serv	280	15	16	–	20	2	–
Thai Dynamite Vegetables & Tofu	1 serv	220	6	16	–	15	3	–
Wontons Crab	4	190	8	13	–	9	0	–
SALAD DRESSINGS AND SAUCES								
Dressing Sesame Ginger	1 serv (2 oz)	170	1	16	–	5	0	–
Lime Vinaigrette	1 serv (2 oz)	230	0	20	–	13	0	–
Sauce Lettuce Wrap	1 serv (2 oz)	70	4	5	–	2	0	–
Sauce Sweet Chili	1 serv (2 oz)	140	0	0	0	34	2	–
Sauce Thai Peanut	1 serv (2 oz)	168	5	11	–	15	1	–
SALADS								
Asian Chopped Chicken w/ Dressing	1 serv	280	24	15	–	13	2	–
Asian Chopped Chicken w/o Dressing	1 serv	200	23	8	–	10	2	–
Pei Wei Spicy Chicken w/ Dressing	1 serv	350	22	16	–	28	2	–
Pei Wei Spicy Chicken w/o Dressing	1 serv	210	22	3	–	23	2	–
Vietnamese Chicken Salad Rolls	3	53	3	3	–	5	1	–

P.F. CHANG'S CHINA BISTRO

DESSERTS								
Banana Spring Rolls	1 serv	814	12	37	–	130	7	–
Cake The Great Wall Of Chocolate	1 serv	2237	20	90	–	376	13	–
Flourless Chocolate Dome Gluten Free	1 serv	572	8	26	–	84	8	–

FOOD	PORTION	CALS	PROT	FAT	CHOL	CARB	FIBER	SOD
Ice Cream Pineapple Coconut	1 serv	111	4	12	–	25	0	–
Mini Dessert Apple Pie	1	170	1	4	–	34	1	–
Mini Dessert Banana Split	1	167	1	6	–	28	1	–
Mini Dessert Carrot Cake	1	295	2	14	–	42	1	–
Mini Dessert Creamy Strawberry Cheesecake	1	239	3	20	–	14	1	–
Mini Dessert Great Wall Of Chocolate	1	336	1	26	–	24	2	–
Mini Dessert S'mores	1	323	3	12	–	50	1	–
Mini Dessert Tiramisu	1	202	3	14	–	15	0	–
Mini Dessert Tres Leche Lemon Dream	1	216	4	8	–	32	1	–
MAIN MENU SELECTIONS								
Almond & Cashew Chicken	1 serv	815	81	30	–	63	5	–
Asian Marinated New York Strip	1 serv	1432	92	86	–	68	2	–
Asian Slaw	1 serv	585	5	57	–	19	5	–
Beef A La Sichuan	1 serv	1172	86	64	–	56	5	–
Beef w/ Broccoli	1 serv	1118	93	65	–	38	7	–
Buddha's Feast Steamed	1 serv	137	8	1	–	29	10	–
Buddha's Feast Stir Fried	1 serv	367	25	5	–	66	10	–
Calamari Salt & Pepper	1 serv	720	33	11	–	118	3	–
Cantonese Scallops	1 serv	408	39	16	–	26	4	–
Cantonese Shrimp	1 serv	330	33	12	–	21	4	–
Cantonese Chow Fun w/ Beef	1 serv	1212	69	38	–	142	5	–
Cantonese Chow Fun w/ Chicken	1 serv	1045	60	23	–	146	5	–
Chang's Spicy Chicken	1 serv	923	56	37	–	88	1	–
Chengdu Spiced Lamb	1 serv	1056	62	75	–	34	5	–
Chicken w/ Black Bean Sauce	1 serv	678	76	23	–	33	1	–
Chow Fun Vegetable	1 serv	878	22	8	–	181	26	–
Chow Mein Combo	1 serv	912	61	34	–	86	6	–
Chow Mein w/ Beef	1 serv	793	54	26	–	84	7	–
Chow Mein w/ Chicken	1 serv	689	49	16	–	84	6	–
Chow Mein w/ Pork	1 serv	898	61	34	–	83	6	–
Chow Mein w/ Shrimp	1 serv	625	41	13	–	84	6	–

FOOD	PORTION	CALS	PROT	FAT	CHOL	CARB	FIBER	SOD
Citrus Soy Salmon w/ Brown Rice	1 serv	1000	69	59	–	42	4	–
Citrus Soy Salmon w/ White Rice	1 serv	1025	70	58	–	49	2	–
Coconut Curry Vegetables	1 serv	686	30	46	–	48	12	–
Crispy Green Beans	1 serv	507	8	28	–	59	8	–
Crispy Honey Chicken	1 serv	867	53	11	–	121	3	–
Crispy Honey Shrimp	1 serv	1061	35	44	–	118	2	–
Dali Chicken	1 serv	1091	91	52	–	53	6	–
Double Pan Fried Noodles Combo	1 serv	1384	68	69	–	118	7	–
Double Pan Fried Noodles w/ Beef	1 serv	1186	53	56	–	112	6	–
Double Pan Fried Noodles w/ Chicken	1 serv	1072	42	47	–	115	7	–
Double Pan Fried Noodles w/ Pork	1 serv	1208	50	60	–	114	7	–
Double Pan Fried Noodles w/ Shrimp	1 serv	1031	37	46	–	115	7	–
Dumplings Peking Pan Fried	1 serv	367	18	23	–	21	1	–
Dumplings Peking Steamed	1 serv	327	18	18	–	21	1	–
Dumplings Shrimp Pan Fried	1 serv	305	21	13	–	25	1	–
Dumplings Shrimp Steamed	1 serv	265	21	8	–	25	1	–
Dumplings Vegetable Pan Fried	1 serv	307	9	11	–	43	2	–
Dumplings Vegetable Steamed	1 serv	267	9	7	–	43	2	–
Eggplant Stir Fried	1 serv	590	10	34	–	64	10	–
Fried Rice Combo	1 serv	1539	68	69	–	154	5	–
Fried Rice w/ Beef	1 serv	1228	58	40	–	150	5	–
Fried Rice w/ Chicken	1 serv	1208	47	44	–	151	5	–
Fried Rice w/ Pork	1 serv	1360	55	57	–	150	5	–
Fried Rice w/ Shrimp	1 serv	1154	40	41	–	149	4	–
Garlic Noodles	1 serv	612	18	11	–	111	6	–
Garlic Snap Peas	1 sm	129	4	7	–	13	4	–
Ginger Chicken w/ Broccoli	1 serv	656	60	26	–	45	7	–

FOOD	PORTION	CALS	PROT	FAT	CHOL	CARB	FIBER	SOD
Ginger Chicken w/ Broccoli Gluten Free	1 serv	677	61	30	–	43	7	–
Ground Chicken & Eggplant	1 serv	792	33	40	–	73	9	–
Harvest Spring Rolls	1 serv	287	6	15	–	30	2	–
Hot Fish	1 serv	1338	60	71	–	111	8	–
Kung Pao Chicken	1 serv	1228	74	79	–	58	8	–
Kung Pao Scallops	1 serv	1136	87	57	–	66	9	–
Kung Pao Shrimp	1 serv	977	60	58	–	58	9	–
Lemon Pepper Shrimp	1 serv	701	36	36	–	59	5	–
Lemon Scallops	1 serv	952	60	28	–	100	3	–
Lemongrass Prawns	1 serv	907	34	58	–	65	4	–
Lettuce Wraps Chicken	1 serv	377	28	12	–	35	5	–
Lettuce Wraps Gluten Free Chicken	1 serv	477	31	12	–	63	5	–
Lettuce Wraps Vegetarian	1 serv	281	25	4	–	37	7	–
Lo Mein Combo	1 serv	1409	66	83	–	98	8	–
Lo Mein w/ Beef	1 serv	1374	67	80	–	94	8	–
Lo Mein w/ Chicken	1 serv	1198	51	67	–	97	8	–
Lo Mein w/ Pork	1 serv	1400	63	54	–	95	8	–
Lo Mein w/ Shrimp	1 serv	1134	43	64	–	97	8	–
Lunch Bowl Almond & Cashew Chicken w/ White Rice	1	955	63	26	–	112	5	–
Lunch Bowl Beef w/ Broccoli w/ Brown Rice	1	844	58	27	–	87	8	–
Lunch Bowl Beef w/ Broccoli w/ White Rice	1	890	59	26	–	99	5	–
Lunch Bowl Buddha's Feast w/ Brown Rice	1	541	23	8	–	101	11	–
Lunch Bowl Buddha's Feast w/ White Rice	1	587	24	6	–	113	7	–
Lunch Bowl Citrus Soy Salmon w/ Brown Rice	1	1047	48	63	–	67	6	–
Lunch Bowl Citrus Soy Salmon w/ White Rice	1	1093	49	62	–	79	2	–
Lunch Bowl Crispy Honey Chicken w/ Brown Rice	1	943	61	13	–	126	6	–
Lunch Bowl Crispy Honey Chicken w/ White Rice	1	989	62	12	–	138	2	–

FOOD	PORTION	CALS	PROT	FAT	CHOL	CARB	FIBER	SOD
Lunch Bowl Moo Goo Gai Pan w/ Brown Rice	1	545	40	8	–	76	7	–
Lunch Bowl Moo Goo Gai Pan w/ White Rice	1	591	41	6	–	88	3	–
Lunch Bowl Pepper Steak w/ Brown Rice	1	820	54	28	–	82	7	–
Lunch Bowl Pepper Steak w/ White Rice	1 serv	968	55	39	–	94	3	–
Lunch Bowl Shrimp w/ Lobster Sauce w/ Brown Rice	1	686	37	25	–	75	6	–
Lunch Bowl Shrimp w/ Lobster Sauce w/ White Rice	1	732	38	23	–	87	2	–
Mongolian Beef	1 serv	1178	96	73	–	29	2	–
Moo Goo Gai Pan	1 serv	661	54	34	–	32	4	–
Mu Shu Chicken	1 serv	715	47	38	–	49	–	–
Mu Shu Pork	1 serv	871	57	50	–	50	25	–
Noodles Dan Dan	1 serv	1087	51	30	–	145	7	–
Noodles Tam's	1 serv	1678	58	93	–	144	6	–
Oolong Marinated Sea Bass	1 serv	521	64	12	–	40	3	–
Orange Peel Beef	1 serv	1568	88	85	–	115	14	–
Orange Peel Chicken	1 serv	1151	61	46	–	127	14	–
Orange Peel Shrimp	1 serv	1010	47	41	–	118	14	–
Pepper Steak	1 serv	971	95	48	–	32	4	–
Philip's Better Lemon Chicken	1 serv	1051	58	42	–	113	5	–
Rice Brown	1 cup	254	5	2	–	53	4	–
Rice Sticks	1 serv	135	0	0	0	33	0	–
Rice White	1 cup	295	6	1	–	64	1	–
Salt & Pepper Prawns	1 serv	844	45	50	–	55	5	–
Seared Ahi Tuna	1 serv	210	26	9	–	9	1	–
Shanghai Cucumbers	1 serv	124	10	6	–	8	4	–
Shrimp w/ Candied Walnuts	1 serv	1225	60	80	–	74	2	–
Shrimp w/ Lobster Sauce	1 serv	480	42	22	–	24	1	–
Sichuan Asparagus	1 sm	97	6	3	–	16	3	–
Sichuan Chicken Flatbread	1 serv	1160	52	80	–	56	4	–

FOOD	PORTION	CALS	PROT	FAT	CHOL	CARB	FIBER	SOD
Sichuan From The Sea Calamari	1 serv	1078	69	36	–	118	4	–
Sichuan From The Sea Scallops	1 serv	1030	70	36	–	98	3	–
Sichuan From The Sea Shrimp	1 serv	728	44	37	–	55	3	–
Singapore Street Noodles	1 serv	572	28	16	–	81	7	–
Singapore Street Noodles Gluten Free	1 serv	566	28	15	–	81	4	–
Spare Ribs Chang's	1 serv	1356	93	89	–	43	1	–
Spare Ribs Northern Style	1 serv	720	49	54	–	6	0	–
Spicy Green Beans	1 sm	234	7	13	–	23	6	–
Spinach w/ Garlic Stir Fried	1 sm	77	7	3	–	9	6	–
Sweet & Sour Chicken	1 serv	764	40	20	–	107	3	–
Sweet & Sour Pork	1 serv	1095	61	46	–	106	3	–
Vegetarian Ma Po Tofu	1 serv	537	40	19	–	51	6	–
Wild Alaskan Sockeye Salmon Steamed w/ Ginger	1 serv	646	60	36	–	23	5	–
Wild Alaskan Sockeye Salmon Steamed w/ Ginger Gluten Free	1 serv	672	60	36	–	30	6	–
Wok Charred Beef	1 serv	941	63	63	–	33	8	–
Wok Seared Lamb	1 serv	1081	62	80	–	29	8	–
Wontons Crab	1 serv	440	19	25	–	32	2	–
SALAD DRESSINGS AND SAUCES								
Dressing Creamy Wedge	1 serv	443	3	43	–	8	1	–
Dressing Signature Ginger	1 serv	483	1	48	–	9	0	–
Sauce Chili Bean	1 serv	81	3	1	–	12	0	–
Sauce Crispy Green Bean	1 serv	451	0	48	–	5	0	–
Sauce Potsticker	1 serv	36	2	1	–	6	0	–
Sauce Shrimp Dumpling	1 serv	24	3	0	0	1	0	–
Sauce Special	1 serv	55	2	1	–	9	0	–
Sauce Spicy Plum	1 serv	110	0	0	0	28	0	–
Sauce Sweet & Sour	1 serv	57	0	0	0	15	0	–
Vinaigrette Mustard	1 serv	66	4	2	–	7	0	–
Vinaigrette Watermelon Citrus	1 serv	240	1	23	–	7	0	–
SALADS								
Bikini Shrimp w/o Dressing	1 serv	192	8	6	–	30	4	–

FOOD	PORTION	CALS	PROT	FAT	CHOL	CARB	FIBER	SOD
Chang's Wedge w/ Chicken w/o Dressing	1 serv	595	57	35	–	12	5	–
Chang's Wedge w/o Dressing	1 serv	244	8	19	–	12	5	–
Chopped Chicken w/o Dressing	1 serv	401	47	14	–	21	5	–
SOUPS								
Chicken Noodle	1 bowl	512	64	13	–	30	2	–
Egg Drop	1 cup	48	1	2	–	7	0	–
Hot & Sour	1 cup	85	5	2	–	11	4	–
Wonton	1 bowl	354	21	10	–	44	3	–
PINKBERRY								
Frozen Yogurt Coffee	½ cup	90	4	0	5	24	0	50
Frozen Yogurt Green Tea	½ cup	50	3	0	5	10	0	50
Frozen Yogurt Original	½ cup	70	3	0	5	14	0	55
PIZZA FUSION								
DESSERTS								
Brownies Gluten Free	½ serv	232	1	16	9	27	1	50
Calzone Chocolate	½	209	5	9	9	30	1	171
Cookies Chocolate Chip	⅓ serv	250	4	13	5	33	3	210
Pastry Strawberry Cheese	1 serv	338	9	10	15	54	2	391
PIZZA								
BBQ Chicken	1 slice	181	8	4	20	26	1	434
Big Kahuna	1 slice	236	12	9	22	26	2	594
Bruschetta	1 slice	159	8	4	10	23	1	255
Cheese	1 slice	167	7	5	10	23	2	359
Eggplant & Mozzarella	1 slice	181	7	6	10	24	2	381
Farmer's Market	1 slice	190	9	6	10	25	2	502
Founder's Pie	1 slice	201	8	7	20	25	2	349
Four Cheese & Sundried Tomato	1 slice	175	8	5	19	26	2	355
Greek	1 slice	204	9	7	12	25	2	442
Pepperoni	1 slice	220	10	9	19	23	2	575
Personal BBQ Chicken	½ pie	272	11	6	30	43	2	635
Personal Big Kahuna	½ pie	365	18	13	33	39	3	930
Personal Bruschetta	½ pie	234	10	5	10	37	2	359
Personal Cheese	½ pie	233	10	6	10	35	2	460

FOOD	PORTION	CALS	PROT	FAT	CHOL	CARB	FIBER	SOD
Personal Eggplant & Mozzarella	½ pie	304	12	11	20	39	4	613
Personal Farmer's Market	½ pie	279	12	8	13	40	3	747
Personal Founder's Pie	½ pie	347	14	14	40	41	3	540
Personal Four Cheese & Sundried Tomato	½ pie	262	12	7	24	39	3	494
Personal Greek	½ pie	299	12	11	13	39	3	571
Personal Pepperoni	½ pie	359	17	15	31	37	2	719
Personal Philly Steak	½ pie	358	19	14	37	42	4	810
Personal Sausage & Tri-Peppers	½ pie	323	15	12	23	39	3	789
Personal Spinach & Artichoke	½ pie	270	12	7	10	41	4	704
Personal Very Vegan	½ pie	321	9	15	0	41	4	539
Philly Steak	1 slice	220	11	8	22	26	3	520
Sausage & Tri-Peppers	1 slice	212	10	8	16	25	2	523
Spinach & Artichoke	1 slice	184	9	5	10	25	2	481
Very Vegan	1 slice	195	6	8	0	27	3	408
SALADS								
Caesar & Roasted Chicken	½ serv	358	9	21	39	28	2	728
Chicken Bruschetta	½ serv	331	11	22	53	22	3	334
Fusion	½ serv	244	5	8	0	20	4	299
Pan Roasted Steak	½ serv	388	18	26	57	22	4	543
Pear & Gorgonzola	½ serv	380	12	34	32	12	4	428
Roasted Beet & Feta	½ serv	320	8	25	17	19	4	602
Side Salad Arugula	1 serv	48	1	4	0	1	0	288
SANDWICHES								
Philly Phusion	½	473	28	23	71	39	3	862
Portabello Grill	½	380	14	20	22	38	3	757
Roasted Chicken	½	357	17	14	56	41	4	722
Roasted Turkey	½	417	26	19	60	35	2	1237
STARTERS								
Flatbread	1 (2 serv)	198	14	2	0	76	4	676
Stuffed Portabello Mushroom	½ serv	140	5	11	6	9	2	506
Trio Of Dips	⅓ serv	191	6	11	10	30	3	491

FOOD	PORTION	CALS	PROT	FAT	CHOL	CARB	FIBER	SOD
PRETZELMAKER								
BEVERAGES								
Breezer Coffee	1 (20 oz)	640	6	21	50	107	0	100
Breezer Mocha	1 (20 oz)	620	6	20	50	106	0	100
Breezer Peach	1 (20 oz)	650	6	20	50	117	0	110
Breezer Raspberry	1 (20 oz)	650	6	20	50	117	0	100
Breezer Strawberry Banana	1 (20 oz)	650	6	20	50	115	0	100
Diet Coke	1 sm (20 oz)	0	0	0	0	0	0	25
Lemonade	1 sm (20 oz)	160	0	0	0	92	0	15
PRETZELS								
Bites	1 med (7.4 oz)	640	13	16	0	112	4	500
Bites	1 sm (5.3 oz)	450	9	11	0	80	3	360
Bites Cinnamon Sugar	1 serv (5.8 oz)	520	9	12	0	95	3	20
Caramel Nut	1 (4.5 oz)	390	7	7	0	74	2	55
Cinnamon Sugar	1 (4.3 oz)	370	7	8	0	68	2	15
Garlic	1 (4.1 oz)	350	7	7	0	64	2	790
Original	1 (4 oz)	340	7	7	0	61	2	220
Parmesan	1 (4.2 oz)	360	9	9	5	61	2	290
Plain	1 (4 oz)	209	7	2	0	61	2	15
PT Pretzel Dog	1 (6 oz)	440	15	27	80	34	1	1120
Ranch	1 (4.1 oz)	240	7	7	0	63	2	930
TOPPINGS								
Cream Cheese	1 serv (1.5 oz)	200	2	20	80	4	0	200
Icing Cream Cheese	1 serv (1.5 oz)	180	1	9	30	22	0	85
Ketchup	2 pkg (0.6 oz)	20	0	0	0	4	0	200
Mustard	2 pkg (0.4 oz)	5	0	0	0	1	0	125
Sauce Caramel	1 serv (1.5 oz)	140	1	0	0	35	0	160
Sauce Cheddar Cheese	1 serv (1.5 oz)	70	1	5	0	6	0	420
Sauce Nacho Cheese	1 serv (1.5 oz)	80	1	5	0	7	0	530

FOOD	PORTION	CALS	PROT	FAT	CHOL	CARB	FIBER	SOD
Sauce Pizza	1 serv (1.5 oz)	30	1	1	0	6	2	250
QUIZNOS								
COOKIES								
Dark Chocolate Chunk	1	380	5	15	25	58	1	300
Double Chocolate Chip	1	370	5	15	0	58	3	230
Oatmeal Raisin	1	340	5	11	25	59	2	290
Snickerdoodle	1	400	3	16	20	59	0	280
SANDWICHES								
Breakfast Bacon Egg Cheddar	1	380	21	21	175	36	4	1030
Breakfast Black Angus Steak & Cheddar	1 sm	330	26	13	180	36	3	950
Breakfast Egg & Cheddar	1	240	12	11	145	35	3	540
Breakfast Garden Vegetable Cheddar	1	250	13	11	145	38	4	540
Breakfast Ham Egg Cheddar	1	290	19	12	165	37	4	1010
Deli Honey Ham & Swiss	1	260	17	4	25	38	4	1020
Deli Oven Roasted Turkey & Cheese	1	250	15	4	20	39	4	1010
Deli Roast Beef & Cheddar	1	230	13	4	10	37	4	450
Deli Tuna Melt	1	500	14	33	40	37	4	630
Sammie Alpine Chicken	1	200	13	6	25	24	1	520
Sammie Balsamic Chicken	1	170	11	4	15	24	1	410
Sammie Bistro Steak Melt	1	180	11	4	15	25	1	490
Sammie Black Angus Steak	1	180	11	4	15	24	1	480
Sammie Italiano	1	240	10	11	25	24	1	710
Sammie Sonoma Turkey	1	160	8	4	10	25	1	580
Sub Baja Chicken w/ Bacon	1 sm	320	25	9	45	37	4	920
Sub Black Angus Steak On Rosemary Parmesan	1 sm	380	30	8	55	46	5	1140
Sub Chicken Carbonara w/ Bacon	1 sm	360	26	10	45	42	3	1010
Sub Classic Club w/ Bacon	1 sm	320	21	9	35	39	5	1270
Sub Classic Italian	1 sm	360	18	15	45	38	4	1220
Sub Honey Bacon Club	1 sm	320	21	9	35	39	5	1270

FOOD	PORTION	CALS	PROT	FAT	CHOL	CARB	FIBER	SOD
Sub Honey Bourbon Chicken	1 sm	260	28	4	35	38	4	700
Sub Honey Mustard Chicken w/ Bacon	1 sm	330	25	9	45	38	4	950
Sub Mesquite Chicken w/ Bacon	1 sm	330	25	9	45	38	4	930
Sub Prime Rib Cheesesteak	1 sm	360	24	11	45	40	4	920
Sub Prime Rib & Peppercorn	1 sm	380	30	8	55	46	5	1140
Sub Steakhouse Beef Dip	1 sm	260	13	6	15	37	4	1070
Sub The Traditional	1 sm	260	16	5	20	39	5	920
Sub Turkey Bacon Guacamole	1 sm	360	21	12	30	43	6	1390
Sub Turkey Ranch & Swiss	1 sm	250	16	4	20	39	5	970
Sub Tuscan Turkey On Rosemary Parmesan	1 sm	300	17	5	20	47	4	1070
Sub Veggie	1 sm	270	10	8	0	41	6	770
SOUPS								
Bread Bowl Chili	1 serv	730	31	22	50	104	8	1680
Bread Bowl Country French	1 serv	720	28	22	45	100	5	1730
Broccoli Cheese	1 cup	150	7	10	25	10	2	800
Chicken Noodle	1 cup	130	6	3	30	18	0	1290
Chili	1 cup	140	9	7	30	12	4	620

RANCH 1

FOOD	PORTION	CALS	PROT	FAT	CHOL	CARB	FIBER	SOD
BEVERAGES								
Barq's Root Beer	1 sm (16 oz)	167	0	0	0	45	0	36
Coca-Cola	1 sm (16 oz)	150	0	0	0	40	0	10
Diet Coke	1 sm (16 oz)	2	0	0	0	0	0	6
Sprite	1 sm (16 oz)	150	0	0	0	40	0	30
CHILDREN'S MENU SELECTIONS								
Kids Meal Chicken Tenders	1 (2 oz)	111	10	4	29	9	0	138
Kids Meal Fries	1 serv (4 oz)	279	4	15	0	31	4	351
Kids Meal Popcorn Chicken	1 (2 oz)	112	9	4	19	10	0	436
MAIN MENU SELECTIONS								
Bowl Chicken Teriyaki	1 (19.3 oz)	504	34	7	69	78	1	3415
Chicken Crispy	1 serv (5 oz)	326	27	15	83	22	1	351
Chicken Grilled	1 serv (3.9 oz)	146	24	6	69	0	0	236

FOOD	PORTION	CALS	PROT	FAT	CHOL	CARB	FIBER	SOD
Chicken On Mixed Greens	1 serv (21 oz)	340	29	19	72	17	7	459
Chicken Popcorn	1 serv (5.5 oz)	325	27	12	55	30	1	1263
Chicken Tenders	1 serv (5.6 oz)	387	35	14	99	32	1	461
Fajita Mix Tomatoes Onion & Carrot	1 serv (3.2 oz)	20	1	0	0	5	1	12
Fajitas Chicken	1 serv (10 oz)	540	30	24	75	53	3	969
Fries	1 med	381	6	21	0	43	6	483
Fries Cheese	1 reg	493	8	27	9	54	6	1129
Green Mix For Sandwiches	1 serv (2.5 oz)	31	1	2	1	2	1	21
Peppers & Onions	1 serv (1.6 oz)	27	0	2	0	3	1	18
Platter Chicken Rice	1 (10.9 oz)	273	28	6	69	28	3	657
Popcorn Chicken	1 sm	325	27	12	55	30	1	1263
Rice	1 serv (4 oz)	97	3	0	0	21	0	395
Sandwich Chicken & Cheese	1 (11.2 oz)	389	33	12	84	39	2	881
Sandwich Chicken Philly	1 (9.2 oz)	410	36	13	79	40	2	777
Sandwich Crispy Chicken	1 (11.4 oz)	711	33	39	103	60	3	950
Sandwich Crispy Spicy Chicken	1 (11.4 oz)	543	34	17	83	68	3	1068
Sandwich Grilled Spicy Chicken	1 (10.3 oz)	363	31	7	69	46	2	951
Sandwich Ranch 1 Classic	1 (9.4 oz)	683	29	47	79	37	2	750
Steamed Vegetables	1 serv (3 oz)	27	2	0	0	6	2	31
Wrap Grilled Chicken Caesar	1 (13.2 oz)	746	44	41	105	55	4	1464
SALAD DRESSINGS AND SAUCES								
Dressing Balsamic Vinaigrette	1 oz	71	0	8	0	1	0	42
Dressing Classic Caesar	1 oz	103	1	11	7	1	0	117
Dressing Salad	1 oz	201	0	22	6	0	0	157
Sauce Ancho Chili Pepper	1 oz	134	1	14	17	1	0	179
Sauce BBQ	1 oz	84	0	4	0	12	0	134
Sauce Honey Mustard	1 oz	110	0	8	0	9	0	95

FOOD	PORTION	CALS	PROT	FAT	CHOL	CARB	FIBER	SOD
Sauce Pepper & Onion Saute	1 oz	143	0	16	0	1	0	192
Sauce Roasted Red Pepper	1 oz	232	0	26	6	0	–	75
Sauce Teriyaki	1 oz	24	1	0	0	5	0	973
SALADS								
Caesar	1 (7 oz)	34	2	1	0	7	4	16
Caesar Grilled Chicken	1 (11.3 oz)	223	28	8	71	13	5	344
Crispy Chicken Club	1 (13.6 oz)	495	30	26	116	29	4	396
Mandarin Chicken	1 (14.5 oz)	553	15	31	–	62	14	176
Mixed Greens w/o Cheese	1 (17 oz)	194	5	14	3	17	7	224
Salad Blend	1 serv (10.3 oz)	45	3	1	0	9	5	26
Southwest Chicken Chop	1 (17.6 oz)	681	33	43	104	44	7	1165
RAX								
BBQ Beef	1	399	–	20	40	43	–	1030
BBQ Sandwich	1	716	–	51	102	37	–	1453
Cheddar Melt	1	346	–	23	41	26	–	539
Deluxe	1	521	–	34	68	34	–	785
Grilled Chicken	1	526	–	33	69	32	–	994
Jr. Deluxe	1	367	–	25	42	25	–	509
Mushroom Melt	1	599	–	37	104	35	–	1688
Philly Melt	1	537	–	32	79	35	–	1296
Regular Rax	1	388	–	22	54	31	–	708
Turkey	1	484	–	32	50	32	–	1286
Turkey Bacon Club	1	680	–	47	76	37	–	1898
RED LOBSTER								
BEVERAGES								
Boston Ice Tea	1 serv	50	–	0	–	12	–	10
Coke	1 serv	100	–	0	–	27	–	35
Diet Coke	1 serv	0	0	0	0	0	0	30
Dr Pepper	1 serv	150	–	0	–	27	–	35
Harbor Cafe Coffee	1 serv	0	0	0	0	0	0	5
Lemonade Light	1 serv	0	–	0	0	0	0	55
Lemonade Raspberry	1 serv	180	–	0	–	30	–	20
Tea Hot or Cold Unsweetened	1 serv	0	0	0	0	0	0	0
Wine Blush	1 glass	120	–	0	–	7	–	20
Wine Red	1 glass	120	–	0	–	7	–	20

FOOD	PORTION	CALS	PROT	FAT	CHOL	CARB	FIBER	SOD
MAIN MENU SELECTIONS								
Artic Char Grilled Broiled or Blackened w/ Broccoli	1 full portion	630	–	29	–	21	–	720
Artic Char Grilled Broiled or Blackened w/ Broccoli	1 half portion	340	–	15	–	13	–	460
Barramundi Grilled Broiled or Blackened w/ Broccoli	1 half portion	230	–	5	–	8	–	270
Barramundi Grilled Broiled or Blackened w/ Broccoli	1 full portion	420	–	10	–	11	–	350
Cobia Grilled Broiled or Blackened w/ Broccoli	1 full portion	760	–	54	–	8	–	310
Cobia Grilled Broiled or Blackened w/ Broccoli	1 half portion	400	–	26	–	6	–	250
Cod Grilled Broiled or Blackened w/ Broccoli	1 full portion	300	–	4	–	10	–	810
Cod Grilled Broiled or Blackened w/ Broccoli	1 half portion	170	–	2	–	8	–	500
Corvina Grilled Broiled or Blackened w/ Broccoli	1 half portion	180	–	2	–	7	–	300
Corvina Grilled Broiled or Blackened w/ Broccoli	1 full portion	320	–	3	–	9	–	420
Flounder Grilled Broiled or Blackened w/ Broccoli	1 half portion	200	–	2	–	8	–	350
Flounder Grilled Broiled or Blackened w/ Broccoli	1 full portion	350	–	3	–	11	–	500
Grouper Grilled Broiled or Blackened w/ Broccoli	1 half portion	210	–	2	–	6	–	280
Grouper Grilled Broiled or Blackened w/ Broccoli	1 full portion	370	–	3	–	6	–	370
Haddock Grilled Broiled or Blackened w/ Broccoli	1 full portion	310	–	3	–	6	–	850
Haddock Grilled Broiled or Blackened w/ Broccoli	1 half portion	180	–	2	–	6	–	520
Lake Whitefish Grilled Broiled or Blackened w/ Broccoli	1 full portion	380	–	5	–	6	–	610
Lake Whitefish Grilled Broiled or Blackened w/ Broccoli	1 half portion	210	–	3	–	6	–	400

FOOD	PORTION	CALS	PROT	FAT	CHOL	CARB	FIBER	SOD
Mahi Mahi Grilled Broiled or Blackened w/ Broccoli	1 full portion	360	–	2	–	7	–	360
Mahi Mahi Grilled Broiled or Blackened w/ Broccoli	1 half portion	200	–	2	–	6	–	270
Monchong Grilled Broiled or Blackened w/ Broccoli	1 full portion	340	–	3	–	9	–	390
Monchong Grilled Broiled or Blackened w/ Broccoli	1 half portion	190	–	2	–	7	–	290
Opah Grilled Broiled or Blackened w/ Broccoli	1 half portion	280	–	12	–	8	–	280
Opah Grilled Broiled or Blackened w/ Broccoli	1 full portion	510	–	24	–	11	–	380
Perch Grilled Broiled or Blackened w/ Broccoli	1 half portion	170	–	2	–	6	–	550
Perch Grilled Broiled or Blackened w/ Broccoli	1 full portion	300	–	4	–	7	–	910
Pompano Grilled Broiled or Blackened w/ Broccoli	1 full portion	430	–	16	–	7	–	430
Pompano Grilled Broiled or Blackened w/ Broccoli	1 half portion	240	–	8	–	6	–	310
Rainbow Trout Grilled Broiled or Blackened w/ Broccoli	1 half portion	220	–	10	–	6	–	380
Red Rockfish Grilled Broiled or Blackened w/ Broccoli	1 full portion	300	–	4	–	10	–	860
Red Rockfish Grilled Broiled or Blackened w/ Broccoli	1 half portion	170	–	3	–	6	–	580
Salmon Grilled Broiled or Blackened w/ Broccoli	1 half portion	270	–	9	–	6	–	310
Salmon Grilled Broiled or Blackened w/ Broccoli	1 full portion	490	–	17	–	6	–	440
Seabass Grilled Broiled or Blackened w/ Broccoli	1 half portion	230	–	6	–	6	–	450
Snapper Grilled Broiled or Blackened w/ Broccoli	1 half portion	210	–	2	–	8	–	330
Sole Grilled Broiled or Blackened w/ Broccoli	1 half portion	140	–	2	–	6	–	860
Tilapia Grilled Broiled or Blackened w/ Broccoli	1 half portion	210	–	3	–	9	–	230

FOOD	PORTION	CALS	PROT	FAT	CHOL	CARB	FIBER	SOD
Tuna Grilled Broiled or Blackened w/ Broccoli	1 half portion	200	–	1	–	7	–	420
Wahoo Grilled Broiled or Blackened w/ Broccoli	1 half portion	220	–	3	–	8	–	340
Walleye Grilled Broiled or Blackened w/ Broccoli	1 half portion	170	–	2	–	7	–	400
RED MANGO								
Blenders Blueberry Moon	1 cup	150	3	2	0	33	1	115
Blenders Captain Berry	1 cup	140	4	1	0	31	2	135
Blenders Green Tea Blueberry	1 cup	130	3	0	0	29	1	115
Blenders Green Tea Honeydew	1 cup	130	3	0	0	29	0	125
Blenders Mango Island	1 cup	150	3	2	0	31	1	115
Blenders Pina Colada	1 cup	160	4	3	0	30	1	120
Blenders Tri-Berry	1 cup	130	3	0	0	30	2	115
Blenders Watermelon Breeze	1 cup	130	3	0	0	29	0	115
Frozen Yogurt All Flavors	½ cup	90	3	0	0	19	0	130
ROBEKS								
FREEZES AND SHAKES								
800 Lb Gorilla	12 oz	375	26	9	27	50	2	216
Freeze Lemon	12 oz	279	2	2	9	60	0	24
Freeze Orange	12 oz	242	9	0	0	56	1	144
Shake Bananasplit	12 oz	302	11	0	0	69	2	168
Shake P-Nut Power	12 oz	422	17	18	0	52	4	288
SMOOTHIES								
Acai Energizer	12 oz	167	2	1	3	36	2	48
Awesome Acai	12 oz	183	34	1	3	42	2	48
Banzai Blueberry	12 oz	175	31	1	3	38	3	24
Berry Brilliance	12 oz	194	30	1	3	45	2	24
Big Wednesday	12 oz	172	1	1	3	40	1	0
Cardio Cooler	12 oz	215	9	1	3	44	3	24
Citrus Stinger	12 oz	194	56	1	3	40	2	24
Cranberry Quest	12 oz	173	24	0	3	40	1	24
Dr. Robeks	12 oz	181	3	1	3	40	3	0
Guava Lava	12 oz	180	20	1	3	42	2	0
Hummingbird	12 oz	185	2	1	3	44	1	0

FOOD	PORTION	CALS	PROT	FAT	CHOL	CARB	FIBER	SOD
Infinite Orange	12 oz	181	4	0	0	42	3	48
Mahalo Mango	12 oz	174	2	1	3	42	1	24
Malibu Peach	12 oz	153	3	0	0	36	1	48
Outrageous Raspberry	12 oz	174	2	1	3	39	2	0
Passionfruit Cove	12 oz	168	2	1	3	38	1	24
Pina Koolada	12 oz	261	39	8	3	46	3	48
Polar Pineapple	12 oz	164	13	1	3	38	1	0
Pomegranate Passion	12 oz	196	4	0	0	48	1	72
Pomegranate Power	12 oz	211	3	0	3	50	1	24
Pro Arobek	12 oz	265	15	1	3	54	3	24
Raspberry Romance	12 oz	172	4	0	0	42	2	48
Robeks MuscleMax	12 oz	202	11	1	15	38	2	24
Robeks Rejuvenator	12 oz	193	5	1	3	43	2	24
South Pacific Squeeze	12 oz	188	2	1	3	42	3	0
Strawnana Berry	12 oz	179	3	0	0	44	2	48
Venice Burner	12 oz	231	9	1	3	46	4	24
Zen Berry	12 oz	190	3	1	0	45	5	24

SAMURAI SAM'S

BOWLS

FOOD	PORTION	CALS	PROT	FAT	CHOL	CARB	FIBER	SOD
Low Carb	1 reg	230	33	4	80	16	5	210
Spicy Beef 'N Broccoli	1 reg	620	26	13	50	97	3	1160
Spicy Beef 'N Broccoli Brown Rice	1 reg	580	26	14	50	85	7	1160
Sumo Brown Rice	1	1022	81	23	214	111	9	1513
Sumo White Rice	1	1083	81	21	214	128	3	1509
Sweet & Sour Dark Chicken	1 reg	610	32	10	85	96	6	200
Sweet & Sour Dark Chicken Brown Rice	1 reg	570	32	12	85	84	9	200
Sweet & Sour White Chicken	1 reg	580	37	5	80	96	6	210
Sweet & Sour White Chicken Brown Rice	1 reg	540	37	6	80	85	9	210
Teriyaki Dark Chicken	1 reg	540	31	10	85	79	2	500
Teriyaki Dark Chicken Brown Rice	1 reg	500	31	11	85	68	12	510
Teriyaki Dark Chicken & Shrimp	1 reg	492	29	6	140	78	2	563

FOOD	PORTION	CALS	PROT	FAT	CHOL	CARB	FIBER	SOD
Teriyaki Dark Chicken & Shrimp Brown Rice	1 reg	451	29	7	290	67	5	565
Teriyaki Dark Chicken & Steak	1 reg	540	27	9	65	83	2	560
Teriyaki Dark Chicken & Steak Brown Rice	1 reg	490	27	10	65	71	5	660
Teriyaki Salmon	1 reg	643	33	3	15	121	3	1223
Teriyaki Shrimp Brown Rice	1 reg	407	28	3	193	65	5	582
Teriyaki Steak	1 reg	530	23	8	50	86	2	810
Teriyaki Steak Brown Rice	1 reg	490	23	9	50	74	5	510
Teriyaki Steak & Shrimp	1 reg	483	26	5	120	77	2	713
Teriyaki Steak & Shrimp Brown Rice	1 reg	442	25	6	120	66	5	715
Teriyaki Veggie	1 reg	363	8	1	0	81	3	393
Teriyaki Veggie Brown Rice	1 reg	323	8	2	0	69	7	395
Teriyaki White Chicken	1 reg	520	37	4	80	79	2	510
Teriyaki White Chicken Brown Rice	1 reg	470	36	5	80	68	5	510
Teriyaki White Chicken & Shrimp	1 reg	478	32	2	127	78	2	567
Teriyaki White Chicken & Shrimp Brown Rice	1 reg	437	32	4	137	67	5	570
Teriyaki White Chicken & Steak	1 reg	520	30	6	65	83	2	660
Teriyaki White Chicken & Steak Brown Rice	1 reg	480	30	7	65	71	5	660
Yakisoba Dark Chicken	1	842	60	24	146	114	6	1154
Yakisoba Dark Chicken & Steak	1	825	54	22	114	113	6	1410
Yakisoba Shrimp	1	677	55	10	330	110	6	1283
Yakisoba Steak	1	809	48	20	83	112	6	1667
Yakisoba Veggie	1	509	19	8	0	110	6	902
Yakisoba White Chicken	1	794	70	14	137	114	6	1169
Yakisoba White Chicken & Steak	1	801	59	17	110	113	6	1410
SALADS AND SIDES								
Crab Rangoon	1 serv	210	7	12	35	20	1	260
Dressing Chinese	1 serv (3.5 oz)	230	0	7	0	44	–	1700

FOOD	PORTION	CALS	PROT	FAT	CHOL	CARB	FIBER	SOD
Dressing Chinese Ginger	1 serv (1 oz)	85	0	5	0	9	0	153
Dressing Oriental	1 serv (1 oz)	70	0	2	0	12	0	180
Egg Roll Grilled Chicken	1	150	7	7	15	17	1	300
Salad Oriental Chicken	1 serv	220	36	4	90	9	3	200
Salad Side	1	10	1	1	0	2	1	5
Salad Toss Sesame Chicken	1	490	41	13	90	57	8	1240
Soup Asian Noodle	1 serv	89	5	2	13	14	1	723
Teriyaki Sauce	1 serv (1 oz)	40	1	0	0	9	0	340
WRAPS								
Teriyaki Dark Chicken	1	670	34	16	75	95	8	1250
Teriyaki Dark Chicken Brown Rice	1	650	34	17	75	90	9	1250
Teriyaki Steak	1	650	27	14	40	101	8	1510
Teriyaki Steak Brown Rice	1	630	27	15	40	95	9	1510
Teriyaki Veggie	1	510	14	8	0	94	8	1130
Teriyaki Veggie Brown Rice	1	490	13	9	0	89	10	1130
Teriyaki White Chicken	1	640	39	11	70	96	8	1260
Teriyaki White Chicken Brown Rice	1	620	39	12	70	90	9	1260
Teriyaki White Chicken & Steak	1	649	33	13	55	95	8	1384
Teriyaki White Chicken & Steak Brown Rice	1	628	33	13	55	89	9	1385

SCHLOTZSKY'S DELI

FOOD	PORTION	CALS	PROT	FAT	CHOL	CARB	FIBER	SOD
CHILDREN'S MENU SELECTIONS								
Pizza Cheese	1 serv	479	18	13	24	73	3	1060
Pizza Pepperoni	1 serv	523	20	17	33	73	3	1246
Sandwich Cheese	1	394	17	15	40	48	2	772
Sandwich Ham & Cheese	1	424	21	16	30	49	2	1147
Sandwich Turkey	1	300	13	5	20	49	2	750
DESSERTS								
Carrot Cake	1 serv	717	7	42	74	80	3	767
Cookie Chocolate Chip	1	160	2	8	20	22	1	160
Cookie Fudge Chocolate Chip	1	160	2	8	25	22	1	190
Cookie Oatmeal Raisin	1	150	2	6	20	22	1	115
Cookie Sugar	1	160	2	7	0	22	0	200

FOOD	PORTION	CALS	PROT	FAT	CHOL	CARB	FIBER	SOD
Cookie White Chocolate Macadamia	1	170	2	9	20	21	1	170
MAIN MENU SELECTIONS								
Salad Caesar	1 serv	103	6	5	6	10	3	289
Salad Garden	1 serv	51	3	1	0	12	4	291
Salad Grilled Chicken Caesar	1 serv	221	53	8	65	12	3	759
Salad Turkey Chef	1 serv	309	26	18	67	14	4	1412
Sandwich Angus Roast Beef & Cheese	1 sm	534	33	22	85	50	2	1424
Sandwich Chicken Breast	1 sm	342	39	4	46	52	3	1341
Sandwich Fresh Veggie	1 sm	342	19	10	22	50	4	751
Sandwich Ham & Cheese	1 sm	508	31	19	80	54	3	2033
Sandwich Smoked Turkey Breast	1 sm	353	20	6	35	52	2	1070
Sandwich The Original	1 sm	559	28	26	85	52	3	1834
Sandwich Turkey	1 sm	602	34	27	96	54	3	1832
Sandwich Turkey Bacon Club	1 sm	561	32	25	83	51	3	1660
Wraps Asian Chicken	1	537	56	12	59	80	5	2143
Wraps Parmesan Chicken Caesar	1	556	61	21	86	61	5	1728

SONIC DRIVE-IN

FOOD	PORTION	CALS	PROT	FAT	CHOL	CARB	FIBER	SOD
ADD-ONS								
Bacon	1 serv (0.5 oz)	70	4	5	15	0	0	260
Cheese	1 serv (0.7 oz)	60	3	5	20	2	0	310
Chili	1 serv (1.2 oz)	50	3	4	10	2	1	160
Green Chilies	1 serv (1 oz)	5	0	0	0	1	0	5
Grilled Onions	1 serv (1 oz)	25	0	2	0	2	1	200
Jalapenos	1 serv (0.7 oz)	5	0	0	0	1	1	280
Slaw	1 serv (1 oz)	45	0	3	5	4	1	45
BEVERAGES								
Barq's Root Beer	1 sm (14 oz)	160	0	0	0	43	0	35
Coca Cola	1 sm (14 oz)	140	0	0	0	39	0	10

FOOD	PORTION	CALS	PROT	FAT	CHOL	CARB	FIBER	SOD
Cream Pie Shake Banana	1 reg (14 oz)	590	7	19	55	98	1	220
Cream Pie Shake Chocolate	1 reg (14 oz)	660	7	19	80	114	0	300
Cream Pie Shake Coconut Cream	1 reg (14 oz)	580	7	20	60	93	0	230
CreamSlush Blue Coconut	1 reg (14 oz)	430	5	13	45	76	0	160
CreamSlush Cherry	1 reg (14 oz)	440	5	13	45	77	0	160
CreamSlush Grape	1 reg (14 oz)	430	5	13	45	76	0	160
CreamSlush Orange	1 reg (14 oz)	430	5	13	45	77	0	160
CreamSlush Strawberry	1 reg (14 oz)	450	5	12	45	84	1	150
CreamSlush Watermelon	1 reg (14 oz)	440	5	13	45	77	0	160
Diet Coke	1 sm (14 oz)	0	0	0	0	0	0	15
Dr Pepper	1 sm (14 oz)	130	0	0	0	37	0	45
Float Barq's Root Beer	1 reg (14 oz)	300	3	8	30	56	0	110
Float Coca Cola	1 reg (14 oz)	290	3	8	30	54	0	95
Float Dr Pepper	1 reg (14 oz)	310	3	8	30	58	0	120
Limeade	1 sm (14 oz)	140	0	0	0	38	0	30
Limeade Cherry	1 sm (14 oz)	170	0	0	0	45	0	35
Limeade Strawberry	1 sm (14 oz)	170	0	0	0	45	0	35
Malt Banana	1 reg (14 oz)	490	7	17	60	78	1	200
Malt Caramel	1 reg (14 oz)	550	7	18	65	90	0	330
Malt Chocolate	1 reg (14 oz)	550	7	17	60	91	0	280
Malt Hot Fudge	1 reg (14 oz)	580	7	22	60	87	1	250
Malt Peanut Butter	1 reg (14 oz)	870	11	36	60	78	0	320

FOOD	PORTION	CALS	PROT	FAT	CHOL	CARB	FIBER	SOD
Malt Peanut Butter Fudge	1 reg (14 oz)	620	9	29	60	83	1	290
Malt Pineapple	1 reg (14 oz)	510	7	17	60	82	0	210
Malt Strawberry	1 reg (14 oz)	520	7	17	60	85	1	210
Malt Vanilla	1 reg (14 oz)	480	7	18	65	72	0	210
Milk 1%	8.5 oz	110	8	3	10	13	0	130
Milk Chocolate 1%	8.5 oz	160	8	3	10	27	0	210
Shake Banana	1 reg (14 oz)	470	7	16	60	76	1	190
Shake Chocolate	1 reg (14 oz)	540	6	16	60	89	0	270
Shake Hot Fudge	1 reg (14 oz)	570	6	21	60	85	1	240
Shake Peanut Butter	1 reg (14 oz)	640	10	34	60	75	0	300
Shake Peanut Butter Fudge	1 reg	610	8	28	60	81	1	280
Shake Pineapple	1 reg (14 oz)	500	6	16	60	80	0	200
Shake Strawberry	1 reg (14 oz)	510	7	16	60	83	1	200
Shake Vanilla	1 reg (14 oz)	470	7	17	65	71	0	200
Sonic Blast Butterfinger	1 reg (14 oz)	580	8	22	60	88	0	240
Sonic Blast M&M's	1 reg (14 oz)	600	8	24	60	88	1	210
Sonic Blast Oreo	1 reg (14 oz)	540	7	21	60	80	1	280
Sonic Blast Reese's Peanut Butter Cup	1 reg (14 oz)	560	9	19	65	89	1	250
Sprite	1 sm (14 oz)	104	0	0	0	37	0	30
Sprite Zero	1 sm (14 oz)	5	0	0	0	0	0	10
BREAKFAST SELECTIONS								
Breakfast Burrito Jr.	1 (4.1 oz)	330	13	21	235	25	2	790
Breakfast Burrito Sausage Egg Cheese	1 (5.9 oz)	480	18	31	325	38	1	1200

FOOD	PORTION	CALS	PROT	FAT	CHOL	CARB	FIBER	SOD
Breakfast Toaster Bacon Egg Cheese	1 (5.6 oz)	530	20	32	325	40	2	1440
Breakfast Toaster Ham Egg Cheese	1 (6.5 oz)	490	24	26	325	40	2	1700
Breakfast Toaster Sausage Egg Cheese	1 (6.8 oz)	620	20	42	340	40	2	1380
CroisSonic Bacon	1 (5.3 oz)	510	18	36	320	29	0	1400
CroisSonic Sausage	1 (6.2 oz)	600	19	46	340	29	0	1340
DESSERTS								
Apple Slice w/ Fat Free Caramel Dipping Sauce	1 serv (3.4 oz)	120	0	0	0	27	2	60
Apple Slices	1 serv (2.4 oz)	35	0	0	0	9	2	0
Banana Split	1 (10.8 oz)	420	4	9	30	80	2	140
Cone Vanilla	1 (4.7 oz)	180	2	6	25	30	0	80
Dish Vanilla	1 (6.5 oz)	240	3	9	35	36	0	100
Sundae Chocolate	1 (8.9 oz)	410	4	13	35	67	0	190
Sundae Hot Fudge	1 (8.9 oz)	440	4	18	35	63	1	170
Sundae Pineapple	1 (8.8 oz)	370	4	13	35	58	0	125
Sundae Strawberry	1 (8.8 oz)	380	4	13	35	61	1	120
MAIN MENU SELECTIONS								
California Cheeseburger	1 (9.3 oz)	690	29	39	80	57	5	1060
Ched 'R' Bites	12 (3 oz)	280	13	15	30	22	1	740
Ched 'R' Peppers	4 (4.2 oz)	330	8	17	25	36	2	1110
Chicken Strip Dinner	1 serv (13.5 oz)	930	36	43	65	100	7	1610
Chicken Strips	2 (2.5 oz)	200	14	11	30	10	1	470
Chili Cheeseburger	1 (7.9 oz)	660	31	35	85	56	5	990
Coney Extra Long Chili Cheese	1 (9 oz)	660	28	39	95	55	4	1860
Coney Regular	1 (5.2 oz)	390	17	23	60	32	2	1090
Corn Dog	1 (2.6 oz)	210	6	11	20	23	2	530
Crispy Chicken Bacon Ranch	1 serv (8.9 oz)	610	30	34	70	48	4	1730
French Fries	1 sm (2.5 oz)	200	2	8	0	30	2	270
French Fries w/ Cheese	1 sm (3 oz)	270	5	13	20	32	2	590
French Fries w/ Chili & Cheese	1 sm (4.1 oz)	300	8	16	25	33	3	540

FOOD	PORTION	CALS	PROT	FAT	CHOL	CARB	FIBER	SOD
Fritos Chili Pie	1 med (4.8 oz)	470	13	32	30	36	3	770
Green Chili Cheeseburger	1 (10 oz)	630	29	31	75	56	5	1070
Grilled Chicken Bacon Ranch	1 serv (8.9 oz)	470	35	22	105	35	3	1620
Hickory Cheeseburger	1 (8.3 oz)	640	28	31	75	61	5	1170
Jalapeno Burger	1 (7.6 oz)	550	25	26	60	53	5	880
Jalapeno Cheeseburger	1 (8.3 oz)	620	28	31	80	54	5	1200
Jr. Bacon Cheeseburger	1 (5 oz)	410	20	23	60	31	3	1060
Jr. Burger	1 (4.1 oz)	310	15	15	35	30	3	610
Jr. Burger Deluxe	1 (4.7 oz)	350	15	20	40	28	3	440
Jr. Double Cheeseburger	1 (6.7 oz)	570	30	35	110	33	3	1290
Jumbo Popcorn Chicken	1 sm (4 oz)	380	18	22	45	27	3	1250
Mozzarella Sticks	1 serv (5 oz)	440	19	22	45	40	2	1050
Onion Rings	1 med (5.5 oz)	440	6	21	0	55	3	430
Pickle-O's	1 serv (4 oz)	310	5	16	0	36	2	1020
Sandwich Breaded Pork Fritter	1 (8.5 oz)	640	22	33	30	66	7	840
Sandwich Crispy Chicken	1 (7.9 oz)	550	22	32	45	46	4	1070
Sandwich Fish	1 (8.6 oz)	650	22	31	40	71	7	1160
Sandwich Grilled Cheese	1 (3.9 oz)	380	12	20	35	39	2	1010
Sandwich Grilled Chicken	1 (7.8 oz)	400	28	19	80	32	3	960
Sonic Bacon Cheeseburger w/ Mayonnaise	1 (9.8 oz)	780	33	48	100	57	5	1300
Sonic Burger w/ Ketchup	1 (8.7 oz)	560	26	26	60	57	5	820
Sonic Burger w/ Mayonnaise	1 (8.7 oz)	650	26	37	70	55	5	720
Sonic Burger w/ Mustard	1 (8.5 oz)	560	26	26	60	54	5	750
Sonic Cheeseburger w/ Ketchup	1 (9.3 oz)	630	29	31	75	59	5	1140
Sonic Cheeseburger w/ Mayonnaise	1 (9.3 oz)	720	29	42	90	56	5	1040
Sonic Cheeseburger w/ Mustard	1 (9.1 oz)	620	29	31	75	55	5	1070
SuperSonic Cheeseburger w/ Ketchup	1 (12 oz)	900	46	53	155	60	5	1540

FOOD	PORTION	CALS	PROT	FAT	CHOL	CARB	FIBER	SOD
SuperSonic Cheeseburger w/ Mayonnaise	1 (12 oz)	980	46	64	165	58	5	1430
SuperSonic Cheeseburger w/ Mustard	1 (11.8 oz)	890	46	53	155	57	5	1480
Thousand Island Burger	1 (8.7 oz)	610	26	32	65	56	5	810
Toaster Sandwich Bacon Cheeseburger	1 (8.5 oz)	670	29	39	90	52	3	1440
Toaster Sandwich BLT	1 (5.2 oz)	500	17	29	40	45	2	950
Toaster Sandwich Chicken Club	1 (9 oz)	740	29	46	80	55	4	1740
Toaster Sandwich Country Fried Steak	1 (8.5 oz)	670	14	37	50	71	4	1370
Tots	1 sm (1.5 oz)	130	1	8	0	13	1	270
Tots w/ Cheese	1 sm (2.2 oz)	190	4	13	20	14	1	590
Tots w/ Chili & Cheese	1 sm (3.2 oz)	220	7	16	25	16	2	540
Wrap Crispy Chicken	1 (8.2 oz)	490	21	23	40	49	3	1280
Wrap Fritos Chili Cheese	1 (8.5 oz)	670	21	39	50	66	4	1420
Wrap Grilled Chicken	1 (8.8 oz)	390	28	14	80	39	2	1420
SALAD DRESSINGS AND SAUCES								
Dressing Honey Mustard	1 serv (1.5 oz)	180	1	16	10	10	0	240
Dressing Italian Fat Free	1 serv (1.5 oz)	40	0	0	0	10	0	450
Dressing Original Ranch	1 serv (1.5 oz)	190	1	20	15	2	0	380
Dressing Original Ranch Light	1 serv (1.5 oz)	110	3	5	10	14	0	590
Dressing Thousand Island	1 serv (1.5 oz)	190	1	19	20	7	0	440
Sauce BBQ	1 serv (1 oz)	45	0	0	0	11	0	390
Sauce Honey Mustard	1 serv (1 oz)	90	0	7	10	7	0	190
Sauce Marinara	1 serv (1 oz)	15	0	0	0	3	1	270
Sauce Ranch	1 serv (1 oz)	140	0	16	10	1	0	210
SALADS								
Crispy Chicken	1 serv (11.4 oz)	340	20	19	50	24	5	970

FOOD	PORTION	CALS	PROT	FAT	CHOL	CARB	FIBER	SOD
Grilled Chicken	1 serv (12 oz)	250	29	10	100	12	3	1070
SOUPER SALAD								
BEVERAGES								
Lemonade	1 (24 oz)	190	0	0	0	49	0	10
Lemonade Mango	1 (24 oz)	220	0	0	0	58	0	10
Lemonade Raspberry	1 (24 oz)	220	0	0	0	58	0	10
Lemonade Strawberry	1 (24 oz)	220	0	0	0	57	0	10
Smoothie Mango	1 tall	250	0	0	0	64	0	0
Smoothie Peach	1 tall	230	0	0	0	62	0	10
Smoothie Raspberry	1 tall	230	0	0	0	62	0	0
Smoothie Strawberry	1 tall	230	0	0	0	60	0	0
DESSERTS								
Blueberry Bread	1 piece	150	3	3	0	29	1	210
Brownies	2 pieces	120	1	5	5	21	0	115
Cornbread	1 piece	170	3	5	0	30	1	350
Cottage Cheese	½ cup	90	13	2	10	5	0	410
Gingerbread	1 piece	180	2	6	0	30	1	290
Peaches	½ cup	70	0	0	0	17	0	10
Pineapple Tidbits	¼ cup	60	0	0	0	15	1	0
Pudding Banana	½ cup	160	2	6	0	26	0	150
Pudding Chocolate	½ cup	170	2	5	0	30	0	115
Soft Serve Cone Chocolate	1	120	1	2	0	22	0	85
Soft Serve Cone Vanilla	1	120	0	3	0	22	0	95
Sponge Cake	4 pieces	80	1	2	5	14	0	160
Strawberry Parfait	½ cup	100	2	2	0	19	0	70
Vanilla Wafers	4	70	1	2	0	13	0	85
Whipped Topping	½ cup	100	0	8	0	8	0	0
PASTA AND PIZZA								
Chicken Alfredo	1 cup	320	19	9	50	40	1	1060
Macaroni & Cheese	1 cup	380	15	18	35	38	1	870
Pizza Slice Cheese	1	70	4	3	5	8	0	125
Pizza Slice Garden	1	80	4	3	5	9	1	125
Pizza Slice Pepperoni	1	90	5	4	10	8	0	190
Pizza Slice Sausage	1	80	4	4	5	9	1	170
Spaghetti & Meatballs	1 cup	280	11	9	15	38	4	700
SALAD DRESSINGS AND SAUCES								
Balsamic Vinegar	1 oz	60	0	0	0	15	0	0

FOOD	PORTION	CALS	PROT	FAT	CHOL	CARB	FIBER	SOD
Bleu Cheese	2 oz	220	2	23	25	1	0	310
Caesar	2 oz	280	4	30	30	4	0	840
Chipotle Ranch	2 oz	280	0	28	10	8	0	480
Fat Free French	2 oz	60	0	0	0	18	1	620
Fat Free Italian w/ Cheese	2 oz	30	0	0	0	6	0	680
Green Goddess	2 oz	260	2	24	10	4	0	580
Honey Mustard	2 oz	240	0	26	20	2	0	460
Mayonnaise	2 tbsp	200	0	22	20	20	0	200
Olive Oil	1 oz	240	0	28	0	0	0	0
Peppercorn Ranch	2 oz	220	1	23	20	2	0	360
Pesto Basil	1 tbsp	45	1	5	0	0	0	100
Ranch	2 oz	220	1	23	20	2	0	360
Reduced Calorie Ranch	2 oz	120	2	11	10	3	0	260
Sauce Alfredo	1½ tbsp	45	2	4	10	2	0	170
Sauce Chipotle Pepper	¼ tsp	0	0	0	0	0	0	30
Sauce Cholula Hot	¼ tsp	0	0	0	0	0	0	5
Sauce Jalapeno Cheese	1 serv (2 oz)	35	1	2	0	5	1	440
Sauce Marinara	1½ tbsp	10	0	0	0	2	0	90
Sauce Meaty Marinara	1½ tbsp	40	1	1	5	2	0	90
Sauce Sriracha Hot	¼ tsp	0	0	0	0	0	0	15
Sour Cream Light	2 tbsp	40	1	3	10	3	0	40
Tangy Oriental	2 oz	160	0	12	0	10	0	760
Thousand Island	1 oz	300	0	30	20	6	0	500
Vinaigrette Cranberry	2 oz	100	0	0	0	24	0	560
Vinaigrette House	2 oz	220	0	22	0	4	0	840
SALADS								
Apple Walnut	1 cup	130	3	11	5	7	1	210
Asian Chicken	1 cup	80	3	3	5	10	2	450
Asian Shrimp	1 cup	100	4	4	20	13	2	470
Buffalo Chicken	1 cup	70	3	6	10	3	1	200
Caesar Chicken	1 cup	90	5	7	15	4	1	340
Caesar Chicken Salsa	1 cup	80	4	5	15	4	1	380
Caesar Shrimp	1 cup	90	4	7	30	3	1	310
California Chicken Salad	⅓ cup	80	5	6	25	4	0	110
Capri	1 cup	50	1	2	0	8	0	540
Chicago Chopped	1 cup	120	4	10	15	3	1	310
Chickpea	⅓ cup	110	3	6	0	11	4	220
Cobb	1 cup	100	4	8	55	2	1	340
Coleslaw Broccoli	⅓ cup	80	1	6	0	6	1	65

FOOD	PORTION	CALS	PROT	FAT	CHOL	CARB	FIBER	SOD
Edamame	⅓ cup	70	4	5	0	4	2	50
Fisherman's Kettle Shrimp & Crab	⅓ cup	120	3	8	15	15	1	300
Gazpacho	⅓ cup	30	0	3	0	3	1	100
Green Goddess Crab	1 cup	70	2	5	5	4	1	240
Italian Antipasto	1 cup	70	2	5	5	3	1	320
Mango Berry	1 cup	110	1	6	0	13	1	75
Marinated Mushrooms	⅓ cup	60	1	7	0	1	0	110
Marinated Oriental Cucumber	⅓ cup	10	0	0	0	2	0	240
Marinated Tomato	1 cup	60	1	2	0	11	1	45
Melon Couscous	⅓ cup	50	1	1	0	10	1	60
Mustard Potato	⅓ cup	80	1	5	25	7	1	280
Paco's Taco	⅓ cup	100	3	5	0	12	2	200
Pasta De Garden	⅓ cup	80	1	5	0	8	0	210
Pasta Fettuccine	⅓ cup	100	2	5	5	11	1	390
Pasta Primavera	⅓ cup	45	1	3	0	4	0	85
Pasta Thai Chicken	⅓ cup	100	3	5	10	11	1	320
Pasta Tuna Skroodle	⅓ cup	130	3	9	10	10	1	135
Red Potato	⅓ cup	50	1	4	0	5	1	125
Rice Florentine	⅓ cup	90	1	5	0	11	0	105
Roasted Mushrooms & Artichokes w/ Feta Cheese	⅓ cup	40	1	3	0	3	1	90
Roasted Vegetables	⅓ cup	20	0	2	0	2	1	125
Salad Of The Sea	⅓ cup	50	2	2	5	6	0	190
Salmon Medley	1 cup	70	4	2	5	10	1	160
Santa Fe Corn	⅓ cup	100	4	4	0	13	3	310
Shrimp & Crab Louie	1 cup	130	5	10	55	5	1	490
Southwest Chicken Chipotle	1 cup	90	3	7	10	4	1	270
Sweet Garden Slaw	⅓ cup	35	0	2	0	4	1	75
Tropical Tuxedo	⅓ cup	60	1	3	0	7	0	150
Tuna Fish	⅓ cup	70	6	5	15	1	0	220
SOUPS								
Adobe Rice & Chicken	1 (5 oz)	100	3	5	25	10	1	540
Alaskan Salmon Chowder	1 (5 oz)	70	3	2	0	9	1	630
Beef Mushroom Barley	1 (5 oz)	80	4	2	5	11	2	510
Beef Noodle	1 (5 oz)	80	4	3	15	10	1	500
Beef Shellini	1 (5 oz)	90	5	3	10	11	1	460

FOOD	PORTION	CALS	PROT	FAT	CHOL	CARB	FIBER	SOD
Beef Stroganoff	1 (5 oz)	120	5	5	15	13	1	820
Black Bean	1 (5 oz)	80	8	2	5	20	11	370
Broccoli Cheese	1 (5 oz)	70	2	2	0	10	1	640
Cajun Gumbo	1 (5 oz)	110	5	4	15	13	1	570
Cauliflower Cheese	1 (5 oz)	70	2	2	0	11	1	650
Cheddar Chicken Broccoli Stew	1 (5 oz)	140	6	6	25	15	2	600
Cherokee Joe Cornbread	1 (5 oz)	70	2	2	0	13	2	950
Chicken Creole	1 (5 oz)	100	5	4	20	12	1	520
Chicken Enchilada	1 (5 oz)	180	6	12	40	13	1	590
Chicken Gumbo	1 (5 oz)	90	4	4	15	10	1	660
Chicken Mushroom Barley	1 (5 oz)	80	5	3	20	9	1	660
Chicken Noodle	1 (5 oz)	80	5	3	25	9	1	620
Chicken Tetrazini	1 (5 oz)	120	6	5	25	13	1	620
Chicken Tortilla	1 (5 oz)	60	4	2	10	7	1	650
Cream Of Asparagus	1 (5 oz)	140	2	10	15	7	1	710
Cream Of Broccoli	1 (5 oz)	60	2	2	0	9	1	620
Cream Of Cauliflower	1 (5 oz)	60	2	2	0	10	1	630
Cream Of Chicken	1 (5 oz)	100	5	5	20	9	1	610
Cream Of Mushroom	1 (5 oz)	80	2	4	0	10	1	480
Holiday Harvest	1 (5 oz)	90	3	6	25	5	0	480
Vegan Split Pea	1 (5 oz)	90	4	1	0	16	5	260
Vegetable Beef	1 (5 oz)	80	4	3	10	11	2	550
Vegetable Cheese	1 (5 oz)	80	2	3	0	12	1	430
Vegetable Lentil	1 (5 oz)	70	5	0	0	16	5	620
Vegetarian Butter Bean	1 (5 oz)	70	6	0	0	21	10	420
Vegetarian Vegetable	1 (5 oz)	50	2	1	0	11	2	320
STARBUCKS								
BAKED SELECTIONS								
Apple Fritter	1	480	4	22	0	64	1	290
Bagel French Toast	1	280	8	1	0	62	2	400
Bagel Multigrain	1	280	10	3	0	60	4	380
Bagel Plain	1	280	10	0	0	62	2	440
Bar Cranberry Bliss	1	320	3	16	45	41	1	260
Bar Toffee Almond	1	400	4	19	50	53	1	340
Brownie Espresso	1	340	4	19	50	40	2	135
Cinnamon Roll	1	470	6	26	45	56	1	350
Cocoa Crispy Square	1	420	5	17	25	66	1	440

FOOD	PORTION	CALS	PROT	FAT	CHOL	CARB	FIBER	SOD
Cookie Chocolate Chunk	1	420	7	20	55	56	6	460
Cookie Coffee Ginger	1	470	6	18	75	70	3	210
Cookie Penguin	1	370	4	18	15	50	tr	280
Cookie Rainbow	1	420	5	19	65	61	1	370
Cookies Mini Black & White	2	240	2	12	40	32	1	160
Croissant Butter	1	370	5	23	65	35	3	310
Doughnut Glazed	1	490	4	23	20	65	1	410
Loaf Banana Nut	1 serv	470	7	24	105	56	2	360
Loaf Iced Lemon	1 serv	500	7	18	140	78	1	440
Loaf Marble	1 serv	410	6	22	130	52	tr	440
Loaf Pumpkin	1 serv	380	5	14	55	59	2	480
Mallorca Sweet Bread	1	420	7	24	20	43	2	560
Muffin Blueberry	1	310	5	11	70	55	1	270
Muffin Pumpkin Cream Cheese	1	490	6	24	85	63	1	470
Muffin Reduced Fat Chocolate	1	290	6	5	75	53	2	460
Muffin Walnut Bran	1	430	8	18	40	62	4	400
Reduced Fat Coffee Cake Banana Chocolate Chip	1	390	5	8	0	76	3	400
Reduced Fat Coffee Cake Blueberry	1 serv	320	4	6	10	54	1	390
Reduced Fat Coffee Cake Cinnamon Swirl	1 serv	290	4	4	5	52	1	330
Reduced Fat Coffee Cake Pumpkin Chocolate Chip	1	300	5	6	0	58	3	270
Rustic Apple Tart	1	190	1	5	0	37	3	80
Scone Blueberry	1	480	7	22	80	64	2	520
Scone Cran Apple Crumb	1	490	7	20	80	74	4	510
Scone Raspberry	1	470	7	21	80	64	2	510
BEVERAGES								
Apple Juice	1 grande	250	0	0	0	64	0	25
Cafe Americano	1 grande	15	1	0	0	3	0	10
Cafe Au Lait Nonfat Milk	1 grande	70	7	0	5	10	0	90
Caffe Mocha No Whip Nonfat Milk	1 grande	220	13	3	5	42	2	125
Caffe Mocha Whip Nonfat Milk	1 grande	290	13	10	30	44	2	135
Cappuccino Nonfat Milk	1 grande	80	8	0	5	12	0	90

FOOD	PORTION	CALS	PROT	FAT	CHOL	CARB	FIBER	SOD
Caramel Apple Cider Whip	1 grande	380	0	8	25	76	0	30
Caramel Apple Spice No Whip	1 grande	310	0	tr	0	74	0	25
Caramel Macchiato Nonfat Milk	1 grande	190	11	1	10	35	0	135
Chocolate Milk Nonfat	1 grande	280	18	3	10	53	2	190
Cinnamon Dolce Creme No Whip Nonfat Milk	1 grande	220	12	0	5	41	0	160
Cinnamon Dolce Whip Nonfat Milk	1 grande	290	13	7	35	43	0	160
Coffee Of The Week	1 grande	5	1	tr	0	0	0	10
Coffee Of The Week Decaf	1 grande	5	1	0	0	0	0	10
Frappuccino Blended Coffee Cafe Vanilla Whip Nonfat Milk	1 grande	430	6	14	55	70	0	240
Frappuccino Blended Coffee Cafe Vanilla Whip Soy	1 grande	430	6	14	55	70	0	240
Frappuccino Blended Coffee Cafe Vanilla No Whip Nonfat Milk	1 grande	310	5	3	15	67	0	230
Frappuccino Blended Coffee Cafe Vanilla No Whip Soy	1 grande	310	5	3	15	67	0	230
Frappuccino Blended Coffee Caramel No Whip Nonfat Milk	1 grande	270	5	4	15	53	0	230
Frappuccino Blended Coffee Caramel No Whip Soy	1 grande	270	5	4	15	53	0	230
Frappuccino Blended Coffee Caramel Whip Soy	1 grande	380	6	15	55	57	0	240
Frappuccino Blended Coffee Cinnamon Dolce No Whip Nonfat Milk	1 grande	260	5	3	15	52	0	220
Frappuccino Blended Coffee Cinnamon Dolce No Whip Soy	1 grande	260	5	3	15	52	0	220

FOOD	PORTION	CALS	PROT	FAT	CHOL	CARB	FIBER	SOD
Frappuccino Blended Coffee Cinnamon Dolce Whip Soy	1 grande	370	6	14	55	55	0	240
Frappuccino Blended Coffee Espresso Nonfat Milk	1 grande	190	4	3	10	38	0	170
Frappuccino Blended Coffee Java Chip No Whip Nonfat Milk	1 grande	340	7	8	15	64	2	230
Frappuccino Blended Coffee Java Chip No Whip Soy	1 grande	190	4	3	10	38	0	170
Frappuccino Blended Coffee Java Chip Whip Nonfat Milk	1 grande	460	7	19	55	67	2	240
Frappuccino Blended Coffee Java Chip Whip Soy	1 grande	460	7	19	55	67	2	240
Frappuccino Blended Coffee Mocha No Whip Nonfat Milk	1 grande	260	6	4	15	54	0	230
Frappuccino Blended Coffee Mocha No Whip Soy	1 grande	260	6	4	15	54	0	230
Frappuccino Blended Coffee Mocha Whip Nonfat Milk	1 grande	380	6	15	55	57	0	240
Frappuccino Blended Coffee Pumpkin Spice No Whip Nonfat Milk	1 grande	290	6	4	15	59	0	260
Frappuccino Blended Coffee Pumpkin Spice No Whip Soy	1 grande	290	6	4	15	59	0	260
Frappuccino Blended Coffee Pumpkin Spice Whip Nonfat Milk	1 grande	400	7	15	55	62	0	280
Frappuccino Blended Coffee Pumpkin Spice Whip Soy	1 grande	400	7	15	55	62	0	280

FOOD	PORTION	CALS	PROT	FAT	CHOL	CARB	FIBER	SOD
Frappuccino Blended Coffee Whip Nonfat Milk	1 grande	370	6	14	55	55	0	240
Frappuccino Blended Coffee White Chocolate Mocha No Whip Nonfat Milk	1 grande	300	6	5	15	59	0	250
Frappuccino Blended Coffee White Chocolate Mocha No Whip Soy	1 grande	300	6	5	15	59	0	250
Frappuccino Blended Coffee White Chocolate Mocha Whip Nonfat Milk	1 grande	410	7	16	55	62	0	270
Frappuccino Blended Coffee White Chocolate Mocha Whip Soy	1 grande	410	7	16	55	62	0	270
Frappuccino Blended Creme Tazo Chai No Whip Nonfat Milk	1 grande	330	10	2	5	67	0	270
Frappuccino Blended Creme Tazo Chai Whip Nonfat Milk	1 grande	570	12	15	60	95	1	330
Frappuccino Blended Creme Vanilla Bean No Whip Nonfat Milk	1 grande	350	11	3	5	72	0	310
Frappuccino Blended Creme Vanilla Bean Whip Nonfat Milk	1 grande	470	12	14	50	75	0	320
Frappuccino Light Blended Coffee Cafe Vanilla Nonfat Milk	1 grande	190	6	1	0	42	3	240
Frappuccino Light Blended Coffee Caramel	1 grande	160	5	2	5	30	3	230
Frappuccino Light Blended Coffee Cinnamon Dolce Nonfat Milk	1 grande	140	5	1	0	29	3	230
Frappuccino Light Blended Coffee Java Chip Nonfat Milk	1 grande	200	6	5	0	36	4	220

FOOD	PORTION	CALS	PROT	FAT	CHOL	CARB	FIBER	SOD
Frappuccino Light Blended Coffee Mocha Nonfat Milk	1 grande	140	6	1	0	29	3	230
Frappuccino Light Blended Coffee Nonfat Milk	1 grande	130	5	1	0	25	3	230
Frappuccino Light Blended Coffee Pumpkin Spice Nonfat Milk	1 grande	150	6	1	0	31	3	240
Frappuccino Light Blended Creme Double Chocolaty Chip Whip Nonfat Milk	1 grande	510	14	19	50	78	2	300
Frappuccino Light Blended Creme Pumpkin Spice No Whip Nonfat Milk	1 grande	360	12	3	5	71	0	350
Frappuccino Light Blended Creme Pumpkin Spice Whip Nonfat Milk	1 grande	470	13	13	50	74	0	360
Frappuccino Light Blended Creme Tazo Green Tea No Whip Nonfat Milk	1 grande	380	11	3	5	78	1	290
Frappuccino Light Blended Creme Tazo Green Tea Whip Nonfat Milk	1 grande	440	11	13	50	71	0	190
Frappuccino Light Blended Creme White Chocolate No Whip Nonfat Milk	1 grande	480	15	7	10	89	0	410
Frappuccino Light Blended Creme White Chocolate Whip Nonfat Milk	1 grande	610	15	19	60	92	0	420
Frappuccino Light Espresso Nonfat Milk	1 grande	110	5	1	0	20	2	180
Hot Chocolate No Whip Nonfat Milk	1 grande	240	14	3	5	48	2	140
Hot Chocolate Whip Nonfat Milk	1 grande	320	14	10	35	50	2	150
Iced Brewed Coffee	1 grande	90	0	0	0	21	0	5
Iced Caffe Americano	1 grande	15	1	0	0	3	0	10
Iced Caffe Latte Nonfat Milk	1 grande	90	8	0	5	13	0	100
Iced Caffe Mocha No Whip Nonfat Milk	1 grande	170	9	3	5	36	2	80

FOOD	PORTION	CALS	PROT	FAT	CHOL	CARB	FIBER	SOD
Iced Caffe Mocha Whip Nonfat Milk	1 grande	290	9	14	45	39	2	90
Iced Caramel Macchiato Nonfat Milk	1 grande	190	10	2	10	34	0	130
Iced Latte Pumpkin Spice No Whip Nonfat Milk	1 grande	220	10	0	5	44	0	170
Iced Latte Pumpkin Spice Whip Nonfat Milk	1 grande	330	11	11	45	48	0	180
Iced Latte Skinny Cinnamon Dolce No Whip Nonfat Milk	1 grande	80	7	0	5	12	0	105
Iced Latte Sugar Free Flavored Syrup Nonfat Milk	1 grande	80	7	0	5	12	0	105
Iced Latte Syrup Flavored Nonfat Milk	1 grande	160	7	0	5	31	0	90
Iced Latte Vanilla Nonfat Milk	1 grande	160	7	0	5	31	0	90
Iced Peppermint White Chocolate Mocha No Whip Nonfat Milk	1 grande	370	10	6	5	72	0	190
Iced Peppermint White Chocolate Mocha Whip Nonfat Milk	1 grande	490	10	17	45	75	0	190
Iced Tazo Latte Black Tea Nonfat Milk	1 grande	170	8	0	0	35	0	100
Iced Tazo Latte Black Tea Soy	1 grande	200	6	3	0	38	1	90
Iced Tazo Latte Chai Nonfat Milk	1 grande	200	8	0	5	44	0	100
Iced Tazo Latte Green Tea Nonfat Milk	1 grande	220	10	5	0	45	1	120
Iced Tazo Latte Green Tea Soy	1 grande	260	7	4	0	48	2	105
Iced Tazo Latte Red Tea	1 grande	200	6	3	0	38	1	90
Iced Tazo Latte Red Tea Nonfat Milk	1 grande	170	8	0	5	35	0	100

FOOD	PORTION	CALS	PROT	FAT	CHOL	CARB	FIBER	SOD
Iced White Chocolate Mocha No Whip Nonfat Milk	1 grande	310	11	6	5	55	0	190
Iced White Chocolate Mocha Whip Nonfat Milk	1 grande	430	11	17	45	59	0	200
Latte Caffe Nonfat Milk	1 grande	130	13	5	5	19	0	150
Latte Cinnamon Dolce No Whip Nonfat Milk	1 grande	210	11	0	5	41	0	135
Latte Cinnamon Dolce w/ Sugar Free Syrup Nonfat Milk	1 grande	130	12	0	5	19	0	170
Latte Cinnamon Dolce Whip Nonfat Milk	1 grande	280	12	7	30	43	0	140
Latte Pumpkin Spice No Whip Nonfat Milk	1 grande	260	14	0	5	50	0	210
Latte Pumpkin Spice Whip Nonfat Milk	1 grande	330	14	7	30	52	0	220
Latte Skinny Caramel No Whip Nonfat Milk	1 grande	130	12	0	5	19	0	170
Latte Skinny Cinnamon Dolce No Whip Nonfat Milk	1 grande	130	12	0	0	19	0	170
Latte Skinny Hazelnut No Whip Nonfat Milk	1 grande	130	12	0	0	19	0	170
Latte Skinny Vanilla No Whip Nonfat Milk	1 grande	130	12	0	5	19	0	170
Latte Syrup Flavored Nonfat Milk	1 grande	200	12	0	5	37	0	140
Milk Nonfat	1 grande	180	18	0	10	26	0	220
Peppermint White Chocolate Mocha No Whip Nonfat Milk	1 grande	420	14	6	5	78	0	230
Peppermint White Chocolate Mocha Whip Nonfat Milk	1 grande	490	14	13	35	80	0	240
Pumpkin Spice Creme No Whip Nonfat Milk	1 grande	270	15	0	5	51	0	230
Pumpkin Spice Creme Whip Nonfat Milk	1 grande	340	15	7	35	53	0	240

FOOD	PORTION	CALS	PROT	FAT	CHOL	CARB	FIBER	SOD
Shaken Black Iced Tea & Lemonade	1 grande	130	0	0	0	33	0	10
Shaken White Iced Tea Blueberry	1 grande	80	0	0	0	21	0	10
Steamed Apple Juice	1 grande	230	0	0	0	56	0	20
Tazo Black Shaken Iced Tea & Lemonade	1 grande	130	0	0	0	33	0	10
Tazo Chai Latte Iced Tea Soy	1 grande	230	6	3	0	47	1	90
Tazo Chai Latte Nonfat Milk	1 grande	200	8	0	5	44	0	95
Tazo Chai Latte Soy	1 grande	230	5	3	0	47	1	85
Tazo Latte Black Tea Nonfat Milk	1 grande	170	7	0	5	34	0	90
Tazo Latte Black Tea Soy	1 grande	190	5	3	0	36	1	75
Tazo Latte Green Tea Nonfat Milk	1 grande	200	8	0	5	42	1	85
Tazo Latte Green Tea Soy	1 grande	220	6	3	0	44	2	75
Tazo Latte Red Tea Nonfat Milk	1 grande	170	7	0	5	34	0	90
Tazo Latte Red Tea Soy	1 grande	190	5	3	0	36	1	75
Tazo Shaken Iced Tea Green	1 grande	80	0	0	0	21	0	10
Tazo Shaken Iced Tea Green & Lemonade	1 grande	130	0	0	0	33	0	10
Tazo Shaken Iced Tea Orange Passion	1 grande	70	0	0	0	19	0	10
Tazo Shaken Iced Tea Passion	1 grande	80	0	0	0	21	0	10
Tazo Shaken Iced Tea Passion & Lemonade	1 grande	130	0	0	0	33	0	10
Tazo Tea	1 grande	0	0	0	0	0	0	0
Vanilla Creme Whip Nonfat Milk	1 grande	270	13	7	35	39	0	160
Vanilla Creme No Whip Nonfat Milk	1 grande	200	12	0	5	37	0	160
Vivanno Blend Banana Chocolate	1 grande	270	21	2	5	44	6	170
Vivanno Blend Orange Mango Banana	1 grande	250	16	2	5	47	5	120

FOOD	PORTION	CALS	PROT	FAT	CHOL	CARB	FIBER	SOD
White Chocolate Mocha No Whip Nonfat Milk	1 grande	360	16	6	10	62	0	260
White Chocolate Mocha Whip Nonfat Milk	1 grande	430	16	13	35	64	0	270
SALADS								
Fiesta	1 (9.4 oz)	320	16	10	20	44	8	930
Fruit & Cheese Plate	1 (8.6 oz)	400	14	20	50	44	2	560
Vegetable Vinaigrette	1 (10.7 oz)	310	8	15	5	40	10	900
SANDWICHES								
Club Chicken Cheddar Bacon w/ Mayo	1	480	31	18	70	48	2	1180
Club Turkey & Avocado	1	390	26	19	65	33	7	1160
Egg Salad On Multigrain	1	470	19	21	340	53	2	810
Turkey & Swiss w/ Mayo	1	310	26	13	55	26	2	1060
TOPPINGS								
Caramel	1 tbsp	15	0	1	0	2	0	5
Chocolate	1 tsp	5	0	0	0	1	0	0
Flavored Sugar Free Syrup	1 pump	0	0	0	0	0	0	0
Flavored Syrup	1 pump	20	0	0	0	5	0	0
Mocha Syrup	1 pump	25	1	1	0	5	0	0
Sprinkles	1 serv	0	0	0	0	0	0	0

STEAK ESCAPE

FOOD	PORTION	CALS	PROT	FAT	CHOL	CARB	FIBER	SOD
BEVERAGES								
Coca-Cola	16 oz	150	0	0	0	40	–	15
Diet Coke	16 oz	0	0	0	0	0	0	30
Lemonade	16 oz	167	0	0	0	44	–	0
Sprite	16 oz	150	0	0	0	39	–	55
SALADS								
Grilled Side	1 serv (5.9 oz)	40	3	1	0	8	–	20
Grilled w/ Chicken	1 serv (11.1 oz)	177	25	5	108	11	–	652
Grilled w/ Ham	1 serv (10.6 oz)	302	19	2	83	8	–	1042
Grilled w/ Steak	1 serv (11.1 oz)	187	23	6	103	11	–	292
Grilled w/ Turkey	1 serv (10.6 oz)	132	19	2	83	8	–	1042

FOOD	PORTION	CALS	PROT	FAT	CHOL	CARB	FIBER	SOD
SANDWICHES								
7 Inch Cajun Chicken	1 (8.6 oz)	408	31	5	55	58	–	1211
7 Inch Capicola Portion	1 serv (1 oz)	31	5	1	14	tr	–	329
7 Inch Chicken Portion	1 serv (3.9 oz)	120	21	4	55	0	0	430
7 Inch Classic Italian Sub	1 (8.4 oz)	471	27	11	49	60	–	1989
7 Inch Ham Portion	1 serv (3 oz)	75	8	1	15	3	–	1020
7 Inch Salami Portion	1 serv (1 oz)	105	6	9	25	0	–	470
7 Inch Steak Portion	1 serv (3.9 oz)	130	19	5	50	0	0	270
7 Inch Turkey Club	1 (7.9 oz)	380	21	2	20	62	–	2040
7 Inch Turkey Portion	1 serv (2.9 oz)	75	8	1	15	3	–	1020
7 Inch Vegetarian	1 (8.8 oz)	311	13	1	0	65	–	733
7 Inch Wild West BBQ	1 (9.6 oz)	455	29	6	50	60	–	1302
Kids Chicken	1 (3.9 oz)	205	12	7	32	29	–	470
Kids Ham	1 (3.7 oz)	183	6	1	13	31	–	765
Kids Steak	1 (3.8 oz)	110	9	3	13	29	–	445
Kids Turkey	1 (3.7 oz)	183	6	1	13	31	–	765
SIDES								
Fries	1 cup (12 oz)	498	8	26	0	67	–	409
Fries	1 cup (32 oz)	996	16	52	0	134	–	818
Fries Kids	1 serv (2.9 oz)	249	4	13	0	34	–	205
Fries Loaded Bacon & Cheddar	1 serv (10.8 oz)	905	18	44	29	88	–	1587
Fries Loaded Ranch & Bacon	1 serv (10.8 oz)	1044	18	71	39	84	–	1398
Kids Chicken Tenders	2 (3.8 oz)	240	15	11	35	21	–	1050
Smashed Potatoes Loaded Bacon & Cheddar	1 serv (16.7 oz)	636	13	26	24	91	–	827
Smashed Potatoes Loaded Ranch & Bacon	1 serv (16.7 oz)	692	14	34	29	87	–	501
Smashed Potatoes Plain	1 serv (13.8 oz)	246	11	0	0	53	–	43
Smashed Potatoes w/ Chicken	1 serv (19.9 oz)	383	33	4	108	56	–	475

FOOD	PORTION	CALS	PROT	FAT	CHOL	CARB	FIBER	SOD
Smashed Potatoes w/ Ham	1 serv (19.4 oz)	338	27	2	83	59	–	1065
Smashed Potatoes w/ Steak	1 serv (19.9 oz)	393	31	5	103	56	–	313
Smashed Potatoes w/ Turkey	1 serv (19.4 oz)	338	27	2	83	59	–	1065
TOPPINGS								
BBQ Sauce	1 serv (1 oz)	40	0	0	0	9	–	252
Brown Mustard	1 serv (1 oz)	0	0	0	0	0	0	340
Cheddar	1 serv (1 oz)	116	8	8	26	1	–	179
Dressing Balsamic Vinaigrette	1 serv (1.5 oz)	90	0	9	0	3	–	350
Dressing Bleu Cheese	1 serv (1.5 oz)	184	2	18	8	3	–	35
Dressing Italian	1 serv (0.5 oz)	51	0	5	0	1	–	248
Dressing Ranch	1 serv (0.5 oz)	83	0	9	5	0	0	137
Lettuce	1 serv (1 oz)	2	1	0	0	0	0	2
Margarine	1 serv (1 oz)	203	0	23	0	0	0	306
Mayonnaise	1 serv (1 oz)	101	0	11	5	0	0	76
Parmesan	1 serv (1 oz)	30	3	2	5	tr	–	120
Peppers Jalapeno	1 serv (1.5 oz)	11	–	–	–	–	–	–
Peppers Mild	1 serv (1.5 oz)	11	0	0	0	4	–	500
Provolone	1 serv (0.75 oz)	80	5	6	15	0	0	190
Sour Cream	1 serv (1 oz)	61	1	6	13	1	–	15
Tomatoes	1 serv (2 oz)	24	2	0	0	2	–	5
White American	1 serv (1 oz)	101	6	9	26	3	–	437

SUBWAY

ADD-ONS AND SALAD DRESSINGS

FOOD	PORTION	CALS	PROT	FAT	CHOL	CARB	FIBER	SOD
American Cheese	1 serv (0.4 oz)	40	2	4	10	1	0	200
Bacon Strips	2	45	3	4	10	0	0	190
Banana Pepper Slices	3	0	0	0	0	0	0	20

FOOD	PORTION	CALS	PROT	FAT	CHOL	CARB	FIBER	SOD
Cheddar	1 serv (0.5 oz)	60	4	5	15	0	0	95
Fat Free Italian	1 serv (2 oz)	35	1	0	0	7	0	720
Fat Free Red Wine Vinaigrette	1 serv (0.7 oz)	30	0	0	1	6	0	340
Jalapeno Pepper Slices	3	<5	0	0	0	0	0	70
Mayonnaise	1 tbsp	110	0	12	10	0	0	80
Mayonnaise Light	1 tbsp	50	0	5	5	tr	0	100
Monterey Cheddar Shredded	1 serv (0.5 oz)	50	3	5	15	1	0	90
Mustard Yellow or Deli	2 tsp	5	0	0	0	tr	0	115
Olive Oil Blend	1 tsp	45	0	5	0	0	0	0
Pepperjack Cheese	1 serv (0.5 oz)	50	3	4	15	0	0	140
Provolone	1 serv (0.5 oz)	50	4	4	10	0	0	125
Ranch	1 serv (2 oz)	320	0	35	29	3	0	560
Ranch Lowfat	1.5 tbsp	120	0	13	11	1	0	210
Red Wine Vinaigrette	1 serv (2 oz)	80	1	1	0	17	0	910
Sauce Chipotle Southwest	1.5 tbsp	100	0	10	8	1	0	220
Sauce Fat Free Honey Mustard	1.5 tbsp	30	0	0	0	7	0	115
Sauce Fat Free Sweet Onion	1.5 tbsp	40	0	0	0	9	0	85
Swiss	1 serv (0.5 oz)	50	4	5	15	0	0	30
Vinegar	1 tsp	0	0	0	0	0	0	0
BREADS								
Hearty Italian	6 inch	220	8	2	0	41	2	470
Honey Oat	6 inch	250	10	4	0	48	5	380
Italian	6 inch	200	7	2	0	38	1	470
Italian Herb & Cheese	6 inch	250	10	5	10	40	2	670
Italian White	1 mini	140	5	2	0	26	1	320
Monterey Cheddar	6 inch	240	10	5	10	39	1	540
Parmesan Oregano	6 inch	220	8	3	0	40	2	620
Wheat	1 mini	140	6	2	0	27	2	240
Wheat	6 inch	200	8	3	0	40	4	360
Wrap	1	190	6	5	0	33	1	470

FOOD	PORTION	CALS	PROT	FAT	CHOL	CARB	FIBER	SOD
DESSERTS								
Apple Slices	1 pkg	35	0	0	0	9	2	0
Cookie Chocolate Chip	1	210	2	10	15	30	1	150
Cookie Chocolate Chip w/ M&M's	1 (1.6 oz)	210	2	10	10	32	tr	100
Cookie Chocolate Chunk	1	220	2	10	10	30	tr	100
Cookie Double Chocolate Chip	1 (1.6 oz)	210	2	10	15	30	1	170
Cookie Oatmeal Raisin	1	200	3	8	15	30	1	170
Cookie Peanut Butter	1	220	4	12	15	26	1	200
Cookie Sugar	1	220	2	12	15	28	tr	140
Cookie White Chip Macadamia Nut	1	220	2	11	15	29	tr	160
Raisins	1 pkg	150	2	0	0	33	2	0
SALADS								
Ham w/o Dressing & Croutons	1 serv	120	12	3	25	14	4	840
Oven Roasted Chicken Breast w/o Dressing & Croutons	1 serv	140	19	3	50	11	4	390
Roast Beef w/o Dressing & Croutons	1 serv	120	13	3	20	12	4	480
Subway Club w/o Dressing & Croutons	1 serv	150	18	4	35	14	4	870
Sweet Onion Chicken Teriyaki w/o Dressing & Croutons	1 serv	210	20	3	50	26	4	780
Turkey Breast	1 serv	110	12	3	20	13	4	580
Turkey Breast & Ham w/o Dressing & Croutons	1 serv	120	14	3	25	14	4	790
Veggie Delight w/o Dressing & Croutons	1 serv	60	3	1	0	11	4	80
SANDWICHES								
6 Inch Chicken & Bacon Ranch	1	580	36	30	100	47	6	1390
6 Inch Cold Cut Combo	1	410	21	17	60	47	5	1530
6 Inch Double Stacked Cold Cut Combo	1	550	31	28	110	49	5	2360

FOOD	PORTION	CALS	PROT	FAT	CHOL	CARB	FIBER	SOD
6 Inch Double Stacked Italian BMT	1	630	34	35	100	49	5	2850
6 Inch Double Stacked Steak & Cheese	1	540	46	18	105	49	7	1500
6 Inch Double Stacked Subway Club	1	420	39	8	65	50	5	2080
6 Inch Double Stacked Sweet Onion Chicken Teriyaki	1	480	43	7	100	65	6	1820
6 Inch Double Stacked Turkey Breast	1	330	28	5	40	48	5	1500
6 Inch Ham	1	290	18	5	25	47	5	1260
6 Inch Italian BMT	1	450	23	21	55	47	5	1770
6 Inch Meatball Marinara	1	560	24	24	45	63	8	1590
6 Inch Oven Roasted Chicken Breast	1	310	24	5	25	48	6	830
6 Inch Roast Beef	1	290	19	5	20	45	5	900
6 Inch Spicy Italian	1	480	21	25	55	45	5	1660
6 Inch Steak & Cheese	1	400	29	12	60	48	6	1110
6 Inch Subway Club	1	320	24	6	35	47	5	1290
6 Inch Subway Melt	1	380	25	12	45	48	5	1600
6 Inch Sweet Onion Chicken Teriyaki	1	370	26	5	50	59	5	1200
6 Inch Tuna	1	530	22	31	45	44	5	1010
6 Inch Turkey Breast	1	280	18	5	20	46	5	1000
6 Inch Turkey Breast & Ham	1	290	20	5	25	47	5	1210
6 Inch Veggie Delite	1	230	9	3	0	44	5	500
Mini Sub Ham	1	180	11	3	10	30	4	710
Mini Sub Roast Beef	1	190	13	4	15	30	4	600
Mini Sub Tuna w/ Cheese	1	320	13	18	30	30	4	690
Mini Sub Turkey Breast	1	190	12	3	15	30	4	670
Softwich Santa Fe Turkey	1	520	33	10	55	78	5	1910
TACO BELL								
Border Bowl Southwest Steak	1 serv	600	28	24	55	68	9	2120
Border Bowl Zesty Chicken	1 serv	640	22	35	30	60	10	1800

FOOD	PORTION	CALS	PROT	FAT	CHOL	CARB	FIBER	SOD
Border Bowl Zesty Chicken w/o Dressing	1 serv	440	21	15	30	57	10	1540
Burrito ½ Lb Beef & Potato	1	530	15	23	30	68	6	1720
Burrito ½ Lb Combo Beef	1	440	21	18	45	51	8	1630
Burrito 7 Layer	1	490	17	18	25	65	9	1350
Burrito Bean	1	350	13	9	6	54	8	1190
Burrito Chili Cheese	1	370	16	16	40	40	3	1060
Burrito Fiesta Chicken	1	360	18	10	30	47	3	1320
Burrito Fiesta Steak	1	370	14	13	25	49	4	1200
Burrito Grilled Stuft Chicken	1	640	34	23	65	73	7	2160
Burrito Grilled Stuft Steak	1	630	30	25	55	72	7	1930
Burrito Supreme Beef	1	420	17	17	40	51	7	1340
Burrito Supreme Chicken	1	400	20	13	45	49	6	1360
Burrito Supreme Steak	1	390	18	14	40	49	6	1250
Chalupa Baja Beef	1	410	13	27	35	30	4	780
Chalupa Baja Chicken	1	390	17	23	40	29	3	800
Chalupa Baja Steak	1	390	15	24	35	28	3	690
Chalupa Nacho Cheese Beef	1	370	12	22	20	32	3	770
Chalupa Nacho Cheese Chicken	1	360	16	18	25	30	2	790
Chalupa Nacho Cheese Steak	1	340	14	19	20	30	2	680
Chalupa Supreme Beef	1	380	14	20	40	30	3	620
Chalupa Supreme Chicken	1	360	17	20	45	29	2	650
Chalupa Supreme Steak	1	360	15	21	40	28	2	530
Cheesy Fiesta Potatoes	1 serv	290	4	17	15	29	2	830
Cinnamon Twists	1 serv	170	1	7	0	26	1	200
Crunchwrap Supreme	1	560	17	24	35	68	5	1430
Crunchwrap Supreme Spicy Chicken	1	540	19	24	35	67	4	1360
Crunchy Taco	1	170	8	25	10	13	3	350
Crunchy Taco Supreme	1	210	9	10	25	15	3	370
Empanada Caramel Apple	1	290	3	14	5	37	1	300
Enchirito Beef	1	360	18	17	50	34	7	1420
Enchirito Chicken	1	340	22	13	50	33	6	1450
Fresco Border Bowl Zesty Chicken w/o Dressing	1 serv	350	19	8	25	51	10	1600

FOOD	PORTION	CALS	PROT	FAT	CHOL	CARB	FIBER	SOD
Fresco Burrito Bean	1 (7.5 oz)	340	12	8	0	56	11	1290
Fresco Burrito Fiesta Chicken	1	330	16	8	25	48	3	1240
Fresco Burrito Supreme Chicken	1 (8.5 oz)	340	18	8	25	50	8	1410
Fresco Burrito Supreme Steak	1 (8.5 oz)	330	16	8	15	49	8	1340
Fresco Crunchy Taco	1 (3.2 oz)	150	7	7	20	13	3	350
Fresco Soft Taco Beef	1 (4 oz)	180	8	7	20	22	3	640
Fresco Soft Taco Grilled Steak	1 (4.5 oz)	160	9	4	15	21	2	600
Fresco Soft Taco Ranchero Chicken	1 (4.7 oz)	170	12	4	25	22	2	740
Gordita Baja Beef	1	340	13	19	35	29	4	780
Gordita Baja Chicken	1	320	17	16	40	28	3	800
Gordita Baja Steak	1	320	15	17	35	27	3	690
Gordita Nacho Cheese Beef	1	300	12	14	25	31	3	770
Gordita Nacho Cheese Chicken	1	280	16	11	25	29	2	800
Gordita Nacho Cheese Steak	1	270	14	12	20	29	2	680
Gordita Supreme Beef	1	310	14	16	40	29	3	620
Gordita Supreme Chicken	1	290	17	12	45	28	2	650
Gordita Supreme Steak	1	290	15	13	40	28	2	530
Guacamole Side	1 serv	70	1	5	0	5	2	180
Mexican Pizza	1	530	20	30	40	46	6	1000
Mexican Rice	1 serv	180	6	7	15	23	1	790
MexiMelt	1 serv	260	15	14	40	22	3	860
Nacho Supreme	1 serv	440	12	26	35	41	7	800
Nachos	1 serv	330	4	21	5	32	2	530
Nachos Bellgrande	1 serv	770	19	44	35	77	12	1280
Pintos 'n Cheese	1 serv	160	9	6	15	19	7	670
Quesadilla Cheese	1	470	19	26	50	39	2	1100
Quesadilla Chicken	1	520	28	28	75	40	3	1420
Quesadilla Steak	1	520	26	28	70	39	3	1300
Salsa Side	1 serv	15	0	0	0	3	0	160
Soft Taco Grande	1	430	19	20	45	43	5	1440
Soft Taco Grilled Steak	1	270	12	16	35	20	2	660
Soft Taco Ranchero Chicken	1	270	14	14	35	21	2	820

FOOD	PORTION	CALS	PROT	FAT	CHOL	CARB	FIBER	SOD
Soft Taco Supreme Beef	1	250	11	13	40	23	3	650
Sour Cream Side	1 serv	80	1	7	25	3	0	30
Taco Double Decker	1	320	14	13	25	38	6	810
Taco Double Decker Supreme	1	370	14	17	40	40	7	820
Taco Spicy Chicken	1	170	10	8	25	20	2	580
Taco Salad Express	1	610	25	32	65	56	14	1420
Taco Salad Fiesta	1	840	30	45	65	80	15	1780
Taco Salad Fiesta w/o Shell	1	470	23	24	65	41	13	1510
Taco Salad Fiesta Chicken	1	790	37	38	75	77	13	1830
Taco Salad Fiesta Chicken w/o Shell	1	430	30	18	75	38	11	1560
Taquitos Chicken Grilled	1 serv	310	18	11	40	37	2	980
Taquitos Steak Grilled	1 serv	310	16	11	35	36	2	870
Tostada	1	240	11	10	15	27	7	730

TACO BUENO

MAIN MENU SELECTIONS

FOOD	PORTION	CALS	PROT	FAT	CHOL	CARB	FIBER	SOD
Bueno Chilada Beef	1 (7.9 oz)	523	24	32	–	42	2	2056
Bueno Chilada Beef w/o Chili	1 (5.5 oz)	412	19	26	–	29	1	1512
Bueno Chilada Beef w/o Queso	1 (5.6 oz)	337	14	18	–	36	2	1147
Bueno Chilada Chicken	1 (7.4 oz)	477	24	26	–	43	2	2090
Bueno Chilada Chicken w/o Chili	1 (5 oz)	366	19	20	–	30	1	1546
Bueno Chilada Chicken w/o Queso	1 (5.1 oz)	290	14	12	–	30	2	1181
Burrito Bean	1 (6.4 oz)	490	15	29	–	45	5	1649
Burrito Bean w/o Cheddar Cheese	1 (5.9 oz)	412	11	23	–	44	5	1528
Burrito Bean w/o Chili	1 (5.2 oz)	434	13	26	–	39	4	1378
Burrito Beef	1 (6.9 oz)	510	23	29	–	41	3	1377
Burrito Beef Potato	1 (4.8 oz)	350	11	21	–	32	3	906
Burrito Beef Potato w/o Queso	1 (4.1 oz)	305	9	17	–	30	3	644
Burrito Beef Potato w/o Sour Cream	1 (4.3 oz)	330	11	18	–	31	3	896
Burrito Beef w/o Cheddar Cheese	1 (6.4 oz)	432	19	22	–	40	3	1255

FOOD	PORTION	CALS	PROT	FAT	CHOL	CARB	FIBER	SOD
Burrito Beef w/o Chili	1 (5.7 oz)	455	20	25	–	36	2	1105
Burrito Big Ol' Beef	1 (10.6 oz)	772	33	46	–	57	3	1833
Burrito Big Ol' Beef w/o Cheddar Cheese	1 (9.6 oz)	615	24	33	–	56	3	1590
Burrito Big Ol' Beef w/o Chili	1 (9.4 oz)	716	31	43	–	51	2	1561
Burrito Big Ol' Beef w/o Sour Cream	1 (9.6 oz)	715	32	40	–	55	3	1814
Burrito Big Ol' Chicken	1 (8.4 oz)	607	31	30	–	53	5	1640
Burrito Big Ol' Chicken w/o Cheddar Cheese	1 (7.4 oz)	450	22	17	–	52	2	1397
Burrito Big Ol' Chicken w/o Sour Cream	1 (7.4 oz)	551	30	24	–	51	2	1621
Burrito Chicken Potato	1 (4.5 oz)	327	11	18	–	33	3	928
Burrito Chicken Potato w/o Queso	1 (3.8 oz)	274	9	14	–	31	3	667
Burrito Chicken Potato w/o Sour Cream	1 (4 oz)	299	11	15	–	32	3	918
Burrito Combination	1 (6.8 oz)	507	19	29	–	43	4	1536
Burrito Combination w/o Cheddar Cheese	1 (6.3 oz)	429	15	23	–	42	4	1414
Burrito Combination w/o Chili	1 (5.6 oz)	452	17	26	–	37	3	1263
Burrito Combination w/o Refried Beans	1 (5.7 oz)	440	18	23	–	40	3	1157
Burrito Party	1 (4 oz)	298	9	18	–	29	3	1041
Burrito Party w/o Cheddar Cheese	1 (3.8 oz)	259	7	14	–	29	3	980
Chimichanger Cheesecake	1 (2 oz)	210	4	11	–	24	1	160
Cinnamon Chips	1 serv (4.5 oz)	676	8	31	–	95	4	254
Corn Tortilla Chips	1 serv (1.5 oz)	219	3	11	–	27	4	25
Guacamole	1 serv (0.9 oz)	55	1	5	–	2	1	128
Jalapenos	1 serv (0.7 oz)	3	0	0	–	1	1	334
Mexican Rice	1 serv (4.2 oz)	469	10	12	–	83	2	1287
Muchaco Beef	1 (5.2 oz)	449	15	25	–	40	3	911

FOOD	PORTION	CALS	PROT	FAT	CHOL	CARB	FIBER	SOD
Muchaco Beef w/o Cheddar Cheese	1 (4.9 oz)	410	13	22	–	40	3	850
Muchaco Beef w/o Refried Beans	1 (4.2 oz)	392	14	20	–	38	2	596
Muchaco Chicken	1 (4.6 oz)	387	17	18	–	40	2	817
Muchaco Chicken w/o Cheddar Cheese	1 (4.4 oz)	348	15	14	–	39	2	756
Nachos Cheese	1 serv (5.5 oz)	572	18	35	–	47	6	1396
Quesadilla Beef	1 (8.5 oz)	823	38	51	–	49	2	1612
Quesadilla Cheese	1 (6.5 oz)	709	30	42	–	48	2	1261
Quesadilla Chicken	1 (7.9 oz)	761	38	44	–	50	2	1658
Quesadilla Kids Cheese	1 (2.2 oz)	219	8	11	–	23	1	462
Quesadilla Mini Cheese	1 (2.7)	274	11	15	–	23	1	533
Refried Beans Powdered	1 serv (6.3 oz)	406	12	34	–	17	5	1905
Refried Beans w/o Cheddar Cheese	1 serv (5.8 oz)	327	8	28	–	16	5	1784
Refried Beans w/o Chili	1 serv (5.1 oz)	360	9	31	–	11	4	1634
Salsa Red	1 serv (2 oz)	14	1	0	–	3	1	366
Soup Tortilla	1 bowl	237	20	11	–	19	2	1430
Soup Tortilla w/o Tortilla Strips & Cheese	1 bowl	148	17	6	–	11	2	1382
Sour Cream	1 serv (1 oz)	57	1	6	–	2	0	19
Taco w/o Cheddar Cheese	1 (1.5 oz)	104	4	7	–	5	0	183
Taco Crispy Beef	1 (2.6 oz)	200	10	14	–	7	0	378
Taco Crispy Chicken	1 (1.9 oz)	140	9	7	–	8	0	368
Taco Crispy Chicken w/o Cheddar Cheese	1 (1.7 oz)	100	7	4	–	7	0	307
Taco Crispy w/o Cheddar Cheese	1 (2.4 oz)	161	7	11	–	6	0	317
Taco Party	1 (1.9 oz)	143	7	10	–	5	0	244
Taco Soft Beef	1 (3.5 oz)	245	11	14	–	18	1	620
Taco Soft Beef w/o Cheddar Cheese	1 (3.2 oz)	206	9	11	–	17	1	559
Taco Soft Chicken	1 (2.9 oz)	184	10	8	–	19	1	610
Taco Soft Chicken w/o Cheddar Cheese	1 (2.5 oz)	145	8	5	–	18	1	540

FOOD	PORTION	CALS	PROT	FAT	CHOL	CARB	FIBER	SOD
Tostada	1 (4.1 oz)	324	11	24	–	18	3	971
Tostada w/o Cheddar Cheese	1 (3.3 oz	207	5	15	–	17	3	789
Tostada w/o Chili	1 (2.9 oz)	269	9	21	–	12	3	699
Tostada w/o Refried Beans	1 (2.5 oz)	234	10	16	–	15	2	467
SALADS								
Nacho Beef	1 (9.3 oz)	759	28	48	–	58	8	1877
Nacho Beef w/o Cheddar Cheese	1 (8.8 oz)	681	24	42	–	57	8	1756
Nacho Beef w/o Chili	1 (6.9 oz)	648	24	41	–	45	6	1334
Nacho Chicken	1 (8.9 oz)	713	28	43	–	59	8	1911
Nacho Chicken w/o Cheddar Cheese	1 (8.4 oz)	634	24	37	–	58	8	1790
Nacho Chicken w/o Chili	1 (6.5 oz)	601	24	36	–	46	6	1368
Taco Beef	1 (12.7 oz)	1043	36	75	–	58	12	1705
Taco Beef w/o Cheddar Cheese	1 (11.7 oz)	886	27	62	–	56	12	1462
Taco Beef w/o Chili	1 (11.5 oz)	987	33	72	–	51	12	1433
Taco Beef w/o Guacamole	1 (11.7 oz)	988	35	70	–	56	11	1577
Taco Beef w/o Sour Cream	1 (11.7 oz)	986	35	70	–	56	12	1686
Taco Beef w/o Tortilla Bowl	1 (9.7 oz)	564	28	45	–	15	2	1383
Taco Chicken	1 (9.6 oz)	838	30	57	–	53	12	1325
Taco Chicken w/o Cheddar Cheese	1 (8.6 oz)	680	21	44	–	52	12	1083
Taco Chicken w/o Guacamole	1 (8.6 oz)	783	29	52	–	51	11	1198
Taco Chicken w/o Sour Cream	1 (8.6 oz)	781	29	51	–	51	12	1307
Taco Chicken w/o Tortilla Bowl	1 (6.6 oz)	359	22	26	–	10	1	1004

TACO JOHN'S

BREAKFAST SELECTIONS

FOOD	PORTION	CALS	PROT	FAT	CHOL	CARB	FIBER	SOD
Breakfast Burrito Bacon	1 (7.6 oz)	550	21	25	250	56	7	1370
Breakfast Burrito Egg	1 (6.6 oz)	420	21	19	270	42	5	730
Breakfast Burrito Egg Bacon	1 (7 oz)	500	26	24	275	43	5	1120
Breakfast Burrito Egg Sausage	1 (8.1 oz)	590	28	34	300	44	6	1050

FOOD	PORTION	CALS	PROT	FAT	CHOL	CARB	FIBER	SOD
Breakfast Burrito Sausage	1 (8.6 oz)	640	23	35	275	56	7	1300
Breakfast Taco Bacon	1 (3.7 oz)	270	10	13	125	25	2	810
Breakfast Taco Sausage	1 (4.2 oz)	310	11	18	135	25	2	770
Scrambler Burrito Bacon	1 (8.6 oz)	550	21	25	250	58	7	1370
Scrambler Burrito Sausage	1 (9.6 oz)	640	21	32	270	58	7	1440
Scrambler Potato Ole Bacon	1 sm (9.4 oz)	630	20	41	260	45	6	1860
Scrambler Potato Ole Sausage	1 sm (10.5 oz)	720	22	50	280	45	6	1780
DESSERTS								
Apple Grande	1 serv (3.4 oz)	270	5	12	5	39	2	420
Choco Taco	1 serv (4 oz)	390	5	20	15	48	1	160
Churro	1 serv (2 oz)	190	2	7	20	15	4	170
Cini-Sopapilla Bites	1 serv (2.6 oz)	210	4	5	0	37	4	320
Giant Goldfish Grahams	1 serv (0.5 oz)	70	1	2	0	11	1	55
MAIN MENU SELECTIONS								
Burrito Bean	1 (6.6 oz)	360	14	9	15	56	9	790
Burrito Beefy	1 (6.6 oz)	440	22	20	50	45	7	860
Burrito Chicken & Potato	1 (8.3 oz)	470	17	19	30	56	7	1220
Burrito Chicken Grilled	1 (8.2 oz)	590	32	29	90	50	6	1510
Burrito Combination	1 (6.6 oz)	400	18	14	35	50	8	830
Burrito Crunchy Chicken & Potato	1 (8.8 oz)	600	20	28	35	65	7	1320
Burrito Grilled Beef	1 (8.2 oz)	600	27	32	75	52	8	1230
Burrito Meat & Potato	1 (8.3 oz)	500	15	23	30	58	8	1100
Burrito Ranch Beef	1 (7.1 oz)	440	17	22	45	45	6	850
Burrito Ranch Chicken	1 (7 oz)	400	19	17	45	44	5	970
Burrito Smothered	1 (11.3 oz)	510	23	20	45	60	10	1310
Burrito Super	1 (8.8 oz)	450	19	18	40	54	9	900
Chili w/o Crackers	1 serv (8 oz)	220	14	11	35	17	4	1240
Chili w/o Crackers & Cheese	1 serv (7.5 oz)	160	10	6	20	17	4	1160
Chilto	1 serv (4.6 oz)	360	15	15	35	40	5	670
Chips & Queso	1 serv (6.7 oz)	430	9	25	20	43	2	940

FOOD	PORTION	CALS	PROT	FAT	CHOL	CARB	FIBER	SOD
Crispy Taco	1 (3.2 oz)	180	9	10	25	13	2	270
Crunchy Chicken w/o Sauce	1 serv (5 oz)	450	29	27	60	24	0	1420
Enchiliada Chili	1 serv (7.6 oz)	310	18	16	50	24	4	1000
Mexi Rolls w/o Nachos	2 pieces (1.9 oz)	130	6	5	10	14	2	190
Mexican Rice	1 serv (6 oz)	250	5	6	0	45	0	1080
Nachos	1 serv (5 oz)	380	6	23	10	38	1	750
Potato Oles	1 sm (5 oz)	430	4	26	0	45	6	1220
Potato Oles Chili Cheese	1 serv (10.7 oz)	590	13	36	25	55	8	2130
Potato Oles Super	1 serv (9.7 oz)	620	14	39	35	53	7	1270
Quesadilla Melt Cheesey	1 (5.6 oz)	440	19	22	55	43	5	1050
Quesadilla Melt Fajita Beef	1 serv (8.6 oz)	540	26	28	70	49	7	1240
Quesadilla Melt Fajita Chicken	1 (8.6 oz)	510	28	23	75	47	6	1360
Refried Beans	1 serv (9.4 oz)	320	18	6	15	47	11	1020
Refried Beans w/o Cheese	1 serv (8.9 oz)	260	14	2	0	47	11	940
Sierra Chicken Sandwich	1 (8.2 oz)	350	23	11	50	37	2	1350
Softshell Taco	1 (4 oz)	220	11	11	25	21	2	580
Super Nachos	1 sm (6.9 oz)	450	12	27	35	38	3	650
Taco Bravo	1 (6.5 oz)	340	15	13	25	40	5	750
Taco Burger	1 (5 oz)	270	14	12	30	28	3	600
Taco Stuffed Grilled	1 (7.4 oz)	560	19	25	40	63	7	920
SALAD DRESSINGS AND TOPPINGS								
Bacon Ranch Dressing	1 serv (1.5 oz)	130	1	10	10	10	0	370
Creamy Italian Dressing	1 serv (1.5 oz)	130	0	15	0	3	0	320
Guacamole	1 serv (2 oz)	90	0	6	0	8	2	115
Hot Sauce	1 serv (1 oz)	10	0	0	0	1	0	125

FOOD	PORTION	CALS	PROT	FAT	CHOL	CARB	FIBER	SOD
House Dressing	1 serv (1.5 oz)	70	0	7	0	2	0	260
Mild Sauce	1 serv (1 oz)	10	0	0	0	1	0	130
Nacho Cheese	1 serv (3 oz)	120	4	9	10	5	0	520
Pico De Gallo	1 serv (1 oz)	10	0	0	0	1	0	90
Ranch Dressing	1 serv (1.5 oz)	140	1	16	20	3	0	350
Salsa	1 serv (2 oz)	20	1	0	0	4	1	220
Sour Cream	1 serv (2 oz)	120	2	12	25	2	0	30
Super Hot Sauce	1 serv (1 oz)	10	0	0	0	1	0	25
SALADS								
Softshell Taco Chicken	1 (4 oz)	190	13	6	30	19	1	700
Taco Chicken w/o Dressing	1 serv (12.7 oz)	480	24	27	65	35	6	1020
Taco Crunchy Chicken w/o Dressing	1 serv (13.4 oz)	660	29	40	70	47	6	1180
Taco w/o Dressing	1 serv (12.7 oz)	520	21	33	60	37	7	860

TACOTIME

FOOD	PORTION	CALS	PROT	FAT	CHOL	CARB	FIBER	SOD
DESSERTS								
Churro Plain	1 (1.5 oz)	205	2	15	20	16	0	1440
Churro w/ Cinnamon & Sugar	1 (2 oz)	245	2	15	20	26	0	1440
Crustos	1 serv	294	6	6	0	58	3	273
Empanada Apple	1 (4 oz)	234	4	7	0	40	2	201
Empanada Cherry	1 (4 oz)	240	4	7	0	41	2	190
Empanada Pumpkin	1 (4 oz)	256	6	8	23	42	2	198
MAIN MENU SELECTIONS								
Burrito Big Juan Chicken	1 (13 oz)	594	35	19	78	68	10	2435
Burrito Big Juan Seasoned Ground Beef	1 (13 oz)	651	30	28	73	71	12	2658
Burrito Big Juan Shredded Beef	1 (13 oz)	633	33	25	64	67	10	2616
Burrito Casita Chicken	1 (12 oz)	494	34	18	85	43	5	2338
Burrito Casita Seasoned Ground Beef	1 (12 oz)	552	29	25	80	46	6	2561
Burrito Casita Shredded Beef	1 (12 oz)	533	31	25	91	42	5	2520

FOOD	PORTION	CALS	PROT	FAT	CHOL	CARB	FIBER	SOD
Burrito Chicken & Black Bean	1 (10 oz)	478	30	16	60	51	9	1219
Burrito Chicken BLT	1 (10 oz)	721	41	41	99	44	8	1642
Burrito Chicken Ranchero	1 (10.8 oz)	654	36	32	80	52	7	1341
Burrito Crisp Chicken	1 (5.5 oz)	336	27	10	42	32	2	566
Burrito Crisp Meat	1 (5.8 oz)	450	23	22	49	36	4	893
Burrito Crisp Pinto Bean	1 (6 oz)	394	13	16	12	50	6	2172
Burrito Soft Meat	1 (6.7 oz)	426	23	16	46	43	8	1095
Burrito Soft Pinto Bean	1 (6.7 oz)	377	14	11	15	54	10	2093
Burrito Veggie	1 (11 oz)	534	18	18	25	74	12	2545
Cheddar Fries	1 sm (6 oz)	374	8	26	23	29	3	877
Cheddar Melt	1 (2.8 oz)	250	11	12	31	25	4	472
Mexi-Fries	1 sm (5 oz)	290	3	19	0	29	2	740
Mexi-Rice	1 serv (4 oz)	87	2	1	0	19	0	401
Nachos Grande	1 serv (16.5 oz)	1132	39	57	90	114	11	4085
Refritos w/ Chips	1 serv (7 oz)	304	14	11	23	35	6	3252
Refritos w/o Chips	1 serv (6.7 oz)	285	13	11	23	32	6	3251
Stuffed Fries	1 sm (5 oz)	321	7	7	14	29	3	705
Taco Crisp Seasoned Ground Beef	1 (4.3 oz)	225	15	12	40	12	2	512
Taco Super Soft Chicken	1 (11 oz)	540	35	18	77	56	10	2354
Taco Super Soft Seasoned Ground Beef	1 (11 oz)	598	30	25	72	59	12	2577
Taco Super Soft Shredded Beef	1 (11 oz)	579	32	25	84	55	10	2535
Taco Value Soft	1 (5.3 oz)	314	18	13	40	28	6	800
Taco ½ Lb Shredded Beef	1 (9 oz)	440	28	18	65	42	7	1218
Taco ½ Lb Soft Chicken	1 (9 oz)	401	30	11	58	43	7	1037
Taco ½ Lb Soft Seasoned Ground Beef	1 (9 oz)	459	25	18	53	46	9	1260
Taco Chips	1 serv (2 oz)	150	3	3	0	27	1	7
SALAD DRESSINGS AND TOPPINGS								
Cheddar Cheese	1 serv (2 oz)	223	14	18	61	1	0	364
Dressing Chipotle Ranch	1 serv (1 oz)	165	1	18	6	1	0	157
Dressing Ranch	1 serv (1 oz)	181	1	20	7	1	–	187
Dressing Thousand Island	1 serv (1 oz)	132	0	12	5	5	0	369
Guacamole	1 serv (1 oz)	50	0	5	0	2	1	125

FOOD	PORTION	CALS	PROT	FAT	CHOL	CARB	FIBER	SOD
Salsa Nuevo	1 serv (1 oz)	8	0	0	0	2	0	131
Salsa Verde	1 serv (1 oz)	6	0	0	0	2	0	149
Sour Cream	1 serv (1.5 oz)	85	1	7	28	1	0	14
SALADS								
Taco Chicken	1 reg (9.2 oz)	351	27	15	58	24	2	899
Taco Seasoned Ground Beef	1 reg (7.8 oz)	396	22	23	53	24	4	860
Taco Shredded Beef	1 reg (7.8 oz)	377	25	22	65	21	2	819
Tostada Delight Chicken	1 (10.5 oz)	565	37	29	100	36	4	2221
Tostada Delight Seasoned Ground Beef	1 (10.5 oz)	623	32	36	95	39	6	2444
Tostada Delight Shredded Beef	1 (10.5 oz)	604	35	36	107	35	5	2402

TCBY

FROZEN YOGURT AND SORBET

FOOD	PORTION	CALS	PROT	FAT	CHOL	CARB	FIBER	SOD
Hand Scooped Butter Pecan Perfection	½ cup	110	4	5	10	14	tr	90
Hand Scooped Chocolate Chocolate Swirl	½ cup	120	4	4	15	19	tr	50
Hand Scooped Chocolate Chunk Cookie Dough	½ cup	160	3	6	15	24	0	75
Hand Scooped Cookies & Cream	½ cup	140	3	4	10	22	0	75
Hand Scooped Cotton Candy	½ cup	120	3	4	15	20	0	60
Hand Scooped Mint Chocolate Chunk	½ cup	140	3	5	10	22	0	55
Hand Scooped Mocha Almond	½ cup	150	3	5	10	22	tr	95
Hand Scooped No Sugar Added Chocolate Chocolate Swirl	½ cup	90	4	1	0	23	6	70
Hand Scooped No Sugar Added Vanilla	½ cup	80	4	1	0	19	5	60

FOOD	PORTION	CALS	PROT	FAT	CHOL	CARB	FIBER	SOD
Hand Scooped No Sugar Added Vanilla Fudge Brownie	½ cup	100	4	2	10	22	5	80
Hand Scooped Pralines & Cream	½ cup	140	3	5	10	23	0	80
Hand Scooped Psychedelic Sorbet	½ cup	290	0	0	0	75	0	30
Hand Scooped Rainbow Cream	½ cup	120	3	4	15	20	0	60
Hand Scooped Rocky Road	½ cup	220	3	7	5	36	1	25
Hand Scooped Strawberries & Cream	½ cup	120	2	3	10	21	0	50
Hand Scooped Vanilla Bean	½ cup	120	3	4	15	19	0	60
Hand Scooped Vanilla Chocolate Chunk	½ cup	140	3	5	10	22	0	55
Soft Serve Frozen Yogurt All Flavors 96% Fat Free	½ cup	140	4	3	15	23	0	60
Soft Serve Frozen Yogurt All Flavors Low Carb	½ cup	110	3	7	25	16	7	60
Soft Serve Frozen Yogurt All Flavors Nonfat	½ cup	110	4	0	<5	23	0	60
Soft Serve Frozen Yogurt All Flavors Nonfat No Sugar Added	½ cup	90	4	0	<5	20	0	35
Soft Serve Sorbet All Flavors Nonfat Nondairy	½ cup	100	0	0	0	24	0	30
SMOOTHIES								
Berrylicious	1 (16 oz)	290	3	3	10	65	3	65
Black 'N Blueberry	1 (16 oz)	280	3	3	10	63	2	65
Mango Tango	1 (16 oz)	330	2	3	10	76	2	65
Mangolada	1 (16 oz)	340	3	6	10	70	2	100
Mondo Mango	1 (16 oz)	310	3	3	10	70	2	65
Pina Paradise	1 (16 oz)	350	3	12	10	58	1	170
Pink Pineapple	1 (16 oz)	340	3	9	10	63	2	135
Straight Up Strawberry	1 (16 oz)	280	3	4	10	44	1	65
Strawberry Bonanza	1 (16 oz)	320	3	4	10	74	2	65
Strawberry Fling	1 (16 oz)	340	3	3	10	78	2	65

FOOD	PORTION	CALS	PROT	FAT	CHOL	CARB	FIBER	SOD
TIM HORTONS								
BAKED SELECTIONS								
Bagel Blueberry	1	270	10	1	0	55	2	470
Bagel Cinnamon Raisin	1	270	10	1	0	55	3	350
Bagel Everything	1	280	10	2	0	53	3	460
Bagel Flax Seed	1	290	10	5	0	53	4	520
Bagel Onion	1	260	9	2	0	53	3	460
Bagel Plain	1	260	9	2	0	52	2	450
Bagel Poppy Seed	1	270	9	2	0	53	3	440
Bagel Sesame Seed	1	270	9	3	0	53	3	430
Bagel Sun Dried Tomato	1	310	9	4	0	59	2	550
Bagel Twelve Grain	1	330	10	9	0	52	6	580
Cinnamon Roll Frosted	1	470	4	25	0	57	2	380
Cinnamon Roll Glazed	1	420	4	23	0	50	2	360
Cookie Caramel Chocolate Pecan	1	230	3	11	20	32	1	290
Cookie Chocolate Chip	1	230	3	9	20	34	1	260
Cookie Oatmeal Raisin Spice	1	220	3	8	25	35	1	200
Cookie Peanut Butter Chocolate Chunk	1	260	5	15	20	28	2	260
Cookie Triple Chocolate	1	250	3	13	30	31	2	220
Cookie White Chocolate Macadamia Nut	1	240	3	12	20	31	1	270
Croissant Butter	1	340	7	18	0	38	1	380
Croissant Cheese	1	370	9	20	15	37	0	410
Danish Cherry Cheese	1	330	5	13	15	46	1	230
Danish Chocolate	1	430	4	24	10	51	1	220
Danish Maple Pecan	1	380	4	20	20	46	1	230
Donut Apple Fritter	1	300	4	11	0	49	2	350
Donut Chocolate Dip	1	210	4	9	0	30	1	190
Donut Chocolate Glazed	1	260	4	10	5	39	2	300
Donut Honey Dip	1	210	4	8	0	33	1	190
Donut Maple Dip	1	210	4	8	0	31	1	200
Donut Old Fashion Glazed	1	320	3	19	10	35	1	230
Donut Old Fashion Plain	1	260	3	19	10	20	1	230
Donut Sour Cream Plain	1	270	3	17	10	27	1	230
Donut Walnut Crunch	1	360	4	23	5	35	1	320
Donut Filled Angel Cream	1	310	4	13	0	46	1	220

FOOD	PORTION	CALS	PROT	FAT	CHOL	CARB	FIBER	SOD
Donut Filled Blueberry	1	230	4	8	0	36	1	210
Donut Filled Boston Cream	1	250	4	9	0	38	1	260
Donut Filled Canadian Maple	1	260	4	9	0	41	1	260
Donut Filled Strawberry	1	230	4	8	0	36	1	220
Honey Cruller	1	320	1	19	50	37	0	220
Muffin Blueberry	1	330	4	11	15	54	2	580
Muffin Blueberry Bran	1	300	6	10	10	53	5	770
Muffin Carrot Wheat	1	400	6	19	10	55	4	580
Muffin Chocolate Chip	1	430	5	16	15	69	2	580
Muffin Cranberry Blueberry Bran	1	290	5	10	10	51	5	710
Muffin Cranberry Fruit	1	350	4	12	15	59	2	560
Muffin Fruit Explosion	1	360	4	11	15	61	2	550
Muffin Raisin Bran	1	360	6	10	10	65	6	790
Muffin Strawberry Sensation	1	350	4	11	15	61	1	580
Muffin Low Fat Blueberry	1	290	4	3	0	62	2	750
Muffin Low Fat Cranberry	1	290	4	3	0	62	2	750
Tea Biscuit Plain	1	250	5	9	0	35	1	590
Tea Biscuit Raisin	1	290	6	10	0	45	2	590
Timbits Apple Fritter	1	50	1	2	0	9	0	55
Timbits Chocolate Glazed	1	70	1	3	0	10	0	75
Timbits Honey Dip	1	60	1	2	0	9	0	50
Timbits Old Fashion Plain	1	70	1	5	5	5	0	60
Timbits Filled Banana Cream	1	60	1	2	0	9	0	65
Timbits Filled Lemon	1	60	1	2	0	9	0	50
Timbits Filled Strawberry	1	60	1	2	0	10	0	50
BEVERAGES								
Cafe Mocha	1 (10 oz)	160	1	7	0	25	1	160
Cappuccino Iced	1 (12 oz)	300	0	15	50	41	0	85
Coffee Decaffeinated Sugar & Cream	1 (10 oz)	75	1	4	15	9	0	15
Coffee Sugar & Cream	1 (10 oz)	75	1	4	15	9	0	15
English Toffee	1 (10 oz)	220	3	6	0	40	0	240
Flavor Shot	1 serv	5	0	0	0	1	0	0
French Vanilla	1 (10 oz)	240	4	7	0	39	0	240
Hot Chocolate	1 (10 oz)	240	2	6	0	45	2	360

FOOD	PORTION	CALS	PROT	FAT	CHOL	CARB	FIBER	SOD
Hot Smoothie	1 (10 oz)	260	5	10	5	39	2	200
Iced Cappuccino w/ Milk	1 (12 oz)	180	3	2	5	39	0	45
Tea Sugar & Milk	1 (10 oz)	50	1	1	5	10	0	20
CREAM CHEESE								
Garden Vegetable	1.5 oz	120	2	11	45	3	1	230
Light Plain	1.5 oz	60	4	5	20	3	0	200
Plain	1.5 oz	130	2	12	50	2	0	180
Strawberry	1.5 oz	120	6	10	40	6	0	160
SANDWICHES								
B.L.T.	1	450	18	18	30	53	2	850
Breakfast Bacon Egg Cheese	1	410	16	25	185	31	1	760
Breakfast Egg Cheese	1	360	13	21	175	30	1	680
Breakfast Sausage Egg Cheese	1	520	19	37	205	30	1	940
Chicken Salad Salad	1	380	21	9	35	55	3	890
Egg Salad	1	390	17	13	245	52	2	780
Ham & Swiss	1	440	28	12	50	56	3	1690
Toasted Chicken Club	1	460	30	7	50	70	2	1170
Turkey Breast	1	390	27	5	10	59	4	1480
SOUPS								
Beef Stew	1 serv (10 oz)	236	17	8	30	25	3	1208
Chicken Noodle	1 serv (10 oz)	120	5	2	20	18	1	880
Chili	1 serv (10 oz)	300	21	16	50	18	5	920
Country Field Mushroom	1 serv (10 oz)	150	3	3	0	28	1	1080
Cream Of Broccoli	1 serv (10 oz)	160	6	9	20	16	1	820
Hearty Vegetable	1 serv (10 oz)	70	4	0	0	14	3	1060
Minestrone	1 serv (10 oz)	120	4	3	0	24	2	940
Potato Bacon	1 serv (10 oz)	180	3	6	0	30	2	1260
Split Pea w/ Ham	1 serv (10 oz)	150	8	3	5	27	5	970

FOOD	PORTION	CALS	PROT	FAT	CHOL	CARB	FIBER	SOD
Turkey Rice	1 serv (10 oz)	120	3	2	0	21	1	1000
Vegetable Beef Barley	1 serv (10 oz)	110	4	2	5	21	2	980
YOGURT								
Low Fat Creamy Vanilla w/ Berries	1 (6 oz)	160	4	3	10	32	2	80
Low Fat Strawberry w/ Berries	1 (6 oz)	150	4	3	10	28	2	75
T.J. CINNAMONS								
Chocolate Twist	1	250	4	12	5	34	2	110
Cinnamon Twist	1	280	3	14	5	33	1	190
Mocha Chill w/ Whipped Cream	1 (12.5 oz)	306	11	7	29	48	1	214
Mocha Chill w/o Whipped Cream	1 (12.5 oz)	264	11	4	17	48	1	214
Original Roll w/o Icing	1	507	10	10	7	73	4	373
Pecan Sticky Bun	1	688	12	22	7	91	5	420
TJ Icing	1 serv (1 oz)	117	1	5	8	18	0	50
TOGO'S								
SALAD DRESSINGS								
Asian	1 serv (2.5 oz)	380	0	33	0	19	0	830
Blue Cheese	1 serv (2.5 oz)	260	2	26	25	3	0	780
Buttermilk Ranch	1 serv (2.5 oz)	250	2	26	20	3	0	890
Caesar	1 serv (2.5 oz)	150	2	12	30	8	0	800
Fat Free Serano Grape Vinaigrette	1 serv (2.5 oz)	90	1	0	0	23	0	290
Low Fat Balsamic Vinaigrette	1 serv (2.5 oz)	90	0	4	0	16	0	780
SALADS								
Asian Chicken w/o Dressing	1 full serv	200	21	9	40	17	3	400
Chicken Caesar w/o Dressing	1 full serv	210	24	6	50	17	3	650

FOOD	PORTION	CALS	PROT	FAT	CHOL	CARB	FIBER	SOD
Cobb w/o Dressing	1 full serv	330	29	20	140	12	6	870
Santa Fe Chicken w/o Dressing	1 full serv	370	27	16	55	33	10	950
Taco w/o Dressing	1 full serv	600	26	39	110	36	9	1190
SANDWICHES								
Albacore Tuna	1 reg	660	30	28	45	73	4	1900
Avocado & Cucumber	1 reg	560	13	25	10	75	9	1340
Black Forest Ham & Cheese	1 reg	670	35	31	80	67	4	2710
Capicolla Dry Salami & Provolone	1 reg	1080	73	59	235	69	4	4980
Cheese	1 reg	800	34	45	90	68	4	2260
Chef's Creations Pacific Cobb	1 reg	710	34	36	70	68	6	2170
Chef's Creations Pastrami Reuben	1 reg	990	52	55	145	67	3	2600
Chicken Salad	1 reg	650	26	29	50	74	5	2010
Egg Salad & Cheese	1 reg	750	31	39	455	70	4	1890
Hot BBQ Beef	1 reg	670	40	19	115	85	3	2010
Hot Meatball	1 reg	690	33	27	70	78	5	2180
Hot Pastrami	1 reg	750	43	33	105	69	4	2280
Hot Roast Beef	1 reg	730	58	25	100	67	4	2410
Hummus	1 reg	650	19	27	15	90	9	1770
Salami & Cheese	1 reg	1100	87	53	295	73	4	6230
Turkey & Avocado	1 reg	640	36	26	55	74	9	1800
Turkey & Cheese	1 reg	670	42	28	80	68	4	2110
Turkey & Cranberry	1 reg	670	34	19	55	95	4	1860
Turkey Bacon Club	1 reg	680	35	32	65	68	4	2210
Turkey Ham & Cheese	1 reg	690	42	29	90	68	4	2430

WHATABURGER

FOOD	PORTION	CALS	PROT	FAT	CHOL	CARB	FIBER	SOD
BEVERAGES								
Barq's Root Beer	1 sm (16 oz)	220	0	0	0	61	0	28
Cherry Coke	1 sm (16 oz)	210	0	0	0	56	0	9
Coca Cola	1 sm (16 oz)	207	0	0	0	56	0	5
Coffee	1 sm (8 oz)	5	0	0	0	1	0	9
Coffee Decafe	1 sm (8 oz)	5	0	0	0	1	0	21
Diet Coke	1 sm (16 oz)	0	0	0	0	0	0	19
Dr Pepper	1 sm (16 oz)	190	0	0	0	51	0	47
Fanta Orange	1 sm (16 oz)	210	0	0	0	56	0	0
Fanta Strawberry	1 sm (16 oz)	230	0	0	0	61	0	0

FOOD	PORTION	CALS	PROT	FAT	CHOL	CARB	FIBER	SOD
Iced Tea Sweetened	1 (34 oz)	430	0	0	0	114	0	0
Iced Tea Unsweetened	1 sm (19 oz)	0	0	0	0	0	0	0
Lemonade Hi-C Poppin' Pink	1 sm (16 oz)	200	0	0	0	51	0	84
Malt Chocolate	1 sm (16 oz)	670	13	15	59	123	2	297
Malt Strawberry	1 sm (16 oz)	670	12	15	59	123	0	250
Malt Vanilla	1 sm (16 oz)	600	13	17	66	98	0	250
Milk Reduced Fat	8 oz	120	8	5	20	11	0	115
Orange Juice Tropicana	1 (10 oz)	140	3	0	0	33	0	0
Powerade Fruit Punch	1 sm (16 oz)	130	0	0	0	33	0	107
Shake Chocolate	1 sm (16 oz)	630	14	16	62	111	2	281
Shake Strawberry	1 sm (16 oz)	630	13	16	62	111	0	234
Shake Vanilla	1 sm (16 oz)	560	14	17	69	87	0	243
Sprite	1 sm (16 oz)	200	0	0	0	51	0	47
CHILDREN'S MENU SELECTIONS								
Kid's Meal Chicken Strips	1 serv	770	22	51	30	53	2	720
Kid's Meal Justaburger	1 serv	570	19	29	33	60	3	862
DESSERTS								
Apple Pie A La Mode	1 serv	520	10	20	37	75	2	413
Apple Pie Hot	1	230	3	11	0	29	2	285
Cinnamon Roll	1	400	6	7	15	80	2	380
Cookie Chocolate Chunk	1 (2 oz)	230	2	11	35	33	1	150
Cookie White Chocolate Chunk Macadamia	1 (2 oz)	250	3	14	30	30	0	130
Peach Pie A La Mode	1 serv	570	10	23	37	82	2	253
MAIN MENU SELECTIONS								
Biscuit	1	300	5	17	0	32	1	644
Biscuit Sandwich Bacon Egg & Cheese	1	500	16	32	232	33	1	1231
Biscuit Sandwich Egg & Cheese	1	450	13	28	224	33	1	1028
Biscuit Sandwich Honey Butter Chicken	1	610	14	38	25	51	1	1072
Biscuit Sandwich Sausage Egg & Cheese	1	690	26	49	247	33	1	1553
Biscuit w/ Bacon	1	355	8	20	8	32	1	847
Biscuit w/ Gravy	1	530	9	36	12	52	1	1823
Biscuit w/ Sausage	1	540	18	37	23	32	1	1169

FOOD	PORTION	CALS	PROT	FAT	CHOL	CARB	FIBER	SOD
Breakfast On A Bun w/ Bacon	1	380	17	22	232	29	1	942
Breakfast On A Bun w/ Sausage	1	570	27	39	247	29	1	1264
Breakfast Platter w/ Bacon	1 serv	730	24	45	460	53	2	1462
Breakfast Platter w/ Sausage	1 serv	930	34	62	475	53	2	1784
Chicken Strips	1	200	9	12	15	11	0	359
Chicken Strips w/ Gravy	4	840	37	54	62	53	0	1858
French Fries	1 sm	260	4	13	0	31	2	26
Gravy White Peppered	1 serv	60	0	5	0	8	0	421
Hashbrown Sticks	4	200	2	12	0	20	1	368
Justaburger	1	329	15	16	33	30	1	862
Onion Rings	1 med	420	5	28	24	36	3	404
Pancakes Plain	1 serv	580	17	8	1	112	5	2170
Pancakes w/ Bacon	1 serv	630	20	12	9	112	5	2373
Pancakes w/ Sausage	1 serv	820	30	20	24	112	5	2695
Sandwich Chicken Strip Honey BBQ	1	1110	45	59	76	102	3	2759
Sandwich Chicken Strip Junior Honey BBQ	1	720	30	41	60	59	1	1904
Sandwich Egg	1	330	14	18	224	29	1	739
Sandwich Grilled Chicken	1	450	33	18	56	45	6	1101
Taquito w/ Bacon & Egg	1	370	17	21	344	27	3	932
Taquito w/ Bacon Egg & Cheese	1	420	19	24	356	27	3	1157
Taquito w/ Potato & Egg	1	430	15	23	336	37	3	912
Taquito w/ Potato Egg & Cheese	1	470	17	27	347	37	3	1137
Taquito w/ Sausage & Egg	1	410	17	24	348	27	3	909
Taquito w/ Sausage Egg & Cheese	1	450	19	28	359	27	3	1134
Texas Toast	1 slice	180	4	8	0	25	1	230
Whataburger	1	640	30	32	65	61	3	1522
Whataburger Double Meat	1	890	47	51	129	61	3	1770
Whataburger Jr.	1	330	15	16	33	32	1	865
Whataburger Triple Meat	1	1140	65	70	192	61	3	2019
Whataburger w/ Bacon & Cheese	1	800	40	45	98	62	3	2257
Whatacatch	1	480	17	30	41	42	2	1013

FOOD	PORTION	CALS	PROT	FAT	CHOL	CARB	FIBER	SOD
Whatacatch Dinner	1 serv	1095	29	92	113	161	8	1661
Whatachick'n	1	530	32	20	46	61	7	1491
SALADS								
Chicken Strips	1 serv	570	21	38	30	34	4	756
Garden Salad	1	60	3	0	0	12	4	56
Grilled Chicken	1 serv	230	23	7	50	19	4	676
WHITE CASTLE								
BEVERAGES								
Barq's Red Cream Soda	1 sm (21 oz)	260	0	0	0	69	0	40
Barq's Root Beer	1 sm (21 oz)	250	0	0	0	68	0	55
Coca Cola	1 sm (21 oz)	220	0	0	0	61	0	10
Coffee Black	1 sm (12 oz)	<5	0	0	0	1	0	0
Crave Cooler Coke	1 sm (21 oz)	150	0	0	0	41	0	15
Diet Coke	1 sm (21 oz)	0	0	0	0	0	0	20
Fanta Orange	1 sm (21 oz)	240	0	0	0	64	0	0
Hi-C Flashing Fruit Punch	1 sm (21 oz)	240	0	0	0	63	0	20
Hot Chocolate	1 sm (12 oz)	220	1	6	0	40	tr	300
Hot Tea	1 sm (12 oz)	0	0	0	0	0	0	0
Iced Tea Sweetened w/ Lemon	1 sm (21 oz)	170	0	0	0	46	0	20
Iced Tea Unsweetened	1 sm (21 oz)	0	0	0	0	0	0	30
Lemonade Raspberry	1 sm (21 oz)	290	0	0	0	78	0	5
Pibb Xtra	1 sm (21 oz)	220	0	0	0	59	0	30
Powerade Mountain Blast	1 sm (21 oz)	140	0	0	0	38	0	139
Sprite	1 sm (21 oz)	220	0	0	0	59	0	50
MAIN MENU SELECTIONS								
Cheeseburger	1	170	7	9	15	15	tr	330
Cheeseburger Bacon	1	200	10	11	20	15	tr	480
Cheeseburger Bacon Double	1	370	19	22	45	23	1	880
Cheeseburger Double	1	300	14	17	30	23	1	590
Cheeseburger Jalapeno	1	180	8	10	20	15	tr	380
Cheeseburger Jalapeno Double	1	320	15	19	40	23	1	680
Chicken Rings	6	210	18	23	80	15	0	670
Clam Strips	1 reg	250	8	22	20	5	0	620
Fish Nibblers	1 reg	280	19	16	30	24	5	820
French Fries	1 reg	310	4	15	0	39	4	250
Mozzarella Cheese Sticks	3	250	10	14	20	22	1	750

FOOD	PORTION	CALS	PROT	FAT	CHOL	CARB	FIBER	SOD
Onion Chips	1 reg	480	7	23	0	62	2	670
Sandwich Chicken Breast w/ Cheese	1	200	12	8	25	21	1	720
Sandwich Chicken Ring	1	180	7	8	35	19	tr	380
Sandwich Chicken Ring w/ Cheese	1	200	8	10	40	19	tr	500
Sandwich Fish w/ Cheese	1	180	9	8	25	19	tr	430
White Castle	1	140	6	7	10	14	tr	210
White Castle Double	1	250	11	13	20	22	1	340
SAUCES AND SPREADS								
Dressing Ranch	1 serv (1 oz)	150	0	17	15	0	0	210
Ketchup	1 pkg	10	0	0	0	3	0	100
Lemon Juice	1 pkg	0	0	0	0	0	0	0
Mayonnaise	1 pkg	60	0	7	5	0	0	55
Sauce BBQ	1 serv (1 oz)	35	0	1	0	8	0	400
Sauce Fat Free Honey Mustard	1 serv (1 oz)	50	0	0	0	12	0	140
Sauce Hot	1 pkg	0	0	0	0	0	0	170
Sauce Marinara	1 serv (1 oz)	15	0	0	0	4	0	260
Sauce Seafood	1 serv (1 oz)	30	0	0	0	7	0	330
Sauce Tartar	1 pkg	30	0	3	0	2	0	115
Sauce Zesty Zing	1 serv (1 oz)	110	0	11	15	3	0	190
WINCHELL'S DONUTS								
Chocolate Bar	1	240	4	16	–	29	–	125
Chocolate Round	1	240	4	16	–	29	–	125
Chocolate Twist	1	240	4	16	–	29	–	125
Croissant	1	260	5	17	–	28	–	280
Glazed Round	1	230	2	15	–	27	–	120
Glazed Twist	1	230	2	15	–	27	–	120
Iced Chocolate	1	230	2	15	–	28	–	220
Traditional	1	215	2	14	–	26	–	215
WORLD WRAPPS								
CHILDREN'S MENU SELECTIONS								
Kid's Bean & Cheese	1	332	18	11	–	36	9	–
Kid's Chicken & Cheese	1	229	15	4	–	25	3	–
Kid's Quesadilla	1	410	19	20	–	39	4	–
Kid's Teriyaki Chicken	1	407	25	6	–	52	4	–

FOOD	PORTION	CALS	PROT	FAT	CHOL	CARB	FIBER	SOD
SALADS								
BBQ Ranch Chicken	1 serv	633	29	48	–	43	15	–
Caesar Blackened Salmon	1 serv	612	27	54	–	9	5	–
Caesar Classic	1 serv	417	9	41	–	7	4	–
California Cobb	1 serv	636	29	62	–	16	6	–
Garden Veggie	1 serv	492	4	51	–	12	15	–
Thai Asian Chicken	1 serv	613	36	36	–	41	15	–
SIDES AND SOUPS								
Chips & Mango Salsa	1 serv	224	3	8	–	34	4	–
Chips & Tomato Corn Salsa	1 serv	184	2	8	–	82	4	–
Potstickers	3	170	8	4	–	24	1	–
Soup Thai Lemongrass	1 cup	256	32	8	–	14	–	–
Soup Tortilla	1 cup	191	8	7	–	26	6	–
Yogurt Parfait	1 serv	281	19	5	–	41	4	–
SMOOTHIES								
Black & Blue	1 (16 oz)	319	2	tr	–	77	3	–
Blue Mango Boost	1 (16 oz)	295	4	1	–	70	5	–
Caribbean C	1 (16 oz)	276	3	1	–	64	3	–
Georgia Peach	1 (16 oz)	343	1	tr	–	86	1	–
Peanut Butter Banana	1 (16 oz)	502	18	17	–	69	4	–
Strawberry Orange Banana	1 (16 oz)	268	3	1	–	61	5	–
Triathlete	1 (16 oz)	341	5	1	–	80	3	–
Tropical Storm	1 (16 oz)	309	6	3	–	72	3	–
WRAPS								
Baja Veggie w/ Cheese Sour Cream Avocado	1 sm	541	18	13	–	89	11	–
Barcelona	1 sm	460	24	11	–	65	4	–
Bean & Cheese	1 sm	452	16	13	–	67	11	–
Bombay Curry Veggie	1 sm	495	12	14	–	81	23	–
Buffalo w/ Shrimp	1 sm	422	18	10	–	65	7	–
Burrito w/ Chicken Cheese Sour Cream Avocado	1 sm	576	26	21	–	66	10	–
Burrito w/ Steak Cheese Sour Cream Avocado	1 sm	573	34	20	–	66	7	–
Caribbean Sole	1 sm	523	23	14	–	80	3	–
Chicken Caesar	1 sm	547	25	30	–	44	5	–
Chicken Parmesan	1 sm	495	32	16	–	53	2	–
Portabello & Goat Cheese	1 sm	391	13	13	–	55	5	–
Samurai Salmon	1 sm	543	22	22	–	65	2	–

FOOD	PORTION	CALS	PROT	FAT	CHOL	CARB	FIBER	SOD
Spicy Southwest Shrimp	1 sm	460	22	8	–	75	8	–
Tequila Lime Shrimp	1 sm	422	18	10	–	65	7	–
Teriyaki Chicken	1 sm	482	25	10	–	73	8	–
Teriyaki Steak	1 sm	497	30	10	–	69	8	–
Teriyaki Tofu & Mushroom	1 sm	387	11	6	–	58	5	–
Texas Roadhouse BBQ Chicken	1 sm	512	27	17	–	64	4	–
Texas Roadhouse BBQ Steak	1 sm	569	28	23	–	64	4	–
Thai Chicken	1 sm	508	30	17	–	58	4	–
YOGEN FRUZ								
Blend It No Sugar Added Vanilla	1 sm	110	4	0	3	24	0	66
Blend It Probiotic Low Fat Chocolate	1 sm	121	3	2	8	22	0	44
Blend It Probiotic Low Fat Vanilla	1 sm	121	4	2	9	22	4	55
Blend It Probiotic Non Fat Vanilla	1 sm	110	4	0	3	24	0	61
Smoothie Dairy Blueberry Breeze	1 sm	180	3	0	0	45	2	38
Smoothie Dairy Peach Berry Sunset	1 sm	150	3	0	0	36	2	45
Smoothie Dairy Strawberry Banana	1 sm	180	3	0	0	42	3	45
Smoothie Non Dairy Raspberry Blast	1 sm	208	2	0	0	51	3	16
Smoothie Non Dairy Tropical Storm	1 sm	224	2	0	0	56	2	16
Smoothie Non Dairy Very Berry	1 sm	192	0	0	0	50	3	16
Top It Probiotic Soft Serve	1 sm	132	5	0	2	28	0	78
YOGURTLAND								
Arctic Vanilla	½ cup (3 oz)	108	3	0	0	24	0	108
Blueberry Tart	½ cup (3 oz)	127	7	0	0	16	0	50
Cafe Con Leche	½ cup (3 oz)	108	3	0	0	24	0	103
Chocolate Mint	½ cup (3 oz)	100	2	0	0	23	0	70
Double Cookies & Cream	½ cup (3 oz)	121	3	0	0	27	0	89

FOOD	PORTION	CALS	PROT	FAT	CHOL	CARB	FIBER	SOD
Dutch Chocolate	½ cup (3 oz)	118	3	0	0	27	0	54
French Vanilla No Sugar Added	½ cup (3 oz)	89	6	0	0	19	0	105
Fresh Strawberry	½ cup (3 oz)	108	3	0	0	24	0	100
Green Tea	½ cup (3 oz)	107	3	tr	0	24	0	104
Heath Bar	½ cup (3 oz)	132	3	3	3	25	0	130
Mango	½ cup (3 oz)	96	2	0	0	22	0	74
Mango Tart	½ cup (3 oz)	127	7	0	0	16	0	50
NY Cheesecake	½ cup (3 oz)	100	3	0	5	23	0	80
Peach	½ cup (3 oz)	100	2	0	0	23	0	70
Peach Tart	½ cup (3 oz)	127	7	0	0	16	0	50
Peanut Butter	½ cup (3 oz)	119	3	3	0	24	0	119
Pineapple Tart	½ cup (3 oz)	127	7	0	0	16	0	50
Pistachio	½ cup (3 oz)	100	3	0	5	22	0	85
Plain Tart	½ cup (3 oz)	108	8	0	0	19	0	40
Strawberry Tart	½ cup (3 oz)	127	7	0	0	16	0	50
Taro	½ cup (3 oz)	102	2	0	0	23	0	136
ZOUP!								
DESSERTS								
Cookie Chocolate Chunk	1	410	4	19	–	57	1	–
Cookie Peanut Butter	1	420	6	21	–	43	1	–
SANDWICHES								
Grilled Turkey Club	½	470	29	28	–	22	1	–
Panini Italian Chicken	½	370	22	21	–	22	1	–
Pesto Three Cheese	1	720	44	42	–	42	2	–
Tuna Melt	1	600	50	23	–	42	2	–
Wrap American Farm	½	435	13	29	–	30	5	–
Wrap Asian	½	615	28	33	–	54	7	–
Wrap Chicken Caesar w/o Dressing	½	505	38	19	–	43	5	–
Wrap Greek w/o Dressing	½	485	15	33	–	33	6	–
Wrap Sonoma	½	595	18	37	–	38	8	–
Wrap Tuna	½	365	28	13	–	35	4	–
Zesty Southwest Turkey	½	310	19	16	–	22	1	–
SOUPS								
Chicken & Dumplings	1 (8 oz)	130	11	3	–	22	1	–
Chicken Potpie	1 (8 oz)	200	13	8	–	21	3	–

FOOD	PORTION	CALS	PROT	FAT	CHOL	CARB	FIBER	SOD
Italian Wedding w/ Turkey Meatballs	1 (8 oz)	120	10	4	–	13	1	–
Jamaican Bay Gumbo	1 (8 oz)	140	12	3	–	20	2	–
Lobster Bisque	1 (8 oz)	260	11	18	–	14	0	–
Pepper Steak	1 (8 oz)	160	11	6	–	19	1	–
Potato Cheddar	1 (8 oz)	210	11	13	–	16	1	–
Sesame Noodle Bowl	1 (8 oz)	80	6	3	–	7	1	–
Shrimp & Crawfish Etouffee	1 (8 oz)	130	10	4	–	17	1	–
Sicilian Pizza	1 (8 oz)	150	6	7	–	18	2	–
Spicy Crab & Rice	1 (8 oz)	110	7	2	–	21	1	–
Turkey Chili	1 (8 oz)	120	11	2	–	19	3	–
Wild Mushroom Barley	1 (8 oz)	108	3	3	–	18	2	–